Review of
DERMATOLOGY

Review of DERMATOLOGY

Seventh Edition

Saurabh Jindal MD DNB DDV (Mumbai)
(Dermatology, Venereology and Leprology)
Consultant—Dr Jindal's Skin and Dental Clinic
Karkardooma, New Delhi, India
Consultant—Dermatology, Max Superspeciality Hospital
Vaishali, Ghaziabad, Uttar Pradesh
Ex-Assistant Professor, Grant Medical College and
JJ Group of Hospitals, Mumbai
Ex-Associate Professor
MGM Medical College
Mumbai, Maharashtra, India

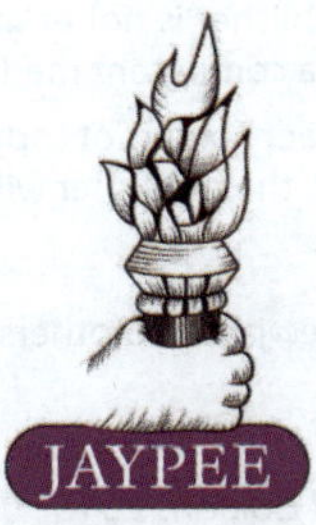

JAYPEE BROTHERS MEDICAL PUBLISHERS
The Health Sciences Publisher
New Delhi | London

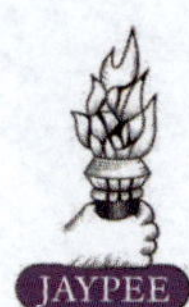

JAYPEE **Jaypee Brothers Medical Publishers (P) Ltd**

Headquarters
EMCA House
23/23-B, Ansari Road, Daryaganj
New Delhi 110 002, India.
Landline: +91-11-23272143, +91-11-23272703
+91-11-23282021, +91-11-23245672
E-mail: jaypee@jaypeebrothers.com

Corporate Office
4838/24, Ansari Road, Daryaganj
New Delhi 110 002, India.
Phone: +91-11-43574357
Fax: +91-11-43574314
E-mail: jaypee@jaypeebrothers.com

Overseas Office
J.P. Medical Ltd
83 Victoria Street, London
SW1H 0HW (UK)
Phone: +44 20 3170 8910
E-mail: info@jpmedpub.com

EU GPSR Authorised Representative
Logos Europe, 9 rue Nicolas Poussin
17000, La Rochelle, France
Phone: +33 (0) 6 67 93 73 78
E-mail: contact@logoseurope.eu

Website: www.jaypeebrothers.com
Website: www.jaypeedigital.com

Inquiries for bulk sales may be solicited at: jaypee@jaypeebrothers.com

Review of Dermatology

First Edition: 2017 *Second Edition: 2018* *Third Edition: 2019*
Fourth Edition: 2020 *Fifth Edition: 2021* *Sixth Edition: 2022*

Seventh Edition: **2025**
Reprint: 2026

ISBN: 978-93-5696-920-9

Printed in India by SDR Printers

Dedicated to

My Family—For giving me the support, encouragement and the space to accomplish this long kept dream

Preface

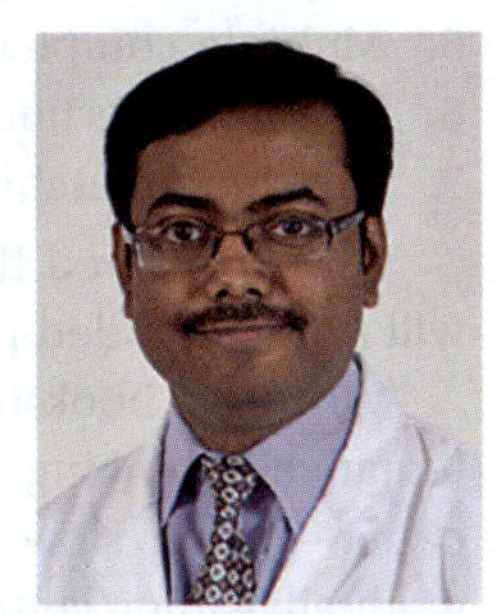

I am now writing the preface for the 7th edition of this long-cherished dream project. The feedback and the love for the previous edition have exceeded my wildest imaginations. It will be no exaggeration to state that almost all questions which came in the last year in national and various state examinations could be solved from this book. That itself is the biggest achievement for this project. Since my undergraduate days I have loved teaching. It has been my 'first true love!' In Latin, the word doctor means 'to teach'. Unsurprisingly then, teaching became my career after my PG days in addition to my clinical work. Through this book, I am attempting to reach students in one more way and complete my identity as a 'doctor'. Teaching has been my calling and energizes me every day, even after **17 years of experience in training students in PGMEE**. I started teaching in coaching classes way back in 2006 and at the time of going to press, I have completed **over 2000 live face-to-face dermatology lectures** in PG entrance coaching classes in the last 17 years to think myself worthy of even writing this book.

Prior to the 1st edition, many of my students had communicated to me the felt-need for a detailed entrance book written by a subject specialist exclusively focusing on dermatology, not just as a portion in 'short subject' guides. Also, with the new pattern of PGMEE, there is increasing emphasis on **image-based MCQs**. This shift away from single line MCQs to clinical case scenarios has made it **essential for you to know images as a part of preparation**. The 'short subject' guides have not been able to keep pace with this change. Unlike in some other books where separate colour plates are provided at the start or at the end of the book away from the actual text, I have given the images their rightful place integrated within the topic itself for a better understanding. Unlike other books where images have been picked up from the internet (on foreign skin), I have used images from my own vast **personal collection of the past 17 years** (I have scrolled through close to 1 TB of images to hand-pick the ones in this book!). This gives an **Indian skin perspective** to learning which is essential in your examinations. The guiding undertone of the book is **'maximum information in minimum time'**. No unnecessary information has been included in this book as dermatology is a short subject in PGMEE. I always used to find **arrow-based flowcharts** very useful for easy recollection during my own PG preparation days. Hence, I have included many of them in my text. Based on students' feedback, I have included a **'Quick revision'** section at the end of each topic for last minute revision before examinations. **'High yield points' and 'Aid to remember'** have been included in the chapters to help you. Putting my thinking cap on, I have made many new mnemonics myself! **MCQs right up to 2024** have been put from all exams.

AIIMS, in July 2019 introduced 7 different MCQs as below:

1. Single best response
2. Multiple True/False
3. Match the following
4. Sequential arrangement
5. Multiple completion
6. Reason/Assertion
7. Extended matching

I have ensured that each chapter has all new pattern MCQs (all 7 different types). You will note an added page at the end of each chapter dedicated to this new pattern.

Writing a book in many ways is like preparing for an entrance examinations. You start tentatively thinking 'Will I be able to do justice to it'—then, starting to plan with pen and paper—taking slow baby steps initially without any momentum-getting into the groove gradually—then getting into a 'zone' with a 'Usain Bolt-like run'—gaining more momentum—hitting the home stretch—and finally crossing the finish line with hands-in-the-air!

After the toil of preparation, I wish for you your own *'hands-in-the-air'* moment on your result day!

All the best! Do let me know your feedback for my book at the mail below.

Dr Saurabh Jindal

drsaurabhdermatology@gmail.com

Acknowledgments

This book has been made possible because of the contribution of a lot of people, few of whom I mention below:

- My wife Dr Shifali Dadu and my daughter Naisha Jindal for their patience and sacrifice, allowing me to ignore them and dive head-on into the book ☺
- My Parents for their persuasion and encouragement
- My Sister Dr Taru Jindal—My one true inspiration in life and for always being there for me
- Shri Jitendar P Vij (Group Chairman), Jaypee Brothers Medical Publishers, who was more than welcoming when I approached him to write this book
- Ms Chetna Malhotra (Senior Director—Professional Publishing, Marketing, and Business Development), for her push and direction
- Ms Ruby Sharma (Business Manager) who was always just a phone call away and ensured timely completion of the project
- Last but certainly not the least—my dear students for prodding me to start and take this endeavour to completion.

How to Use this Book

- *Category 1:* For students having good amount of time at their hands—"Prospective study"—Start from theory of chapter first, then MCQs and then explanation of MCQs. Revise at the end of the chapter by reading "Quick revision"
- *Category 2:* For students having moderate amount of time at their hands—"Prospective study of 5 star and 4 star chapters"—Start from theory of chapter first, then MCQs and then explanation of MCQs. Revise at the end of the chapter by reading "Quick revision"
- *Category 3:* For students having very less amount of time at their hands—"Retrospective study"—Start by seeing images of each chapter with the legends below it, then go straight to MCQs and then explanation of MCQs (page numbers of the theory page relevant to the said MCQ have been provided in the MCQ answer page). Revise at the end of the chapter by reading "Quick revision".

Contents

*****	**Most Important**
****	**Very Important**
***	**Important**

Recent Questions and Answers with Explanation

INI-CET November 2024

1. Which organism does not cause urethritis in males:

a. Trichomonas vaginalis
b. Mycoplasma genitalium
c. Neisseria gonorrhoeae
d. Gardenella vaginalis

Ans. (d) Gardenella vaginalis

Gardenella vaginalis causes bacterial vaginosis and not urethritis.

2. A woman presents with foul smelling discharge. Her cervix appears normal. Whiff test is positive. The diagnosis is:

a. Bacterial vaginosis
b. Candidiasis
c. Trichomonas vaginitis
d. Chlamydial infection

Ans. (a) Bacterial vaginosis

All the features are s/o bacterial vaginosis.

3. Topical drug used for onychomycosis treatment is:

a. Griseofulvin
b. Tavaborole
c. Capsofungin
d. Itraconazole

Ans. (b) Tavaborole

Tavaborole topical solution, 5% is a novel, boron-based pharmaceutical approved by the Food and Drug Administration (FDA) in July 2014 for the treatment of toenail onychomycosis caused by *Trichophyton rubrum* and *T. mentagrophytes.*

Griseofulvin and Itraconazole are not available in topical forms.

4. Incorrect regarding Behcet's disease is:

a. Ulcers on dorsum of penile shaft
b. More in Crohn's disease than ulcerative colitis
c. Pathergy test is positive
d. Bilateral pan uveitis

Ans. (b) More in Crohn's disease than ulcerative colitis

People with Behcet's disease have a state of altered tissue reactivity in response to minor trauma. The pathergy test is a nonspecific hypersensitivity skin reaction induced by needle prick that is performed to look for evidence of this phenomenon. Pathergy lesions are generally manifested clinically by erythematous induration at the location of skin trauma, which may remain as papules or progress to sterile pustules.

Genital ulcers/panuveitis are other features.

5. Which occurs due to bare foot walking through inoculation through soil?

a. Madura mycosis
b. Coccidioides immitis
c. Toxocara canis
d. Cryptococcosis

Ans. (a) Madura mycosis

6. A gardener who resides in sub-Himalayan area came with nodules on the forearm. Which is the causative agent?

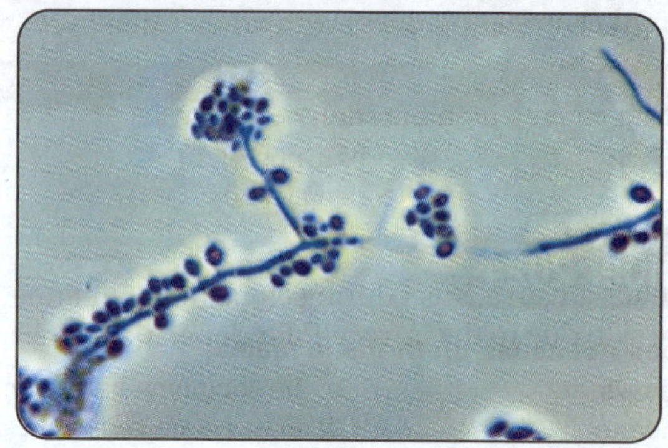

a. Sporothrix schenckii
b. Cryptococcosis
c. Blastomycosis
d. Madurella mycetomatis

Ans. (a) Sporothrix schenckii

Gardner's occupation is a clue to the diagnosis of sporotrichosis.

INI-CET May 2024

7. Which type of vitiligo is progressive initially then becomes static?

a. Focal vitiligo
b. Segmental vitiligo
c. Acrofacial vitiligo
d. Mixed vitiligo

Ans. (b) Segmental vitiligo

People with segmental vitiligo have rapid color loss on one side of the body. After 6–12 months, segmental vitiligo tends to stabilize, meaning that the color loss stops. Once it stops, most people with segmental vitiligo do not develop new patches or spots.

8. Match the following:

Column A	Column B
1. Patch test	a. Contact dermatitis
2. Slit skin smear	b. Leprosy
3. Biopsy	c. Lupus vulgaris
4. KOH	d. Tinea corporis

Select the correct answer given below code:

a. 1-c, 2-a, 3-b, 4-d
b. 1-a, 2-c, 3-b, 4-d
c. 1-a, 2-b, 3-c, 4-d
d. 1-b, 2-c, 3-a, 4-d

Ans. (c) 1-a, 2-b, 3-c, 4-d

9. Which does not cause annular plaque?

a. Pityriasis rosea
b. Tinea corporis
c. Urticaria
d. Porokeratosis

Ans. (c) Urticaria

Pityriasis rosea has annular lesions on trunk in a Christmas tree pattern. Tinea corporis has annular scaly itchy lesions. Porokeratosis is a precancerous skin lesion that presents with small, round-shaped lesions (annular plaques) with an elevated border. Urticaria has wheals and not annular lesions on skin.

10. Which anti-leprosy drug causes pigmentation?

a. Rifampicin
b. Dapsone
c. Clofazimine
d. Ofloxacin

Ans. (c) Clofazimine

The most frequent cutaneous adverse effect during clofazimine treatment is the brownish-red hyperpigmentation of the skin due to the intracellular deposition of drug-derived crystals.

11. Which STD is drug resistant?

a. Syphilis
b. Gonorrhea
c. Chancroid
d. Donovanosis

Ans. (b) Gonorrhea

Gonorrhea has developed resistance to nearly all the antibiotics used for its treatment. Currently, cephalosporins are still effective to treat this infection.

INI-CET November 2023

12. A 45-year-old male comes with recurrent blisters and oral ulcers for 3 years. The histology is as shown. Diagnosis is:

a. Pemphigus vulgaris
b. Dermatitis herpetiformis
c. Bullous pemphigoid
d. Linear IgA disease

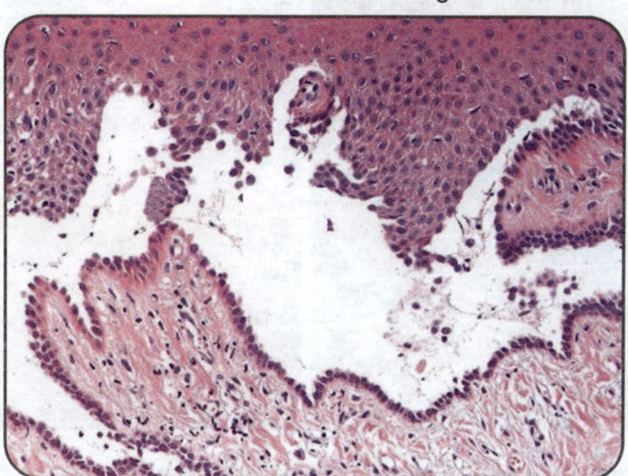

Ans. (a) Pemphigus vulgaris

The image shows a suprabasal blister with row of tombstones appearance and is seen in pemphigus vulgaris. Recurrent blisters and oral ulcers also point to the same diagnosis.

13. A patient comes with skin lesions. Investigation is as shown. What test is this?

a. Indirect immunofluorescence
b. Direct immunofluorescence
c. Immunohistochemistry
d. FISH

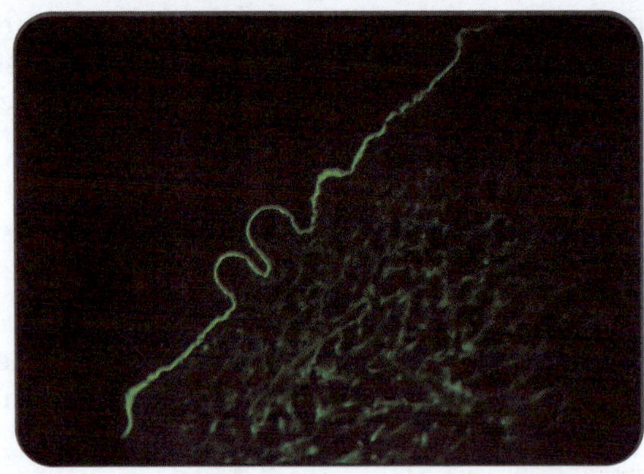

Ans. (b) Direct immunofluorescence

Direct immunofluorescence is a one step procedure that involves application of fluoresceinated antibodies to a frozen section of the skin. This test determines the deposition of immunoreactants in the patient's tissue. Biopsy specimens are examined for *in vivo* deposits of serum proteins.

14. A 25-year-old patient comes with lesions on trunk as shown. The correct option here would be:

a. Pityriasis rosea-collarette scale-Christmas tree pattern
b. Lichen planus-Flexures-Wickham's striae
c. Lichen planus-collarette scales-Christmas tree
d. Seborrheic dermatitis-Wickham's striae-Christmas tree pattern

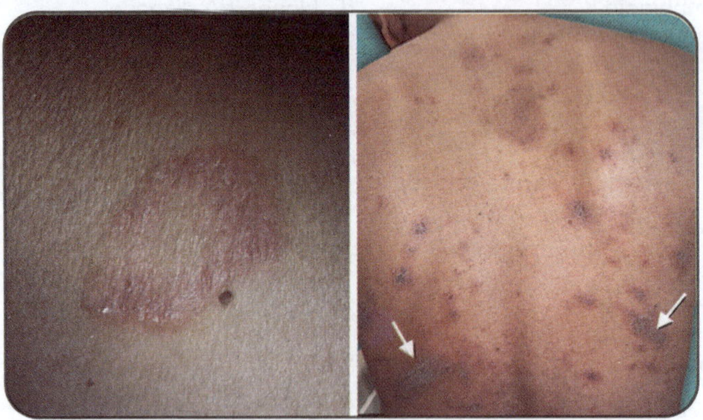

Ans. (a) Pityriasis rosea-collarette scale-Christmas tree pattern

Note the truncal lesions in an inverted V shape (right image) s/o pityriasis rosea. The left sided image shows herald patch of pityriasis rosea. Collarette scale is seen in this disease. Christmas tree pattern refers to the V shaped pattern as the lesions come along the rib lines.

15. A 12-year-old obese girl comes with discoloration of neck and axilla as shown. What risk factor is associated with this?

a. Metabolic syndrome
b. Vitamin B12 deficiency
c. Lichen planus
d. Rubbing

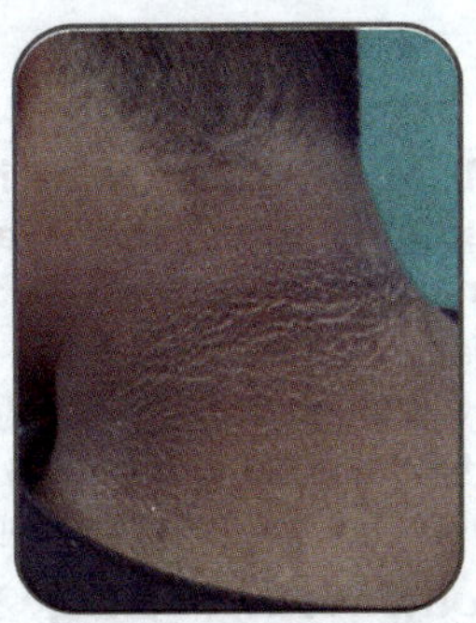

Ans. (a) Metabolic syndrome

The image shows ribbed appearance along with blackness of the neck suggestive of acanthosis nigricans. Similar lesions would be expected in the armpits, groins, knuckles and even the face. This is suggestive of insulin resistance and metabolic syndrome.

16. An immunocompromised individual presents with a corrugated white lesion on the side of the tongue which does not wipe off. The cause would be:

a. EBV b. HSV 1 c. Candida d. HHV 8

Ans. (a) EBV

Hairy leukoplakia (HL) is associated with Epstein-Barr virus (EBV), also known as human herpesvirus 4. It occurs most commonly in people infected with HIV. Hairy leukoplakia is often asymptomatic and presents as a non-tender whitish plaque along the lateral border of the tongue.

17. An 18 days old baby was brought with neonatal meningitis and has vesicles over trunk and upper limb. Mother had genital ulcers 1 year back but they have resolved now. The biopsy of vesicles shows multinucleate giant cells. The diagnosis is:

a. Herpes simplex virus type 2 b. MCV
c. HPV d. Varicella

Ans. (a) Herpes simplex virus type 2

Herpes simplex virus (HSV) and varicella zoster virus (VZV) infections induce the formation of intraepidermal vesicles containing acantholytic cells and multinucleated giant cells in the skin. Tzanck smear is most commonly used to diagnose cutaneous herpetic infections. If left untreated, HSV-2 can lead to neonatal herpes encephalitis, meningitis, brain damage and cerebral palsy.

18. A obese female with BMI 29, hirsutism score of 6, irregular menses comes to you. Her testosterone level was 0.36 ng/dL. You will advise all *except*:

a. Lifestyle modification b. Anti androgens, OCP with lifestyle modification
c. Counselling about future risk of metabolic syndrome
d. OCP only

Ans. (d) OCP only

Only OCP will not be effective since it will not help deal with the main pathology of insulin resistance.

19. Recombinant HPV vaccine is made from which antigen:

a. E1 and E2 b. E6 and E7 c. L1 d. L2

Ans. (c) L1

INI-CET May 2023

20. A 26-year-old women with BMI of 30 comes with infertility since 6 years along with hirsutism and acne. On ultrasound, polycystic ovaries was found. Ferriman-Gallwey score was 10. The next line of management would be:

a. Finasteride + metformin + ovulation induction
b. Weight reduction + metformin + clomiphene
c. Weight reduction + metformin + urinary gonadotropins
d. Weight reduction + try spontaneous, if fails go for induction

Ans. (d) Weight reduction + try spontaneous, if fails go for induction

An obese female with infertility, hirsutism and acne likely has PCOD. USG confirms it. Ferriman-Gallwey score is for hirsutism. Weight reduction is itself often solves the problem. If not, then induction would be planned.

21. A 50-year-old patient on nivolumab has pruritic and urticarial lesions. Histopathology shows subepidermal blister and IgG and C3 deposition along the dermoepidermal junction. Which of the following matches with given history and immunofluorescence?

a. Pemphigus vulgaris
b. Pemphigus foliaceus
c. Bullous pemphigoid
d. Dermatitis herpetiformis

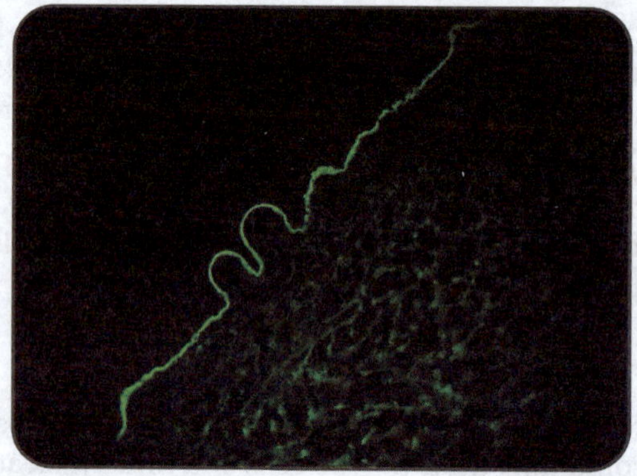

Ans. (c) Bullous pemphigoid

The image shows linear deposits on the DEJ. This is s/o bullous pemphigoid. Pruritic and urticarial lesions are also s/o BP.

22. Match the following:

Disease	Wood's lamp
a. Vitiligo	1. Pink
b. Erythrasma	2. Green
c. Tinea capitis	3. Yellow
d. Pityriasis versicolor	4. Coral red
	5. White
	6. Blue

a. a1, b3, c2, d4
b. a5, b4, c2, d3
c. a3, b1, c4, d2
d. a6, b2, c3, d1

Ans. (b) a5, b4, c2, d3

23. A 34-year-old multiparous patient with multiple sexual partners comes with painless ulcer on genitals. The first test to be done here will be:

a. Scrapping from ulcer
b. VDRL
c. HIV ELISA
d. Giemsa stain

Ans. (a) Scrapping from ulcer

The diagnosis seems to be primary syphilis due to painless ulcer on genitals. VDRL would usually be negative at such early stages.

24. A lady comes with white vaginal discharge not staining undergarments. She is on oral contraceptive pills. The Ph of vagina is acidic and lactobacillus is normal. There is no itch or soreness. The likely cause is:

a. Bacterial vaginosis
b. Candidiasis
c. Chlamydia
d. Physiological

Ans. (d) Physiological

Physiological vaginal discharge will be non-itchy, non-smelly and does not stain undergarments. Ph is normal (acidic). *Lactobacillus* is also normal. So the answer is d.

25. A patient of bacterial vaginosis comes with grey white discharge. She has clue cells. The best description of this cell is:

a. Epithelial cells coated with bacteria
b. Cells with flagella
c. Epithelial cells coated with bacteria
d. Filamentous organisms

Ans. (a) Epithelial cells coated with bacteria

Clue cells are cells in the vagina (vaginal epithelial cells) that appear fuzzy without sharp edges under a microscope as they are coated with bacteria. This is seen in bacterial vaginosis.

INI-CET November 2022

26. A 24-year-old diabetic male presents with bilateral brown pigmentation in axilla and groin. Which of the following is the correct match?

a. Wood's lamp examination showing green fluorescence
b. Wood's lamp examination showing yellow fluorescence
c. Wood's lamp examination showing blue fluorescence
d. Wood's lamp examination showing coral red fluorescence

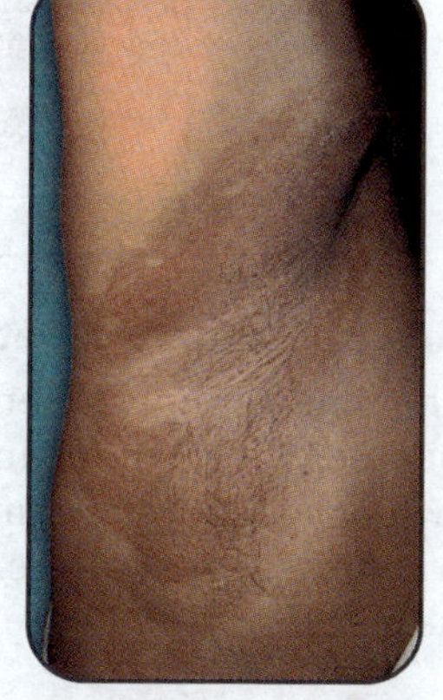

Ans. (d) Wood's lamp examination showing coral red fluorescence

The diagnosis is erythrasma. Wood's lamp would show coral red fluorescence. Yellow fluorescence is seen in pityriasis versicolor. Green fluorescence is seen in tinea capitis.

27. The mechanism of action of finasteride is:

a. Aromatase inhibitor
b. 5-Alpha reductase inhibitor
c. Androgen receptor blocker
d. CYP 17 A1 inhibitor

Ans. (b) 5-Alpha reductase inhibitor

28. Vesicular lesions are seen in:

a. Hand, foot mouth disease
b. Roseola
c. Dengue
d. Measles

Ans. (a) Hand, foot mouth disease

Hand-foot-and-mouth disease is a mild, contagious viral infection common in young children. Symptoms include ulcers in the mouth and a vesicular rash on the hands and feet. Hand-foot-and-mouth disease is caused by a coxsackie virus. Roseola/dengue/measles all are macular, red, non-vesicular rashes.

29. A child presents with multiple lesions on thigh and genital area. Some lesions have umbilication. Histology is as shown. What is being shown?

a. Donovan body
b. Tzanck cell
c. Koilocyte
d. Henderson-Peterson body

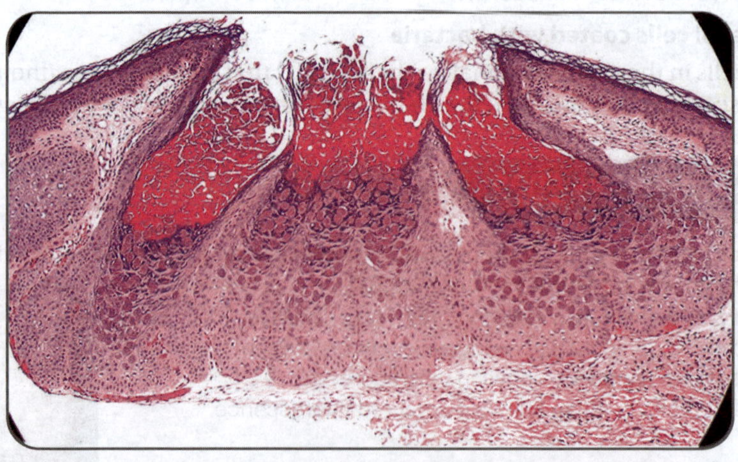

Ans. (d) Henderson-Peterson body

The image shows Henderson-Peterson body seen in molluscum disease. Umbilicated papules (seen more in children) will have this histology. Koilocytes are seen in warts (which will not have umbilicated lesions). Donovan body will be seen in donovanosis and will have genital ulcers. Tzanck cell is an acantholytic cell seen in diseases like pemphigus, herpes.

30. A farmer presents with linear lesions as shown. All the following can cause this spread along lymphatics *except*:

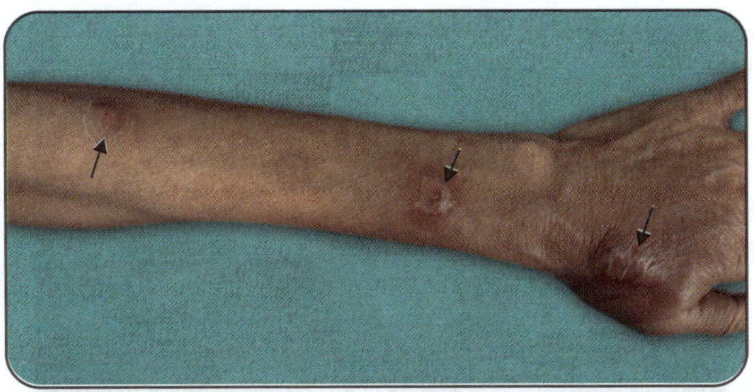

a. Sporothrix
b. Nocardia
c. Staphylococcal aureus
d. Mycobacterial marinum

Ans. (c) Staphylococcal aureus

Sporotrichosis presents as linear lesions along the lymphatics. It is often seen in farmers or gardeners after a thorn prick. Mycobacterial marinum is often similar in those with water contact like swimmers/fish handlers. Nocardia also causes similar lesions.

31. A patient presents with fever and a black eschar as shown. The likely diagnosis is:

a. Rocky mountain spotted fever
b. Scrub typhus
c. COVID 19
d. Malaria

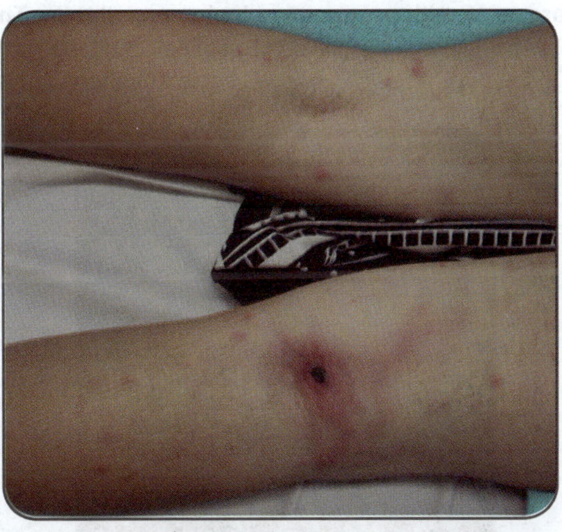

Ans. (b) Scrub typhus

Scrub typhus, also known as bush typhus, is a disease caused by bacteria called *Orientia tsutsugamushi*. Scrub typhus is spread to people through bites of infected chiggers (larval mites). The most common symptoms of scrub typhus include fever, headache, body aches, and rash which typically starts a black eschar at the site of the chigger bite.

32. **A female with a history of Raynaud's phenomenon, skin thickening and breathlessness presents with skin lesions as shown in the image. Which of the following best represents it?**

a. Leucoderma
b. Vitiligo
c. Contact allergy
d. Salt and pepper pigmentation

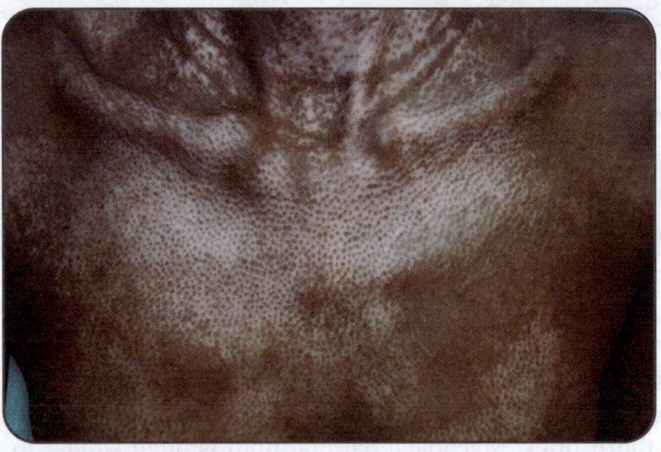

Ans. (d) Salt and pepper pigmentation

A classic cutaneous manifestation of systemic sclerosis is the "salt-and-pepper appearance". The presence of salt-and-pepper appearance in conjunction with sclerosis of skin provides strong evidence for pointing the diagnosis toward systemic sclerosis.

33. **A 60-year-old man presents with progressive lesions as shown. The diagnosis is:**

a. Squamous cell cancer
b. Basal cell cancer
c. Melasma
d. Discoid lupus erythematosus

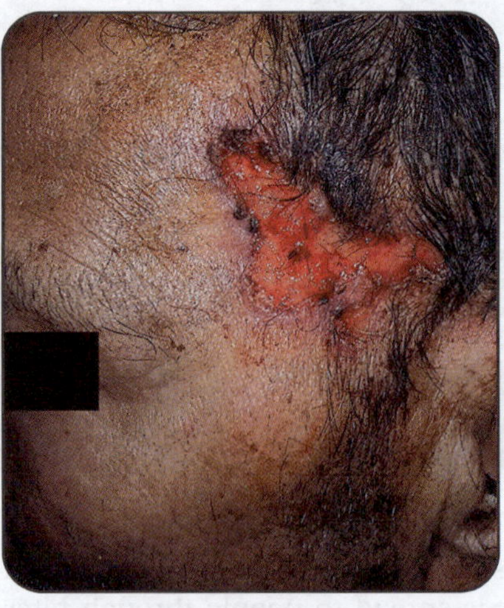

Ans. (b) Basal cell cancer

This is the classical rodent ulcer seen on the face in patients of basal cell cancer.

34. A patient presented to you in the OPD with blackening of the hands after a recent episode of amoebic dysentery for which he took medication. What can be the reason for such a condition?

a. Allergic contact dermatitis
b. Fixed drug eruption
c. Maculopapular rash
d. Atopic dermatitis

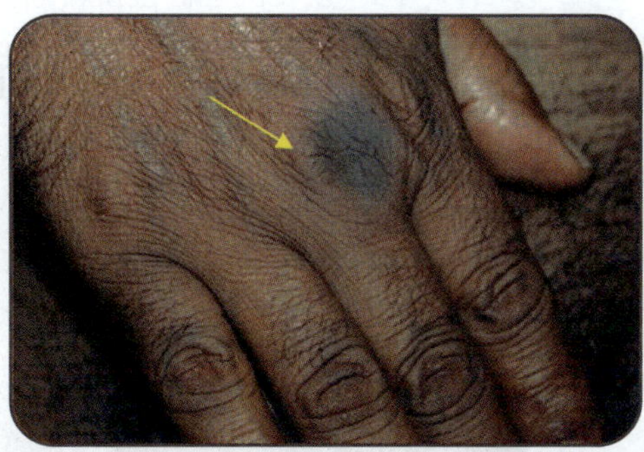

Ans. (b) Fixed drug eruption

Note the dermal pigmentation in the form of greyish patches. This is often seen in patients with fixed drug eruption. The patients suffering from amoebic dysentery would have taken possibly metronidazole/tinidazole/ornidazole all of which can create this eruption.

35. Which of the following is a scarring alopecia?

a. Alopecia areata
b. Telogen effluvium
c. Androgenetic alopecia
d. Frontal fibrosing alopecia

Ans. (d) Frontal fibrosing alopecia

Frontal fibrosing alopecia (FFA) is a condition that causes hair loss on the front and sides of your scalp. Hair loss may also occur on eyebrows, eyelashes and other body parts. An autoimmune reaction, genetics or hormones may cause FFA. Scarring is permanent here.

36. A farmer comes with nodular lesions on foot. The microscopy is as shown. Pick the true statement.

a. Blood invasion is common in those with hematological malignancy
b. Dimorphic organism
c. Does not involve fascia, tendon, muscles
d. These are dead fungi engulfed by macrophages

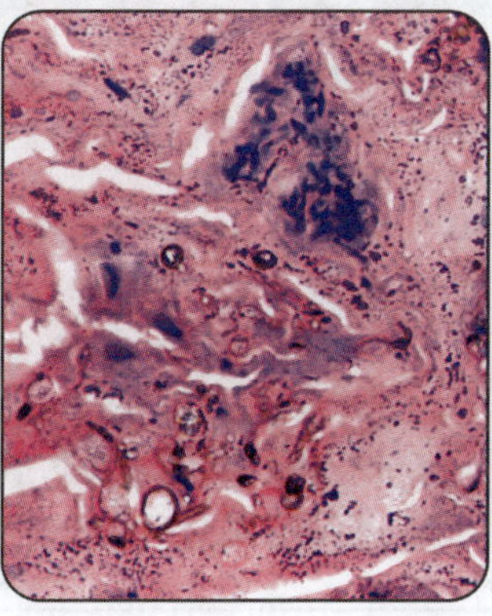

Ans. (c) Does not involve fascia, tendon, muscles

The image shows sclerotic bodies seen in chromoblastomycosis. These are pigmented brown bodies as shown in the image. This infection does not involve the fascia, tendons and muscles which is more likely with mycetoma. Dimorphic fungus indicates fungi which are present in both mold and yeast forms and is seen in sporotrichosis.

37. A patient presents with recurrent itchy, erythematous plaques over scalp and sacral area. There is history of joint pains. Nail findings are as shown. The likely diagnosis is:

a. Psoriasis
b. Lichen planus
c. Alopecia areata
d. Tinea

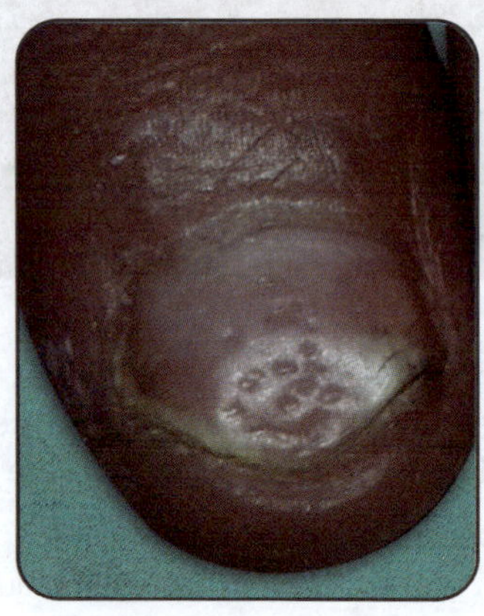

Ans. (a) Psoriasis

Scalp and sacral area lesions along with nail involvement are suggestive of psoriasis. The image shows nail pitting, salmon patch and onycholysis.

INI-CET May 2022

38. A patient with satellite skin lesion presents to you. He also has one hypopigmented lesion and one thickened feeder nerve. The treatment best suited would be:

a. Packet A × 12 months
b. Packet B × 12 months
c. Packet A × 6 months
d. Packet B × 6 months

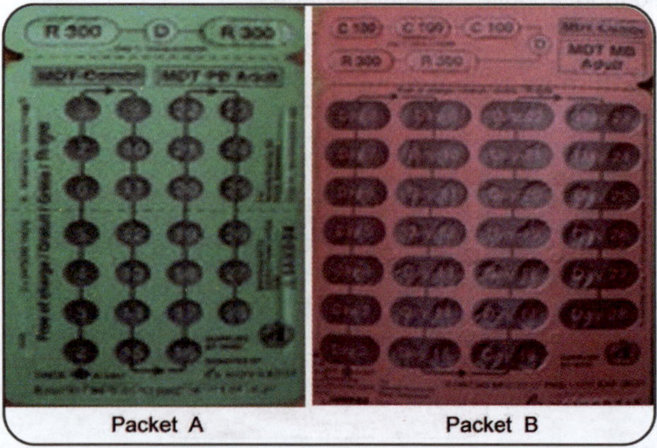

Packet A Packet B

Ans. (b) Packet B × 12 months

Single lesion and single thick nerve suggests MB Hansen for which the current guidelines suggests MDT with 3 drugs for 12 months.

39. Match the options in column A with the correct options in B:

Scale	Disease
a. Silvery	1. Pityriasis Rosea
b. Branny	2. Psoriasis
c. Mica	3. Pityriasis versicolor
d. Collarette	4. Pityriasis lichenoides chronica

Ans. a-2, b-3, c-4, d-1

40. A pregnant female had type 2 lepra reaction. Best treatment for her would be:

a Add steroids
b. Stop MDT and give steroids
c. Thalidomide
d. Azathioprine

Ans. (a) Add steroids

Steroid is the DOC for lepra 2 reactions.

41. A forest worker has a history of warty/cauliflower lesion on foot. His histology is as shown. The histology image is of:

a. Broad base non-capsulated
b. Splendore-Hoeppli phenomenon
c. Encapsulated budding yeast
d. Sclerotic body

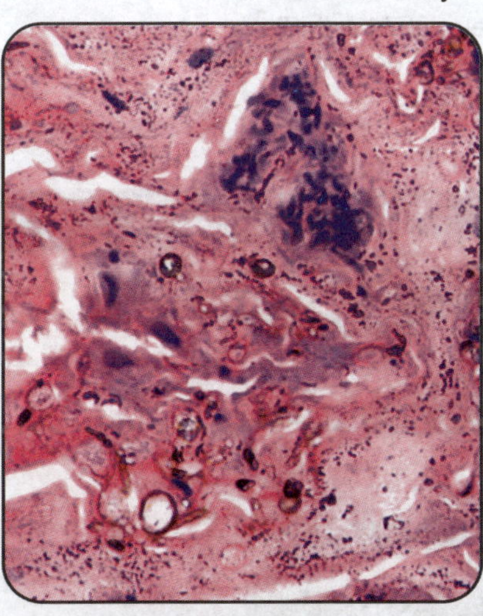

Ans. (d) Sclerotic body

The diagnosis in this question is chromoblastomycosis which shows sclerotic pigmented bodies on microscopy.

42. A patient has lesions as shown. Patient mentioned that a spider crawled in that area while sleeping. The diagnosis is:

a. Allergic dermatitis
b. Irritant dermatitis
c. Herpes zoster
d. Chickenpox

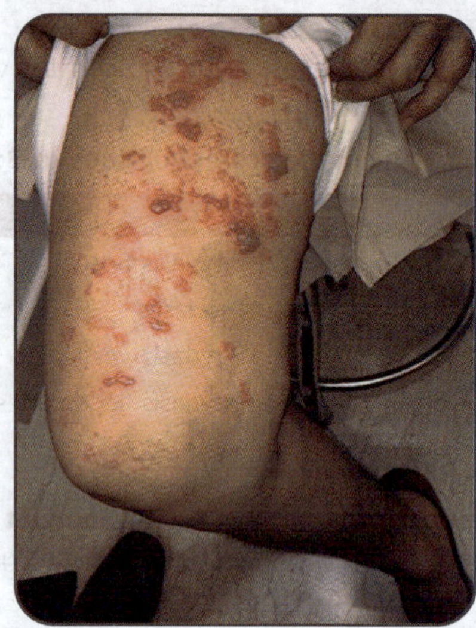

Ans. (c) Herpes zoster

We have to ignore the incorrect history of spider crawl. The lesions are dermatomal vesicles in herpes zoster.

43. A 10 year presents with arthritis of knee and lesions on the hand as shown. The diagnosis is:

a. Nodules in Juvenile Rheumatoid Arthritis
b. Gottron's papules in Juvenile dermatomyositis
c. Systemic lupus erythematosus
d. Sclerodactyly

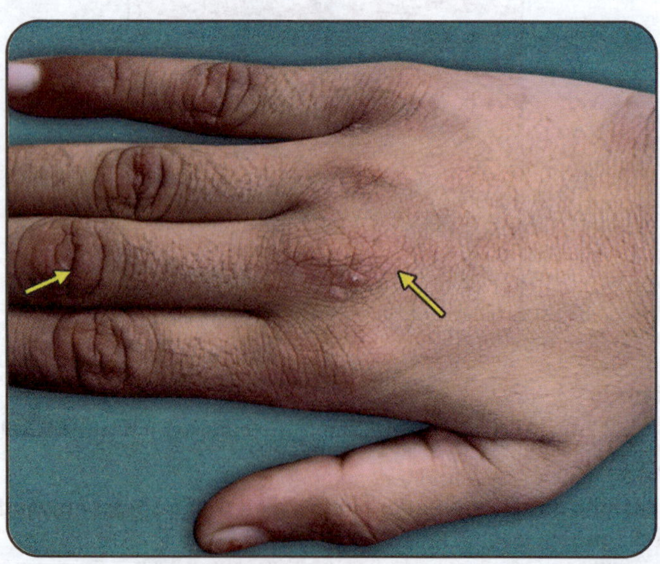

Ans. (b) Gottron's papules in Juvenile dermatomyositis

INI-CET November 2021

44. A patient from Bihar had history of very high grade fever. He later developed symmetrical lesions on his back without any nerve thickening and without any sensation loss. The diagnosis is:

a. Tuberculoid leprosy
b. Lepromatous leprosy
c. Post kala azar dermal leishmaniasis
d. Pityriasis versicolor

Ans. (c) Post kala azar dermal leishmaniasis

Bihar is endemic for both leprosy and leishmaniasis. History of fever (past visceral leishmaniasis), absent nerve thickening and sensory loss points to PKDL.

45. A patient presents with lesions as shown. All of the following can be used for treatment of this patient *except*:

a. Topical benzoyl peroxide
b. Topical fluocinolone
c. Topical tazarotene
d. Oral retinoic acid

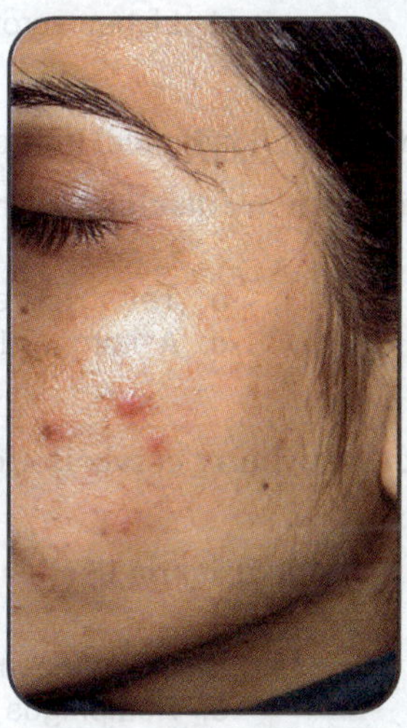

Ans. (b) Topical fluocinolone

The diagnosis is acne. Fluocinolone is a topical steroid which would exacerbate acne. All others are used for treatment.

46. A patient has not been given any specific treatment for his leprosy. Pick the true statement:

a. 50% cases resolve spontaneously after bacillus exposure
b. Spontaneous remission more in children than adults
c. Indeterminate leprosy resolves more spontaneously than tuberculoid
d. Most cases do not resolve spontaneously

Ans. (c) Indeterminate leprosy resolves more spontaneously than tuberculoid

Indeterminate leprosy typically resolves in most cases. Option a is incorrect (almost 95% patients resolve spontaneously without treatment).

47. Asymptomatic lesions occurred in a child with lesions on dorsal hand and shaft of penis as shown.

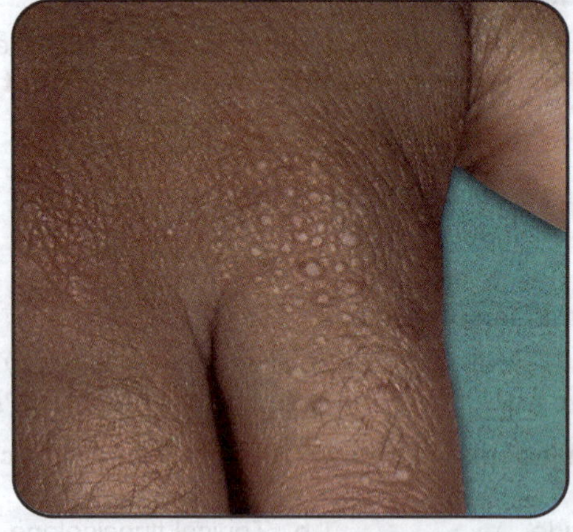

The diagnosis is:

a Lichen planus
b. Scabies
c. Lichen nitidus
d. Lichen scrofulosorum

Ans. (c) Lichen nitidus

Asymptomatic lesions on the site mentioned is typical for lichen nitidus.

48. A female comes with profuse vaginal itchy discharge. She has strawberry cervix on examination. The treatment is:

a. Metronidazole
b. Tetracycline
c. Aciclovir
d. Azithromycin

Ans. (a) Metronidazole

Profuse vaginal itchy discharge with strawberry cervix is s/o trichomonal vaginitis. The DOC is metronidazole.

49. A 65-year-old man comes with itching, urticaria like lesions and bullae on red as well as normal skin. The diagnosis is:

a. Dermatitis herpetiformis
b. Bullous pemphigoid
c. Linear IgA disease
d. Pemphigus

Ans. (b) Bullous pemphigoid

Old age, urticaria like lesions, bullae with itch on red and normal skin—all are strongly s/o bullous pemphigoid.

50. A 20-year-old female, unmarried with history of irregular menses and hirsutism. USG shows increased ovarian volume of 30 mL and 40 mL for ovaries. The initial treatment options are:

A. Oral contraceptive pills
B. Laparoscopic ovarian drilling
C. Lifestyle modification, weight reduction
D. Spironolactone

a. ABC
b. ABD
c. ACD
d. BCD

Ans. (c) ACD

The initial treatment would be oral contraceptive pills, lifestyle modification, weight reduction and spironolactone. Laparoscopic ovarian drilling would not be first line.

51. A farmer comes with history of thorn prick. Lesion occur along the lymphatic drainage as shown. The diagnosis is:

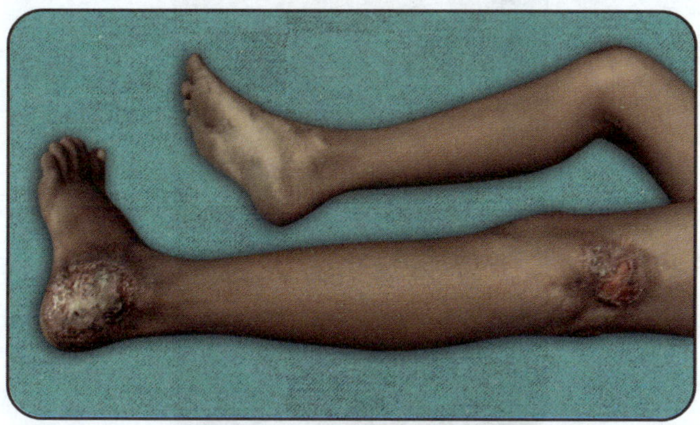

a. Cryptococcus
b. Sporotrichosis
c. Blastomycosis
d. Chromoblastomycosis

Ans. (b) Sporotrichosis

The image, farmer with thorn prick history, lymphatic lesions are all s/o sporotrichosis.

52. A 60-year-old patient comes with painful lesions on back. The image is as shown. The diagnosis is:

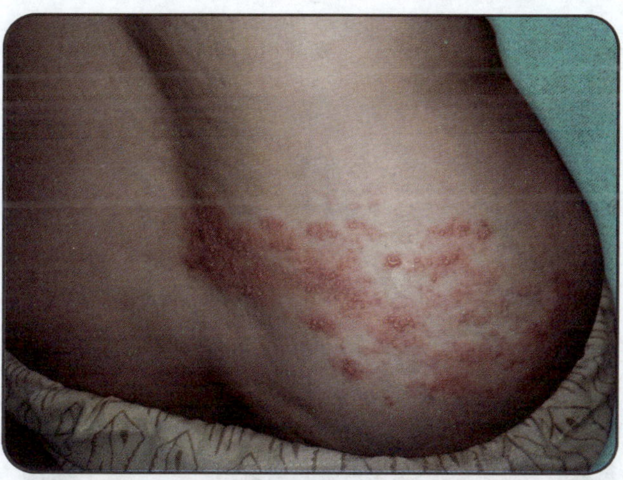

a. Psoriasis
b. Herpes zoster
c. Pyoderma
d. Pemphigus

Ans. (b) Herpes zoster

The image is of herpes zoster with dermatomal vesicles in an elderly person.

INI-CET July 2021

53. A female comes with unilateral lesions as shown in the image. She also has Leucotrichia. The diagnosis is likely to be:

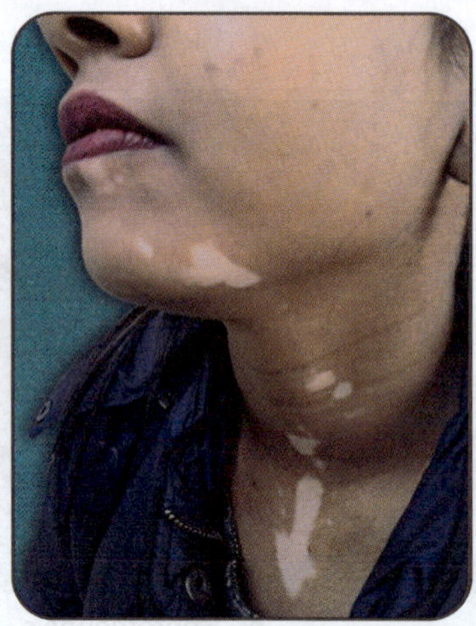

a. Segmental vitiligo
b. Focal vitiligo
c. Piebaldism
d. Nevus depigmentosus

Ans. (a) Segmental vitiligo

The image is of segmental vitiligo. Leucotrichia is also s/o vitiligo.

54. An adult presents with itchy hyperpigmented plaque with exudation on the flexure of the elbow and back of knee as shown. The diagnosis is:

a. Psoriasis
b. Atopic dermatitis
c. Dermatitis herpetiformis
d. Pemphigus

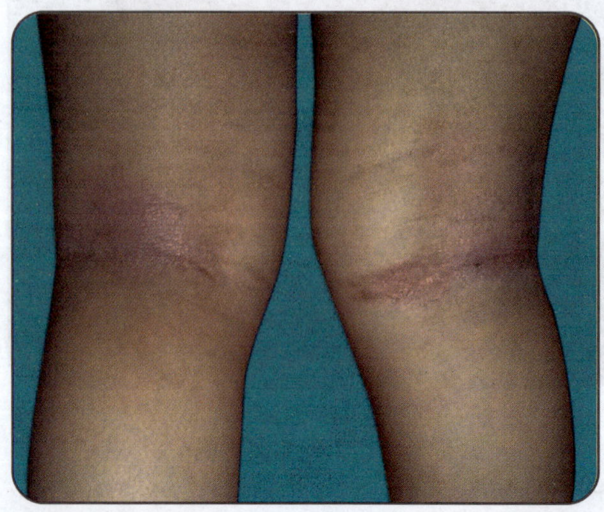

Ans. (b) Atopic dermatitis

Hyperpigmented plaque with exudation on the flexure of the knee in the image is s/o atopic dermatitis.

55. A patient presents with lesions as shown. The diagnosis is:

a. Borderline leprosy
b. Borderline lepromatous leprosy
c. Lepromatous leprosy
d. Histoid leprosy

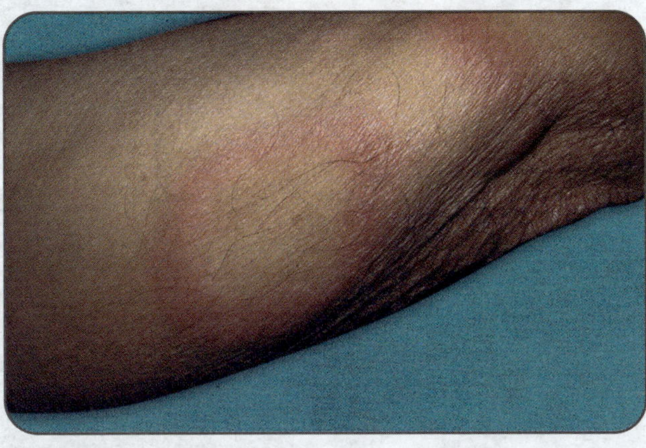

Ans. (a) Borderline leprosy

Punched out lesions/annular lesions in the image is s/o borderline Hansen.

56. A patient comes with lesions. A biopsy was done and the image as shown was found on histology.

a. Mycosis fungoides
b. Lepromatous leprosy
c. Pemphigus
d. Leishmaniasis

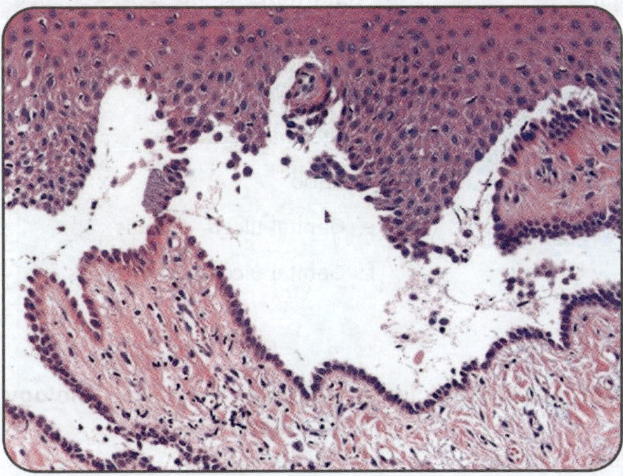

Ans. (c) Pemphigus

The histology is classical of suprabasal blister of pemphigus vulgaris.

57. A child comes with patchy hair loss, itching and scaling on the scalp as shown. The next best step is:

a. KOH mount
b. Giemsa staining
c. Biopsy
d. Tzanck smear

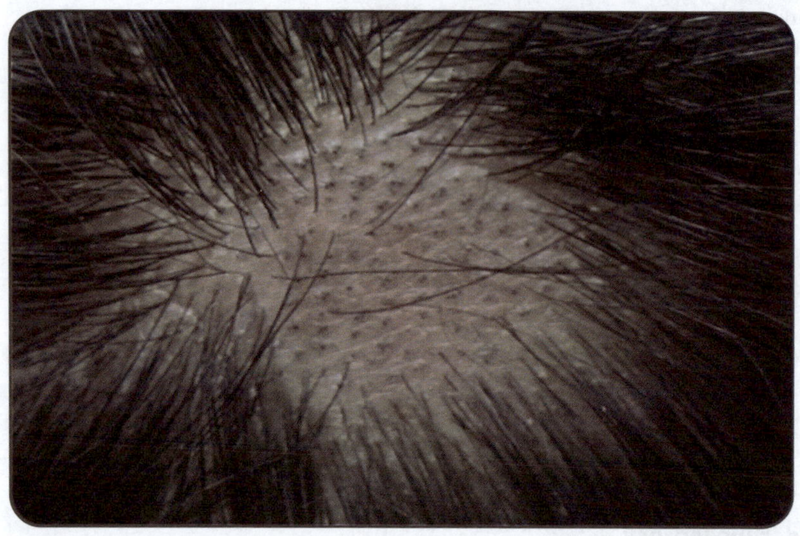

Ans. (a) KOH mount

The image is of black dot tinea capitis. Next best test is KOH.

58. Match the following:

STD kit	Conditions used
1. Green	a. Lower abdominal pain
2. Grey	b. Vaginal discharge
3. Yellow	c. Urethral discharge
4. White	d. Bubo
	e. Genital ulcer—Herpes
	f. Genital ulcer—Non herpes

Ans. 1-b, 2-c, 3-a, 4-f

59. A patient comes with painful vesicles on genitals. The histopathology finding will be:

a. Tzanck cells
b. Pund cells
c. Henderson-Peterson bodies
d. Koilocytes

Ans. (a) Tzanck cells

Painful vesicles on genitals is s/o herpes genitalis for which Tzanck smear is done which would show Tzanck cells.

NEET August 2024

60. A 27 years has moth eaten alopecia, grey, moist groin lesions and an asymptomatic macular rash. What is the causative organism?

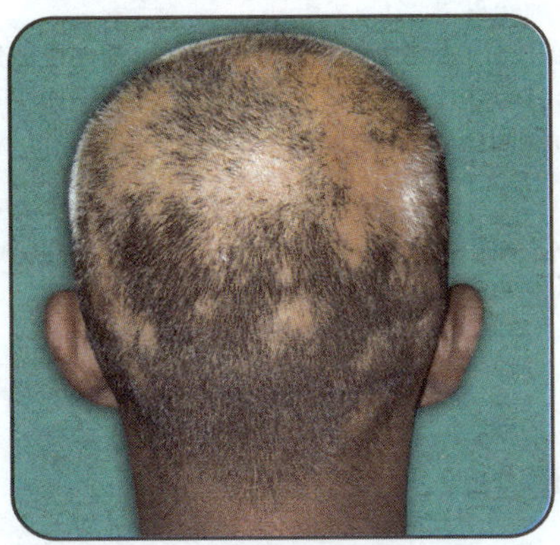

a. Hemophilus
b. Klebsiella
c. Treponema
d. Herpes simplex

Ans. (c) Treponema

The image shows moth eaten alopecia. Grey, moist groin lesions would be condyloma lata. Secondary syphilis also has asymptomatic macular skin rash. So, the cause is treponema.

61. A patient presents with painful nodules on arms and legs with nerve involvement in the ulnar nerve path. The diagnosis is:

a. Tuberculoid leprosy with lepromin positive
b. ENL with lepromin negative
c. Lepromatous leprosy with lepromin positive
d. Scrofuloderma

Ans. (b) ENL with lepromin negative

Painful nodules on limbs would be s/o ENL. ENL is a type of lepra reaction seen on the LL spectrum and hence would be lepromin negative. TT leprosy would not be nodular. Lepromatous leprosy would have painless nodules, not painful and it is lepromin negative. Scrofuloderma is a type of non healing sinus due to TB.

62. A patient comes with box shape or square shaped appearance on biopsy. The diagnosis is:

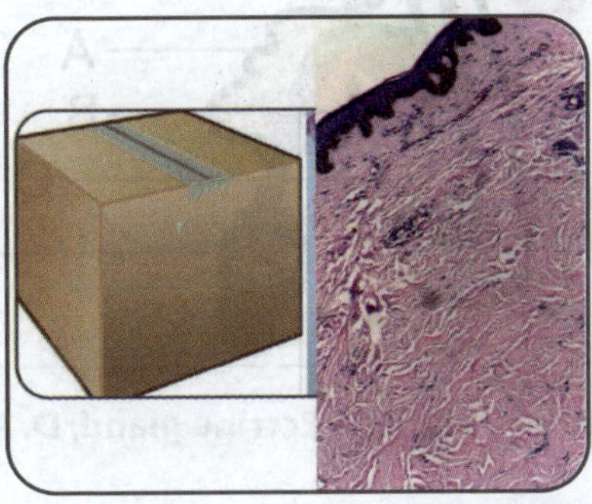

a. Lichen planus
b. Lichen amyloidosis
c. Morphea
d. Lichen nitidus

Ans. (c) Morphea

Biopsy from morphea (localized scleroderma) is squared off at the edges, giving the appearance of box-shaped (or boxed dermis appearance). This boxing of the dermis happens due to the marked sclerosis of collagen throughout the reticular dermis and extending to the septa of subcutaneous fat.

63. A patient has itchy lesions on his skin with blistering along with gut issues. What other findings will be seen?

a. Anti-TTG antibody
b. Anti-nuclear antibody
c. Anti-Sm antibody
d. Anti-Desmoglein antibody

Ans. (a) Anti-TTG antibody

Dermatitis herpetiformis (DH) is an autoimmune blistering skin disorder that is associated with intestinal gluten sensitivity. Epidermal transglutaminase (TGe) and closely related tissue transglutaminase (tTG) are considered to be autoantigens in DH, because a majority of DH patients have IgA specific for transglutaminase.

64. Label the slide:

a. A. Sebaceous gland, B. Apocrine, C. Eccrine gland, D. Hair shaft
b. A. Eccrine, B. Apocrine, C. Hair shaft, D. Sebaceous gland
c. A. Sebaceous gland, B. Hair shaft, C. Eccrine gland, D. Apocrine gland
d. A. Eccrine, B. Sebaceous, C. Hair shaft, D. Apocrine

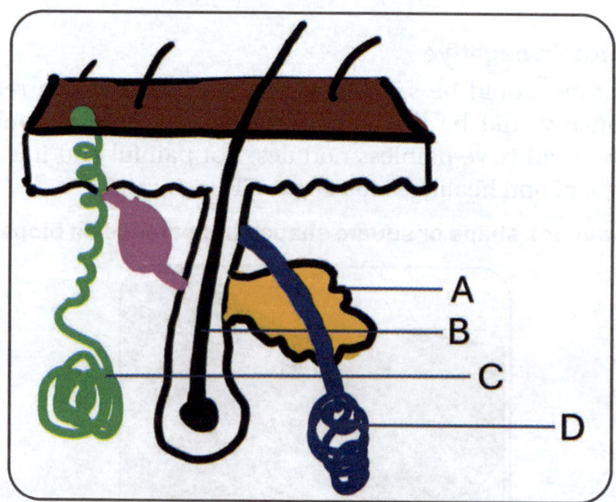

Ans. (c) A. Sebaceous gland, B. Hair shaft, C. Eccrine gland, D. Apocrine gland

65. A patient has genital grouped vesicles. The likely organism is:

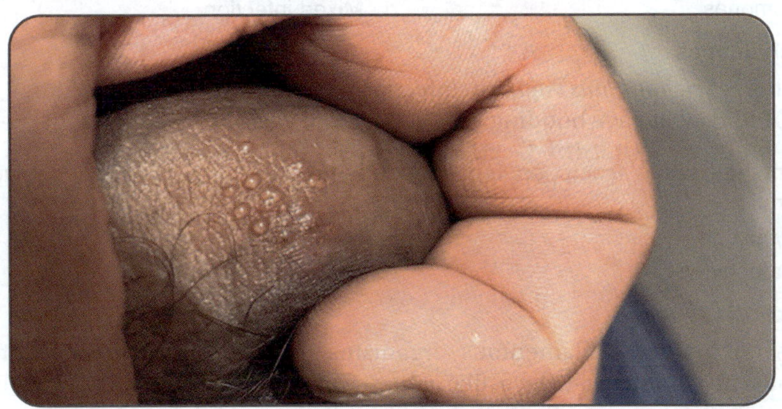

a. Herpes
b. Hemophilus
c. Klebsiella
d. Treponema

Ans. (a) Herpes

Grouped vesicles indicate Herpes genitalis. Haemophilus will cause non-vesicular ulcers. *Klebsiella* would create bleeding ulcers without vesicles. *Treponema* would be painless ulcers.

66. A patient has orange hue skin lesions and hyperkeratotic palms and soles. Biopsy shows alternating parakeratosis and orthokeratosis. The diagnosis is:

a. Pityriasis rubra pilaris
b. Follicular psoriasis
c. Keratosis follicularis
d. Reactive arthritis

Ans. (a) Pityriasis rubra pilaris

Pityriasis rubra pilaris is an uncommon skin condition characterized by orange colored patches with scaling, clear areas of normal skin, and thick palms and soles. Hair follicles with keratin plugging is a characteristic sign. Biopsy shows alternating parakeratosis and orthokeratosis.

67. A female with dysuria and vaginal discharge presents to you. The smear shows as follows. The likely diagnosis is:

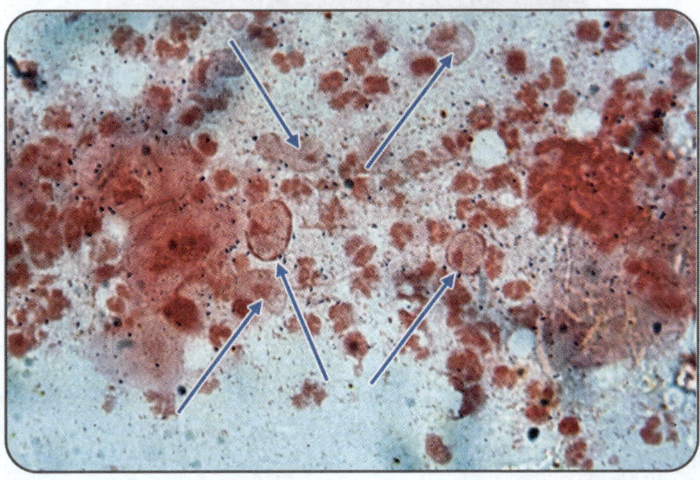

a. Candida
b. Bacterial vaginosis
c. Trichomonas
d. Mixed infection

Ans. (c) Trichomonas

The image shows *Trichomonas vaginalis* infection. Dysuria and vaginal discharge supports the diagnosis. Candida will have budding yeasts. Bacterial vaginosis will have clue cells.

68. A patient has sinus tracts on foot with filamentous organisms on smear. The likely organism is:

a. Sporothrix
b. Nocardia
c. Dermatophytes
d. Candida

Ans. (b) Nocardia

Sinus tracts on foot with filamentous organisms on smear is suggestive of mycetoma. Actinomycotic mycetoma will have filamentous organisms. The causes can be nocardia, actinomyces or streptomyces. Sporothrix will be linear nodules and sinuses with asteroid bodies on smear. Dermatophytes will not have sinus tracts. Candida will have itchy red or white areas clinically without sinus tracts.

69. An adolescent male shows the following acne lesions. Which is the best effective drug for this condition?

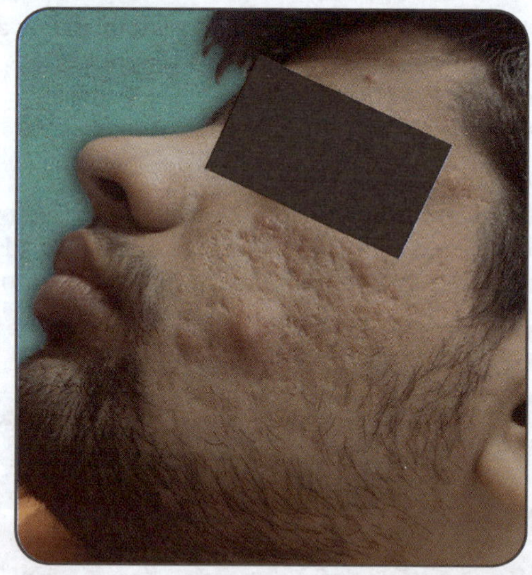

a. Minocycline
b. Doxycycline
c. Isotretinoin
d. Topical dapsone

Ans. (c) Isotretinoin

The image shows primarily comedonal acne. This acne would need a keratolytic agent like retinoids. Here, the best answer is isotretinoin. Minocycline, doxycycline and dapsone are mainly bactericidal.

70. A 60-year-old person has completed his treatment of leprosy. Many years later he presents with a punched out painless ulcer on his sole. What is the management?

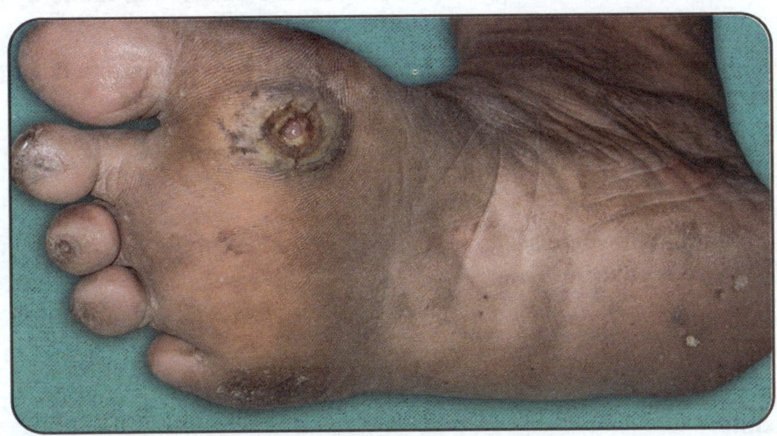

a. Ask him to bear less weight on that leg
b. Restart MDT
c. Amputation
d. Intense debridement and iv antibiotics

Ans. (a) Ask him to bear less weight on that leg

The image shows trophic ulcers on pressure bearing sites on the foot. This is common in peripheral neuropathy seen in lepromatous leprosy. The best treatment is to reduce weight on that leg to allow the ulcer to heal. MDT would not help as this ulcer is due to nerve damage and not due to living organisms (patient has already completed his treatment earlier). Antibiotics will not help as there is no infection here. The ulcer is mainly due to absent sensations and consequent ulceration due to unnoticed traumas and pressure.

71. A patient presents with skin lesions and vesicular buccal mucosa lesions. His immunofluorescence is as shown. The diagnosis is:

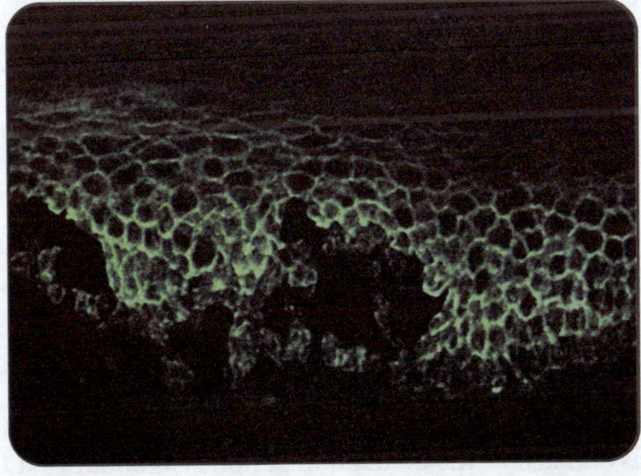

a. Bullous pemphigoid
b. Pemphigus
c. Dermatitis herpetiformis
d. Linear IgA disease

Ans. (b) Pemphigus

Skin and buccal mucosa lesions suggest pemphigus. The direct immunofluorescence shows fishnet appearance further supporting a diagnosis of pemphigus.

72. A child presents with multiple patchy hair loss areas with scales and itching. Sister also had similar lesions. The diagnosis is:

a. Alopecia areata
b. Tinea capitis
c. Pediculosis capitis
d. Pyoderma

Ans. (b) Tinea capitis

Patchy hair loss with itching and scales is suggestive of tinea capitis which can often crossover to contacts in the house like her sister.

73. A patient with multiple sexual exposures has gonorrhea. The treatment is:

a. Aciclovir
b. Doxycycline
c. Cefixime
d. Penicillin

Ans. (c) Cefixime

The CDC guidelines support the use of cefixime in the treatment of gonorrhea. There is now MDR strains of gonorrhea. Hence, cefixime is important in the management.

NEET March 2023

74. Which vitamin deficiency causes diarrhea, dermatitis, and dementia?

a. Vitamin C deficiency
b. Vitamin B3 deficiency
c. Vitamin B6 deficiency
d. Vitamin B12 deficiency

Ans. (b) Vitamin B3 deficiency

The diagnosis is Pellagra which is a triad of diarrhea, dermatitis, and dementia. Pellagra is caused because of cellular deficiency of niacin, resulting from an inadequate dietary supply of niacin and tryptophan mostly seen in chronic alcoholics, and in patients with gastrointestinal diseases or severe psychiatric disturbances. The cutaneous changes include erythema and scaling on sun exposed areas with a "butterfly" eruption on face and a well-marginated eruption on the front of the neck ("Casal's necklace"). Oral nicotinamide is given initially as 100–300 mg daily in 3–4 doses until improvement in acute symptoms, then slowly tapered to 50 mg BD or TDS. Oral nicotinamide is preferred over niacin/nicotinic acid as it does not precipitate flushing, itching and burning commonly seen with ingestion of niacin in large doses.

75. A 5-year-old child presents to OPD with fever, rash, and Koplik spots. What is the most probable diagnosis?

a. Measles
b. Diphtheria
c. Rotavirus
d. Cytomegalovirus

Ans. (a) Measles

Measles is a highly contagious, serious airborne disease caused by a virus that can lead to severe complications and death. The incubation period lasts about 10–14 days, then the fever appears up to over 40°C accompanied with cough, coryza, and conjunctivitis. Pathognomonic for this pathology are Koplik spots, which occur the day before the onset of the rash and persist for 2 or 3 days. Koplik spots appear as bluish-white lesions, slightly raised by 2–3 mm, on a reddened base and are identifiable on the oral mucosa at the level of the first molar but may also occur at the level of the soft palate. The rash lasts 3–7 days, in some cases followed by a fine scaling. Initially, the areas involved are those of the face, with a subsequent distribution in 2–3 days of the caudal skull (erythematous macules of 3–8 mm subsequently confluent); instead, a cough can persist for up to 10 days. Accompanying these signs are other symptoms, such as photophobia from iridocyclitis, headache, abdominal pain, and mild generalized lymphadenopathy. The combination of generalized maculopapular rash, fever (≥38°C), and either cough, coryza, or conjunctivitis has a high sensitivity (75–90%) for diagnosis.

76. What ocular complication is this patient likely to suffer from?

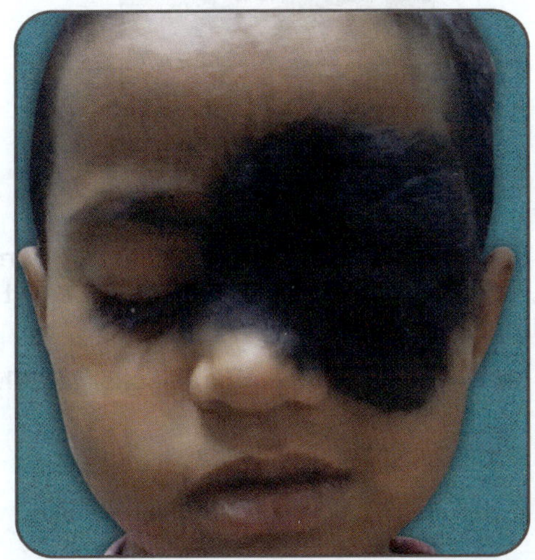

Source: https://europepmc.org/article/MED/2537888

a. Malignant melanoma
b. Basal cell carcinoma
c. Squamous cell carcinoma
d. Hemangioma

Ans. (a) Malignant melanoma

This is a large congenital melanocytic nevus (CMN). The most common complication is malignant transformation of the melanocytes. Malignant melanomas may develop in any patient with CMN, although the risk is higher in patients with large lesions >20 cm in size, or with multiple CMNs.

77. A 30-year-old sexually active male presents with a painless ulcer around the perineum and genital region associated with non-tender lymphadenopathy. Most likely diagnosis would be:

a. Donovanosis
b. Syphilis chancre
c. Lymphogranuloma venereum
d. Chancroid

Ans. (b) Syphilis chancre

Syphilis chancre will present as painless ulcers and painless lymph nodes. Donovanosis will not have lymphadenopathy. LGV will have tender lymphadenopathy. Chancroid will have painful ulcer and painful lymphadenopathy.

78. A male with a history of hair dye use presented with the following features. What is the most likely causative agent?

a. Paraphenylenediamine
b. Nickel
c. Cobalt Chloride
d. Monobenzyl ether of hydroquinone

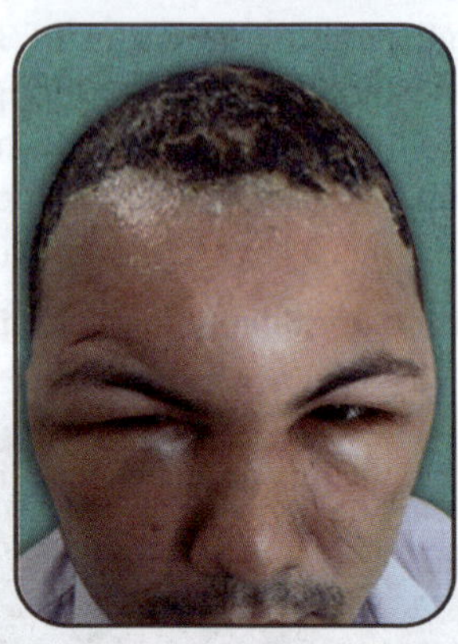

Ans. (a) Paraphenylenediamine

Paraphenylenediamine in hair dyes can cause allergic contact dermatitis in many patients. This can present as edema, itching, and inflammation. Monobenzyl ether of hydroquinone is a cause of ACD to rubber slippers.

79. A female presented to an STI clinic with vaginal discharge. What is the kit used for the treatment of this?

a. Red
b. Blue
c. Grey
d. Green

Ans. (d) Green

The green kit covers cases of vaginal discharge. It has fluconazole and Secnidazole and covers candida, trichomonas and bacterial vaginosis. Red kit is for genital ulcers due to herpes. Blue kit for genital ulcers non herpetic. Grey kit is for urethral discharge and cervical discharge.

80. A HIV-positive patient with low CD4 count presented with umbilcated nodules and lung involvement. What is the most likely diagnosis?

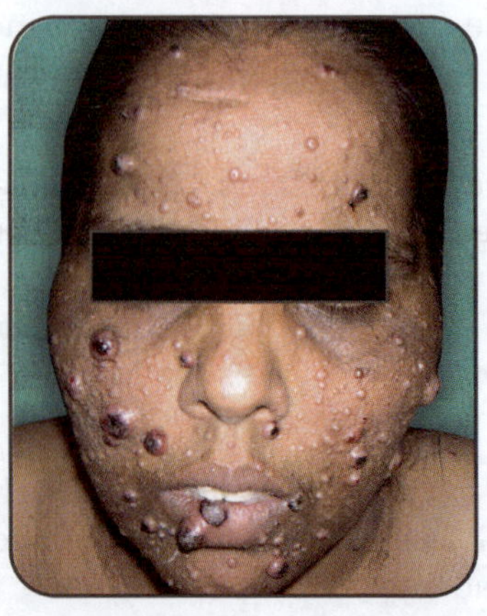

a. Hypersensitivity due to TB
b. Cryptococcus
c. Disseminated Molluscum contagiosum
d. Histoplasmosis

Ans. (d) Histoplasmosis

The leisure shown seems to be a disseminated case of nodules on the face some of them seem to be umbilicated. Differential diagnosis for an umbilicated lesion in HIV would be molluscum, cryptococcosis or histoplasmosis. Since the question mentions lung involvement, the answer would be histoplasmosis. Cryptococcosis would have CNS involvement and can similar lesions while molluscum also has similar lesions but will have no internal systemic involvement.

81. A 35-year-old obese woman presented with acne as given in an image which is not responding to antibiotics and isotretinoin, what's the next step?

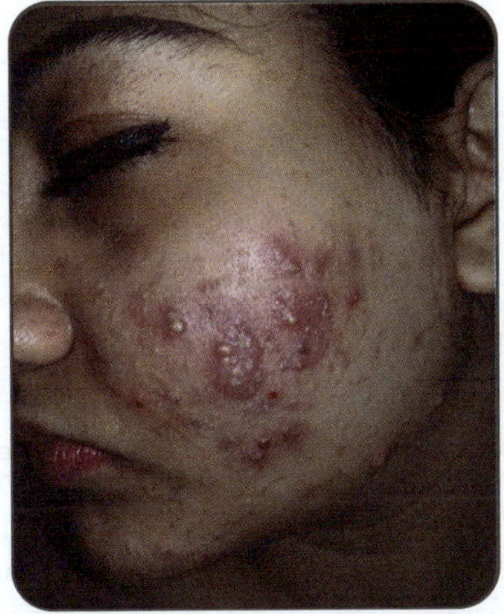

a. Look for dietary triggers
b. Investigation to rule out causes of hyperandrogenism
c. Check for antibiotic resistance
d. Look for drug triggers

Ans. (b) Investigation to rule out causes of hyperandrogenism

Whenever an acne does not respond to the standard drugs like antibiotics and isotretinoin, its important to rule out hormonal causes, especially in an obese person.

NEET May 2022

82. A patient aged 30 years has a history of COVID, 8 months back. She presents with hair loss since 4 months. The diagnosis is:

a. Telogen effluvium
b. Trichotillomania
c. Female pattern androgenic alopecia
d. Anagen effluvium

Ans. (a) Telogen effluvium

This is post-COVID acute telogen effluvium which typically starts after 3–4 months of COVID.

83. A patient presents with cauliflower like growths on foot. The histology is as shown: The diagnosis is:

a. Mycetoma
b. Sporotrichosis
c. Chromoblastomycosis
d. Cutaneous blastomycosis

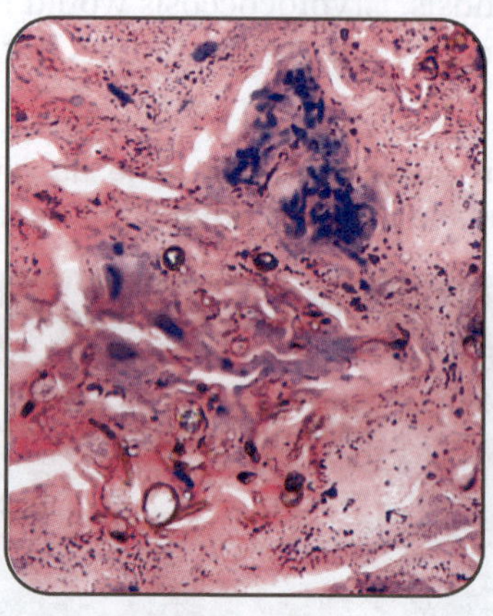

Ans. (c) Chromoblastomycosis

This is the sclerotic pigmented body of chromoblastomycosis.

84. A patient presents with irregular nail pitting, subungual hyperkeratosis and oil drop sign. The diagnosis is:

a. Psoriasis
b. Lichen planus
c. Alopecia areata
d. Atopic dermatitis

Ans. (a) Psoriasis

The described nail changes are typical of psoriasis.

85. A 65-year-old patient comes with erosions on nasolabial area with history of local erosion. The histology is as shown. The diagnosis is:

a. Squamous cell carcinoma
b. Basal cell carcinoma
c. Melanoma
d. Mycosis fungoides

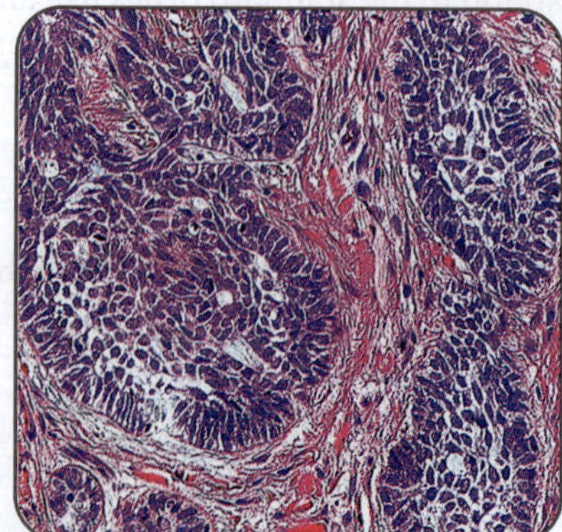

Ans. (b) Basal cell carcinoma

The histology is typical of basal cell carcinoma (BCC) with basaloid tumor cells. Also the question mentions nasolabial area erosion in an elderly man which again supports a diagnosis of BCC.

86. A patient of leprosy presents with painful lesions around eyes and center of forehead as shown. The likely nerve involved will be:

a. Trigeminal
b. Facial
c. Orbital
d. Abducent

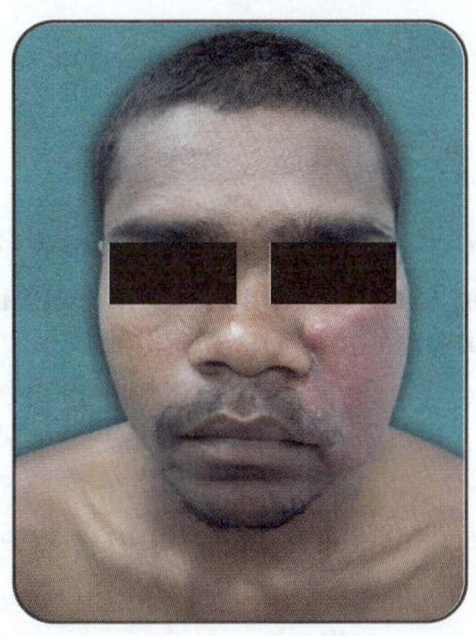

Ans. (b) Facial

Facial nerve involvement is common in Hansen's, especially with lesions around the eyes.

87. A lady with a body mass index of 30 shows with following physical finding on neck. The likely underlying cause will be:

a. Metabolic syndrome
b. Hypothyroidism
c. Lichen planus
d. Addison's disease

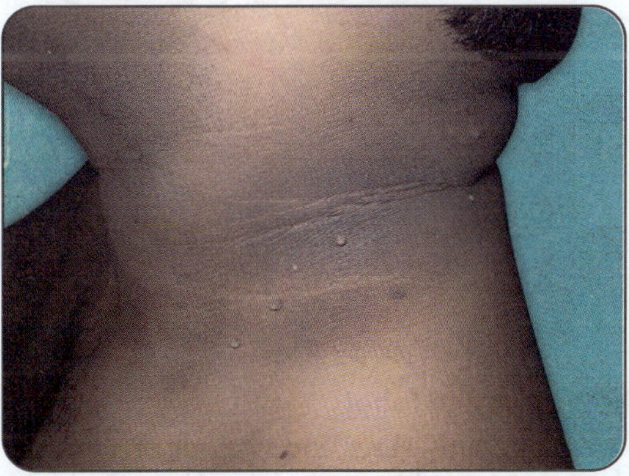

Ans. (a) Metabolic syndrome

This is an image of acanthosis nigricans which is due to metabolic syndrome.

88. A patient with anogenital wart comes to you. Histology shows squamous cell atypia. The high risk HPV causing this will be:

a. HPV 2
b. HPV 18
c. HPV 5
d. HPV 11

Ans. (b) HPV 18

89. A wrestler complaints of itch in axilla. The lesions show central clearing. The organism produced red, velvety colonies in culture. They had pencil shaped macroconidia and abundant microconidia. Diagnosis is:

a. Trichophyton rubrum
b. Trichophyton mentagrophytes
c. Trichophyton schoenleinii
d. Trichophyton tonsurans

Ans. (a) Trichophyton rubrum

The diagnosis is tinea with central clearing. T. rubrum causes red, velvety colonies.

90. A military person staying in a crowded basement gets itchy rash on body sparing the palm and sole. Lice was found on him. The diagnosis is:

a. Rickettsia akari
b. Rickettsia conorii
c. Rickettsia typhi
d. Rickettsia prowazekii

Ans. (d) Rickettsia prowazekii

The rash sparing palms and soles caused by a louse is s/o epidemic typhus caused by Rickettsia prowazekii.

91. A 45-year-old farmer has foot swelling and sinuses on foot. Microscopy of granule is shown. Pick the correct statement:

a. Caused by both bacteria and fungi
b. Do not invade deeper tissues
c. Hematogenous spread
d. Splendore-Hoeppli phenomenon

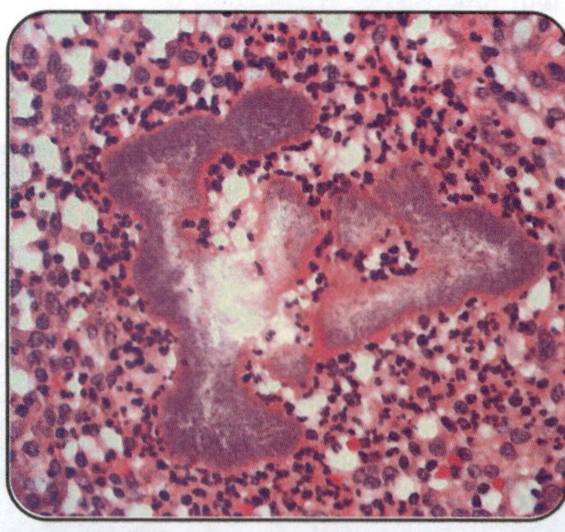

Ans. (a) Caused by both bacteria and fungi

The diagnosis is mycetoma with grains, sinus and swelling on foot. It is caused both by bacteria and fungi. It does invade deep tissue like underlying bone. It does not have hematogenous spread. Splendore-Hoeppli phenomenon is seen in sporotrichosis and not mycetoma.

NEET September 2021

92. A patient has raw skin lesions and flaccid blisters which crust on drying up. He shows a suprabasal blister on histology. The diagnosis is:

a. Pemphigus foliaceus
b. Pemphigus vulgaris
c. Erythema multiforme
d. Pemphigus vegetans

Ans. (b) Pemphigus vulgaris

Flaccid blisters with suprabasal blisters are s/o pemphigus vulgaris.

93. A 10-year-old girl present with the condition as shown. She has a dog as a pet. The diagnosis is:

a. Folliculitis
b. Abscess
c. Kerion
d. Epidermoid cyst

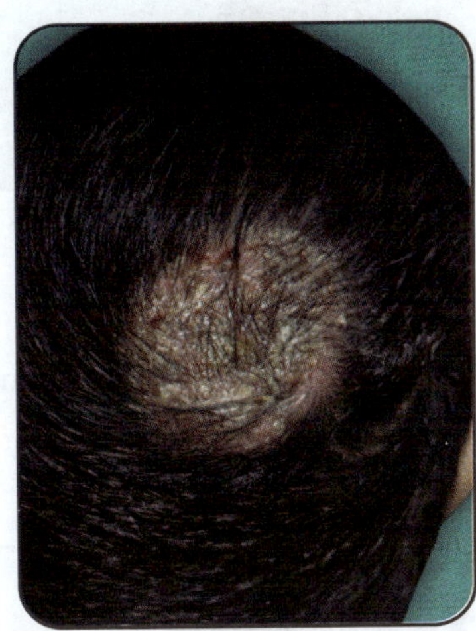

Ans. (c) Kerion

The diagnosis is kerion. Pointers in the question are the child and pet transmission of dermatophytes (zoophilic mode of transmission).

94. Hair perforation test positive on microscopy. The likely dermatophyte would be:

a. Trichophyton mentagrophyte
b. Microsporum audouinii
c. Microsporum gypseum
d. Epidermophyton floccosum

Ans. (a) Trichophyton mentagrophyte

Hair perforation test is an in vitro hair perforation test to help distinguish the isolates of dermatophytes, typically Trichophyton mentagrophytes. The test is performed by placing an organism into a Petri dish containing hair. T. mentagrophytes produce marked localised areas of pitting and marked erosion in the hair shaft whereas those of T. rubrum do not.

95. A patient with leprosy and type 1 lepra reaction with tender nerves is on MDT. There are no systemic features. Next line of management would be:

a. Continue MDT with corticosteroids
b. Stop MDT and give steroids
c. Continue MDT with thalidomide
d. Stop MDT and give thalidomide

Ans. (a) Continue MDT with corticosteroids

Corticosteroid is the DOC for Type 1 lepra reaction with neuritis. MDT always to be continued.

96. A patient has paronychia followed by lesions as shown. The treatment would be:

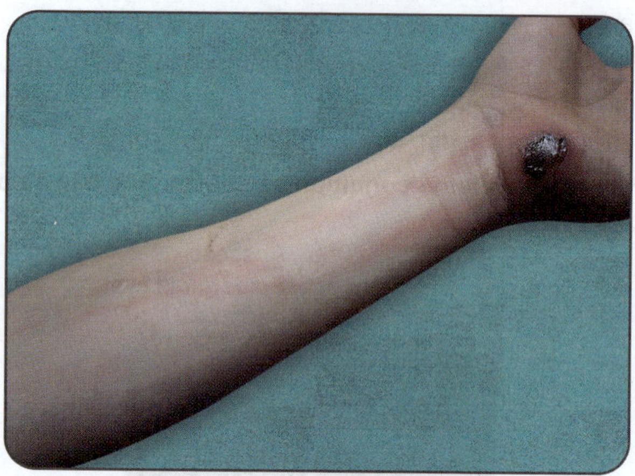

a. Co-amoxiclav
b. Metronidazole
c. Amikacin
d. Norfloxacin

Ans. (a) Co-amoxiclav

Acute paronychia is likely bacterial. The image shows lymphangitis secondary to bacteria.

97. A patient with sexual exposure has history of purulent urethral discharge as shown in the image. The most common organism was asked:

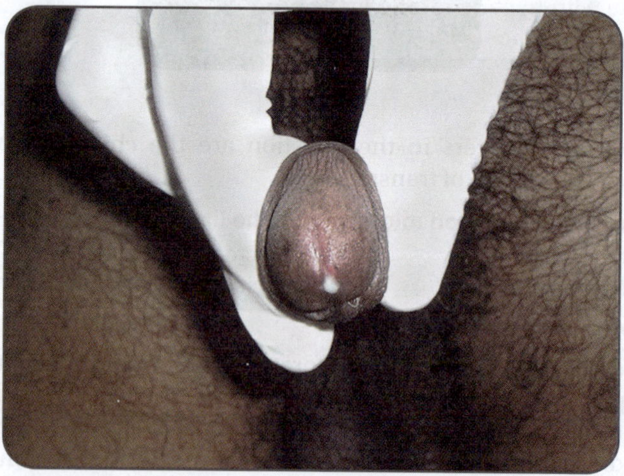

a. Gonorrhea
b. Herpes
c. Ureaplasma
d. Escherichia coli

Ans. (a) Gonorrhea

Purulent discharge from urethra after sexual exposure is s/o gonorrhea.

98. A patient eats maize as staple diet. He presents with rash around neck since 1 year. He also has diarrhoea. The likely deficiency is:

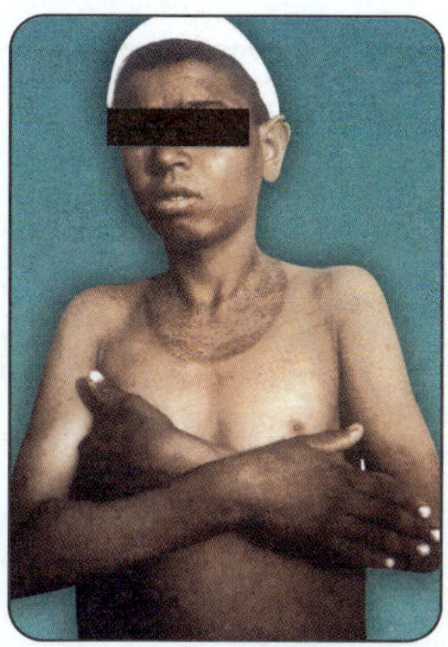

a. Vitamin A
b. Vitamin C
c. Niacin
d. Vitamin B12

Ans. (c) Niacin

Pellagra is a clinical syndrome characterized by a photo distributed rash developing into a chronic dermatitis, gastrointestinal manifestations and neurologic and psychiatric disturbances and traditionally these symptoms remembered as classic four Ds: the Dermatitis, Diarrhea, Dementia, and rarely Death if it is untreated. People who consumed maize as their staple diet were more prone to pellagra as maize is poor in tryptophan and hence niacin.

99. A patient presents with hyperkeratotic lesions on the elbow as shown. He also has night blindness. The likely diagnosis is:

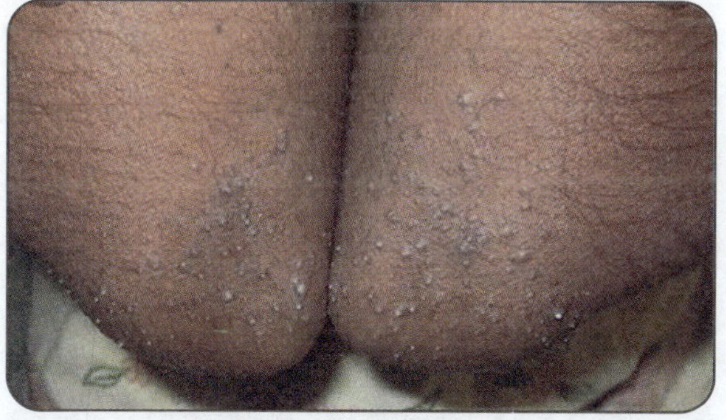

a. Keratosis pilaris
b. Phrynoderma
c. Psoriasis
d. Darier's disease

Ans. (b) Phrynoderma

Phrynoderma is a form of follicular hyperkeratosis that is associated with nutritional deficiencies. This form of dermatosis can be caused by isolated deficiencies of vitamins A, B complex, C and E. Adjunctive symptoms, such as cheilitis, glossitis, blepharitis, night blindness, diarrhea, muscle weakness and neuritis, may develop when hypovitaminosis A is predominant relative to other vitamin deficiencies.

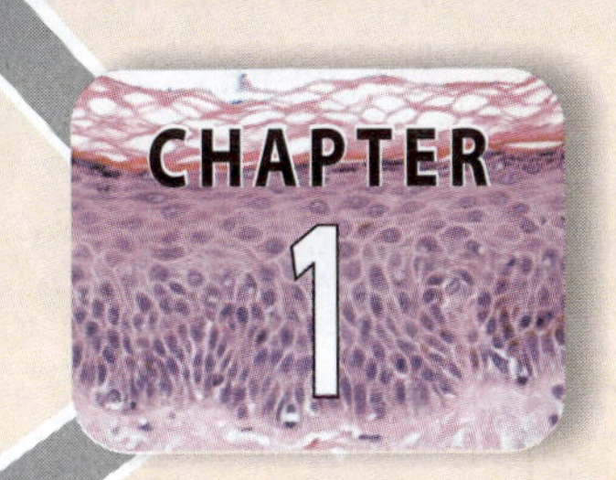

Anatomy and Physiology of Skin

INTRODUCTION

Human skin (the largest organ of the body) consists of three layers:

1. **Epidermis**—Superficial stratified, squamous layer.
2. **Dermis**—Underlying layer consisting of connective tissue with a dermal-epidermal junction (DEJ) basement membrane separating the two.
3. **Subcutaneous fat (panniculus)**—Consisting of **fat lobules** (containing adipocytes) and **fat septae** (fibrous tissue).

Attached into the skin are **appendages, also called as adnexae** (literally, appendage = attachment). **Pilosebaceous unit (pilo = hair), nail and sweat glands** are included in the term "appendages". Sweat glands are **apocrine** (present in axillae, perineum, areolae) opening into the pilosebaceous unit or **eccrine** which open directly onto the skin surface (Fig. 1).

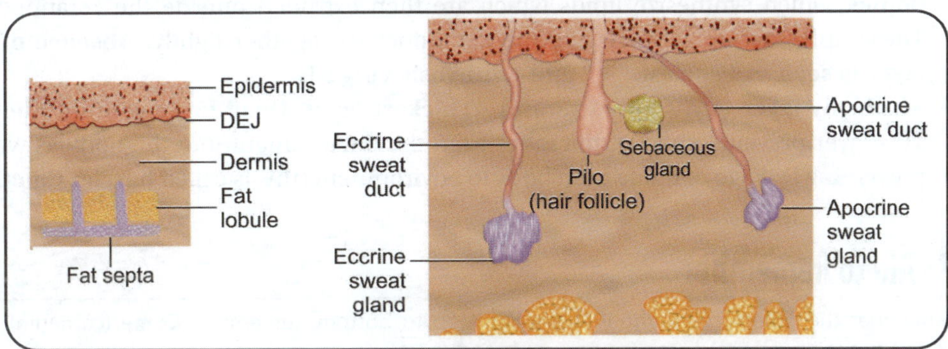

Fig. 1: Schematic architecture of skin

EPIDERMIS

- **Thickest on the palms and soles** (approximately 1.5 mm), **thinnest on the eyelid** measuring less than 0.1 mm.
- Derived from **ectoderm** (dermis is derived from mesenchyme).
- Contains **keratinocytes, melanocytes, Langerhans cells and Merkel cells.**
- **Four layers** from bottom to top—**Stratum basale (SB), stratum spinosum (SS), stratum granulosum (SG), stratum corneum (SC)** (Fig. 2)
  - **SB (basal layer-stratum basale)**—Dividing layer, columnar cells
  - **SS (prickle layer-stratum spinosum)**—The intercellular attachments, also called **desmosomes**, are most prominent here. These desmosomes appear like spines on microscopy—hence called the **prickle layer.**

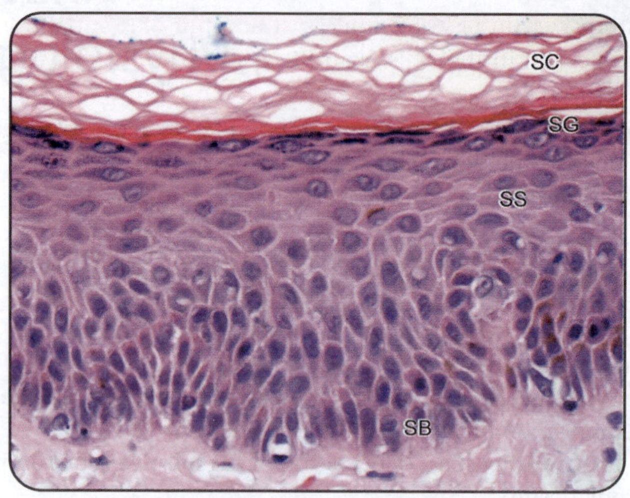

Fig. 2: Normal histology of the skin

- **SG-Granular layer (stratum granulosum)**—Layer is called granular as it has **keratohyaline granules**. Also this layer contains **lamellar bodies** (also called **Odland bodies**) which synthesize lipids which are then extruded outside the keratinocytes. These lipids act as glue sticking the keratinocytes together tightly. **Absence of this layer is seen in Psoriasis(MCQ) and Ichthyosis vulgaris.**
- **SC-Horny layer (stratum corneum)—Thickest layer. Dead layer without nucleus.** This layer prevents entry of microbes from the environment into the body as well as preventing leakage of fluids from body to environment (this is called **barrier function**).

Aid to Remember

To remember the order of epidermal layers from top to bottom, remember: **Come** (corneum) **lets** (lucidum) **get** (granulosum) **some** (spinosum) **bread** (basal)

- On the palms and soles, a **clear zone called stratum lucidum** is seen above the granular layer. This layer has **degenerated keratinocytes**
- The term **Malpighian layer** includes both spinous and basal layers

Keratinocytes

- The cells are named after its intermediate filament called **keratin** which provides mechanical strength to this cell (strength is required for resisting daily trauma and mechanical pressures on the epidermis).
- Keratinocytes divide and generate the upper layers. **Transit time/Turnover time** is the time it takes for basal cells to reach the skin surface and shed. **Best answer would be 28 days**

******Note:* **If 28 days is not in the MCQ option, next best answer is 40–56 days**

- More the need for strength, more the need for keratin. Since SC requires the maximum strength, maximum keratin is in SC and least amount of keratin is in SB. This process of increasing the keratin in the cells from SB upwards to SC is called **keratinization of epidermis** (Fig. 3).
- As function of SC is protection and it does not divide, it sheds off its nucleus. In contrast, SB divides and needs a nucleus. Hence, as the basal cells go up, gradually in 4 weeks, the **nucleus is lost** and hence, stratum corneum is non-nucleated (Fig. 4).

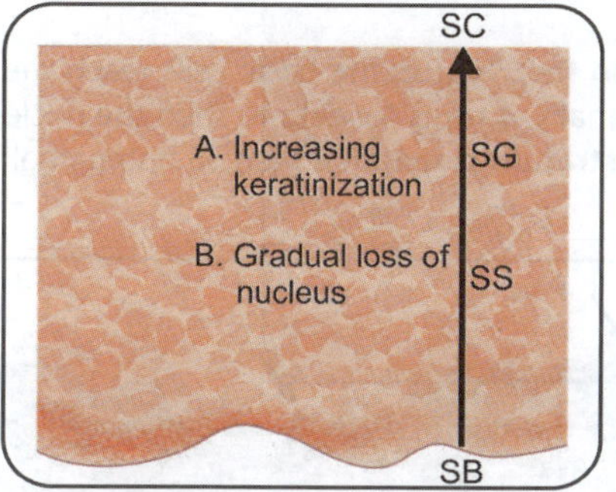

Fig. 3: Changes in the epidermis as cells move up from SB to SC

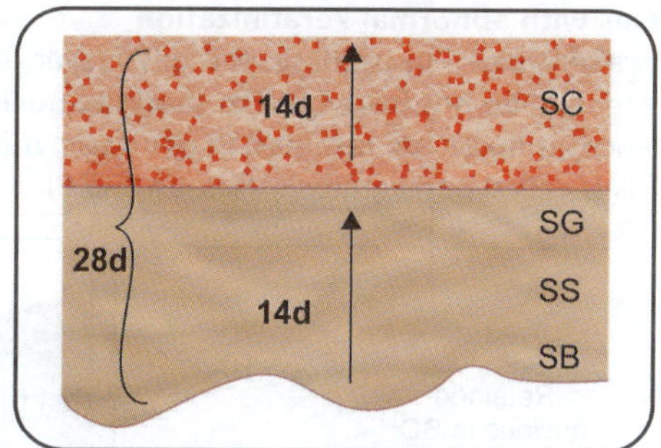

Fig. 4: Keratinocyte travel times—From SB to bottom of SC = 14 days, and from bottom of SC to the top of SC = 14 days

- **90–95% of all epidermal cells are keratinocytes.**
- **Original residents in epidermis. In contrast, melanocytes, Langerhans cells and Merkel's cells are immigrants(MCQ).**
- There is a change in the keratin filaments (K) from basal to upper layers—**K5 and K14—basal layer, K1 and K10—suprabasal layers.**

Note:* Mutations in the genes for keratins 5 and 14 are associated with **epidermolysis bullosa simplex—EBS (more information on EBS in chapter 9).

- Since it would be better to **intermingle and enmesh the keratin filaments** for even more strength in the epidermis, keratin filaments tend to join together in the upper epidermis. **Filaggrin does this** (Fig. 5). Since upper layers require more strength than lower layers, filaggrin synthesis is in **upper layers (starting from the granular layer up to the corneal layer)**. In the granular layer, the **keratohyaline granules contain these filaggrin molecules (Hence, granular layer is called granular)**.

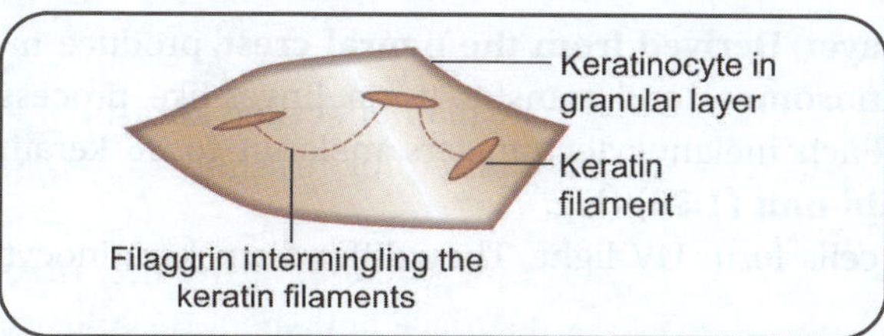

Fig. 5: Role of filaggrin in keratinization

Aid to Remember

Filaggrin = fil = filament, aggr = aggregating, in = protein (hence filaggrin aggregates keratin filaments)

High Yield Points

Diseases with abnormal keratinization

- **Parakeratosis**—In psoriasis, the basal layer divides **too fast**. Hence, the basal cells reach the SC faster and **do not have time to shed the nucleus** (normally, it takes 4 weeks to shed the nucleus). Hence, as nuclei are **retained in psoriasis, nucleated stratum corneum** is seen on histopathology. **This is called parakeratosis** (Figs. 6A and B).

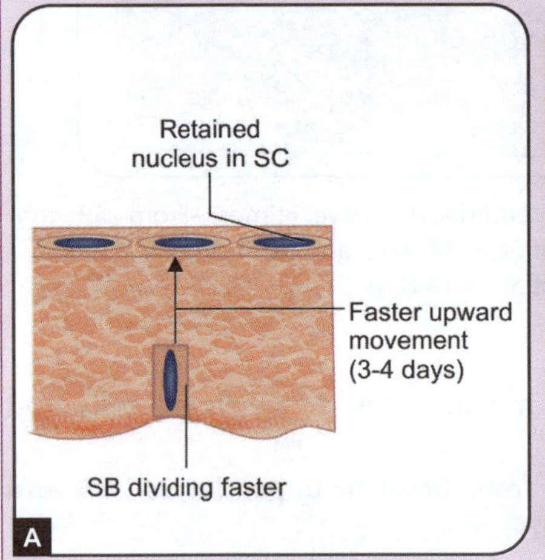

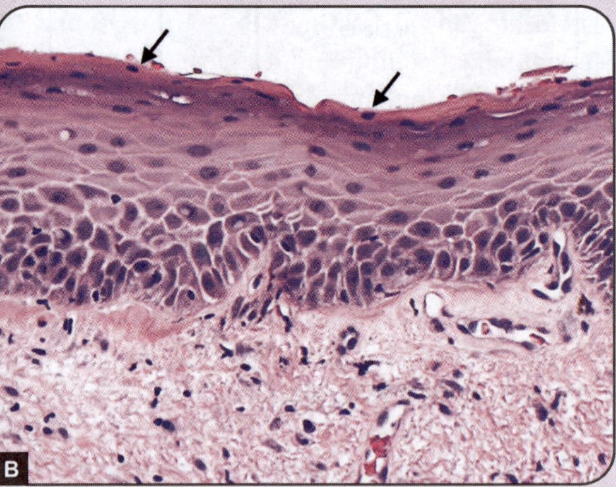

Figs. 6A and B: Parakeratosis: Note the retained nuclei in the corneum (black arrows)

- **Dyskeratosis**—This is defined as **premature keratinization in the epidermis** (prominent keratinization occurs in the lower epidermis itself here, whereas normally prominent keratinization occurs in upper epidermis). Seen in **Darier's disease.** Such cells are round and lose attachments to the surrounding cells (acantholytic cells). Therefore, **dyskeratosis is often associated with acantholysis** (separation of cells in the epidermis with formation of circular keratinocytes).

Melanocytes

- Present in **basal layer. Derived from the neural crest,** produce melanin, package it in **organelles (melanosomes)** and transfer it via finger-like processes called **dendrites** to keratinocytes. Each melanocyte transfers melanin to 36 keratinocytes forming the **epidermal-melanin unit (1:36)** (Fig. 7).
- Melanin protects cells form UV light. They differ from keratinocytes by possessing **no desmosomes.**

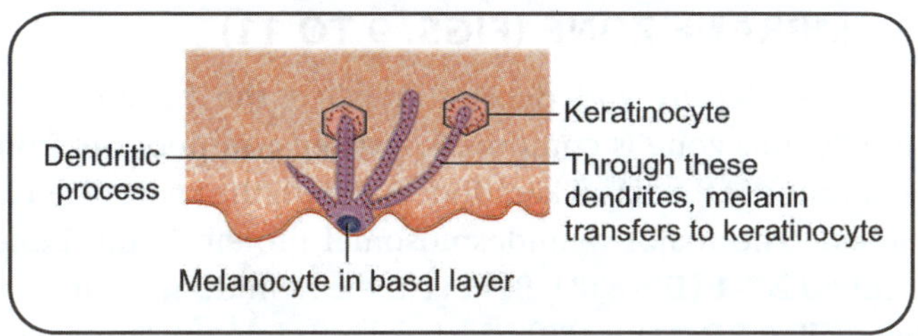

Fig. 7: Schematic representation of melanin transfer into keratinocytes

Langerhans Cells

- Derived from **bone marrow**
- Dendritic cells expressing **CD45, HLA-DR and CD1c**
- Role in adaptive immune responses in the skin since they are **antigen-presenting cells** (APC) processing antigens and transporting them to local lymph nodes

Merkel Cells

- Seen **amongst the basal keratinocytes** (Fig. 8A). **Contain desmosomes**
- Derivation of this cell is controversial-evidence supports both differentiation from epidermal keratinocytes as well as migration from the neural crest
- **Slow-adapting touch receptors**[(MCQ)]

  At the boundary between the epidermis and dermis (dermo-epidermal junction) are finger-like upward projections called the **dermal papilla**. Similarly, there are downward projections into the dermis called the **epidermal rete ridges** (Fig. 8B).

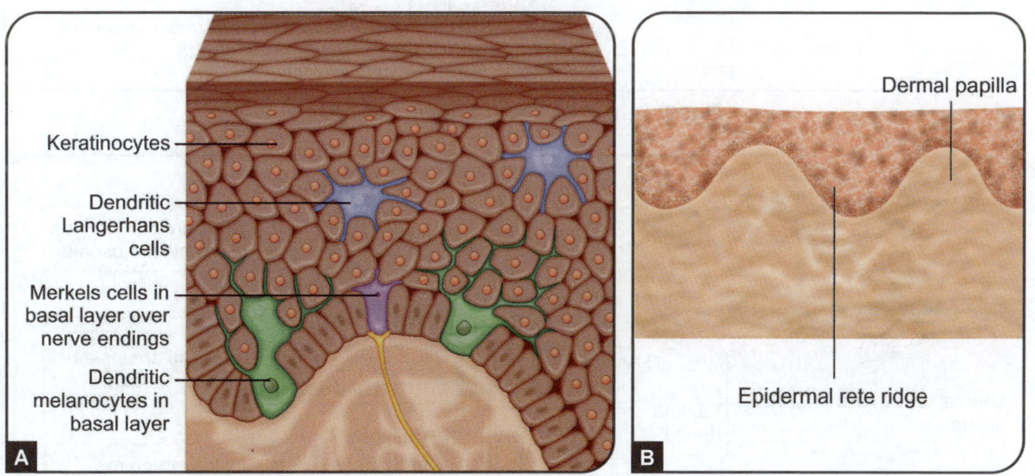

Figs. 8A and B: Schematic representation of epidermis (A) and DEJ (B)

BASEMENT MEMBRANE ZONE (FIGS. 9 TO 11)

The junction between epidermis and dermis is called **the basement membrane zone (BMZ)**. Ultrastructurally, this zone is composed of **three components from top to bottom.**

1. The plasma membranes of the basal keratinocytes with the specialized attachment plates (**hemidesmosomes**). The major hemidesmosomal protein is the **bullous pemphigoid antigen 1, also called BP-1 (BP-230)**. BP-1 is in the hemidesmosome and attaches below to another protein **called BP-2** (BP-180) which extends into the lamina lucida layer below.
2. **Dermoepidermal junction (DEJ)**—It is divided into the upper lamina lucida and the lower lamina densa. **Type IV collagen** is the major component of lamina densa. In the lamina lucida, structures called **anchoring filaments** exist. These anchoring filaments connect the basal keratinocytes above to the lamina densa below and enclose the proteins **BP-2** (also called Type XVII collagen) **and another protein called laminin.**
3. **Anchoring fibers** (attaches the lamina densa above to the underlying connective tissue below in dermis)—**Type VII collagen** is the major protein in the anchoring fiber.

   Blistering diseases in the DEJ and dermis are due to problems in some components of the diagram shown above.

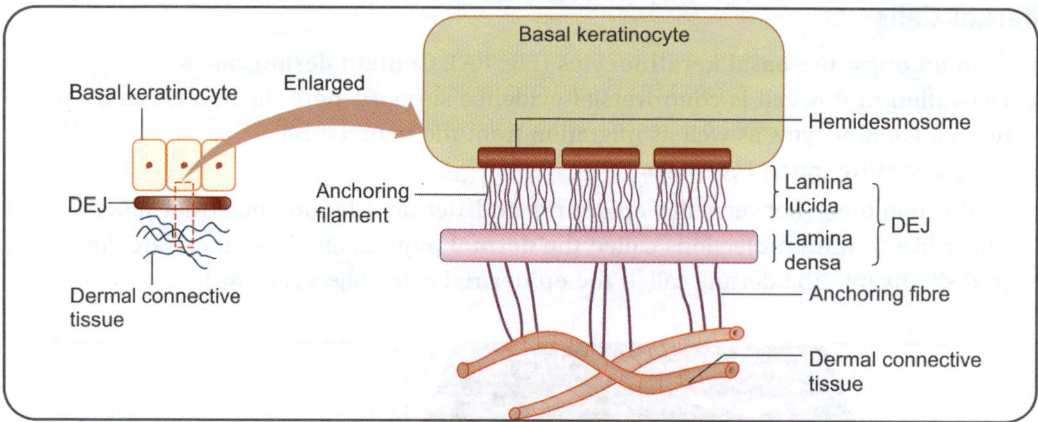

Fig. 9: Schematic representation of DEJ

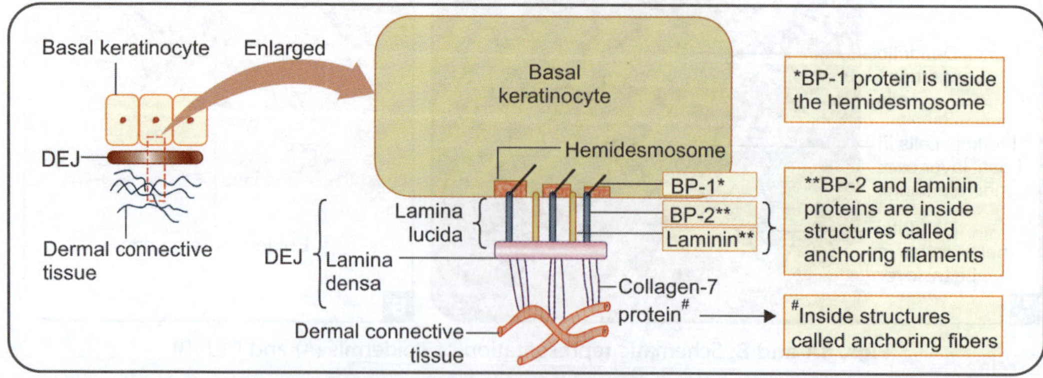

Fig. 10: Schematic representation of DEJ

Diseases*	Target
Bullous pemphigoid (BP)	IgG antibodies against BP-1 or BP-2 (BP-2 > BP-1)
Linear IgA disease (LAD)	IgA antibodies against BP-2
Epidermolysis bullosa junctional (EBJ)	Absent laminin since birth
Epidermolysis bullosa dystrophica (EBD)	Absent collagen 7 since birth
Epidermolysis bullosa acquisita (EBA)	IgG antibodies against collagen 7

*More details on these blistering diseases in chapter 9

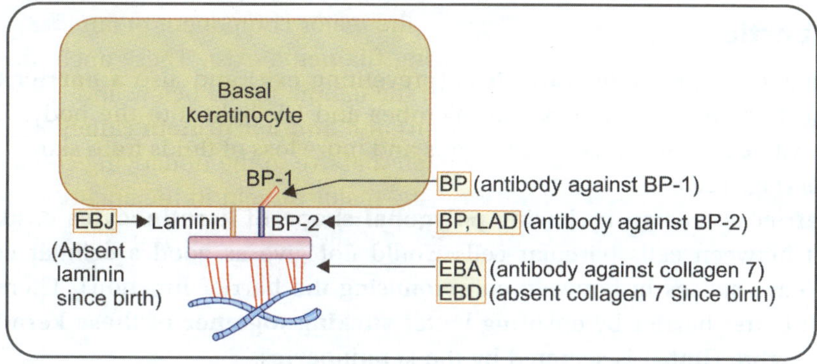

Fig. 11: Schematic representation of DEJ

*The orange boxes indicate the names of diseases and the arrows point to the target of that disease

Dermis: The dermis is subdivided into the **papillary dermis** (part of dermis in the papilla) and a **reticular dermis** (mainly consist of collagen I and collagen III fibers, elastic fibers and matrix).

SUBCUTANEOUS FAT (PANNICULUS)

It is divided into lobules by vascular fibrous septa. The subcutaneous fat may contain large number of mast cells. **Rupture of mast cells in this subcutaneous fat causes the disease angioedema** (Rupture of mast cells in dermis causes the disease **urticaria**).

SWEAT GLANDS

Eccrine sweat glands	Apocrine sweat glands
• Distributed almost **all over the body** (most dense on palms, soles) • Absent on vermilion border of lips, nailbeds, labia minora, glans penis, inner aspect of prepuce	• Localized distribution (**axillae, perineum, and areolae**) • Decapitation secretion • Odor because of skin's bacteria; otherwise odorless
Opens directly on skin	**Opens into hair follicles**
Under sympathetic **cholinergic** control	Under sympathetic **adrenergic** control
Eccrine diseases—e.g. Miliaria, Hyperhidrosis	**Apocrine diseases**—e.g. Hidradenitis suppurativa, Fox-Fordyce disease, Bromhidrosis, etc.

Aid to Remember

Apocrine—Series of letter **A**—**A** = **A**xilla, **A** = **A**reola, **A** = **A**drenergic supply, **A**pex of cell falls off during secretion (decapitation)

Eccrine—Rhymes with word acral—palm and sole distribution, e**CC**rine—**C** = **C**holinergic supply

PHYSIOLOGICAL FUNCTIONS OF SKIN

Barrier Function

- Epidermis is a **barrier to water loss** (preventing exit) and also **a barrier to prevent entry of harmful substances** like microbes and UV light into the body. Loss of this barrier will lead to increase of infections and more loss of fluids from skin, e.g. in burns patients (Fig. 12C).
- This barrier is created by having **polygonal shape of keratinocytes** ensuring better **contact** between cells (circular cells would not give as good a cellular contact and would leave spaces in between compromising the barrier function). There would be an even better barrier by ensuring better **sticking together of these keratinocytes**—Hence, a **glue (lipid)** is secreted by the keratinocytes.
- It has traditionally been compared to a **brick and cement model** where bricks are synonymous with keratinocytes and cement is the glue (Fig. 12A).
- The glue (**technically called intercellular cement**) is composed of sticky lipids (ceramide, squalene, etc.). **Lamellar granules (Odland bodies)** which appear in the **upper spinous and the granular layers** produce this intercellular cement (Fig. 12B).

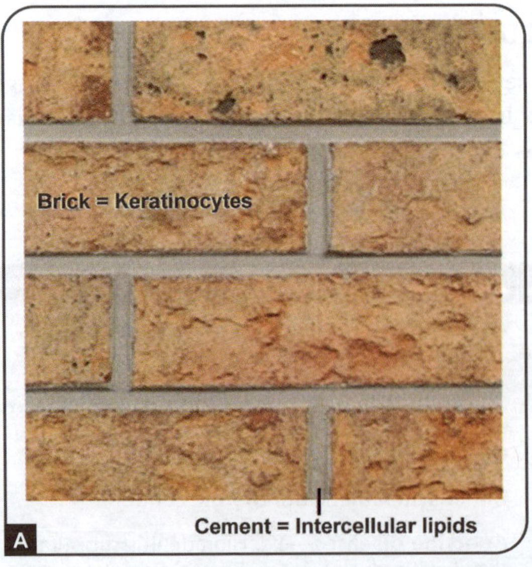

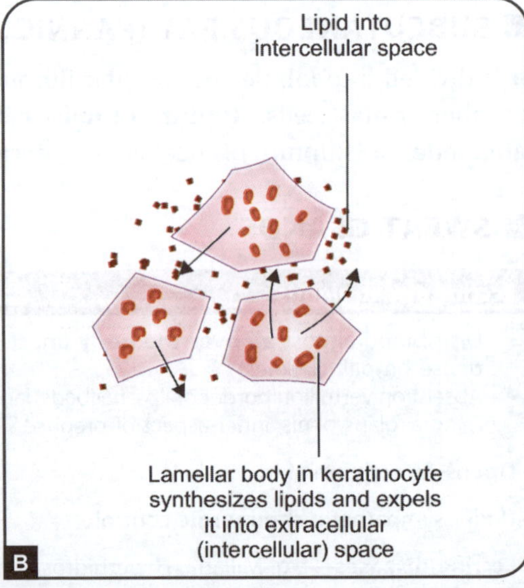

Figs. 12A and B

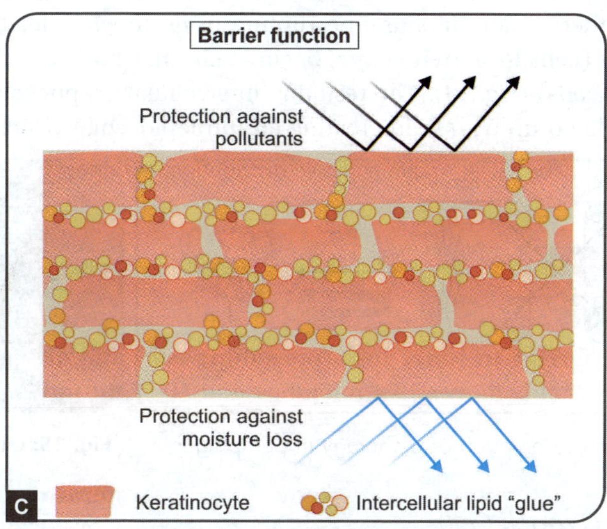

Figs. 12A to C: Barrier function

Barrier Loss

As per the above discussion, barrier loss can either be due to **problems in the keratinocytes (brick damage)** or **problems in the glue (cement collapse)**.

Problems in Keratinocytes (Brick Damage)

The problems in keratinocytes can arise from:

1. Damage to intercellular junctions called **desmosomes** (desmosomes are responsible for maintaining keratinocyte shape and adhesion to each other)
2. Primary destruction of the keratinocyte itself (**cytolysis**)
3. Problems in **calcium pump** (this pump transports calcium from extracellular into intracellular space in keratinocyte—This intracellular calcium is important for proper keratinocyte function as well as desmosome function).

Damage to Intercellular Junctions (Desmosomes)

- Desmosomes are the major intercellular junctions in skin. They join adjacent keratinocytes. Desmosomes contain desmoglein proteins (Fig. 13)

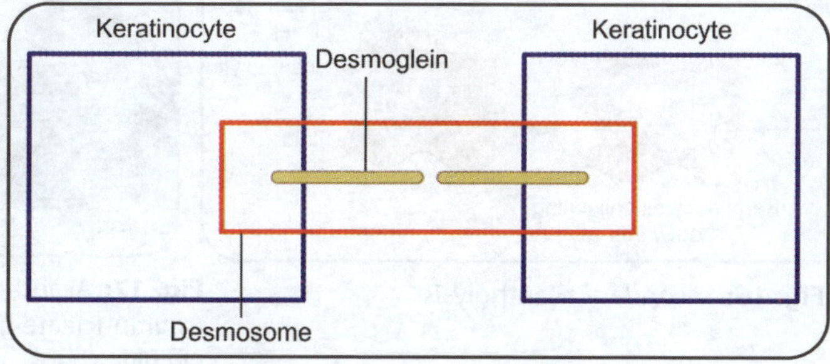

Fig. 13: Desmosomal architecture

- In **pemphigus**, there is an autoimmune rupture of desmoglein leading to separation of the keratinocytes (**cells lose their shape, become circular and are called as acantholytic cells or Tzanck cells**) (Fig. 14). The resulting intercellular empty space between circular keratinocytes is filled up with fluid creating an intraepidermal vesicle (Fig. 15).

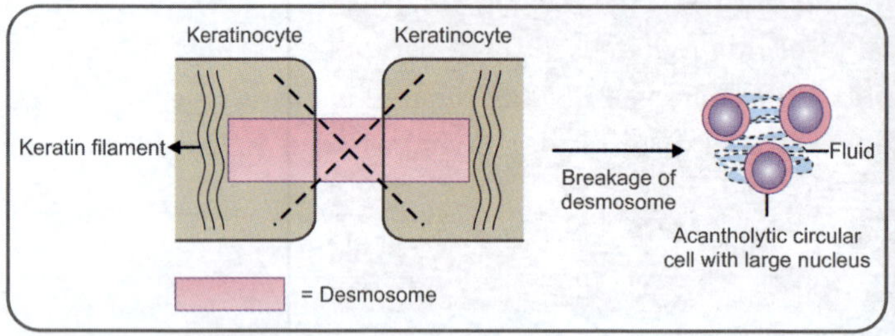

Fig. 14: Schematic representation of pathology in pemphigus

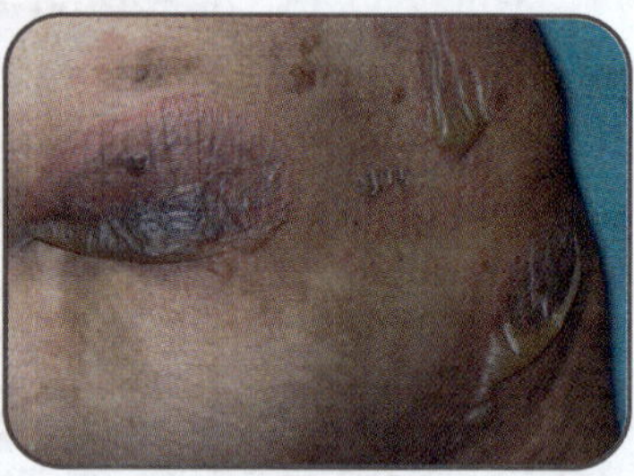

Fig. 15: Clinical image of blisters in pemphigus

Acantholytic Cell (Tzanck Cell)

- A **large rounded keratinocyte** with an **enlarged nucleus and absent nucleoli**. The cytoplasm is more prominent peripherally on the cell membrane, leading to a **perinuclear halo**.
- **Acantholysis** process of formation of an acantholytic cell. It may be a primary event (**primary acantholysis**) or a secondary phenomenon (**secondary acantholysis**).

Primary acantholysis	Secondary acantholysis
When the initial problem is rupture of the desmosome → causing circular cells (hence, desmosomes damaged first → then keratinocyte changes shape)	When the initial problem is not with desmosome, but ballooning of the keratinocyte → causing circular cells (hence, keratinocytes changes shape first)
Seen in 1. **Pemphigus**—Autoimmune damage of desmosome 2. **Staphylococcal scalded skin syndrome (SSSS)**—Staphylococcal toxin damaging the desmosome 3. **Darier's disease**—Genetic defect in desmosome 4. **Hailey-Hailey disease**—Genetic defect in desmosome	**Seen in viral infections (herpes) (Figs. 16 and 17)**

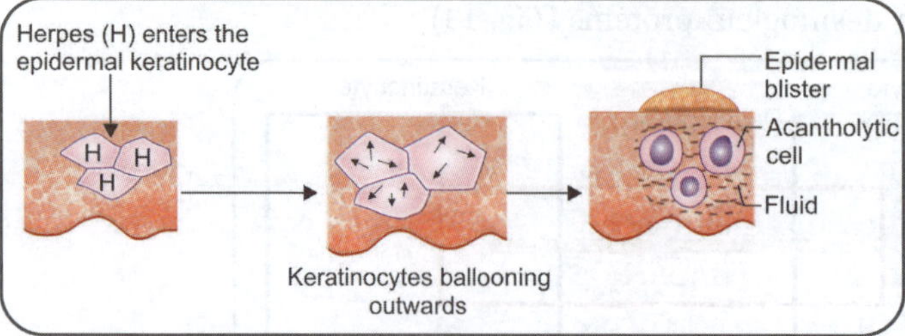

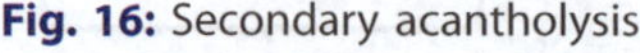

Fig. 16: Secondary acantholysis

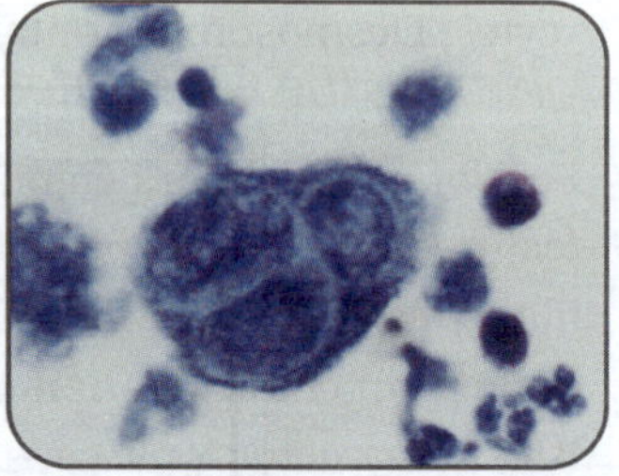

Fig. 17: Acantholytic cell in herpes (multinucleate giant cell)—Note the circular shape, multiple nuclei and the peripheral rim of cytoplasm

Cytolysis

Due to **genetic keratin defects in keratinocytes**, the keratinocytes become **fragile** (remember that keratin gives cellular strength) and **break easily with even minimal trauma (cytolysis)**. This will lead to **separation of cells** from each other, leading to fluid accumulation in epidermis. Such cytolysis in basal layer due to defect in basal keratins (K5 and K14) is seen in **Epidermolysis Bullosa Simplex-EBS (hence, EBS has blister in basal layer). Similar cytolysis in granular layer (hence, blister in granular layer) is seen in epidermolytic hyperkeratosis** (Fig. 18).

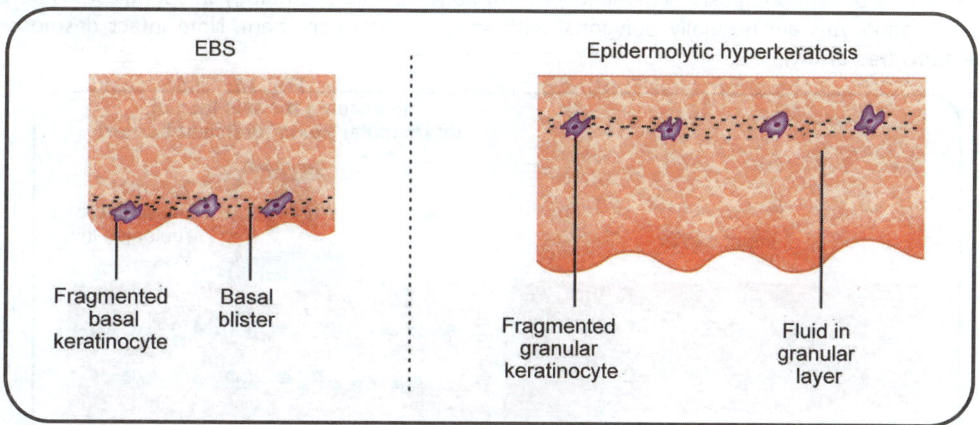

Fig. 18: Cytolysis

Problems in Calcium Pump

Desmosomes are calcium dependent. This calcium is pumped into cells by the **calcium ATPase pump**. Hence, if there is a mutation with this pump, due to less intracellular calcium, desmosomes malfunction leading to separation of epidermal keratinocytes i.e. acantholysis. This occurs in **Darier's disease and Hailey-Hailey disease**.

Problems in the Glue (Intercellular Cement)

- Loss of intercellular cement (containing ceramide, squalene, fatty acids) is an important feature in **eczema**. This small gap creates a barrier function disturbance. This gap then fills up with fluid—**this is called intercellular edema or spongiosis**. The fluid can ooze out of skin clinically (**hence oozing an important sign of acute eczema**) (Figs. 19A and B). These microscopic gaps also allows entry of organisms in to skin (**patients with atopic eczema have more infections, especially staphylococcal infection**). Also in eczema, to replace this loss of ceramide, moisturizers containing ceramide are often given to replace this intercellular cement (Fig. 20).

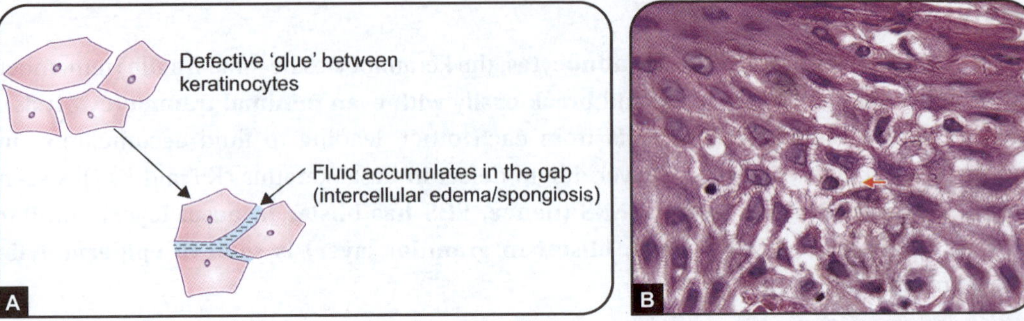

Figs. 19A and B: (A) Spongiosis: Schematic and histology; (B) Histopathology in spongiosis: Note epidermal keratinocytes are normally polygonal with space in between them. Note intact desmosomal connections (red arrow)

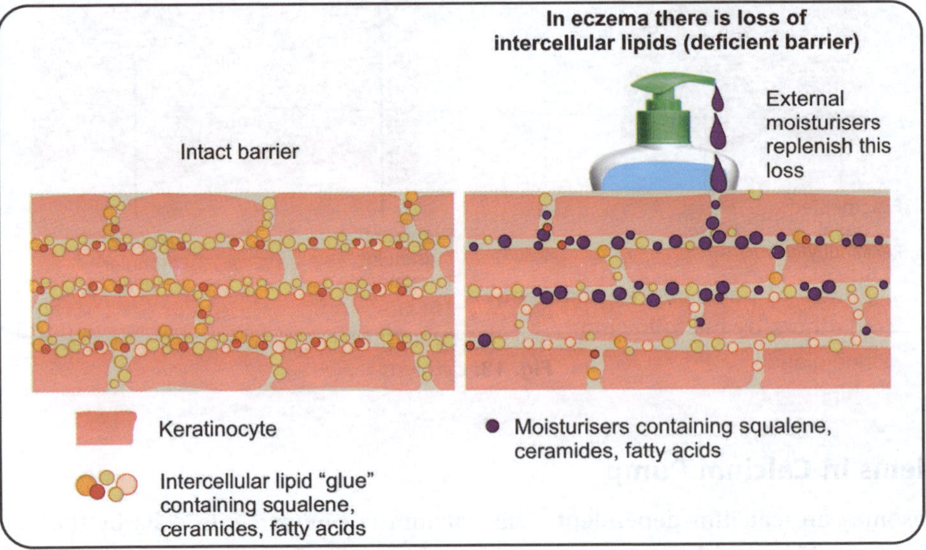

Fig. 20: Schematic representation of barrier loss and repair in eczema

Other Functions of Skin

A. Vitamin D synthesis from UVB light exposure onto skin
B. Immune function: Contributed by **Langerhans cells and keratinocytes**
C. **Receptors in skin:**

Type	Anatomy	Function
Free nerve endings	Nonencapsulated nerve endings	Pain, temperature, crude touch
Meissner's corpuscles(AIIMS Nov 18)	Encapsulated; in dermal papillae	Touch, pressure
Pacinian corpuscles	Encapsulated; deep dermis	Deep pressure, vibration
Merkel's disks	Encapsulated; basal epidermis	Touch
Ruffini's corpuscles	Encapsulated; oriented along stretch lines	Sensation of cutaneous stretching

QUESTIONS

1. Desmosomes are helpful in connecting: *(NEET Pattern)*
a. Keratinocytes
b. Melanocytes
c. Dermis and epidermis
d. Langerhans cells

2. Spongiosis involves:
a. Stratum basale
b. Stratum corneum
c. Stratum granulosum
d. Stratum spinosum

3. In which of the following conditions does parakeratosis most frequently occur?
a. Actinic keratosis
b. Seborrheic keratosis
c. Molluscum contagiosum
d. Basal cell carcinoma

4. Sweat glands of palm can be differentiated from others by the following:
a. Apocrine glands
b. High chloride content
c. Secretion stimulated by emotional stimuli
d. Adrenergic mediators control the secretion

5. Acantholysis is seen in all *except*:
a. Pemphigus vulgaris
b. Darier's disease
c. Staphylococcal scalded skin syndrome
d. Bullous pemphigoid

6. Acantholysis is seen in:
a. Epidermis
b. Dermis
c. Dermoepidermal junction
d. Subcutaneous tissue

7. Acantholysis is due to destruction of:
a. Epidermis
b. Subepidermis
c. Basement membrane
d. Intercellular substance

8. Melanocytes are present in:
a. Stratum corneum
b. Stratum basale
c. Stratum granulosum
d. Dermis

9. Layer of skin with maximum desmosome interconnection is depicted by which arrow? *(AIIMS Nov 17)*
a. A b. B
c. C d. D

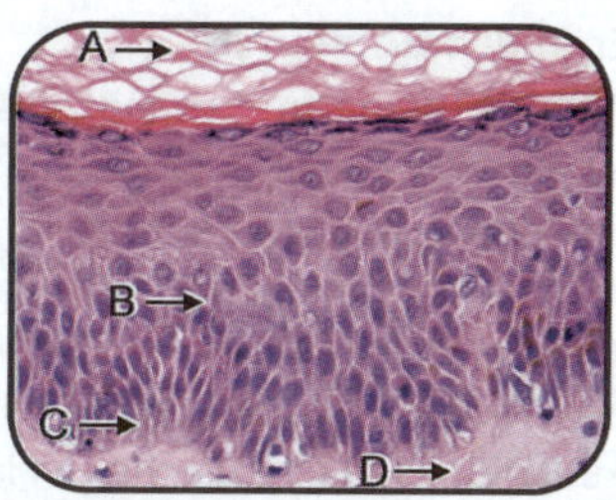

10. Desmosomes are associated with: *(PGI May 17)*
a. Lichen planus pemphigoides
b. Cardiac arrhythmia
c. Pemphigus
d. Psoriasis
e. Lichen planus

11. Meissner's corpuscles are found in: *(AIIMS Nov 18)*
a. Stratum lucidum b. Stratum basale
c. Papillary dermis d. Reticular dermis

New Questions

12. The following statements are true/false regarding receptors in skin:
a. Meissner's corpuscles are encapsulated and in epidermis
b. Merkel's disks are touch receptors
c. Free nerve endings are encapsulated
d. Pacinian corpuscles are in deep dermis
e. Ruffini's end organs are for perception of stretching

13. Arrange the following structures in skin in the order of top to bottom (from most superficial to deepest):

1. Desmoglein
2. Hemidesmosome
3. Collagen 7
4. Laminin

a. 1, 2, 3, 4
b. 2, 1, 4, 3
c. 2, 1, 3, 4
d. 1, 2, 4, 3

14. Assertion: Desmosomes are damaged in pemphigus
Reason: Pemphigus has autoimmunity against desmoglein

a. Both assertion and reason are true and reason is correct explanation of assertion
b. Both assertion and reason are true but reason is not correct explanation of assertion
c. Assertion is true and reason is false
d. Assertion is false and reason is true
e. Both Assertion and reason are false

15. Match items in column A with best alternative in column B:

Column A	Column B
1. Pemphigus 2. Eczema 3. Epidermolysis Bullosa simplex 4. Hailey-Hailey disease	a. Spongiosis b. Calcium pump mutation c. Cytolysis d. Ballooning degeneration e. Desmoglein destruction f. Staphylococcal toxin damage

16. Select the items in column A with corresponding column B. Select the correct answer from given code below:

Structure	Function
a. Desmosome	1. Keratin 5 and 14 formation
b. Basal Keratinocytes	2. Antigen presentation
c. Merkel cell	3. Intercellular junctions
d. Langerhans cell	4. Touch receptors

a. a1, b2, c3, d4
b. a4, b3, c2, d1
c. a3, b1, c4, d2
d. a2, b1, c4, d3

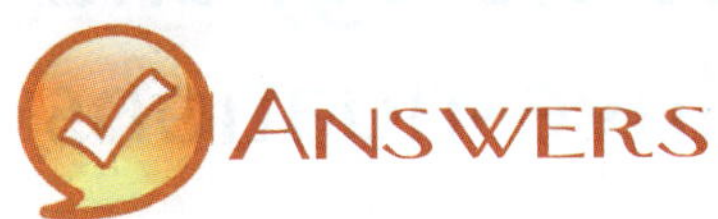

ANSWERS

1. **Ans. (a) Keratinocytes** *(Ref: Fitzpatrick's Textbook, 8th edn, Page 2281)*
2. **Ans. (d) Stratum spinosum** *(Ref: Fitzpatrick's Textbook, 8th edn, Page 45)*
3. **Ans. (a) Actinic keratosis** *(Ref: Rook's Textbook of Dermatology, 9th edn, Page 142.2)*
4. **Ans. (c) Secretion stimulated by emotional stimuli** (See page 8 for explanation)
5. **Ans. (d) Bullous pemphigoid** (See page 11 for explanation)
6. **Ans. (a) Epidermis** (See page 11 for explanation)
7. **Ans. (d) Intercellular substance** (See page 11 for explanation)
8. **Ans. (b) Stratum basale** (See page 5 for explanation)
9. **Ans. (b)** The letter **B** is pointing to the spinous layer which has the most prominent desmosomes (See page 1 for explanation)
10. **Ans. (b) Cardiac arrhythmia (c) Pemphigus;** Pemphigus is classically associated with autoimmune desmosomal dysfunction. Desmosomes are also necessary for mechanically coupling and reinforcing cardiomyocytes. Intercellular communication via cardiac desmosomes is essential for proper cardiac function.
11. **Ans. (c) Papillary dermis** (See page 14 for explanation)

New Answers

12. **Ans. a-False; b-True; c-False; d-True; e-True**
13. **Ans. (d) 1, 2, 4, 3**
14. **Ans. (a) Both assertion and reason are true and reason is correct explanation of assertion**
15. **Ans. 1-e; 2-a; 3-c; 4-b**
16. **Ans. (c) a3, b1, c4, d2**

CHAPTER 2

Skin Lesions, Morphology, Histopathology and Investigations

CLASSIFICATION OF SKIN LESIONS

When skin diseases are described, the lesions which come first are called as **primary lesions** and those that occur on top of primary lesions are called as **secondary lesions.**

Primary Lesions

Features	<1 cm*	>1 cm*
Flat	Macule	Patch
Solid elevation	Papule	Plaque, nodule
Clear fluid	Vesicle	Bulla
Pus filled	Pustule	Pustule

**Note:* Some consider 0.5 cm as the dividing line

1. **Macule**(MCQ)—These are **flat, circumscribed changes in skin color <1 cm in size**. These macules may be hyperpigmented, hypopigmented or depigmented (Fig. 1). The level of melanin in the hyperpigmented lesions can be differentiated by their color as below:

Level of melanin	Clinical color (due to Tyndall effect and light scattering from the melanin residing in various layers)
Epidermis	Brown
Upper dermis	Purple (violaceous)
Lower dermis	Blue, slate gray

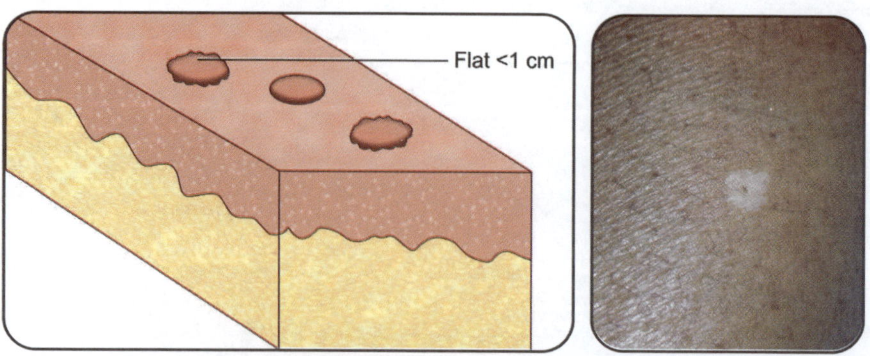

Fig. 1: Hypopigmented macule

2. **Patch**—basically a large macule >1 cm in diameter (Fig. 2)

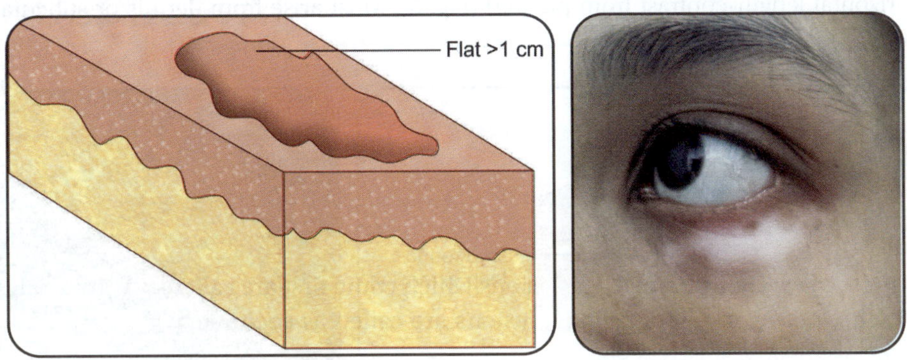

Fig. 2: Depigmented patch

3. **Papule**—Solid elevations with no visible fluid <1 cm in size
Flat topped papules(MCQ)—Lichen planus, **Umbilicated papule**(MCQ)—Molluscum contagiosum (Fig. 3)

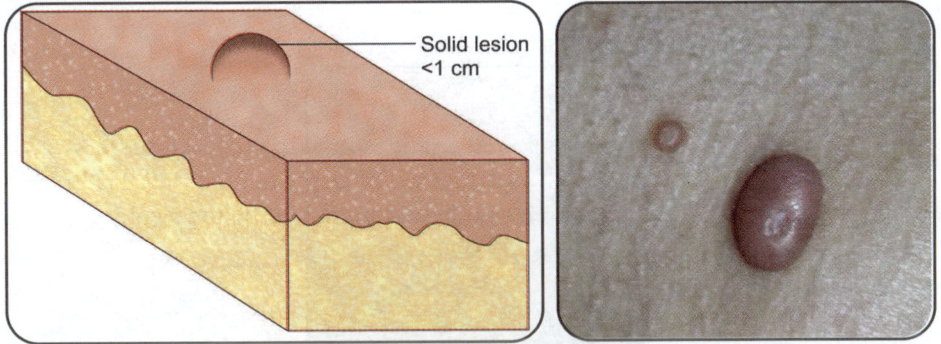

Fig. 3: Erythematous papules

4. **Plaque**—Confluence of many papules creates an elevated lesion >1 cm (horizontal length > vertical depth) (Fig. 4)

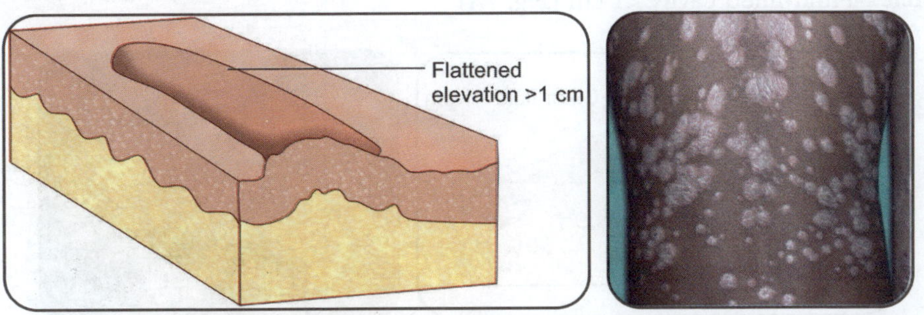

Fig. 4: Erythematous scaly plaques (psoriasis)

5. **Nodule**—Solid, round or ellipsoidal palpable lesion that has a diameter >1 cm (vertical depth > horizontal length-contrast from plaque) (Fig. 5). Most arise from dermis or subcutaneous tissue

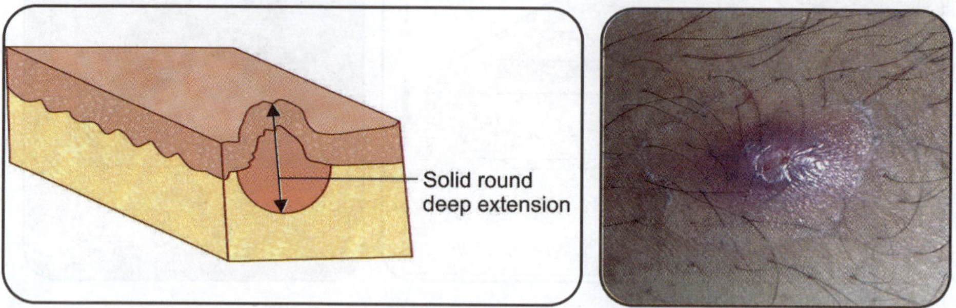

Fig. 5: Erythematous nodule: Note only the "tip of the iceberg" is seen

6. **Tumor**—Masses on skin >2 cm in diameter
7. **Wheal**—Transient elevated edematous lesions. Result of edema produced by the escape of plasma through vessel walls in the upper portion of the dermis. **Classical of urticaria** (Fig. 6)(MCQ)

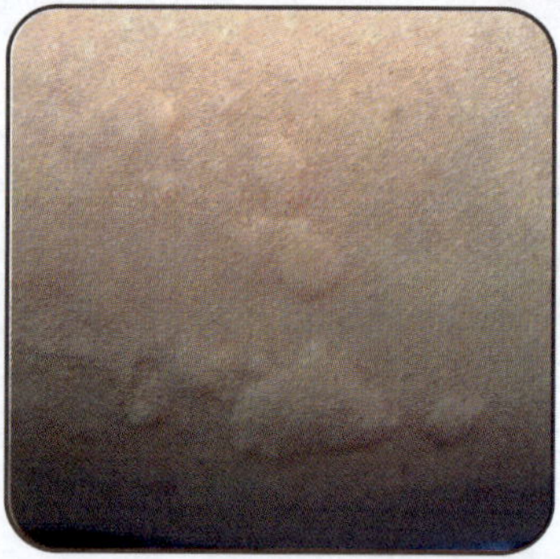

Fig. 6: Wheals—Edematous, elevated plaques

8. **Vesicle**—Fluid-filled cavity <1 cm (Fig. 7A)

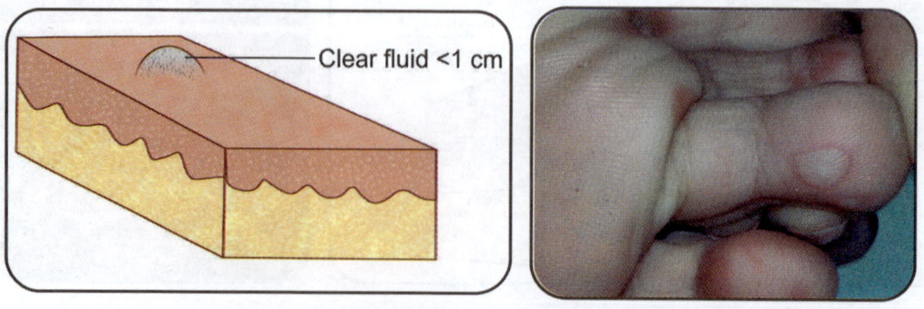

Fig. 7A: Vesicle

9. **Bulla**—Larger vesicle >1 cm (Fig. 7B)

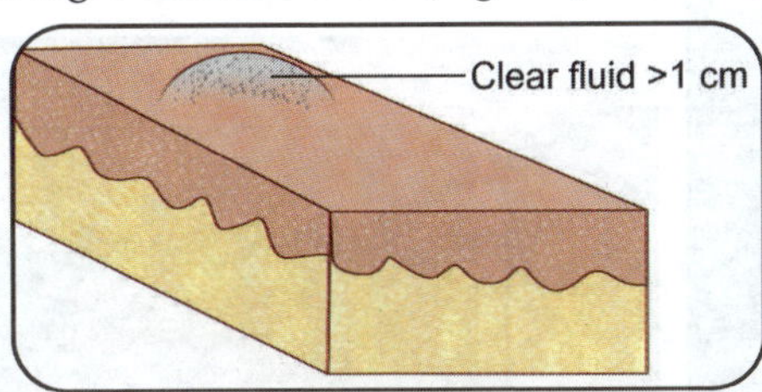

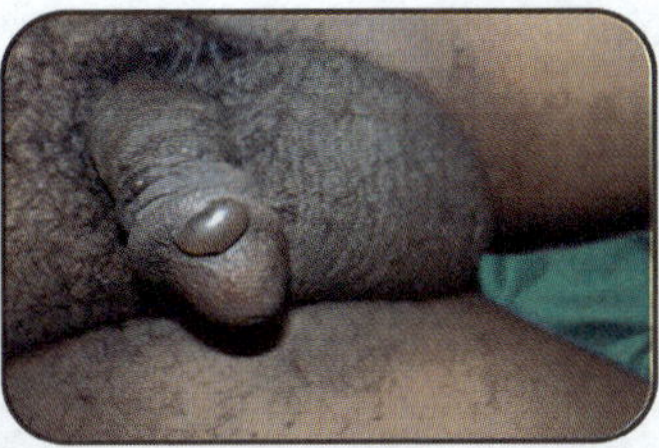

Fig. 7B: Bulla in fixed drug eruption

Depending on the clinical character of the blister, histopathological levels of fluid accumulation in the skin can be judged, as given in the table below. **All epidermal blisters are flaccid while DEJ/dermal blisters are tense.**

Level of Fluid Collection and their Clinical Correlation

Epidermal		
Subcorneal (immediately below corneum, granular)	**Rest of the epidermis (spinous layer, suprabasal and basal layers)**	**DEJ and dermal**
Very flaccid (so fragile that blisters rupture and are almost **never seen clinically**)	Flaccid but lesser than subcorneal blisters (Hence, less fragile and intact loose blisters may **sometimes be seen clinically**) (Fig. 8A)	Tense blisters (hence, intact blisters are usually seen clinically) (Fig. 9A)
Rupture **very** easily. Presents not as erosions but as **crusts/scales** (usually no visible erosions) (see Figs. 5A and B, Chapter 9)	Rupture easily. **Presents as erosions** (Fig. 8B)	Do not rupture easily as they are tense
Do not heal with scars	Do not heal with scars	Heals with scars and milia
Heals with normal skin	**Heals with hyperpigmentation** (Fig. 8B)	**Heals with hypopigmentation** (Fig. 9B)
E.g. Pemphigus foliaceus, Staphylococcal scalded skin syndrome (SSSS), bullous impetigo	E.g. Pemphigus vulgaris, Toxic epidermal necrolysis	E.g. Bullous pemphigoid

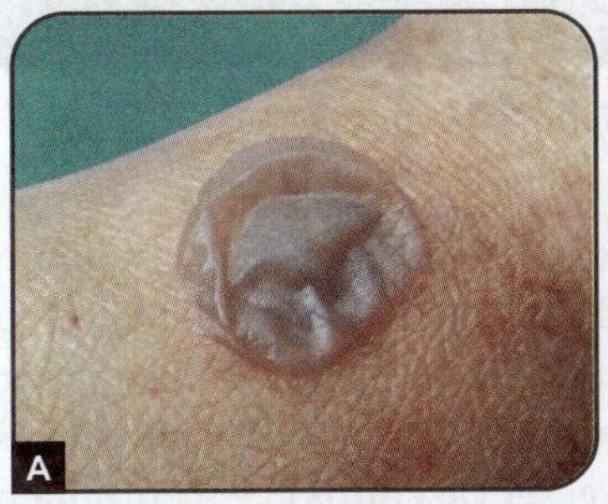

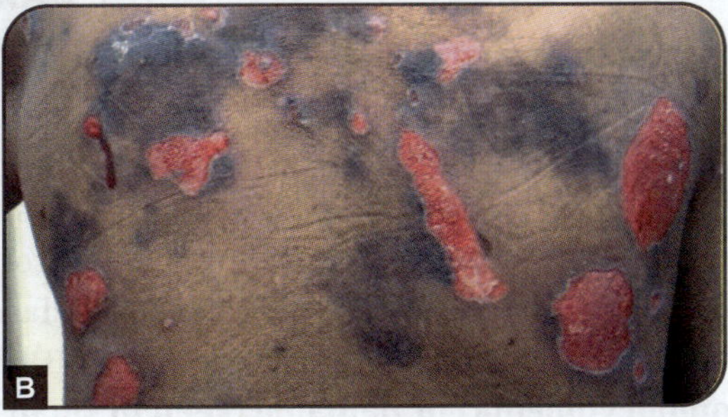

Figs. 8A and B: (A) Epidermal level (suprabasal)—flaccid blisters (pemphigus vulgaris); (B) Epidermal level (suprabasal)—erosions (after rupture of flaccid blisters) healing with hyperpigmentation (pemphigus vulgaris)

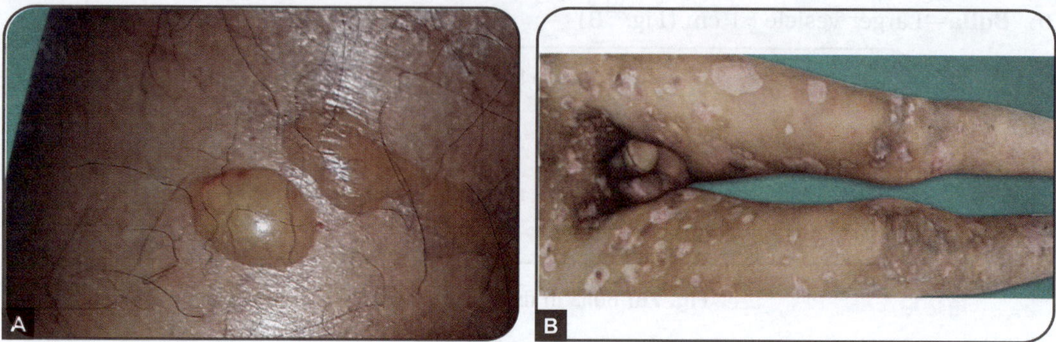

Figs. 9A and B: (A) DEJ/Dermal level—Tense blisters; (B) DEJ/Dermal level—blisters healing with hypopigmentation

10. **Pustule**: Raised area in the epidermis or hair containing pus. An abscess is a localized accumulation of pus very deep in the dermis or subcutaneous tissue.
    - **Lakes of pus** (when individual pustules fuse to form **flat sheets of pus)—seen in generalized pustular psoriasis (von Zumbusch type)** (Fig. 10)
    - **Hypopyon sign** (when a horizontal pus level can be seen inside the blister cavity)—seen in **bullous impetigo (for image, see Figure 9B in Chapter 4)**

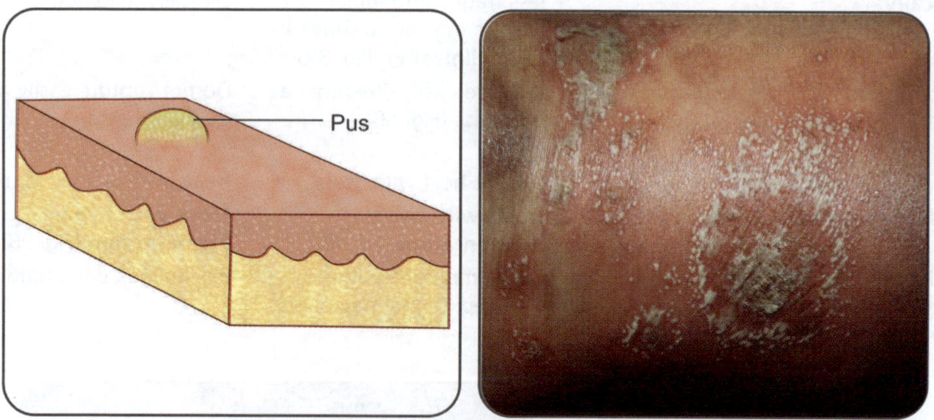

Fig. 10: Pustules, many fusing to form "lakes of pus"

11. **Purpura**—Red blood cells exiting from vessels into skin or mucous membranes. Both erythema and purpura look red in appearance. They can be differentiated by pressing the lesion with a **glass slide (test is called diascopy). If the redness disappears—it is erythema; if it stays, it is purpura** (Fig. 11B). Purpura can be **non-palpable (seen in thrombocytopenia) or palpable (seen in small vessel vasculitis).**[MCQ] Purpura can also be differentiated on size: **Petechiae** are small, pinpoint macules while **ecchymoses** are larger, bruise-like patches (Fig. 11A)

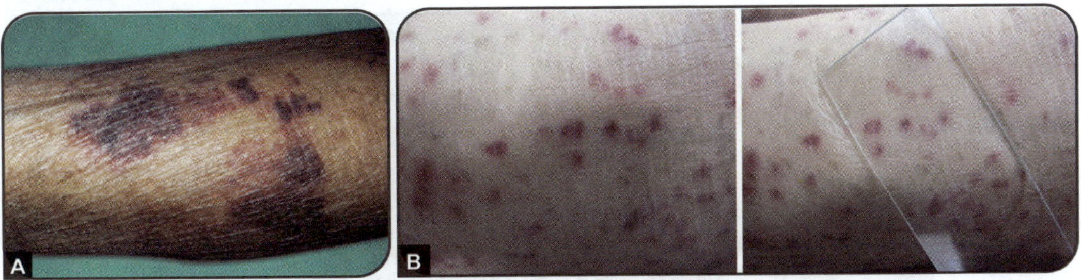

Figs. 11A and B: (A) Ecchymosis; (B) Purpura—lesions remain the same even after diascopy

Special Lesions

1. **Burrow**(MCQ)—A wavy, thread like tunnel through the stratum corneum as a site of entry for the **scabies mite** (image in Chapter 7)
2. **Comedone**(MCQ)—occlusion of hair follicle by keratin and lipids. Two types: **1. Open/black comedone ("black head")**: When the keratin plug in the pilosebaceous duct is open to the surface, the content oxidizes and becomes black, **2. Closed/white comedone ("white head")**—when the keratin plug in the pilosebaceous duct is deep inside and is closed to air hence their is no oxidization. Seen in **acne, hidradenitis suppurativa** (image in Chapter 11).

Secondary Lesions

A. **Scale (exfoliation)**—Visible exfoliation of skin is a scale. It is the result of defects in normal keratinization of the epidermis.

Types of Scales and Associated Diseases

Silvery/mica like—Seen in Psoriasis(MCQ) (Figs. 4 and 12A)	**Yellow, greasy scale**—Seen in Seborrheic dermatitis (For image, see Chapter 10-Figs. 23B and C)	**Wickham's striae**(MCQ)—Lacy white pattern overlying purple papules/plaques in lichen planus on putting oil on them (Fig. 12C)	**Powdery, branny, fine scales**—Seen in Pityriasis versicolor (Pityriasis = powder) (For image, see Chapter 5-Figs. 3A to D)
Collarette scale(MCQ)—Seen in Pityriasis rosea ("Collar"= something on the periphery, "ette" = small- Hence small peripheral scale") (Fig. 12B)	**Leaf like**—Seen in Pemphigus foliaceous (Folia = leaf) (For image, see Chapter 9-Figs. 5 and 6)	**Fish-like scales**—Seen in Ichthyosis vulgaris (Icthyos = fish) (Fig. 12D)	

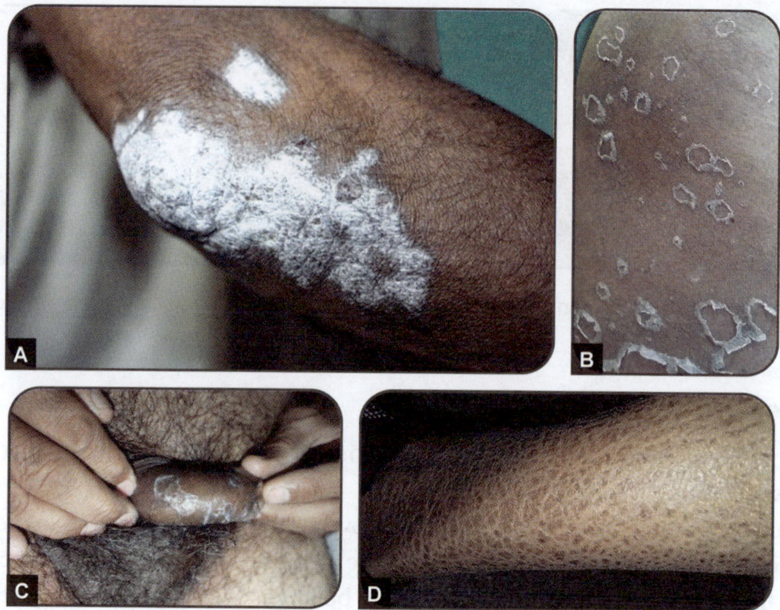

Figs. 12A to D: (A) Silvery scale on elbow extensors—Psoriasis; (B) Collarette scale; (C) Net-like, lacy pattern on putting oil (Wickham's striae) in lichen planus; (D) Fish-like scales—Ichthyosis vulgaris

B. **Crust (scab)**—Dried exudate (dried serum, pus, or blood), mixed with epithelial and sometimes bacterial debris.
   - **Golden-yellow, honey-colored crust**(MCQ)—seen in **non-bullous impetigo** (Fig. 13B)
   - **Hemorrhagic crust**(AIIMS May 15)—seen in **toxic epidermal necrolysis (TEN)** (Fig. 13A)

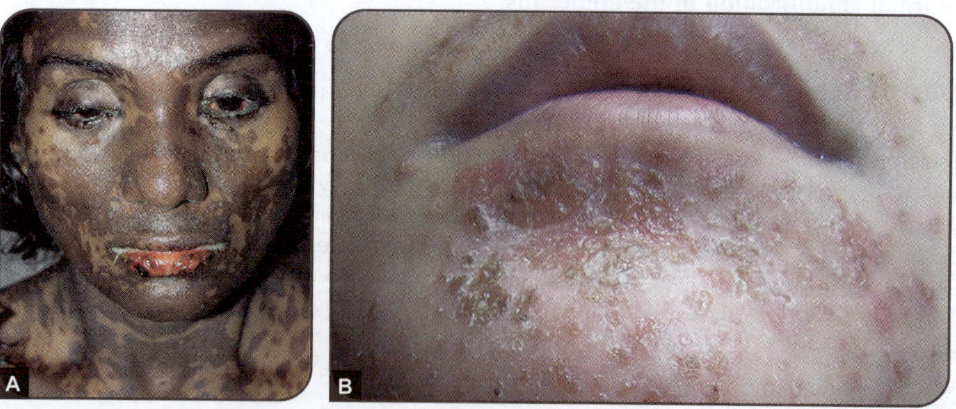

Figs. 13A and B: (A) Hemorrhagic crust on lips in TEN; (B) Honey colored crust-nonbullous impetigo

C. **Excoriations (scratch marks)**—Due to itching and scratching, scratch marks erode the epidermis/upper dermis. Almost all itchy skin diseases (except lichen planus) cause excoriations.

D. **Erosions, ulcer, fissure**

Erosion—raw lesions due to loss of **only the epidermis**. Hence, it does not leave scars (Fig. 14B).

Ulcer—raw lesions due to loss of **epidermis and dermis**. As injury is in DEJ and dermis, it heals with scars.

- **Undermined ulcers**—seen in cutaneous TB (Fig. 14D), pyoderma gangrenosum, chancroid(MCQ)
- **Punched out/trophic ulcers**—seen in peripheral neuropathy (DM, lepromatous Hansen's) (Fig. 14C)
- **Ulcers with rolled, beaded, pearly edge**—seen in basal cell carcinoma (For image, see Chapter 16, Figures 3B to D).

Fissure—Linear crack in the skin (Fig. 14A)

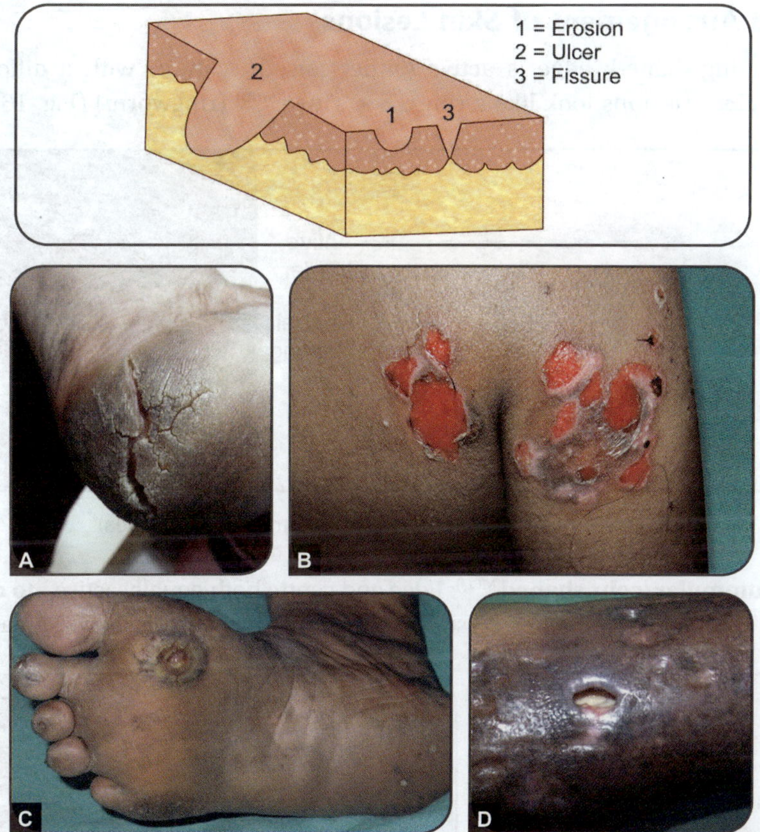

Figs. 14A to D: (A) Fissure; (B) Erosions (this was a case of pemphigus vulgaris); (C) Trophic ulcer—punched out vertical ulcer in Hansen's disease with peripheral neuropathy; (D) Undermined ulcer—cutaneous TB

E. **Scar:** Scar is the end result of a dermal or deeper injury with new connective tissue formation.

F. **Lichenification (lichen simplex chronicus):** In chronic itchy diseases, repeated rubbing of the skin induces a reactive process in the skin called as lichenification (Fig. 15).

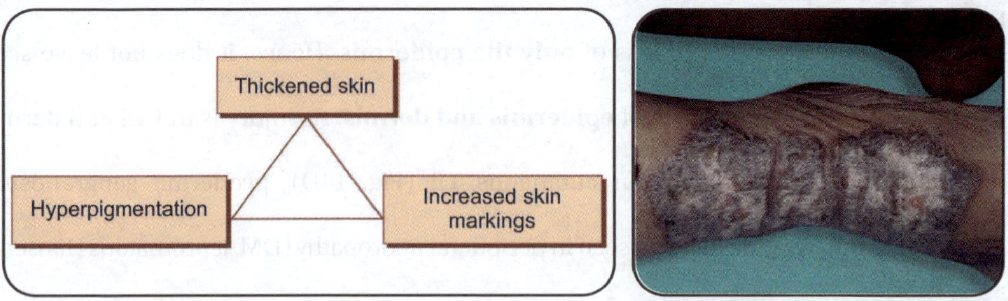

Fig. 15: Lichenification—Hyperpigmented, thickened plaque with increased skin markings on the ankle

Shapes and Arrangement of Skin Lesions

1. **Annular**—Ring-shaped; edge is active (either raised, scaly or with a different color), **central is clear** (lesions look like a ring). E.g. Tinea(MCQ) (ringworm) (Fig. 16)

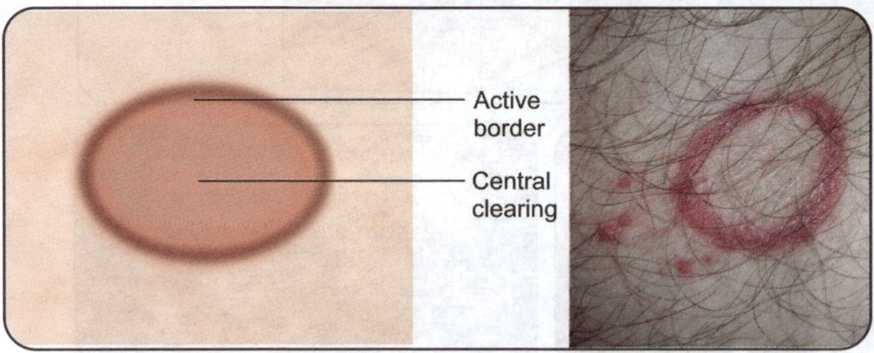

Fig. 16: Annular scaly plaque with central clearing (tinea)

2. **Discoid/nummular/coin-shaped**(MCQ): Edge and centre both equally active, **no central clearing.** "Disc"= coin, "oid"= like—e.g. Discoid lupus erythematosus, discoid eczema (Fig. 17)(MCQ)

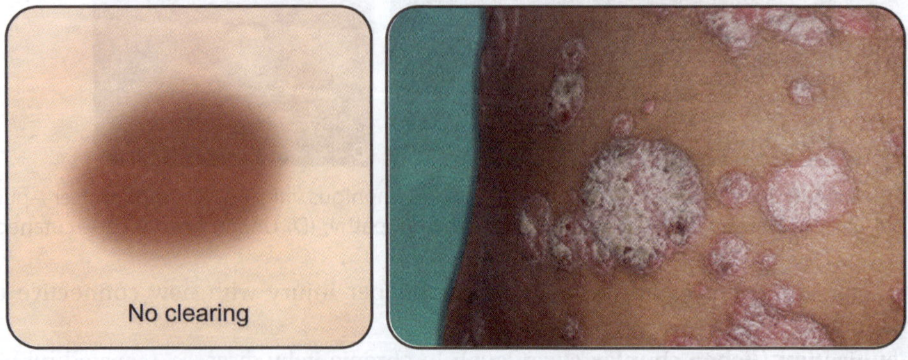

Fig. 17: Discoid scaly plaque

3. **Isomorphic/Koebner's phenomenon**(MCQ): Development of lesions in previously normal skin that has been subjected to trauma (like scratching, injury, friction, surgical incisions). The new lesions resemble the initial lesion ("**iso**" means same, "**morphic**" means morphology)

True-in auto-immune disorders	False (Pseudo)-in viral infections
Psoriasis (Fig. 18A)	Wart (verruca) (For image, see Chapter 6, Figure 11A)
Lichen planus (Fig. 18B)	Molluscum contagiosum (Fig. 18D)
Vitiligo (Fig. 18C)	

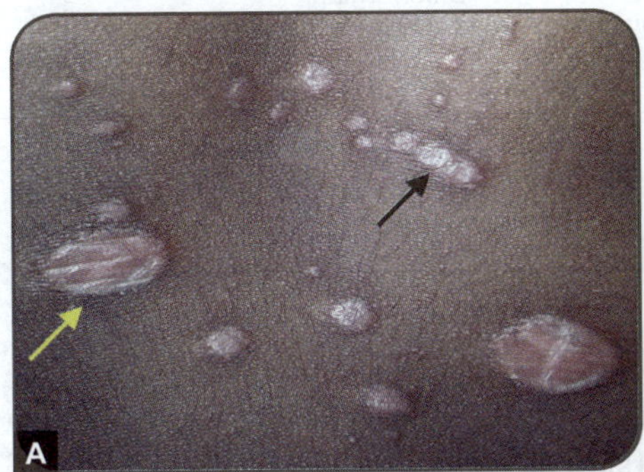

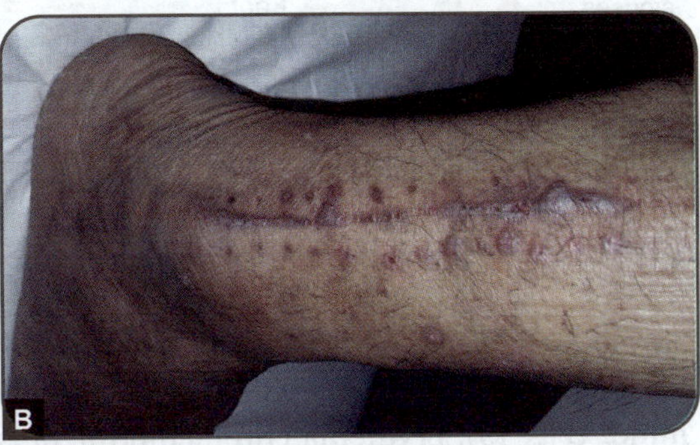

Figs. 18A and B: (A) Erythematous plaque with silvery scale in psoriasis (yellow arrow), Koebner's phenomenon on scratching (black arrow); (B) lesions of lichen planus coming in a surgical incision site

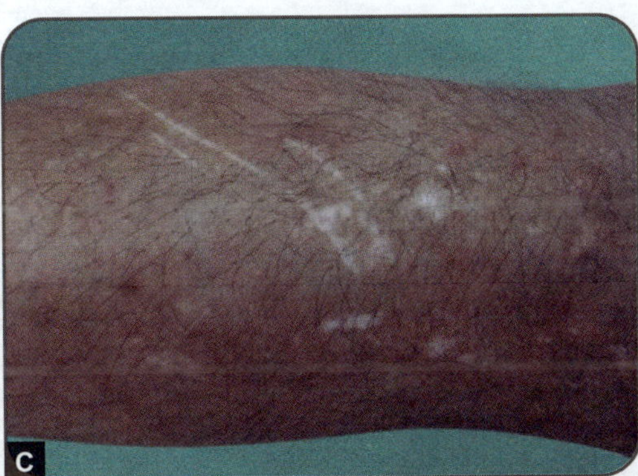

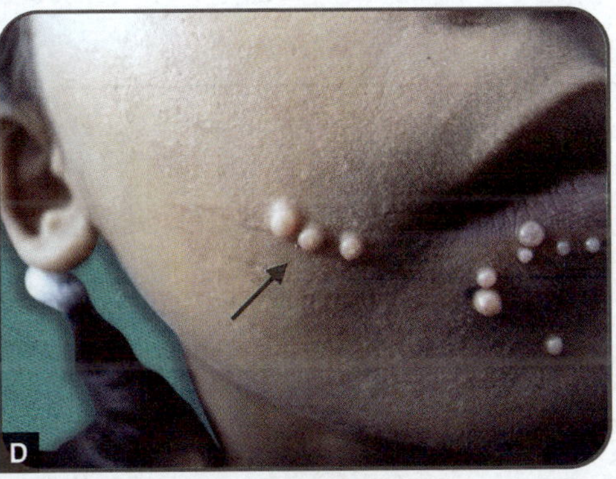

Figs. 18C and D: (C) Depigmented vitiligo lesions increasing with Koebner's phenomenon; (D) Molluscum papules increasing linearly on trauma (black arrow)

4. **Linear nodules and discharging sinuses along lymphatics** (for images and more details, refer to Chapter 5-Figs. 21A and B)—Lesions are nodular and are distributed linearly along lymphatics. They burst creating sinuses along these lymphatics. Seen in:
   - **Sporotrichosis**—caused by *sporothrix schenckii*
   - **Fish Tank granuloma (swimming pool granuloma)**—caused by *Mycobacterium marinum*

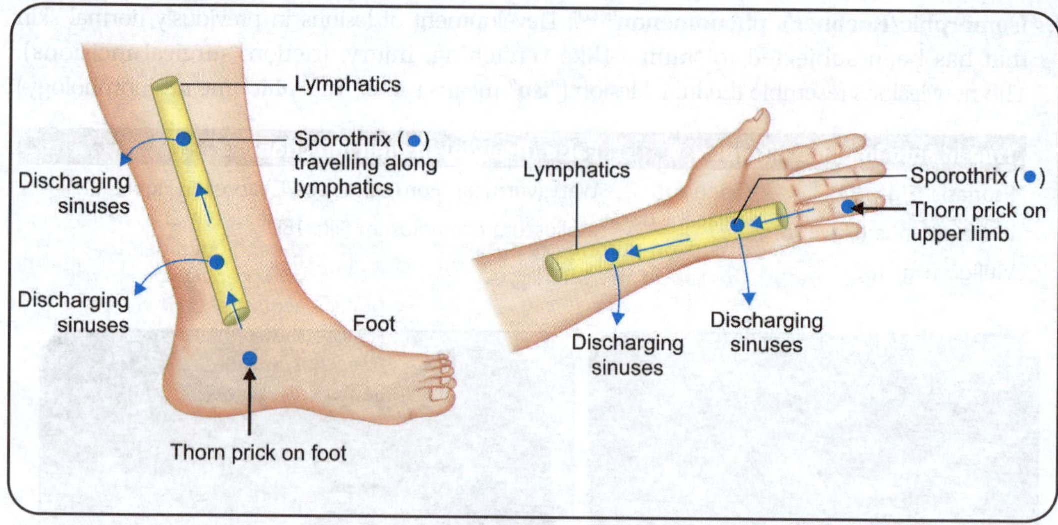

5. **Target lesions/iris lesions/Bull's eye lesions** (more details in Chapter 14)
Lesions resemble **targets with at least 3 distinct zones**. Seen in Erythema multiforme minor (Fig. 19), Erythema chronicum migrans (skin sign of Lyme's disease).

> **Note:* **Targetoid lesions** (atypical target lesions) having 2 zones are seen in **Stevens-Johnson syndrome (SJS), toxic epidermal necrolysis (TEN)**

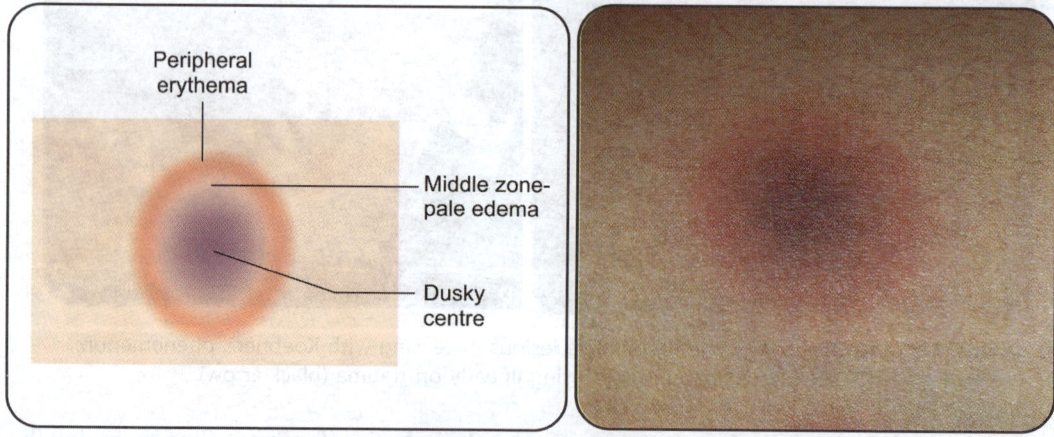

Fig. 19: Target lesions

6. **Dermatomal**—along a spinal or cranial nerve root. These lines are oriented horizontally on trunk (along intercostal nerves), longitudinally along limbs (along peripheral nerves) or cranial nerves. Seen in **Herpes zoster.**(MCQ)

Selected Signs

Name	Description	Disease
Asboe-Hansen sign(MCQ)	A pen mark is made at the margin of the blister—Extension of a blister to adjacent unblistered skin occurs on putting pressure **on the top of the blister**	**Positive in both subepidermal and epidermal blisters:** • **Rounded extension of the blister:** Seen in subepidermal blisters (e.g. bullous pemphigoid, dermatitis herpetiformis, epidermolysis bullosa acquisita, epidermolysis bullosa dystrophica, etc.) • **Irregular angulated edge:** Pemphigus vulgaris ***Note:** This sign is negative in subcorneal blisters as they are very fragile and cannot be pushed (e.g. Staphylococcal scalded skin syndrome, Pemphigus foliaceous)
Bulla spread sign(MCQ) **(Lutz sign)** (Image in Chapter 9-Figs. 8A and B)	Similar to Asboe-Hansen sign, a pen mark is made at the margin of the blister—Here however, the pressure is put from **one side of the blister**. The blister then extends toward the other side	Same as above
Nikolsky sign (Image in Chapter 4-Fig. 10B)	Lateral pressure on normal skin around a blister results in separation between the layers of epidermis and the epidermis moves under the finger and then shears off	**Positive only in epidermal blisters. Clinical sign of acantholysis. Seen in:** • **Pemphigus** • **Staphylococcal-scalded skin syndrome** (SSSS) • **Toxic epidermal necrolysis** (in TEN, it is called **pseudo-Nikolsky sign** as there is no acantholysis but epidermal separation due to death of epidermal cells) • **Hailey-Hailey disease** (sometimes)
Apple-jelly sign/Apple jelly nodule(MCQ) (Image in Chapter 4-Fig. 5D)	A yellowish tinge produced from pressure on the lesion with a glass slide (Diascopy)	Granulomatous diseases like **Lupus vulgaris, Leishmaniasis, Sarcoidosis**
Auspitz sign(MCQ) (Image below) (Figs. 20A and B)	Pinpoint bleeding when lesions are scrapped off (**Grattage** refers to this scratching action)	**Psoriasis, Darier disease, Actinic keratosis**

Contd...

Contd…

Name	Description	Disease
Carpet tack sign(MCQ) (Image in Chapter 14-Fig. 1C)	When scales are removed, the undersurface of the scales have attached horny plugs which once occupied dilated follicles on skin surface below	**Discoid lupus erythematosus,** Seborrheic dermatitis
Darier sign(MCQ) (Image in Chapter 17-Fig. 2C)	When a pigmented lesion is rubbed with a rounded end of a pen, urticarial wheal is produced confined to the pigmented lesion	**Urticaria pigmentosa** (a type of mastocytosis) Other causes: Histiocytosis, Leukemia, Xanthogranuloma
Gottron sign(MCQ) (Image in Chapter 14-Fig. 3C)	Flat pink to violaceous erythema on metacarpal or interphalangeal joints, olecranon, patellae, or malleoli	**Dermatomyositis**
Heliotrope sign (Image in Chapter 14-Fig. 3A)	Flat pink to violaceous erythema over periorbital area	**Dermatomyositis**
Shawl sign (Image in Chapter 14-Fig. 3B)	Erythema over upper back and shoulders (shawl distribution)	**Dermatomyositis**

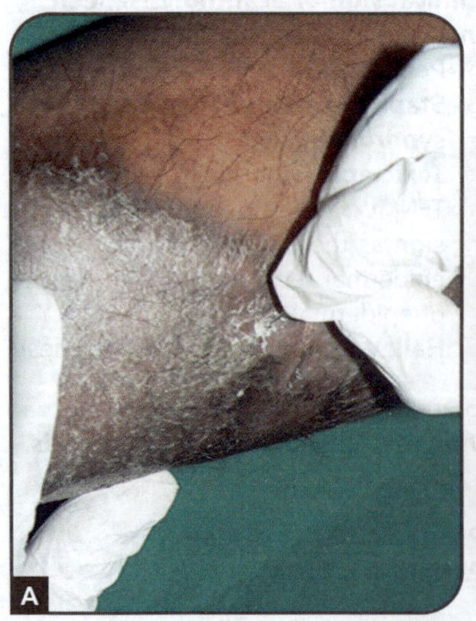
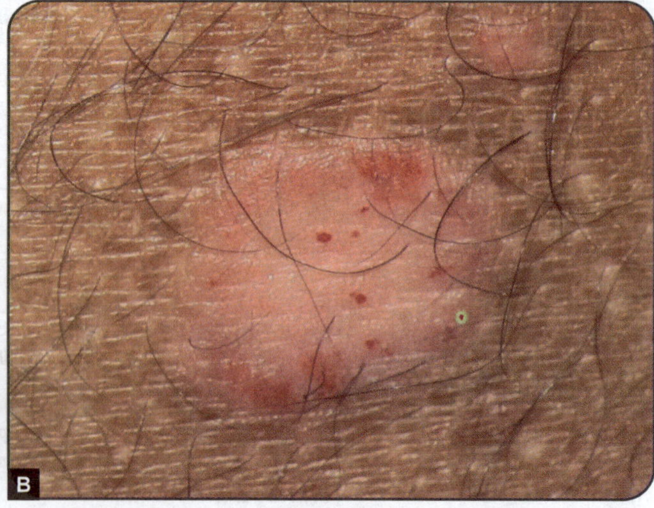

Figs. 20A and B: (A) Psoriasis lesion being scrapped (grattage) to demonstrate Auspitz sign; (B) Pin point bleeds of Auspitz sign (Note—scales have been removed by grattage)

Basic Histopathology of Skin

1. **Colloid body (Civatte body/Cytoid body)**—degenerated dead keratinocytes seen as eosinophilic hyaline ovoid bodies in lower epidermis and dermis. **Seen in lichen planus, lupus erythematosus**
2. **Epidermotropism**—migration of malignant lymphocytes from the dermis into the epidermis. Seen in mycosis fungoides (a type of cutaneous T-cell lymphoma)
3. **Grenz zone**—this comes from the German word for "border". Applies to a narrow zone of normal dermis between the epidermis and the underlying affected dermis. **Seen in leprosy (toward the lepromatous spectrum)**
4. **Hypergranulosis**—this refers to an increase in thickness of the granular layer of the epidermis. **Seen in lichen planus** (Fig. 21A)
5. **Hyperkeratosis**—increased thickness of the stratum corneum
6. **Parakeratosis**—nucleated stratum corneum. Seen in psoriasis (Fig. 21B), actinic keratosis
7. **Spongiform pustule of Kogoj**—accumulation of neutrophils in the stratum spinosum in psoriasis (Fig. 21B)
8. **Munroe's microabscess**—accumulation of neutrophils in the stratum corneum in psoriasis
9. **Papillary tip microabscess**—accumulation of neutrophils in the dermal papilla in dermatitis herpetiformis (Fig. 21C)
10. **Pautrier's microabscess**—accumulation of groups of malignant lymphocytes in the epidermis in cutaneous T-cell lymphoma (mycosis fungoides)
11. **Spongiosis**—also known as intercellular edema, and describes the widening of intercellular spaces between keratinocytes due to fluid accumulation. Seen in eczema (Fig. 21D)
12. **Acantholysis**—Details in Chapter 1

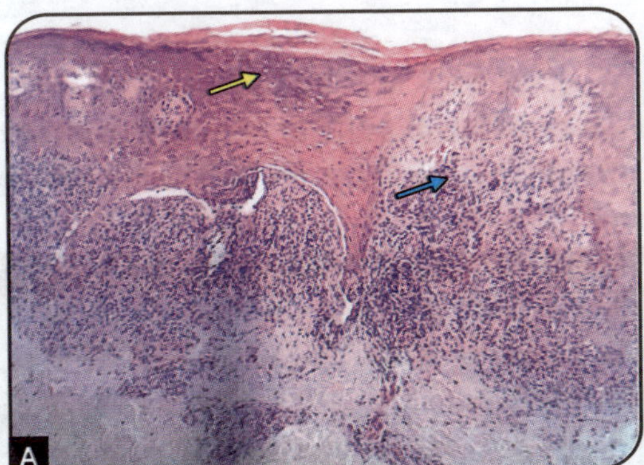

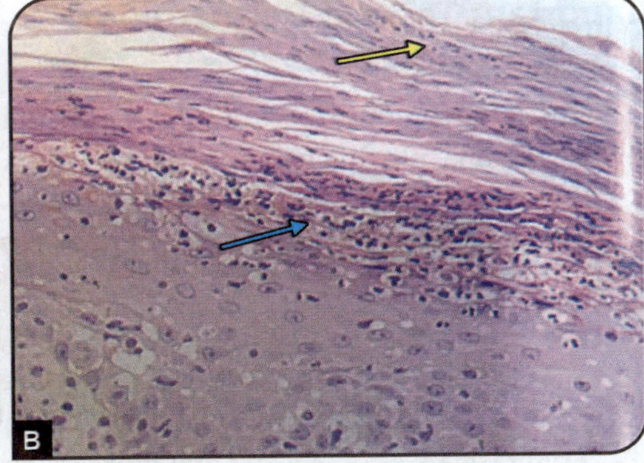

Figs. 21A and B: (A) Histopathology of lichen planus—Hypergranulosis (yellow arrow) and band of lymphocytes under epidermis (blue arrow); (B) Histopathology in psoriasis- Note the parakeratosis (yellow arrow) and spongiform pustule of kogoj (blue arrow)

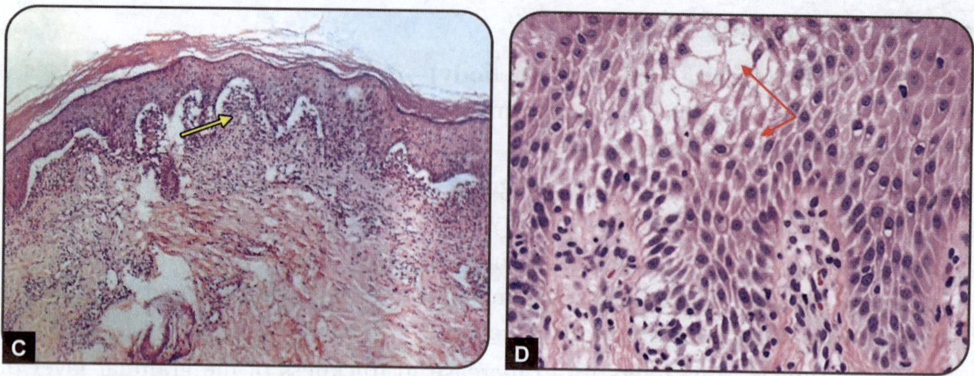

Figs. 21C and D: (C) Papillary tip microabscess in dermatitis herpetiformis (yellow arrow); (D) Spongiosis. Not the increased intercellular space between keratinocytes (red arrows)

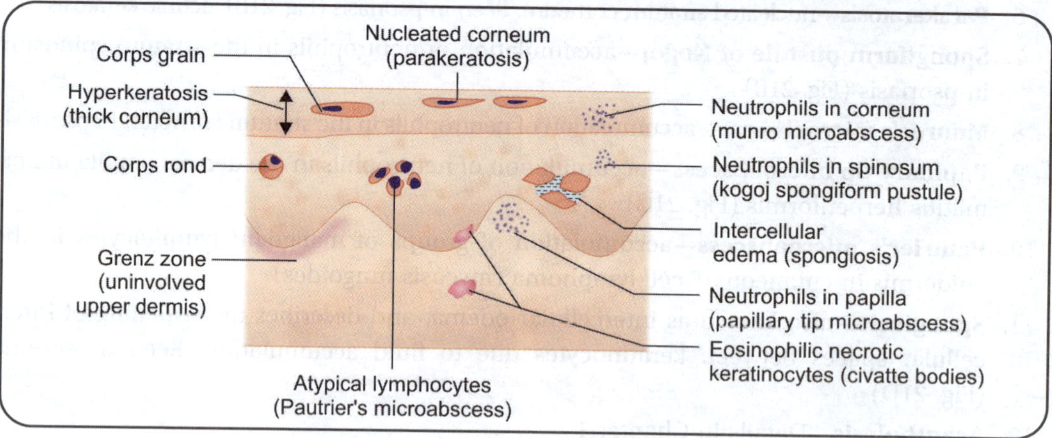

Important Tests in Dermatology

1. **Wood's light**(MCQ)

   This is a type of ultraviolet light from a lamp called Wood's lamp from which all rays except 365 nm have been blocked by a Wood's 9% (nickel oxide + barium silicate) filter.

Disease	Color on Wood's light
Tinea capitis(MCQ)	Yellow-green/Blue-green fluorescence associated with tinea capitis caused by microspora species. Tinea capitis caused by trichophyton species is negative on woods lamp [exception being favus caused by T. schonleinii (positive on woods lamp)] (Fig. 22C)
Erythrasma(MCQ)	**Coral pink**(MCQ) (due to porphyrins) (Fig. 22D)
Pityriasis versicolor(MCQ)	**Faint yellow**(MCQ) (due to porphyrins) (Fig. 22B)
Pseudomonas	Yellowish green

Contd...

Contd…

Disease	Color on Wood's light
Scabies	Fluorescein solution fills the burrows and fluoresces on Wood's light
Porphyria	Urine, feces, blister fluid fluoresce red or pink
Vitiligo	Ivory or milky-white (Fig. 22A)
Melanin disorders	Epidermal melanin disorders become more prominent, dermal melanin disorders become less prominent
Ash leaf macules in tuberous sclerosis	Difficult to see on naked eye examination, these ash-leaf macules become more prominent and are easily seen (bluish white color)
Differentiation between epidermal and dermal melanin	Epidermal melanin becomes more prominent, while dermal melanin becomes less prominent after woods lamp

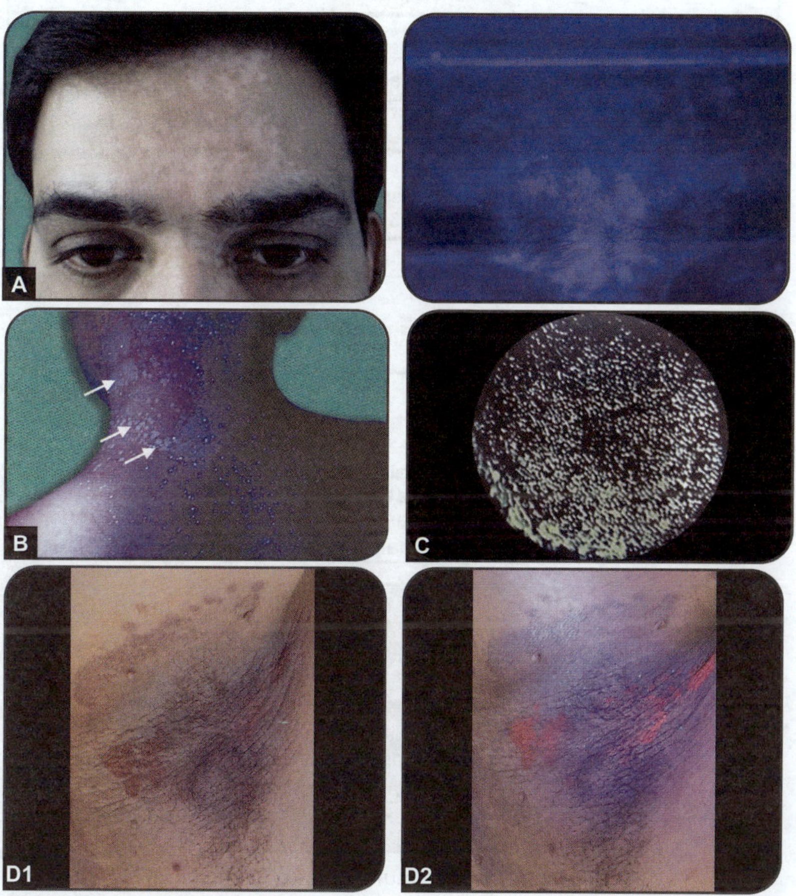

Figs. 22A to D: (A) Vitiligo lesions become whiter and makes even subclinical lesions more prominent on Wood's lamp; (B) Faint yellow fluorescence in pityriasis versicolor (white arrows); (C) Tinea capitis—Green fluorescence; (D) Erythrasma (D1: clinically as red/brown asymptomatic patch in axilla and D2: coral red fluorescence)

2. **Diascopy**
When a glass slide is pressed onto the skin, it compresses blood out of small vessels and due to resulting vasoconstriction allows evaluation of other colors of skin.

Disease	Color
Lupus vulgaris(MCQ)	Yellowish nodules called **"apple-jelly"** nodules Other causes of "apple-jelly" nodules—sarcoidosis, leishmaniasis

3. **Tzanck smear**
Blister fluid and floor of the blister is stained with Giemsa or Wright stain (the Papanicolaou staining method can also be used)

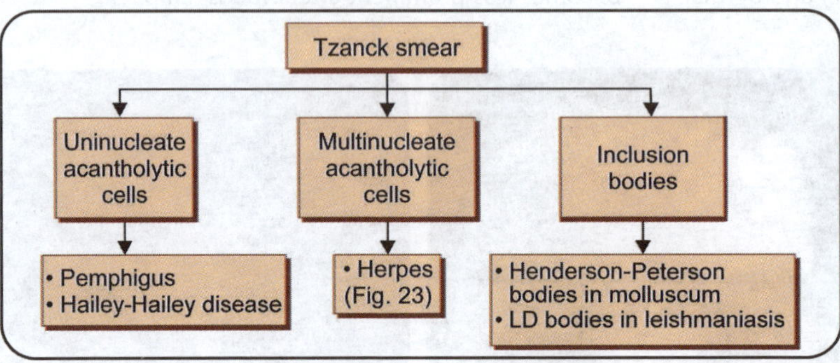

Note*—Tzanck smear is negative in bullous pemphigoid**(MCQ)

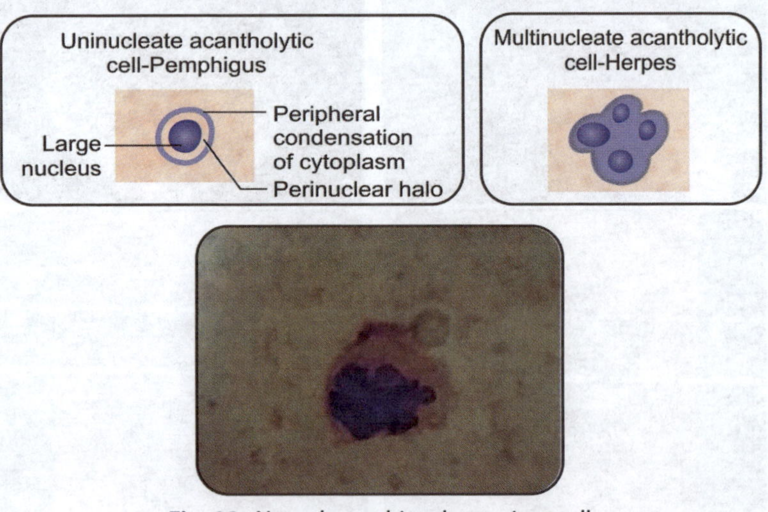

Fig. 23: Note the multinucleate giant cell

4. **Skin Prick test**
A small quantity of the test solution is placed on the skin and a prick is made through it with a sharp needle. The size of the wheal and flare are measured after 15 minutes.

Used to detect food-induced urticaria.

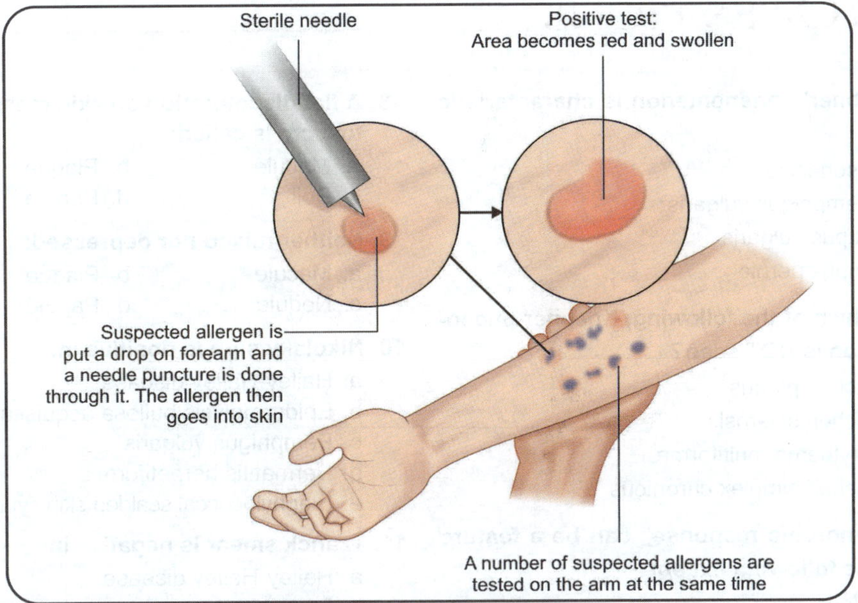

5. **KOH mount**
   Useful in:
   - Pityriasis versicolor—spherical yeast in clusters (looking like grapes or meatballs), with short filaments (resembling banana or spaghetti)— **"banana and grapes"** or **"spaghetti and meatballs"** appearance of *Malassezia* (Fig. 24A)
   - Cutaneous dermatophytosis (tinea) and cutaneous candidiasis—**hyphae or pseudo-hyphae with yeasts**
   - Dermatophytes of hair—fungal spores within the hair shaft (endothrix) or outside the hair shaft (ectothrix)
   - Bacterial vaginosis—the vaginal fluid is put on a slide with 10% KOH—fishy odor **("whiff" test)**
   - Mites—*Sarcoptes scabiei* mites in scabies (Fig. 24B)
   - Deep fungal infection—chromoblastomycosis—shows brown colored pigmented bodies **(called muriform/sclerotic/copper-penny/medlar bodies)**(JIPMER 16)

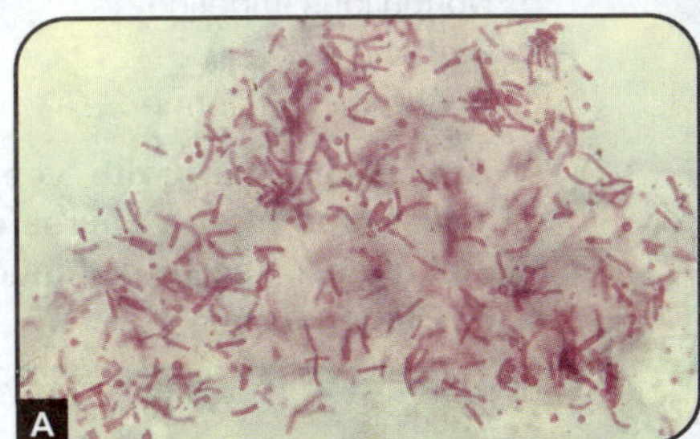

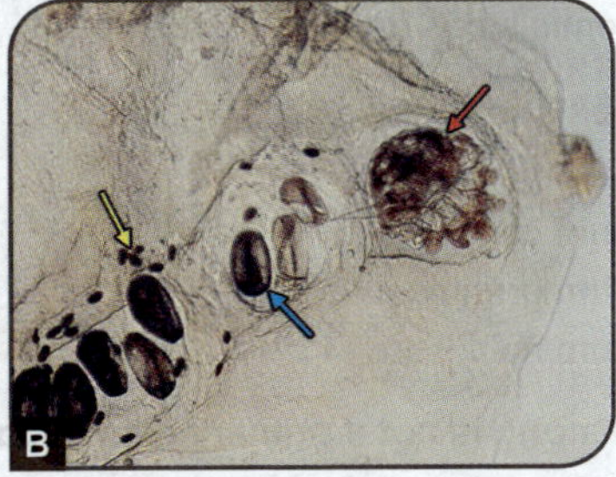

Figs. 24A and B: (A) Note the hyphae (like spaghetti) and yeasts forms (like meat balls); (B) Scabies mite (red arrow), eggs (blue arrow) and fecal pellets (yellow arrow)

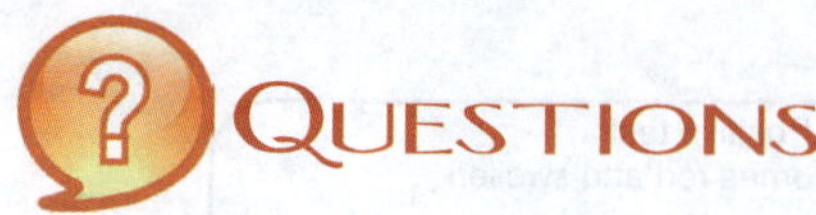

QUESTIONS

1. **Koebner's phenomenon is characteristic of:**
   a. Psoriasis
   b. Pemphigus vulgaris
   c. Lupus vulgaris
   d. Lupus pernio

2. **In which of the following, Koebner phenomenon is NOT seen?**
   a. Lichen planus
   b. Lichen sclerosis
   c. Erythema multiforme
   d. Lichen simplex chronicus

3. **"Isomorphic response" can be a feature of the following *except*:**
   a. Warts
   b. Tinea
   c. Psoriasis
   d. Molluscum contagiosum

4. **Pseudoisomorphic phenomenon is seen in:**
   a. Psoriasis
   b. Lichen planus
   c. Vitiligo
   d. Plane warts

5. **Carpet-tack sign is seen in:**
   a. Lupus vulgaris
   b. Lupus pernio
   c. Discoid lupus erythematosus
   d. Systemic lupus erythematosus

6. **Spongiosis involves:**
   a. Stratum basale
   b. Stratum corneum
   c. Stratum granulosum
   d. Stratum spinosum

7. **Which among is not a primary skin lesion?**
   a. Plaque b. Macule
   c. Abscess d. Scale

8. **A flat discoloration on skin measuring up to 1 cm is called:**
   a. Macule b. Plaque
   c. Boil d. Papule

9. **Neither raised nor depressed:**
   a. Macule b. Plaque
   c. Nodule d. Papule

10. **Nikolsky sign is positive in:**
    a. Hailey-Hailey disease
    b. Epidermolysis bullosa acquisita
    c. Pemphigus vulgaris
    d. Dermatitis herpetiformis
    e. Staphylococcal scalded skin syndrome

11. **Tzanck smear is negative in:**
    a. Hailey-Hailey disease
    b. Pemphigus
    c. Bullous pemphigoid
    d. Herpes

12. **A child presents with the following skin lesion on chin. The diagnosis would be:**

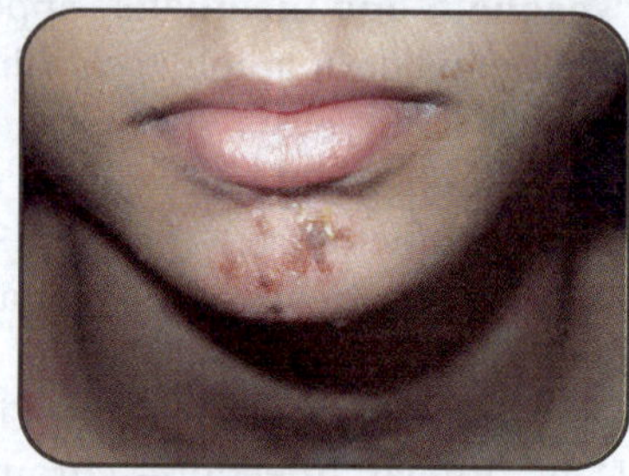

    a. Bullous pemphigoid
    b. Nonbullous impetigo
    c. Pemphigus
    d. Erythema multiforme

13. **A 70-year-old man with vesicular rash on lower limb after a course of steroids. Tzanck smear shows multinucleate giant cells. Diagnosis is:**
    a. Varicella zoster virus infection
    b. Vaccinia
    c. Molluscum
    d. Mycobacterium tuberculosis

14. A lady presents with bilateral buccal reticulate white streaks. Pain increases on spicy food intake. Patient gives no h/o tobacco but shows amalgam on 3rd molar. The diagnosis would be:
a. Lichen planus b. Leukoplakia
c. Aphthous stomatitis
d. Candida

15. Linear discontinuation of skin is called as:
a. Ulcer b. Excoriation
c. Erosion d. Fissure

16. Asboe-Hansen sign is negative is:
a. Pemphigus vulgaris
b. Bullous pemphigoid
c. Stevens-Johnson syndrome
d. Staphylococcal scalded skin syndrome

17. Munroe microabscess is positive in:
a. Psoriasis b. Lichen planus
c. Lupus vulgaris d. Impetigo

18. Psoriasis is characterized by:
a. Darier's sign b. Auspitz sign
c. Nikolsky sign d. Bohr's sign

19. Civatte bodies are seen in:
a. Seborrheic dermatitis
b. Lichen planus
c. Psoriasis
d. Acanthosis nigricans

20. Wickham's striae are seen in:
a. Lichen planus
b. Lichen aureus
c. Lichen nitidus
d. Lichen sclerosus et atrophicus

21. Coin-shaped eczema is:
a. Nummular eczema
b. Atopic eczema
c. Infantile eczema
d. Endogenous eczema

22. Type of scale in pityriasis rosea is:
a. Mica-like b. Powdery
c. Silvery d. Collarette

23. Target lesions in acral areas are seen in:
a. Stevens-Johnson syndrome
b. Erythema multiforme
c. Toxic epidermal necrolysis
d. Lichen planus

24. Coral red color on Wood's lamp is seen in:
a. Pityriasis versicolor
b. Amyloidosis
c. Melasma
d. Erythrasma

25. The causative organism for erythrasma is:
a. Corynebacterium b. Staphylococcus
c. Streptococcus d. Pseudomonas

26. Apple-jelly nodules are seen in:
a. Tuberculosis verrucosa cutis
b. Tuberculous gumma
c. Scrofuloderma
d. Lupus vulgaris

27. Gottron's papule is seen in:
a. Dermatomyositis
b. Scleroderma
c. Mixed connective tissue disorder
d. Pemphigus vulgaris

28. Wood's lamp is diagnostic of:
a. Tinea capitis b. Candidiasis
c. Onychomycosis d. Kala-azar

29. A patient presents with urticaria. She suspects some food item to be involved. The test for her would be:
a. Patch test b. Prick test
c. Serum IgE d. Skin biopsy

30. A patient presents with blisters on skin. His Tzanck smear shows cells as shown below. The true statement is:

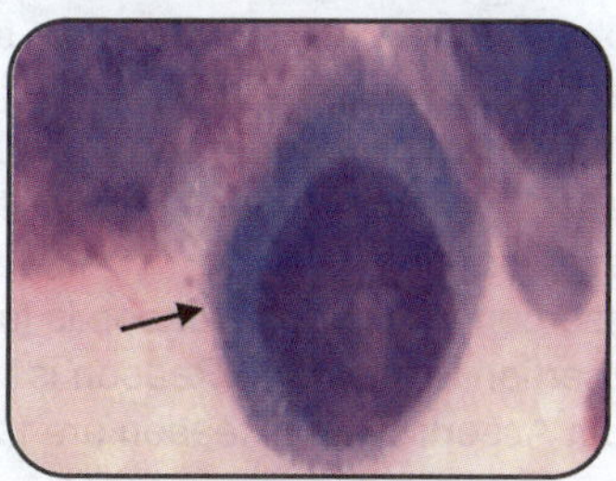

a. Seen in herpes
b. Hypochromatic nucleus
c. Perinuclear halo
d. Due to keratin mutation

31. A patient presents with lesions as shown. The scale is:

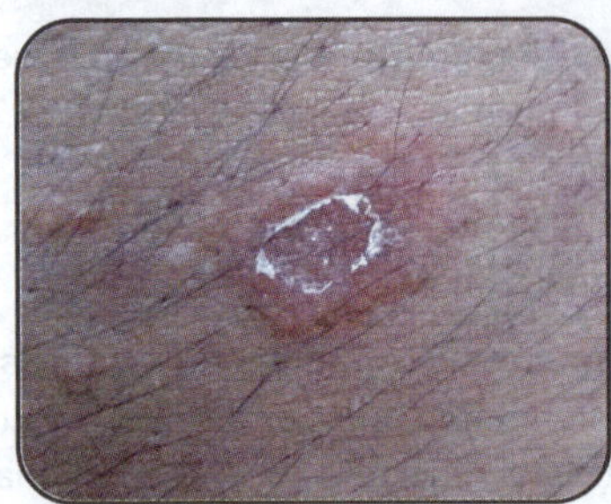

a. Powdery b. Silvery
c. Mica like d. Collarette

32. The following statements are true/false regarding the utility of KOH mount in skin diseases:

a. Bacterial vaginosis
b. Tinea
c. Lupus vulgaris
d. Scabies
e. Pityriasis versicolor

33. Arrange the following blisters in skin in the order of level of fluid collection (from most superficial to deepest):

1. Bullous pemphigoid
2. Pemphigus foliaceous
3. Pemphigus vulgaris
4. Burns

a. 1, 2, 3, 4 b. 2, 3,1, 4
c. 2, 1, 3, 4 d. 1, 2, 4, 3

34. Assertion: Nikolsky sign is seen in pemphigus
Reason: Pemphigus has flaccid blisters

a. Both Assertion and Reason are true and Reason is correct explanation of Assertion
b. Both Assertion and Reason are true but Reason is not correct explanation of Assertion
c. Assertion is true and Reason is false
d. Assertion is false and Reason is true
e. Both Assertion and Reason are false

35. Assertion: Pityriasis versicolor has faint yellow color on Wood's lamp examination
Reason: Malassezia is a perifollicular commensal releasing azelaic acid:

a. Both Assertion and Reason are true and Reason is correct explanation of Assertion
b. Both Assertion and Reason are true but Reason is not correct explanation of Assertion
c. Assertion is true and Reason is false
d. Assertion is false and Reason is true
e. Both Assertion and Reason are false

36. Check the histological terms and their associated diseases:

a. Colloid body- Erythema multiforme
b. Epidermotropism- Subcutaneous mycosis
c. Spongiosis- Eczema
d. Parakeratosis- Lichen planus

1. If a, b, c are correct
2. If a and c are correct
3. If b and d are correct
4. If all four (a, b, c, & d) are correct

37. Match items in column A with best alternative in column B:

Column A	Column B
1. Papule	a. Fluid filled lesion <1 cm
2. Plaque	b. Solid palpable lesion that has a diameter <1 cm
3. Wheal	c. Flat, circumscribed change in skin color <1 cm in size
4. Macule	d. Masses on skin >2 cm in diameter
	e. Transient elevated edematous lesion
	f. Horizontally elevated lesion >1 cm in size

New Questions

38. Match the following:

1. Crust	a. Thickening with hyperpigmentation
2. Ulcer	b. Dried exudate on the skin surface
3. Lichenification	c. Clear fluid filled lesion
4. Bulla	d. Loss of epidermis with partial or complete loss of dermis

A. 1-a, 2-b, 3-c, 4-d B. 1-d, 2-c, 3-b, 4-a
C. 1-b, 2-d, 3-a, 4-c D. 1-b, 2-c, 3-a, 4-d

39. Select the items in column A with corresponding column B. Select the correct answer from given code below:

Scale	Disease
a. Collarette	1. Pityriasis versicolor
b. Fish like	2. Seborrheic dermatitis
c. Greasy, yellow	3. Ichthyosis
d. Branny	4. Pityriasis rosea

A. a1, b2, c3, d4
B. a4, b3, c2, d1
C. a3, b1, c4, d2
D. a2, b1, c4, d3

40. The below instrument is frequently used in dermatology. The name of this instrument is:

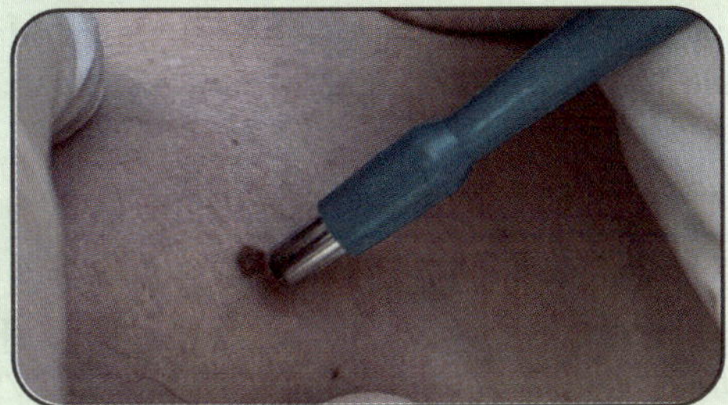

a. Woods lamp
b. Spatula
c. Curette
d. Punch biopsy

41. Identify the phenomenon of the lesion below. This phenomenon is seen in all diseases *except*:

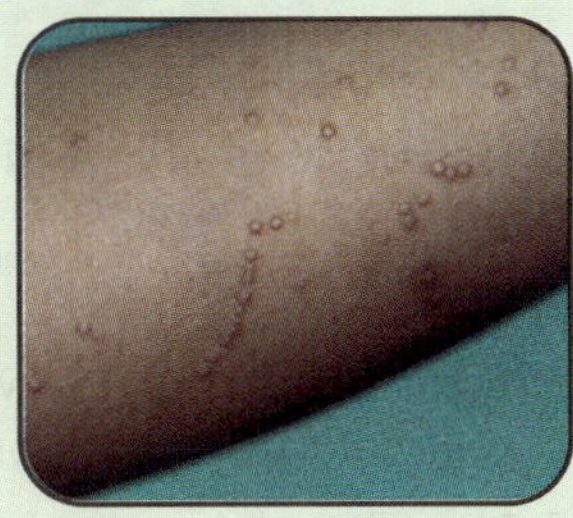

a. Psoriasis
b. Eczema
c. Lichen planus
d. Warts

42. The below instrument is used for diagnosis. See the instrument and mention the condition where it would not be helpful?

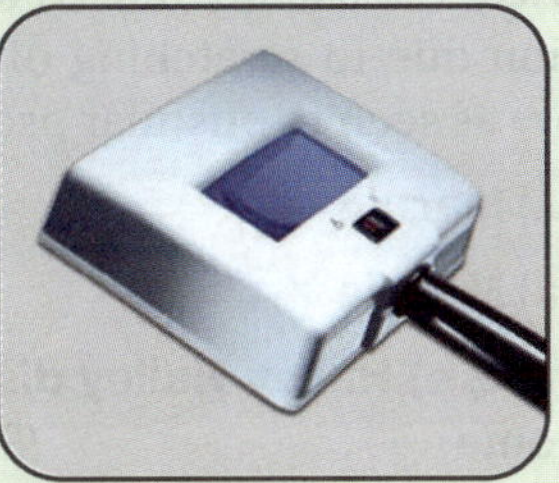

a. Tinea corporis
b. Scabies
c. Tuberous sclerosis
d. Erythrasma

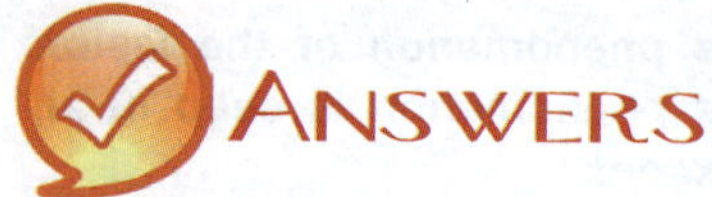

1. **Ans. (a) Psoriasis** *(Ref: Andrew's Textbook, 11th edn, Page 193)*
2. **Ans. (d) Lichen simplex chronicus** *(Ref: Rook's Textbook of Dermatology, 9th edn, Page 123.3)*
3. **Ans. (b) Tinea** *(Ref: Rook's Textbook of Dermatology, 9th edn, Page 123.2-3)*
   Even though the response in warts and molluscum are more appropriately labeled as pseudo-koebner's phenomenon, they can be considered in this question.
4. **Ans. (d) Plane warts** *(Ref: Rook's Textbook of Dermatology, 9th edn, Page 123.2)*
5. **Ans. (c) Discoid lupus erythematosus** (See page 32 for explanation)
6. **Ans. (d) Stratum spinosum** *(Ref: Fitzpatrick's Textbook, 8th edn, Page 45)*
7. **Ans. (d) Scale** (See pages 18-27 for explanation)
   An abscess is usually due to secondary changes over a primary lesion (e.g. secondary infection due to scratching of an itchy papule in scabies) though sometimes it can be primary as seen in pustular psoriasis.
8. **Ans. (a) Macule** *(Ref: Rook's Textbook of Dermatology, 9th edn, Page 4.11)*
9. **Ans. (a) Macule** *(Ref: Rook's Textbook of Dermatology, 9th edn, Page 4.11)*
10. **Ans. (a, c, e) Hailey-Hailey disease; Pemphigus vulgaris; Staphylococcal scalded skin syndrome** *(Ref: Mckee's pathology of skin, 4th edn, Pages 152,167,242,792)*
    Nikolsky sign is positive in SSSS, pemphigus, hailey-hailey disease (sometimes), toxic epidermal necrolysis (pseudo-nikolsky sign).
11. **Ans. (c) Bullous pemphigoid** *(Ref: Rook's Textbook of Dermatology, 9th edn, Page 3.25)*
12. **Ans. (b) Nonbullous impetigo** *(Ref: Fitzpatrick's Textbook, 8th edn, Page 2130)*
    The image is showing a honey-colored crust in non bullous impetigo.
13. **Ans. (a) Varicella zoster virus infection** *(Ref: Rook's Textbook of Dermatology, 9th edn, Page 3.26)*
    A vesicular rash on lower limbs in an old man on steroids indicates herpes zoster triggered by immunosuppression (more details will be in the chapter on viral infections).
14. **Ans. (a) Lichen planus** *(Ref: Fitzpatrick's Textbook, 8th edn, Page 35)*
    Reticulate white streaks on buccal mucosa indicate oral lichen planus. Dental amalgam is a trigger (more details in topic of lichen planus in chapter 10).
15. **Ans. (d) Fissure** (See page 26 for explanation)
16. **Ans. (d) Staphylococcal scalded skin syndrome** (See page 31 for explanation)
17. **Ans. (a) Psoriasis** (See page 34 for explanation)
18. **Ans. (b) Auspitz sign** *(Ref: Fitzpatrick's Textbook, 8th edn, Page 40)*
19. **Ans. (b) Lichen planus** *(Ref: Rook's Textbook of Dermatology, 9th edn, Page 3.35)*
20. **Ans. (a) Lichen planus** *(Ref: Fitzpatrick's Textbook, 8th edn, Page 35)*

21. **Ans. (a) Nummular eczema** *(Ref: Fitzpatrick's Textbook, 8th edn, Page 38)*

22. **Ans. (d) Collarette** (See page 24 for explanation)

23. **Ans. (b) Erythema multiforme** (See page 29 for explanation)

24. **Ans. (d) Erythrasma** *(Ref: Rook's Textbook of Dermatology, 9th edn, Page 4.20)*

25. **Ans. (a) Corynebacterium**

26. **Ans. (d) Lupus vulgaris** (See page 37 for explanation)

27. **Ans. (a) Dermatomyositis** (See page 33 for explanation)

28. **Ans. (a) Tinea capitis** *(Ref: Rook's Textbook of Dermatology, 9th edn, Page 4.20)*

29. **Ans. (b) Prick test**

30. **Ans. (c) Perinuclear halo**

    Herpes will have multinucleate giant cells not uninucleate cells as shown in the MCQ. Acantholytic cells have hyperchromatic nucleus, perinuclear halo, rim of cytoplasm

31. **Ans. (d) Collarette** (See page 24 for explanation)

32. **Ans. a-True; b-True; c-False; d-True; e-True**

33. **Ans. (b) 2, 3, 1, 4**

    Burns have dermal blisters

34. **Ans. (b) Both Assertion and Reason are true but Reason is not correct explanation of Assertion**

35. **Ans. (b) Both Assertion and Reason are true but Reason is not correct explanation of Assertion**

    Faint yellow color in pityriasis versicolor is due to porphyrin released by malassezia, not due to azelaic acid.

36. **Ans. (2) If a and c are correct**

    Epidermotropism is seen in mycosis fungoides, not subcutaneous mycosis. Parakeratosis is seen classically in psoriasis, not LP.

37. **Ans. 1-b; 2-f; 3-e; 4-c**

New Answers

38. **Ans. (c) 1-b, 2-d, 3-a, 4-c**

39. **Ans. (b) a4, b3, c2, d1**

40. **Ans. (d) Punch biopsy**

41. **Ans. (b) Eczema**

42. **Ans. (a) Tinea corporis**

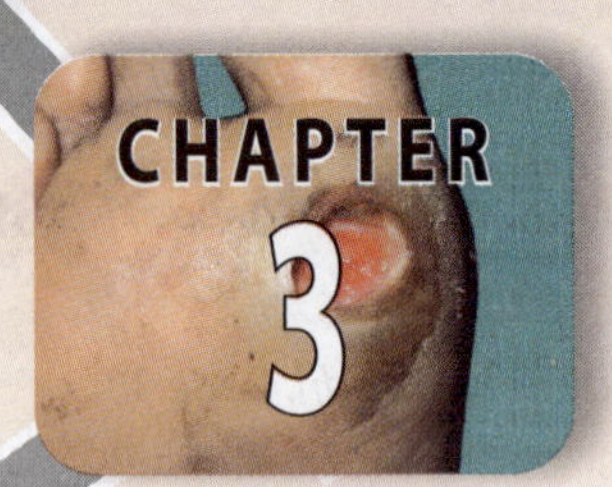

Hansen's Disease

ORGANISM

Mycobacterium leprae grows **best at 30°C** which is below the core temperature in humans. Hence, lesions localizes to **cooler superficial areas** of the body (**e.g. ear lobes, nose, testes, liver**) and superficial cooler nerves **(e.g. ulnar, facial, etc.)** rather than deeper warmer nerves.

Classification

- **Ridley-Jopling classification**(AIIMS): Based on four criteria:
  1. Clinical
  2. Bacteriological (slit skin smear-SSS)
  3. Histological (skin biopsy) and
  4. Immunological (lepromin testing)

  This classification classifies leprosy into five types—(1) TT (tuberculoid), (2) BT (borderline tuberculoid), (3) BB (borderline-borderline), (4) BL (borderline lepromatous), (5) LL-polar (lepromatous-polar).

  *There is also a pole between LL-polar and BL called LL-subpolar

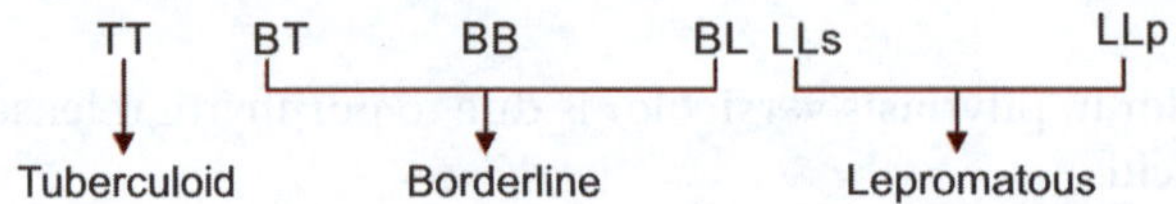

**Note:* Ridley-Jopling classification does not include the indeterminate and the pure neural types of Hansen's disease.

Pathogenesis

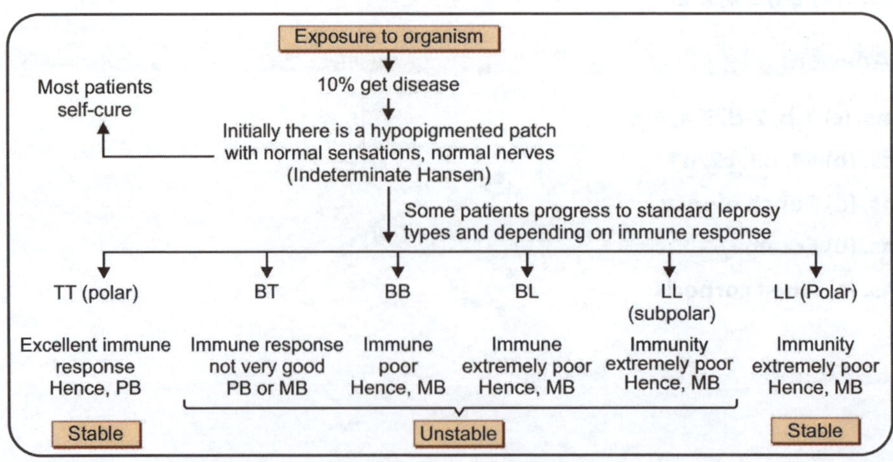

* BB is the most unstable leprosy
* Stable leprosy does not change or shift immunologically, while unstable leprosies can shift between each other

Disease Behavior

- TT has the best T cell immunity (Th-1 cellular response) and hence tuberculoid granulomas form on histology in TT. Many bacilli are killed by these efficient T-cells. Hence, TT is a paucibacillary (PB) leprosy. In LL, there is absent T cell immunity and high B cell immunity (Th-2 cellular response). Since B cells cannot kill lepra bacilli, numerous bacilli persist mainly in macrophages. Hence, LL is a multibacillary (MB) leprosy. These macrophages are called foam cells. Without treatment, immunity gradually slides downwards towards LL side-this is called **downgrading direction**. Hence, during downgradation, tuberculoid granulomas reduce and foam cells increase on histology. TT is a stable leprosy and does not downgrade. BT, BB, BL can downgrade towards the lepromatous pole. Downgradation can occur till LL-subpolar (LLs). LLs does not downgrade to LL-polar (LLp).
- On treatment, due to killing of bacilli, immunity improves and is logically then called upgradation. When T cell immunity improves after treatment, it is called Type 1 lepra reaction. When B cell immunity improves after treatment, it is called Type 2 lepra reaction. After treatment in BT and BB—T cell immunity increases and hence they show type 1 lepra reaction. After treatment in LL (more accurately LLs)—B cell immunity increases and shows type 2 lepra reaction. BL has the worst of both worlds—in some cases of BL, T cells increase after treatment (Type 1 lepra), some cases show B cell upgradation (type 2 lepra). TT and LLp are stable poles and do not usually show reactions.

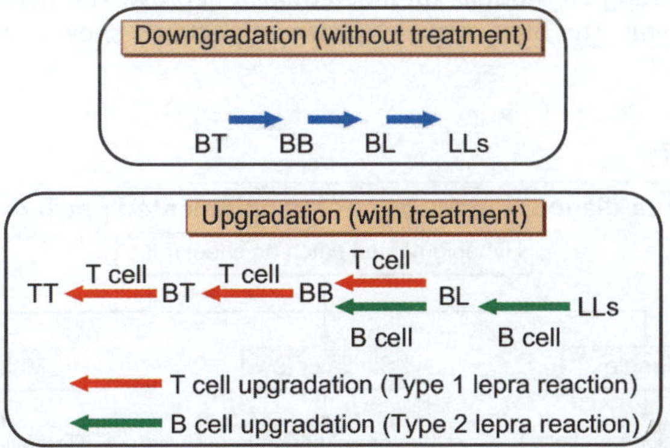

Types of Leprosy

1. **Indeterminate Hansen's disease**(MCQ)
   - The immune system is yet to determine the appropriate response to the invading bacillus. An early form of leprosy.

- Many patients will **self-heal** in some time. Some downgrade to standard leprosy types (TT, BT, BL, LL). Present as **solitary, ill-defined, hypopigmented macule or patch usually on cheeks**, arms, thigh, buttocks (Fig. 1A)(MCQ)
- **Normal sensations.**(MCQ) **Peripheral nerves not enlarged**(MCQ)
- Histology shows **periadnexal and perineural lymphocytic infiltrate**(MCQ) (without granulomas). **No or very few bacilli** are seen on biopsy (Fig. 1B).

Aid to Remember

"In-determinate" meaning immunity has not yet determined what it wants to do (unsure). Hence, no granuloma formation and only early lymphocyte accumulations (under-developed leprosy). So nerves are yet to enlarge and normal sensations.

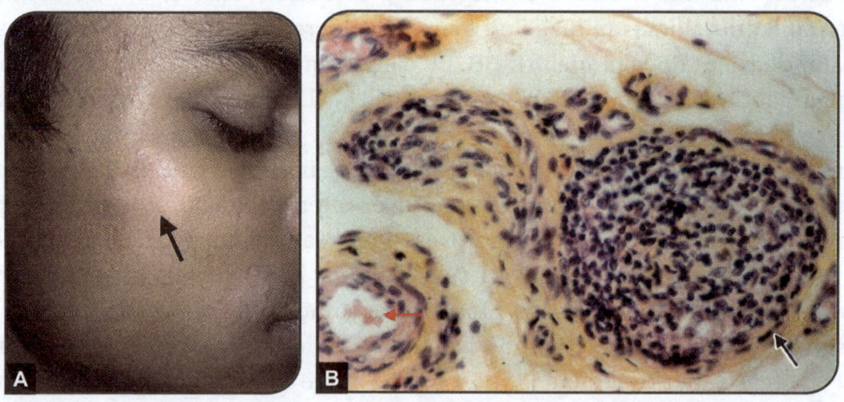

Figs. 1A and B: (A) Indeterminate Hansen's—Faint hypopigmented ill-defined patch on zygomatic area (arrow). Sensations, sweating are normal; (B) Indeterminate leprosy. The nerve in a neurovascular unit is replaced by lymphocytes. The black and red arrows respectively show a stretched perineurium and blood vessel (H & E × 400)

High Yield Points

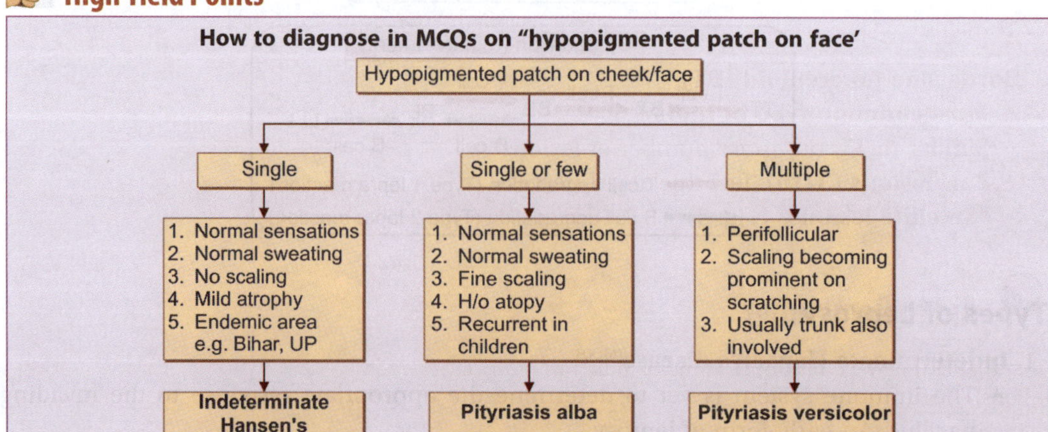

2. **Tuberculoid leprosy (TT)**
   - **Tuberculoid granuloma** forms in dermis and cutaneous nerves (Th-1 disease). **Excellent cell-mediated immune response**
   - Nerve granulomas compress the nerves causing compression symptoms. Usually only **one nerve** is compressed by the granuloma. Hence, **single nerve is thickened and single lesion occurs on skin (1 skin lesion, 1 thickened nerve).** Sometimes up to 3 lesions may be seen (Figs. 2A and B).
   - Nerve compression leads to **sensory loss, sweating loss and hypopigmentation** (sometimes erythematous) in the localized solitary area of the skin supplied by that nerve.
   - The typical lesion is a plaque with a well-defined, hypopigmented (sometimes erythematous) **and elevated border**. **Well-defined borders** indicate good immunity (Hence, **LL will have ill-defined borders**).

Aid to Remember

T (tea) is served in a cup and saucer (saucer lesion in TT)

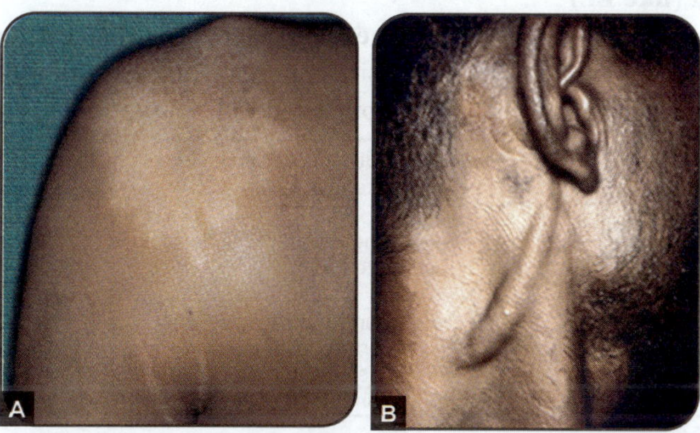

Figs. 2A and B: (A) TT—Single well-defined, hypopigmented, dry, anesthetic patch on shoulder; (B) A Single thickened greater auricular nerve in a case of TT Hansen's (the skin lesion was on the face)—not visible in the image

3. **Borderline tuberculoid (BT)**
   - **Most common type in India**(MCQ)
   - Similar to TT, but more number of lesions
   - **Few lesions (3–10)**, few thickened nerves
   - **"Satellite lesions"** (Fig. 3)(MCQ)

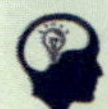

Aid to Remember

BharaT (भारत)—BT **commonest** in India. India has many **satellite** countries around it (BT has satellite lesions)

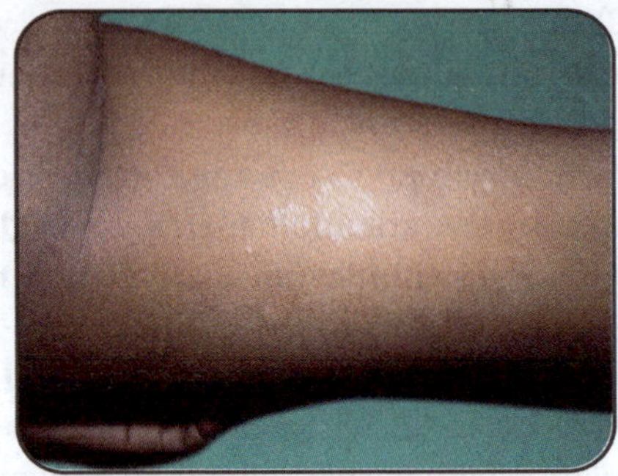

Fig. 3: Satellite lesion in BT

4. **Mid-borderline, borderline-borderline Hansen (BB)**
   - **Many lesions but countable (10–30)** and many thickened nerves
   - Lesions start crossing the midline more and more
   - Since it is in the middle of the spectrum, it shares features of both TT and LL. **Hence, 2 borders are visible**(MCQ)**—Inner border is well-defined (like TT) and outer border is ill-defined (like LL)**
   - **Inverted saucer (/‾\)/Swiss-cheese/Punched out/Dimorphic lesions/ Annular.**(AIIMS May 15)(MCQ) Punched out lesions indicate areas of normal skin at the center of the plaque, as if leprosy has been "punched out" of that area (Figs. 4A to C).

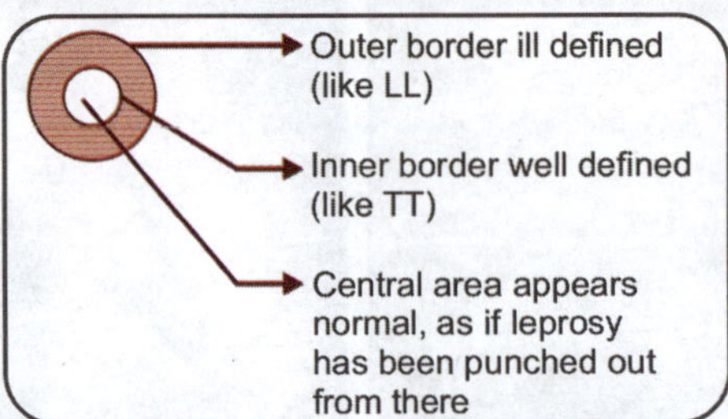

   - Sensations improve, sweating improves (as patient moves from TT towards LL, granuloma size reduces and more foam cells form. Hence, compression on nerves reduces and hence sensations and sweating improves)
   - **Most unstable form**(MCQ)

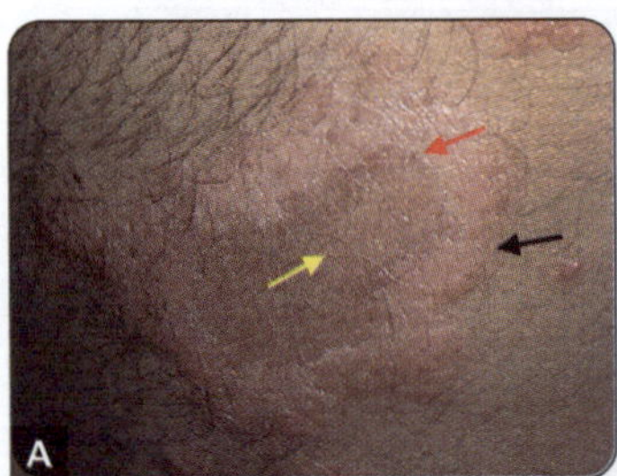

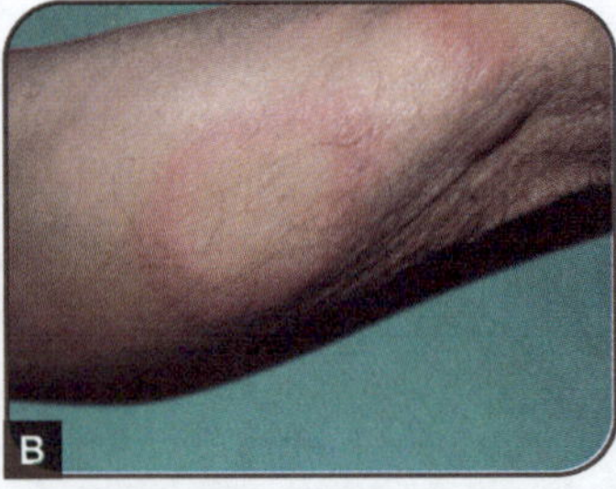

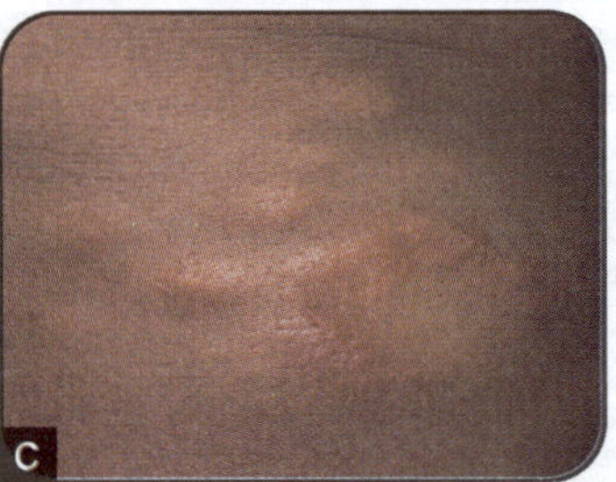

Figs. 4A to C: BB Hansen—(A) Punched out lesion in BB. Note the outer ill-defined edge (black arrow), inner well-defined edge (red arrow) and the punched-out centre (yellow arrow); (B) Annular lesions with central "punched-out" appearance; (C) Annular lesions—multiple lesions

5. **Borderline lepromatous (BL)**
   - **Numerous small lesions (uncountable)** and numerous thickened nerves (Figs. 5A and B)
   - As numerous lesions occur, they tend to cross the midline more and more and hence become **almost completely symmetrical**(MCQ) (perfect symmetry will be seen only in LL)
   - Sensations and sweating return to **almost normal**(MCQ) (very less compression of nerves as more foam cells and less granuloma formation)
   - **Inverted saucer (/‾\)/Swiss-cheese/punched out/dimorphic lesions**

High Yield Points

- Both BB and BL give inverted saucer lesions. Hence, the term "borderline" which includes both BB and BL is used. Both BB and BL are unlikely to be in the options for a question on inverted saucer lesion as it is present in both. Hence, the term borderline would be the best answer.

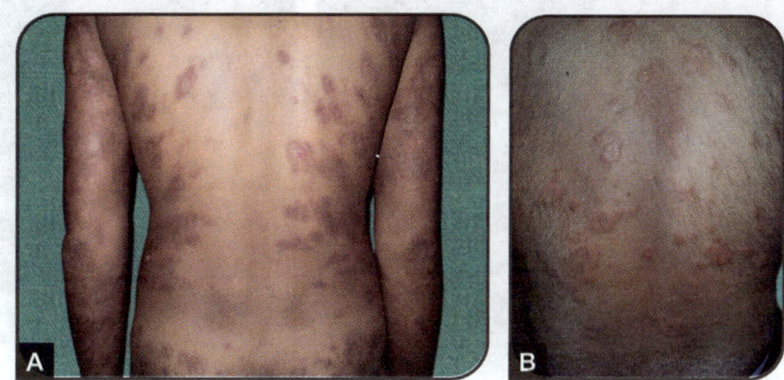

Figs. 5A and B: (A) BL—Multiple almost symmetrical erythematous lesions; (B) Multiple almost symmetrical lesions on trunk. This patient downgraded from BB without treatment

6. **Lepromatous leprosy (LL)**
   - **Lepra cells (foam cells)** predominate on biopsy **(Th-2 disease). IL-4, IL-10 are prominent**
   - Diffuse infiltration of skin with **ill-defined borders** (no immune response. Hence, diffuse dissemination of bacilli)
   - Nodules and infiltration thicken the skin causing prominence of skin folds (called **"leonine leprosy"**) (Figs. 6A and B)
   - **Perfectly symmetrical lesions. No granuloma forms, hence no nerve compression.** Hence, **normal sensations and normal sweating** in skin in the initial phase. Gradually, the nerves are invaded by bacilli. Hence, peripheral nerves are only very slowly damaged over time causing **peripheral neuropathy** and **glove and stocking anesthesia** (Fig. 6C).
   - **Earliest sign of LL—Nasal stuffiness and epistaxis.** Nasal discharge from untreated LL patients are the **main source** of infection in the community.
   - Other features—**Ear lobe infiltration** ultimately causing in later stages enlarged, loose, pendulous ear lobules called **buddha ears,** madarosis, gynecomastia (due to testicular involvement), saddle nose, **nasal septal perforation** (Figs. 6B, 7A and B).

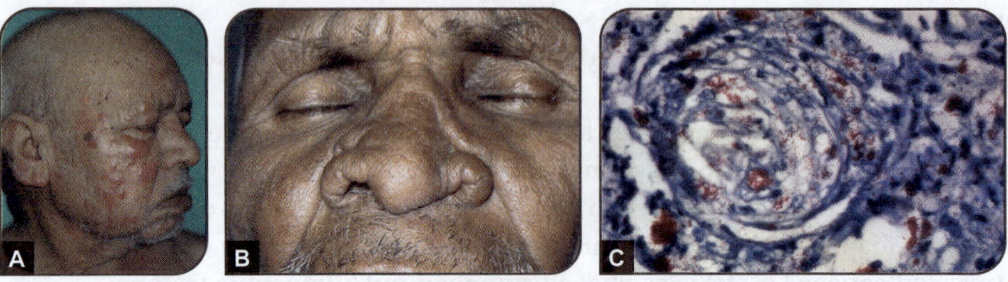

Figs. 6A to C: (A) LL—Nodular infiltrated erythematous nodules with ear lobe involvement. (B) LL—Note the collapsed bridge of nose and lateral madarosis; (C) LL—Horizontal section of the nerve showing infiltration of nerve by AFB (showing as red in this special stain)

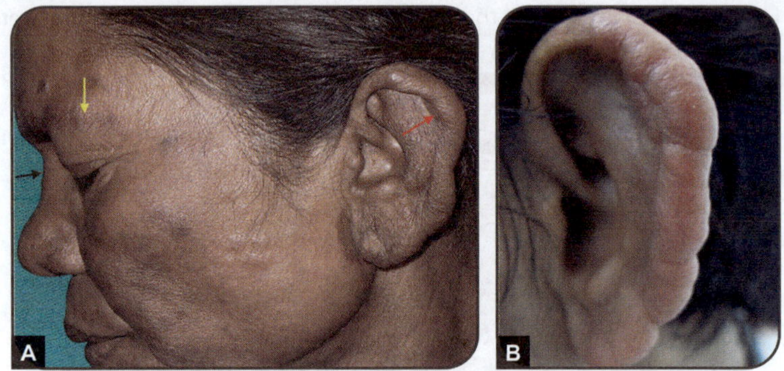

Figs. 7A and B: LL—(A) Collapse of bridge of nose (black arrow), lateral madarosis (yellow arrow), ear lobe infiltration (red arrow), infiltrated nodules; (B) infiltrated ear lobes

- On histopathology, **foam cells (dermal histiocytes full of lepra bacilli)** are seen in the dermis. The uppermost part of the dermis (papillary dermis) is however uninvolved. This zone of clearing is called **grenz zone** (grenz zone is best seen in LL) (Figs. 12C and D).

Aid to Remember

- **LL has many L**
  L = **L**eonine facies, **L** = **L**epra cells on histology, **L** = **L**oss of lateral eyebrows, **L** = **L**oss of nasal bridge, **L** = **L**eaves upper dermis intact (grenz zone), **L**oss of peripheral sensations, **L** = **L**obe (ear lobe) involved, **L** = **L**ots of bacilli (multibacillary)

Histoid Leprosy

- Type of LL usually with **dapsone resistance** (sometimes de-novo).
- More common in earlier times when only dapsone monotherapy used to be given.
- Shiny papules and nodules with **intervening normal skin** (Figs. 8A and B).
- Skin biopsy-shows **spindle shaped** foam cells.

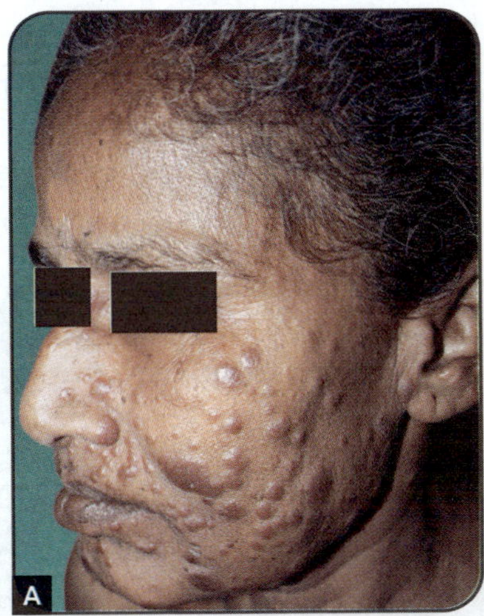

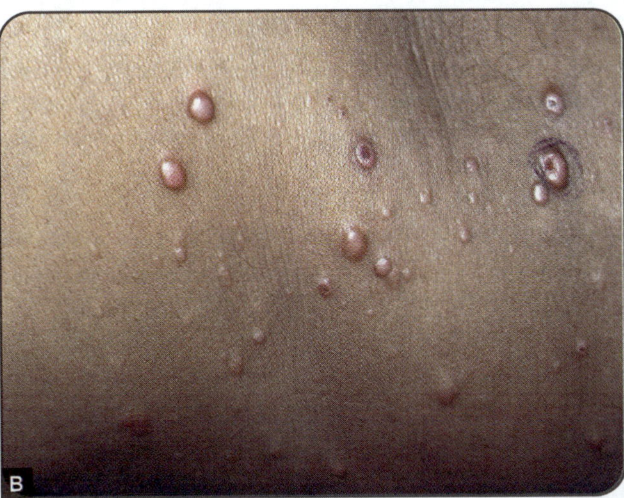

Figs. 8A and B: Histoid Hansen—(A) Shiny papules, nodules and plaques with intervening normal skin; (B) Shiny papules with normal intervening skin

Nerve Involvement in Leprosy

- **100%** patients have nerve involvement (Fig. 9)
- Towards TT side—fast compression loss of nerve function. Nonsymmetrical involvement. No glove and stocking anesthesia
- Towards LL side—slower invasion of peripheral nerves (**peripheral neuropathy causing glove and stocking anesthesia**).(MCQ) Symmetrical involvement. **Trophic ulcers** due to lack of peripheral sensations (Fig. 10)
- If skin not clinically involved, only nerves involved—**pure neural Hansen**(MCQ)
- **Order of sensory loss = Hot and cold differentiation > cold > hot > light touch > pain > deep touch**

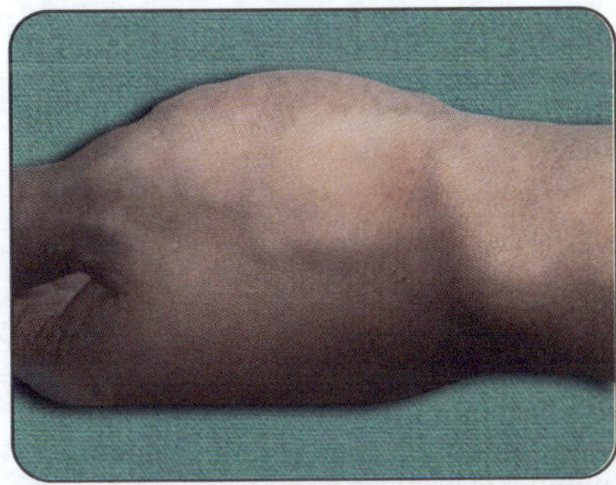

Fig. 9: Thickened radial cutaneous nerve at wrist in a case of pure neural Hansen's

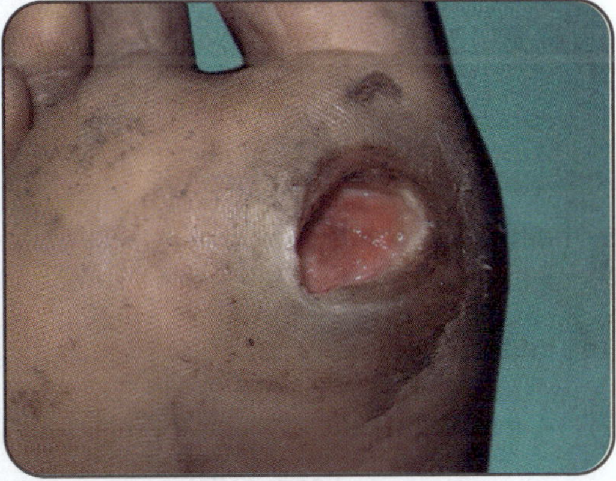

Fig. 10: Trophic ulcer

Eye Involvement in Leprosy

- 7th nerve involvement—corneal erosions, exposure keratitis, iridocyclitis (Fig. 11A), lagophthalmos (Fig. 11B)
- In BL and LL cases, the iris can show **micro-granuloma deposits of leprosy ("iris pearls").**(MCQ)

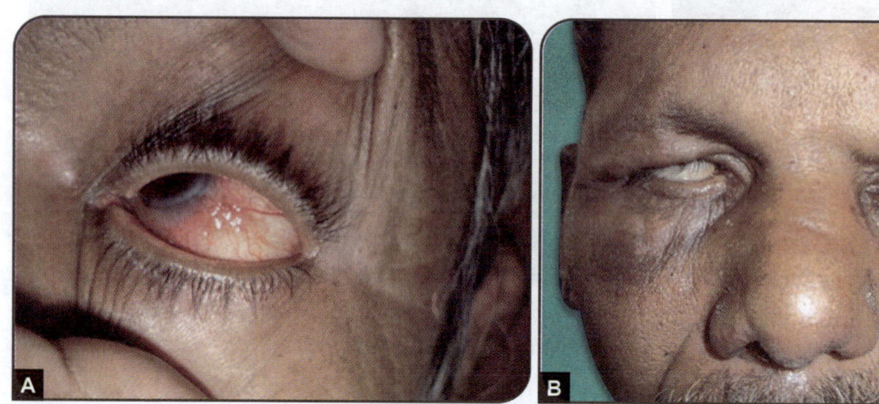

Figs. 11A and B: (A) Perilimbal redness of eye, suggestive of iridocyclitis in a patient with LL leprosy and Type 2 reaction; (B) Untreated lepromatous leprosy with bilateral lagophthalmos

Systemic Involvement in Leprosy

- Renal involvement—Secondary amyloidosis is the most common renal lesion. Amongst glomerulonephritis—**Mesangioproliferative glomerulonephritis** > MPGN > MPN(MCQ)
- CNS, female reproductive system, lungs, prostrate, breasts are not involved.

High Yield Points

Between ovary and uterus, if one option to be selected for uninvolved site, choose uterus > ovary

Histopathology in Leprosy

- Routine HE stains as well as special stain (**fite-faraco stain**) are used
- As patient moves from TT to LL, tuberculoid granulomas reduce and **foam cells, grenz zone formation** and number of bacilli increases. **Foam cells** are called so as they have lipids in them which look foamy on histology

$$TT \xrightarrow[\text{Foam cells, grenz zone and number of bacilli increases}]{\text{Tuberculoid granuloma size reduces}} LL$$

Indeterminate	TT	BT	BB	BL	LL
Absent granuloma(MCQ) Perineural, periadnexal, perivascular lymphocytes(MCQ)	**Dermal tuberculoid granulomas** (arranged around nerves)(MCQ) (Fig. 12A)	Similar to TT, but less tuberculoid granulomas. Grenz zone clear zone in papillary upper dermis starts to form. Early foam cells	Similar to BT, tuberculoid granulomas even less prominent. Grenz zone more prominent. More foam cells	Prominent foam cells. Prominent grenz zone. Large number of organisms arranged in clumps. Perineural fibroblast proliferation forming an **"onion skin"** or **"onion peel"** in cross-section, is typical(MCQ)	**Only foam cells/ Virchow's cells/ Lepra cells (dermal histiocytes laden with bacilli).**(MHCET 01) **Most prominent Grenz zone.** AFB typically abundant and are seen as round clumps **("globi")**(MCQ) (Figs. 12B to D)

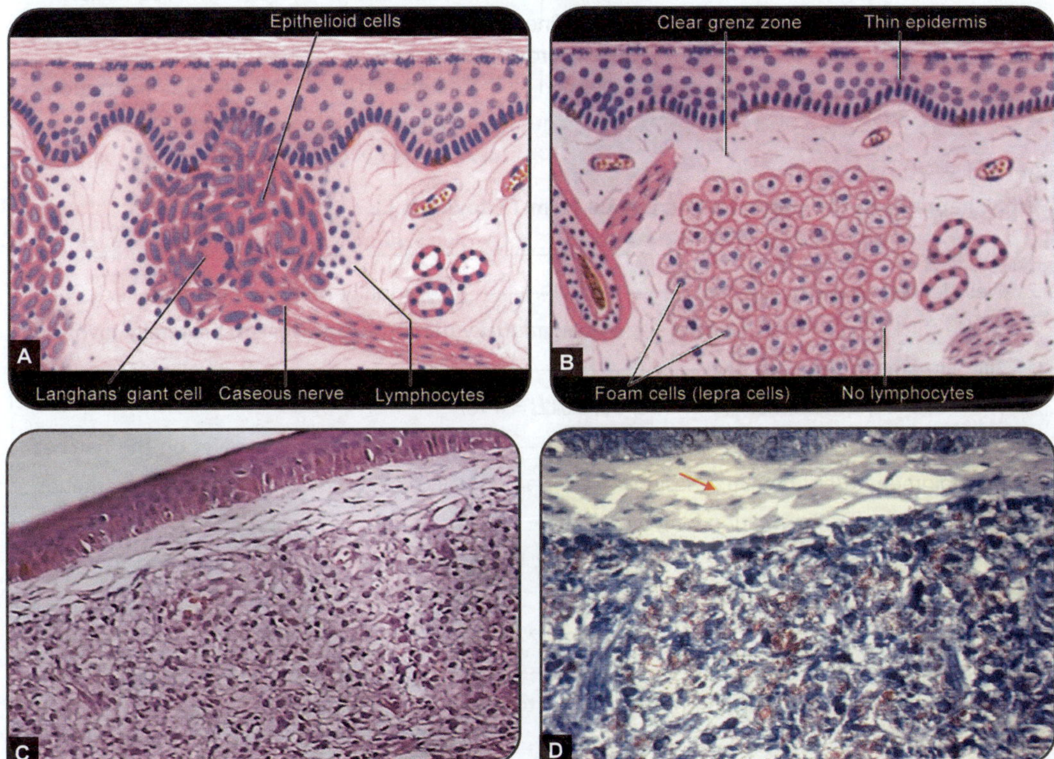

Figs. 12A to D: (A) Schematic representation of histopathology findings in TT; (B) Schematic representation of histopathology findings in LL; (C) Histopathology of LL. Note the numerous foam cells in the dermis and the clear grenz zone separating the epidermis from the dermis; (D) Special stain for AFB (AFB is seen stained red) in LL. Note the clear grenz zone without the bacilli (red arrow)

High Yield Points

How to arrive at the diagnosis of leprosy in an MCQ?

TT	BT	BB	BL	LL
1. **Single lesion** 2. **Single thick nerve** 3. **Well-defined borders**	1. **Satellite lesion/few lesions** 2. Few non-symmetrical nerve thickenings and non-symmetrical patches	1. **Punched out lesions/ Swiss-cheese lesions/ Inverted-saucer lesions** 2. Multiple lesions but countable 3. Inner border of lesions-Well-defined, Outer border-ill-defined	1. **Multiple lesions,** uncountable 2. Almost symmetrical on both sides of midline 3. Multiple, bilaterally thick nerves 4. Punched out lesions/ Swiss-cheese lesions/ Inverted-saucer lesions	1. **Multiple lesions/ diffuse infiltration/ nodules** 2. **Perfectly symmetrical** on both sides of midline 3. **Glove and stocking anesthesia** 4. No hypopigmentation 5. Normal sensations on patches in early stages 6. Ear-lobe infiltration 7. Trophic ulcers

What happens in the patient as he moves from TT towards LL

1. Number of lesions ⟶ gradually increase
2. Well-defined, elevated margins ⟶ gradually margins becomes ill-defined
3. Single thickened nerve, unilateral ⟶ gradually more nerves involved, bilaterally involved
4. Slit Skin Smear (SSS) negative ⟶ gradually SSS positive
   (TT = SSS -ve, BT = either -ve or +ve, BB/BL/LL = +ve)
5. Anesthetic lesions ⟶ gradually sensations recover on the patches
6. Hypopigmented/erythematous lesions ⟶ gradually more erythema, less hypopigmentation
   (LL has no hypopigmentation, only erythema)
7. Tuberculoid granuloma ⟶ gradually, tuberculoid granulomas reduce and foam cells and grenz zone formation increases
8. Large lesions ⟶ gradually become smaller and more numerous
9. Dry lesions ⟶ Shiny lesions
   (Shiny lesion occurs as sweating recovers due to lesser compression on nerves)

Reactions in Leprosy

- **Type 1 lepra reactions (also called as reversal/upgrading)**
- **Type 2 reactions also called as "Erythema Nodosum Leprosum" (ENL)**

Type 1 reaction	Type 2 reaction (ENL)
Occurs any time during treatment and within 3 years after treatment	May occur prior, with or after MDT
• Primarily cell mediated • **Type 4 hypersensitivity**(MCQ)	• Primarily humoral • **Type 3 hypersensitivity.**(MCQ) Immune complexes deposits in various tissues and also vessels (leukocytoclastic vasculitis) • **Cytokine involved-TNF-α**
Mainly in the borderline spectrum (BT,BB,BL). Most severe in BL	Most in LL (50%)(MCQ) > BL (15%)
Inflammation of existing lesions(MCQ) (Red, painful, edematous skin lesions) and/or red painful inflamed **nerves (neuritis)** (Figs. 13A and 15).(MCQ) Sudden neuritis can lead to permanent nerve damage. **Nerve abscesses can form (most in BT)** (Fig. 14)(MCQ). Sometimes the type 1 reaction can be severe and can cause ulceration of overlying skin. The ulcerative type 1 reaction is called Lazarine leprosy (Fig. 13B)	**New, tender, red, papules or nodules on extremities and face** (Fig. 16)(MCQ) (existing lesions do not change)
No systemic inflammation—no fever	**Systemic inflammation**—fever, arthralgia, conjunctivitis, keratitis, iritis, synovitis, nephritis, hepatosplenomegaly, orchitis, and generalized lymphadenopathy
Treatment of skin reaction • NSAIDs • **Oral steroids-DOC**(MCQ) -1 mg/kg prednisolone tapered in 12 weeks (WHO guideline)	**Treatment** • NSAIDs (for mild ENL) • **Oral steroids- DOC**(MCQ) • Thalidomide(MCQ) • Clofazimine
Treatment of neuritis • Splinting of limb(MCQ) • Oral steroids-DOC MCQ) **Treatment of Nerve abscess**(MCQ) • Nerve abscess-m/c seen in ulnar nerve • Only oral steroids may not be enough. Incision and drainage decompresses the nerve and restores nerve function(MCQ)	**Treatment for 1st episode ENL** Prednisolone 1 mg/kg gradually tapered over 12 weeks is the DOC **Treatment for recurrent/chronic ENL** • **Option 1:** Prednisolone + Thalidomide • **Option 2:** Prednisolone + Clofazimine

Note: WHO does not support the use of Thalidomide due to risk of phocomelia and peripheral neuropathy.

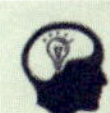

Aid to Remember

Total will be five—Type 1 lepra is type 4 hypersensitivity, type 2 lepra is type 3 hypersensitivity

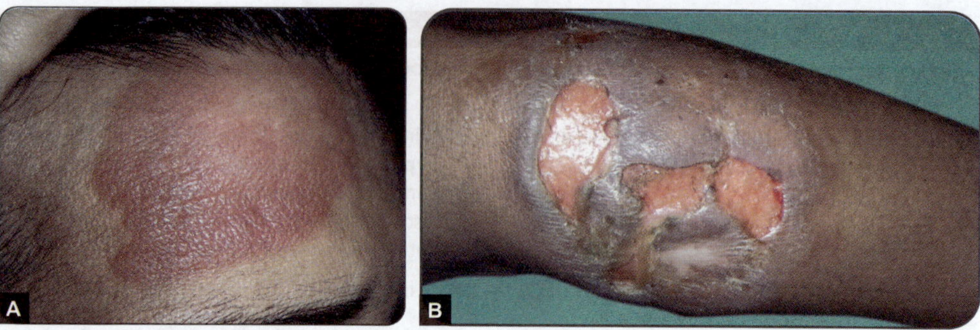

Figs. 13A and B: Type 1 lepra reaction—edematous, tender erythema over an established leprosy lesion

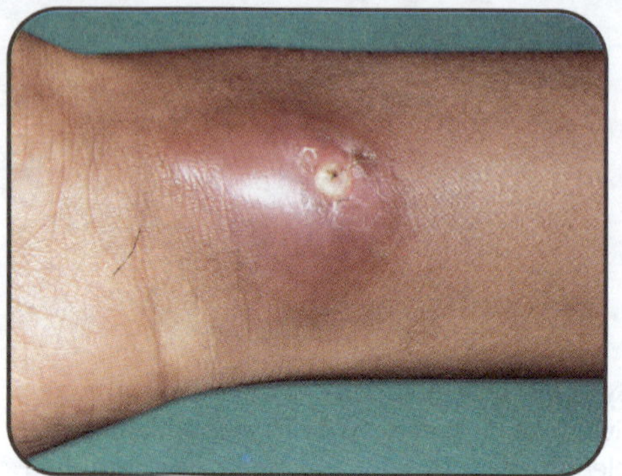

Fig. 14: Neuritis with nerve abscess

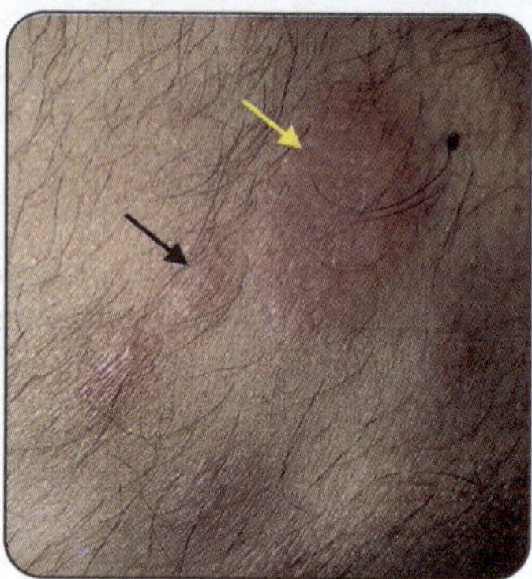

Fig. 15: Type 1 lepra reaction in a case of BT. Note the edema, redness on the main lesion (yellow arrow) and satellite lesions of BT (black arrow)

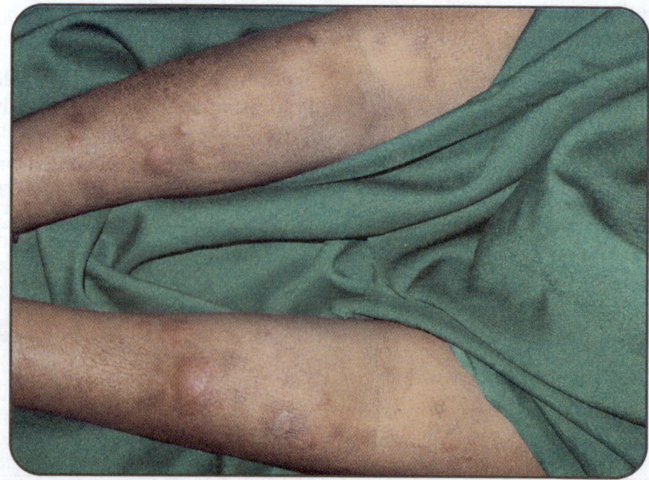

Fig. 16: ENL—tender, erythematous subcutaneous nodules on extremities

DIAGNOSIS

- **WHO definition of leprosy:** In an endemic country, an individual should be regarded as having leprosy if he or she shows **one or more** of the following cardinal signs:
  - Hypopigmented or reddish skin lesions with definite sensory loss
  - Thickened nerves
  - Positive skin smears

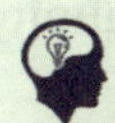

Aid to Remember the Cardinal Signs

LEProsy-**L** = Loss of sensation, **E** = Enlarged nerves, **P** = Positive AFB on smear

- **Usually skin biopsy is done to confirm diagnosis (nerve biopsy in cases of pure neural Hansen)**
- **Slit skin smear (SSS)**(AIIMS 06,03)
  - Slits are made on skin with a blade and stained for AFB (the number of sites vary- **WHO says ideally 4 sites, minimum 3 sites—one ear lobe and two active lesions**).
  - On AFB staining, 3 staining patterns are seen—**Solid bacilli (S) = Viable organisms, Fragmented (F) = Dead bacilli, Granular (G)= Dead bacilli**

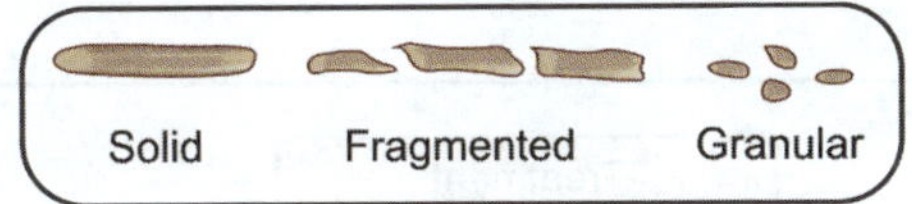

Bacterial index (BI)	Morphological index (MI)
Count S + F + G (dead+ living) The results are reported on a 0–6 scale. This is an indicator of the **total bacillary load of the patient**. Hence, **remains positive after therapy**	Count only S- solid bacilli (living) This is reported as percentage (e.g. 50% means 50% bacilli are alive). As it counts the living bacilli hence a **better indicator of treatment efficacy and drug resistance**. It **becomes negative after therapy**

  - The monitoring of the response to treatment can be done by an annual BI (**BI reduces by 1+ every year on treatment** e.g. if BI is 4+ to begin with, it becomes 3+ after 1 year of treatment. After this stage, BI reduces automatically by 1+ every year even without treatment)
  - **Diagnosing relapse after completion of treatment**—BI increases by 2+ from previous baseline value
  - SSS negativity is called **paucibacillary (PB) and positivity is called multibacillary (MB)**
  - As SSS sample is a superficial nick with a blade and not a deep sample, hence, many patients with significant number of bacilli in deep dermis will be declared SSS negative (false negative). **Thus, histological biopsy examination is the gold standard for diagnosis and not SSS**.

High Yield Points

- **Best site for SSS in untreated cases—Ear lobes**(MCQ)
- **Best site for SSS in treated cases—dorsa of fingers**(MCQ)
- SSS can only detect bacilli if they are **>10,000/gm of tissue.**(MCQ) **Hence, SSS is negative in TT, Indeterminate Hansen's, pure neural Hansen**

- **Lepromin test**—Intradermal injection of antigen is done to assess cell mediated immunity (CMI)
  - A **prognostic test** that is very helpful in classifying leprosy (negative lepromin—lepromatous side, positive lepromin—tuberculoid side)
  - **Cannot be used for diagnosis**(MCQ) as it is positive in normal people as well
  - Readings: 1. Fernandez response—within 48 hours
    2. Mitsuda response—at 4 weeks- better indicator of CMI
- FNAC of nerves—Specially for pure neural leprosy. Aspirate is stained for cells, bacilli.

TREATMENT

Most patients come with established nerve damage and hence, hypoesthesia, color change **may remain even after treatment.** The patient needs to be counseled about persistence of these features even after treatment.(MCQ)

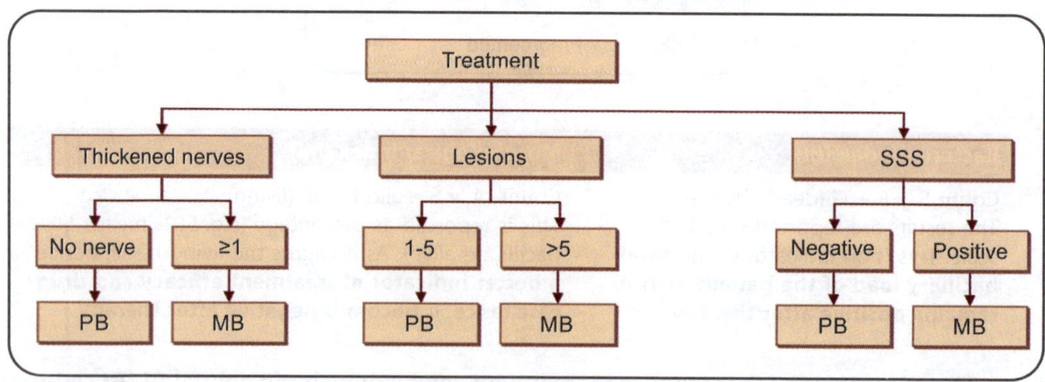

*Rifampicin is the **most important antileprosy drug**(MCQ) and is strongly bactericidal (Dapsone and Clofazimine have only a weak bactericidal action). It kills all viable bacilli in **4 days after a single dose.**

WHO Recommended Packet for Multidrug Therapy

*ROM therapy—rifampicin + ofloxacin + minocycline (ROM) was earlier given for single lesion leprosy, but is no longer used in the Indian programme as it has more failure rates
*According to WHO—Follow-up surveillance period after MDT is not required

Age group	Drug	Dosage and frequency	Duration	
			MB	PB
Adult (Fig. 17)	Rifampicin	600 mg once a month	12 months	6 months
	Clofazimine	300 mg once a month and 50 mg daily		
	Dapsone	100 mg daily		
Children (10–14 years)	Rifampicin	450 mg once a month	12 months	6 months
	Clofazimine	150 mg once a month, 50 mg daily		
	Dapsone	50 mg daily		
Children <10 years old or <40 kg	Rifampicin	10 mg/kg once month	12 months	6 months
	Clofazimine	6 mg/kg once a month and 1 mg/kg daily		
	Dapsone	2 mg/kg daily		

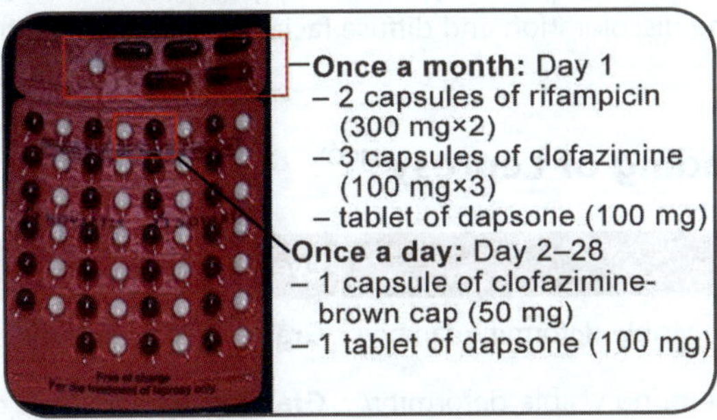

Fig. 17: Leprosy packet—Adult

Drugs in Leprosy

1. Dapsone:
   - Weakly bactericidal
   - Side-effects: Anemia, Dapsone hypersensitivity syndrome (5th week syndrome—Erythroderma + Fever + Lymphadenopathy + Hepatitis after 5 weeks of taking dapsone) (Fig. 18A)
2. Rifampicin
   - Powerful bactericidal
   - Cornerstone of leprosy management
   - Because of slow growth rate of *M. leprae* doubling in number only in 12 days, once monthly rifampicin suffices
3. Clofazimine
   - Made of an orange colored dye
   - Weakly bactericidal
   - Side-effects: Ichthyosis (Fig. 18B). The most common side effect is discoloration and darkening of skin (reversible on drug discontinuation-for image of skin discoloration, see Chapter 13-Fig. 6E)
   - Both anti-leprosy and anti-reactional (for ENL)

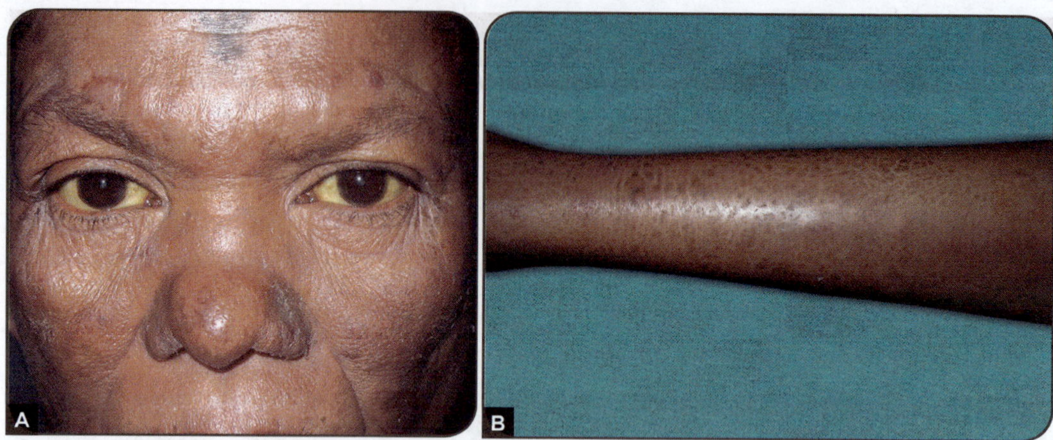

Figs. 18A and B: (A) Icterus due to dapsone hypersensitivity syndrome in an LL patient (Note the saddle nose, madarosis, clofazimine discoloration and diffuse facial infiltration); (B) Ichthyosis due to clofazimine

WHO Disability Grading of Leprosy(MCQ)

Hands and feet	Eyes
Grade 0: No anesthesia, no visible deformity/damage	**Grade 0:** No eye problem due to leprosy
Grade 1: Anesthesia present, no visible deformity/damage	**Grade 1:** Eye problem due to leprosy, but vision not severely affected (vision 6/60 or better)
Grade 2: Visible deformity present (Figs. 19A and B)	**Grade 2:** Severe visual impairment (vision less than 6/60, cannot count fingers), lagophthalmos, iridocyclitis, and corneal opacities

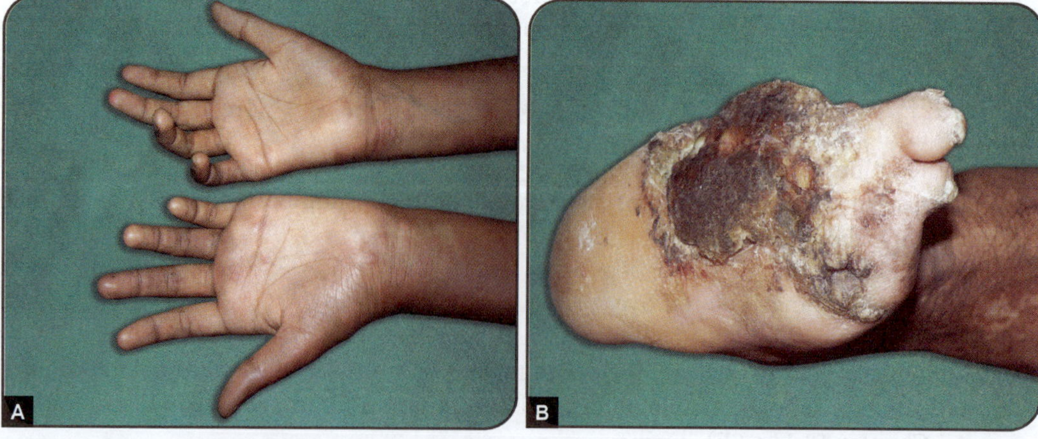

Figs. 19A and B: (A) Grade 2 deformity—claw hand; (B) Grade 2 deformity—deformed foot

High Yield Points

How to differentiate from all other hypopigmented diseases in MCQs?

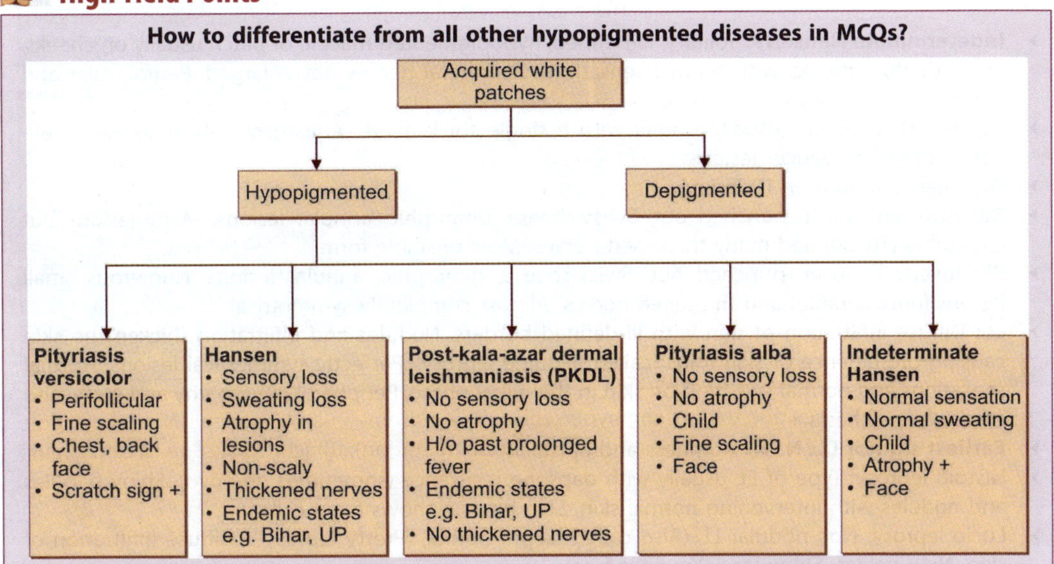

High Yield Points

High yield points in Hansen's disease

- M/c peripheral nerve involved = Ulnar (UL), posterior tibial (LL) (overall-ulnar > posterior tibial).
- M/c cause of nerve abscess- BT
- M/c nerve for abscess- Ulnar
- M/c deformity = Claw hand
- M/c Cranial nerve involved = Facial (1st to be involved- olfactory)
- M/c Hansen in India = BT
- M/c internal organ involved= Testis (male), liver (female)
- M/c nerve taken for biopsy-Radial cutaneous > Sural
- Order of sensory loss = Hot and cold differentiation > cold > hot > light touch > pain > crude touch
- Sensation never lost-Proprioception, vibration
- Internal organs not involved = Female reproductive system (uterus least involved > ovary-sometimes involved), CNS, lungs, GIT, prostrate

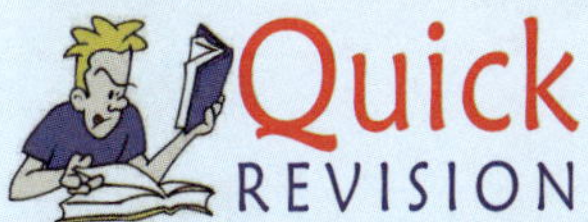

- Hansen's localizes to cooler superficial areas of the body (e.g. ear lobes, nose, testes, liver, ulnar nerve, facial nerve, etc.)
- **Ridley-Jopling classification:** TT (Tuberculoid), BT (borderline tuberculoid), BB (mid borderline), BL (borderline lepromatous), LL (lepromatous). BT—m/c in India
- Tuberculoid downgrades towards LL without treatment. Lepromatous upgrades towards TT with treatment (upgrading, reversal or type 1 lepra reaction)

Contd...

Contd...

- **Indeterminate Hansen's:** Solitary, ill-defined, hypopigmented macule or patch usually on cheeks, arms, thigh, buttocks with normal sensations. Peripheral nerves not enlarged. Perifollicular and perineural lymphocytes on biopsy'
- **TT:** 1–3 skin lesions (usually single) with a single thick nerve. Anesthesia, absent sweat, well-defined borders, Saucer lesions
- **BT:** satellite lesions. 3–10 lesions
- **BB:** inverted saucer, punched out, Swiss-cheese, dimorphic, annular lesions. Many lesions but countable (10–30) and many thickened nerves. Most unstable form
- **BL:** inverted saucer, punched out, Swiss-cheese, dimorphic, annular lesions. Numerous small lesions (uncountable) and thickened nerves. Almost completely symmetrical
- **LL:** Diffuse infiltration of skin with ill-defined borders. Nodules and infiltration thicken the skin causing prominence of skin folds (called "leonine leprosy').Perfectly symmetrical lesions. Normal sensations and normal sweating on skin in the initial phase. Peripheral neuropathy and glove and stocking anesthesia +"
- **Earliest sign of LL:** Nasal stuffiness and epistaxis
- Histoid leprosy: Type of LL usually with dapsone resistance (sometimes de-novo). Shiny papules and nodules with intervening normal skin. Skin biopsy- shows foam cells
- Lucio leprosy: Non-nodular LL (Also called "Lepra Bonita', "Pretty leprosy')- Diffuse infiltration of skin. No wrinkles, Shiny face (Younger face)
- Renal involvement: Mesangioproliferative glomerulonephritis. CNS, female reproductive system, lungs, Prostrate, Breast are not involved
- Type 1 lepra reaction: Upgrading. Type 4 hypersensitivity. Redness, pain and edema of existing skin lesions after MDT is started. Oral steroid-DOC
- **Type 2 lepra reaction (ENL):** Type 3 hypersensitivity. New painful, red nodules on extremities, unrelated to MDT. No change of existing leprosy lesions. Vasculitis on histology. Oral steroid-DOC. Oral thalidomide is more effective and faster but still not DOC. Nerve abscess—incision and drainage
- **SSS:** Positive if >10,000 bacilli/gm tissue. BI = Living + Dead, MI = Only living bacilli
- **MB-MDT- 3 drugs:** Clofazimine+ Rifampicin + Dapsone (12 months). **PB-MDT- 2 drugs**—Dapsone + Rifampicin (6 months)

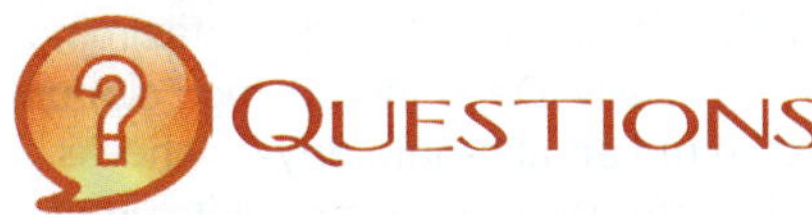

QUESTIONS

1. Leprosy does not involve:

a. CNS
b. Cornea
c. Testis
d. Skin

2. Skin smear is negative in which leprosy?

a. Borderline
b. Neuritic
c. Lepromatous
d. Borderline lepromatous

3. Most common type of leprosy in India:

a. BT
b. TT
c. BL
d. Indeterminate leprosy

4. Virchow's cells are seen in:

a. Henoch-Schonlein purpura
b. Toxic epidermal necrolysis
c. Congenital syphilis
d. Leprosy

5. Lepra cell is a:

a. Plasma cell
b. Neutrophil
c. Lymphocyte
d. Histiocyte

6. Satellite lesions are seen in:

a. Tuberculoid leprosy
b. Lepromatous leprosy
c. Borderline tuberculoid leprosy
d. Histoid leprosy

7. A patient of leprosy presents with lesions as shown. The likely diagnosis is:

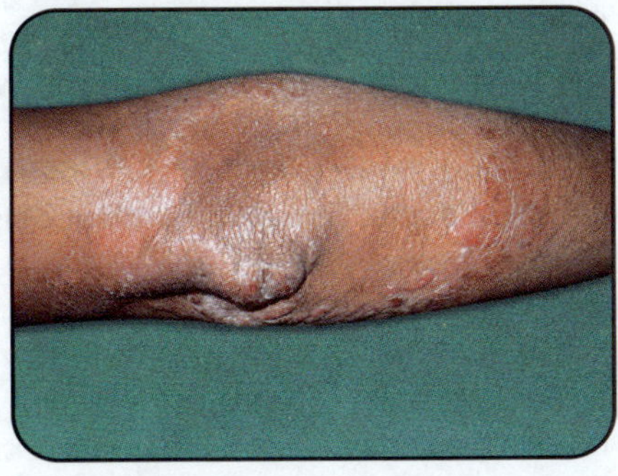

a. LL Hansen
b. Indeterminate Hansen
c. BB Hansen
d. BT Hansen

8. Nerve abscess is most seen in:

a. TT
b. BT
c. BB
d. LL

9. All are true about lepromatous leprosy *except:*

a. Presence of globi
b. Subepidermal free zone
c. Decreased cell mediated immunity
d. Presence of granulomas subdermally

10. A 45-year-old male had multiple hypoesthetic mildly erythematous large plaques with elevated margins on trunk and extremities. His ulnar and lateral popliteal nerves on both sides were enlarged. The most probable diagnosis is:

a. Lepromatous leprosy
b. Borderline tuberculoid leprosy
c. Borderline leprosy
d. Borderline lepromatous leprosy

11. Multiple hypoesthetic, hypopigmented macules on right lateral forearm with numerous acid-fast bacilli is indicative of:

a. Tuberculoid leprosy
b. Lepromatous leprosy
c. Indeterminate leprosy
d. Borderline leprosy

12. In leprosy which of the following is not seen?

a. Abnormal EMG
b. Voluntary muscle wasting
c. Decreased proprioception
d. Decreased response to tactile sensation
e. Increased response to tactile sensation

13. Earliest sensation to be lost in Hansen's disease is:

a. Pain
b. Touch
c. Vibration
d. Temperature

14. Nerves are not thickened in:
a. Tuberculoid leprosy
b. Lepromatous leprosy
c. Indeterminate leprosy
d. Borderline tuberculoid leprosy

15. A single hypopigmented anesthetic patch with satellite lesion on forearm. Likely diagnosis is:
a. Indeterminate leprosy
b. Borderline tuberculoid leprosy
c. Neuritic leprosy
d. Lupus vulgaris

16. All lesions are seen in leprosy *except:*
a. Erythematous macule
b. Hypopigmented patch
c. Vesicles
d. Patches

17. All are features of lepromatous leprosy *except:*
a. Gynecomastia b. Madarosis
c. Saddle nose
d. Early nerve involvement

18. A patient of leprosy presents with lesions as shown. The likely diagnosis is:

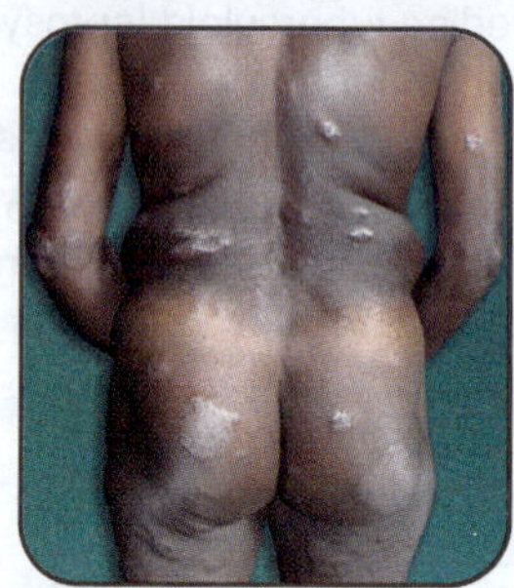

a. BL Hansen
b. Indeterminate Hansen
c. TT Hansen
d. BT Hansen

19. A 12-year-old child presented with 4 hypopigmented patches on back and 4 patches on forearm with loss of sensation. Treatment regimen would be: *(AIIMS May 2017)*
a. Monthly rifampicin-600 mg, clofazmine-300 mg. Daily dapsone-100 mg, clofazimine-50 mg
b. Monthly rifampicin-450 mg, clofazimine-150 mg. Daily Dapsone-50 mg, clofazimine 50 mg an alternate days
c. Monthly rifampicin 450 mg, clofazimine-150 mg. Daily- Dapsone 50 mg, clofazimine 50 mg
d. Monthly rifampicin 600 mg, Dapsone 100 mg

20. In leprosy neural involvement occurs in what percentage of patients?
a. 30% b. 60%
c. 90% d. 100%

21. Iris pearl is seen in:
a. Leprosy b. Sarcoidosis
c. Tuberculosistso d. Chloasma

22. A known case of lepromatous leprosy was initiated on treatment. She developed painful erythematous papules with fever and lymphadenopathy. What is the likely reactional state?
a. Type 1 lepra reaction
b. Type 2 lepra reaction
c. Lucio's phenomenon
d. Lupus pernio

23. Lepromin test is positive in which leprosy:
a. Lepromatous
b. Indeterminate
c. Histoid
d. Tuberculoid

24. Features of leprosy: *(PGI May 2017)*
a. Leonine facies
b. Saddle nose
c. Small ear lobe
d. Lagophthalmos
e. Microstomia

25. A 16-year-old student reports with multiple hypopigmented macules on trunk and limbs. All of the following tests are useful in making a diagnosis of leprosy *except:*
a. Sensation testing
b. Lepromin test
c. Skin smears
d. Skin biopsy

26. ENL is seen in which form of leprosy:

a. Indeterminate
b. BT
c. LL
d. BL
e. BB

27. The main cytokine involved in erythema nodosum leprosum (ENL) reaction is:

a. Interleukin-2
b. Interferon-gamma
c. Tumor necrosis factor–alpha
d. Macrophage colony stimulating factor

28. Type-1 lepra reaction is commonly seen in:

a. Histoid leprosy
b. Lepromatous leprosy
c. Borderline lepromatous leprosy
d. Polyneuritic leprosy

29. The following drug is used for the treatment of type II lepra reaction *except*:

a. Chloroquine
b. Thalidomide
c. Cyclosporine
d. Corticosteroid

30. DOC for lepra II reaction is:

a. Steroids
b. Thalidomide
c. Clofazimine
d. Dapsone

31. Drug of choice for ENL in a post-menopausal female is:

a. Thalidomide
b. Steroids
c. Clofazimine
d. Analgesics

32. A patient of leprosy presents with lesions as shown since past 7 days. The lesion is painful though there is no fever. The DOC would be:

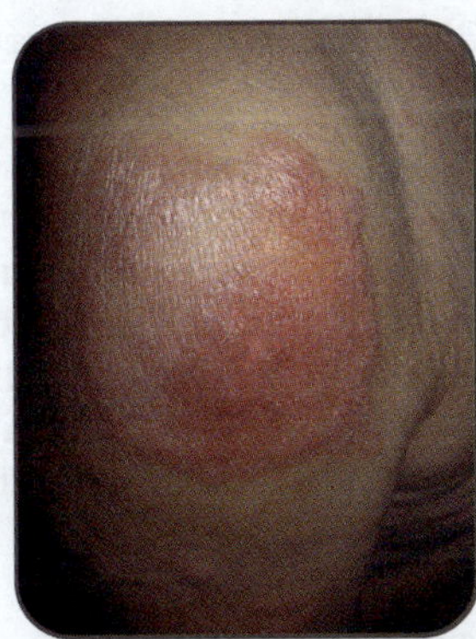

a. Thalidomide
b. Clofazimine
c. Dapsone
d. Corticosteroids

33. Reversal lepra reaction shows no response to:

a. Azathioprine
b. Cyclosporine
c. Glucocorticoids
d. Thalidomide

34. Antileprotic drug also used in lepra reaction is:

a. Rifampicin
b. Dapsone
c. Ciprofloxacin
d. Clofazimine

35. Lucio reaction is seen in: *(NEET Pattern)*

a. TB
b. Leprosy
c. Syphilis
d. LGV

36. Duration of treatment in multibacillary leprosy according to WHO is:

a. 6 months
b. 1 year
c. 2 years
d. 5 years
e. Lifelong

37. Under leprosy eradication programme the management of single lesion is:

a. Single dose of rifampicin and dapsone
b. Rifampicin, Dapsone and Clofazimine for 6 months
c. Rifampicin, ofloxacin and minocycline single dose
d. Rifampicin and minocycline for 6 months

38. Treatment of severe ulnar neuritis in borderline tuberculoid leprosy is:

a. MDT only
b. MDT + steroid
c. Wait and watch
d. MDT + thalidomide

39. Best method of treatment of ulnar never abscess in case of leprosy is:

a. High dose of steroid
b. Incision and drainage
c. Thalidomide
d. High dose clofazimine

40. The most effective drug against M. leprae is:

a. Dapsone
b. Rifampicin
c. Clofazimine
d. Prothionamide

41. WHO regimen for PB leprosy is:

a. Dapsone, Rifampicin—6 months
b. Dapsone, Rifampicin, Clofazimine—6 months
c. Dapsone, Clofazimine—6 months
d. Rifampicin, Clofazimine—6 months

42. The Ridley-Jopling classification for leprosy is based on which of the following parameter:

a. Clinical, bacteriological, immunological, histological
b. Histopathological, clinical, therapeutic
c. Histopathological, epidemiological, therapeutic
d. Histopathological, clinical, epidemiological

43. A 50-year-old male from Bihar came with symmetrical juicy papules and nodules with hypopigmentation on face and trunk. There was no hypoesthesia and nerve thickening. There was fever a few years back. The likely diagnosis is: *(AIIMS May 15)*

a. Lepromatous leprosy
b. Post-kala-azar dermal leishmaniasis
c. Borderline lepromatous leprosy
d. Mycosis fungoides

44. An 8-year-old boy from Bihar presents with a 6 month h/o an ill defined hypopigmented slightly atrophic macule on the face. The most likely diagnosis is:

a. Pityriasis alba
b. Indeterminate leprosy
c. Morphea
d. Calcium deficiency

45. An 8-year-old boy from Tamil Nadu presents with a white, non-anesthetic, non-scaly hypopigmented macule on his face. Likely diagnosis is:

a. Pityriasis alba
b. Pityriasis versicolor
c. Indeterminate leprosy
d. Neuritic leprosy

46. Commonest nerve involved in leprosy is: *(AIIMS)*

a. Ulnar b. Median
c. Radial d. Sciatic

47. Leprosy affects all organs *except:*

a. Eyes
b. Nerves
c. Uterus
d. Ovary

48. Tuberculoid leprosy is characterized by:

a. Non-caseating granuloma in skin
b. Subepidermal free zone
c. Bacilli in skin
d. Unstable disease

49. Skin biopsy in indeterminate leprosy is characterized by:

a. Periappendageal bacilli
b. Periappendageal lymphocytes
c. Perivascular lymphocytes
d. All of the above

50. Cell mediated immunity is maximally suppressed in:

a. Indeterminate b. BT
c. LL d. TT

51. Lepromin test is used for:

a. Diagnosis
b. Treatment
c. Prognosis
d. Epidemiological investigation

52. The following test is not used for diagnosis of leprosy:

a. Lepromin test
b. Skin slit smear
c. Fine needle aspiration cytology
d. Skin biopsy

53. Not true about lepromin test is:

a. It is diagnostic
b. Negative in infants <6 months
c. Used to classify
d. BCG vaccination may convert negative to positive

54. A 27-year-old patient was diagnosed to have borderline leprosy and started on multibacillary multidrug therapy. Six weeks later, be developed pain in the nerves and redness and swelling of the skin lesion. The management of his illness should include all of the following *except:* *(AIIMS)*

a. Stop anti-leprosy drug
b. Systemic corticosteroids
c. Rest to the limbs affected
d. Analgesics

55. A patient of leprosy presents with painful ulcerated lesion on the wrist as shown. He has recently been started on MDT for leprosy. The DOC would be:

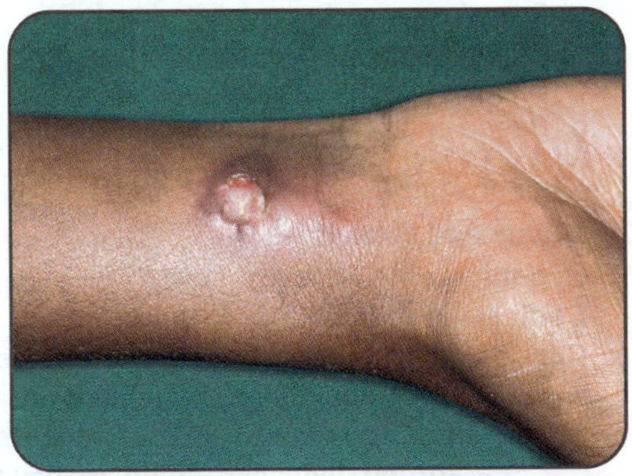

a. Choloquine b. Clofazimine
c. Dapsone d. Corticosteroids

56. Manifestation of ENL includes all of the following *except:*

a. Pancreatitis b. Fever
c. Hepatitis d. Arthritis
e. Cutaneous nodules

57. A patient of leprosy presents with painful lesions on arms as shown. He is also febrile. He is a given a drug which increases the numbness of the hands and feet. The likely drug is:

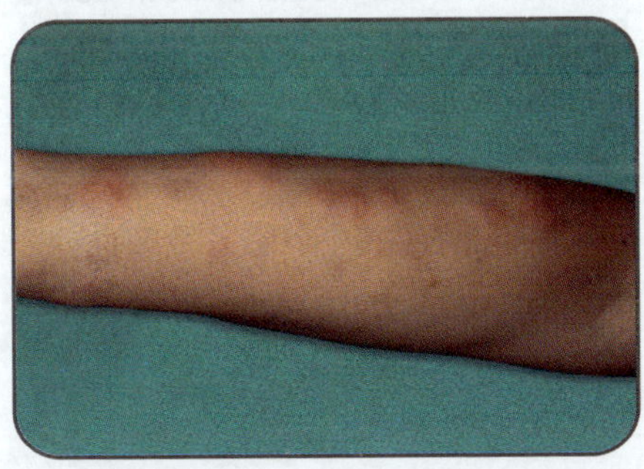

a. Clofazimine b. Rifampicin
c. Thalidomide d. Prednisolone

58. The following drug is not used for the treatment of type 2 lepra reaction:

a. Chloroquine b. Thalidomide
c. Cyclosporine d. Corticosteroids

59. Most potent antileprotic drug is: *(AIIMS)*

a. Rifampicin b. Dapsone
c. Clofazimine d. Norfloxacin

60. A patient of lepromatous leprosy is started on treatment. He develops ENLs with fever. He reports a change in her skin color after therapy as shown in the image. The likely drug responsible for this is:

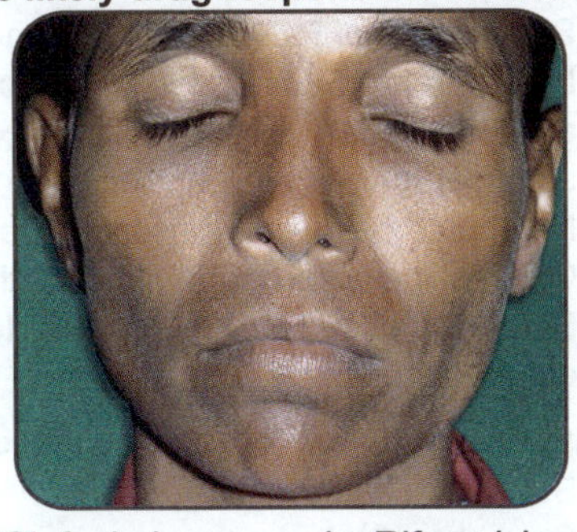

a. Clofazimine b. Rifampicin
c. Thalidomide d. Prednisolone

61. Skin pigmentation and ichthyosis-like side effects are seen in:

a. Rifampicin b. Clofazimine
c. Dapsone d. Steroid

62. Antibiotic against leprosy organism is: *(AIIMS May 2017)*

a. Ciprofloxacin b. Ofloxacin
c. Erythromycin d. Amoxicillin

63. Thalidomide is not used in:

a. ENL
b. Behcet's syndrome
c. HIV associated oral ulcers
d. HIV associated neuropathy

64. All are true statement regarding leprosy *except:*

a. Paucibacillary leprosy means person having 1-5 skin lesions and/or only one nerve involvement
b. Regular MDT means patient received 2/3rd of month of treatment schedule
c. Lepra reaction if not treated can lead to permanent deformities
d. Immunoprophylaxis have no role in leprosy

65. Indeterminate Hansen's is diagnosed by:
a. Skin biopsy
b. Slit skin smear
c. Hypopigmented patch
d. Sensory loss

66. Patient with a single anesthetic hypopigmented patch on forearm. What is true?
a. Single dose of ROM can be given
b. Left untreated, blindness, nasal collapse and testicular atrophy are expected sequelae
c. He should be given Dapsone, Rifampicin, Clofazimine for a period of 6 months
d. Serology or PCR are helpful tests in diagnosis

67. Drug of choice for recurrent ENL is:
a. Steroids
b. Steroids + Clofazimine
c. Steroids + dapsone
d. Cyclosporine

68. All the following are modes of transmission of leprosy *except:*
a. Breast milk
b. Insect bite
c. Transplacental spread
d. Droplet transmission

69. Babloo, a 5-year-old presents with small hypopigmented macules on his cheek. Some of his classmates also have similar lesions. The diagnosis is: *(AIIMS)*
a. Pityriasis rosea
b. Pityriasis versicolor
c. Indeterminate Hansen's
d. Pityriasis alba

70. Which of the following is classical of borderline leprosy?
a. Extensive glove and stocking anesthesia
b. Inverted saucer lesions
c. Erythema nodosum leprosum
d. Facial lesions

71. Leprosy causes:
a. Membranous glomerulonephritis
b. Focal segmental glomerulonephritis
c. Membrano proliferative glomerulonephritis
d. Diffuse glomerulonephritis

New Questions

72. The following statements are true/ false regarding the Ridley-Jopling classification in leprosy:
a. Based on microbiology criteria
b. Based on clinical criteria
c. Based on histology criteria
d. Based on treatment response criteria
e. Based on immunology criteria

73. Theme and Focus:
Hypopigmented Lesion
Clinical vignette:
Case 1. A 30-year-old patient presents with many hypopigmented lesions on trunk. Many patients around him also seem to have similar complaints. There is no previous significant past history. On examination, his lesions are non-scaly. Wood's lamp examination is negative. The diagnosis is likely to be:
Case 2. A 5 years old child presents with faint hypopigmented lesion on face. There is mild scaling. He also falls sick frequently and has frequent asthmatic episodes. The diagnosis is likely to be:
Choose the diagnosis of both scenarios from the options listed below:
a. Pityriasis versicolor
b. Pityriasis rosea
c. Psoriasis
d. Post-kala azar dermal leishmaniasis
e. Vitiligo
f. Borderline Hansen
g. Mycosis fungoides
h. Pityriasis alba

74. Assertion: Lepromin test is positive in tuberculoid leprosy
Reason: Lepromin detects T cell immune status in leprosy
a. Both Assertion and Reason are true and Reason is correct explanation of Assertion

b. Both Assertion and Reason are true but Reason is not correct explanation of Assertion
c. Assertion is true and Reason is false
d. Assertion is false and Reason is true
e. Both Assertion and Reason are false

75. Assertion: Slit skin smear is negative in TT leprosy
Reason: TT is a paucibacillary leprosy
a. Both Assertion and Reason are true and Reason is correct explanation of Assertion
b. Both Assertion and Reason are true but Reason is not correct explanation of Assertion
c. Assertion is true and Reason is false
d. Assertion is false and Reason is true
e. Both Assertion and Reason are false

76. Check the MDT schedule in adult leprosy and mark the correct options:
a. Rifampicin-600 mg once a month supervised
b. Clofazimine-300 mg once a month supervised
c. Dapsone-50 mg once a day unsupervised
d. Clofazimine-50 mg once a day unsupervised
1. If a, b, d are correct
2. If a and b are correct
3. If b and d are correct
4. If all four (a, b, c, & d) are correct

77. Match items in column A with best alternative in column B:

Column A	Column B
1. LL 2. BL 3. Indeterminate Hansen 4. BT Hansen	a. Inverted saucer lesions b. No skin involvement c. Satellite lesions d. Ear lobe infiltration e. Single thick nerve f. Not included in Ridley-Jopling classification

78. Pick the features of leprosy:
1. Itching along lesions
2. Painless ulcers
3. Glove and stocking anesthesia
4. Polygonal lesions
a. 1, 2 and 3 correct
b. 2 and 3 are correct
c. 1 and 4 are correct
d. Only 3 correct

79. A 45-year-old male had multiple hypoesthetic mildly erythematous large plaques on trunk and extremities. His ulnar and lateral popliteal nerves on both sides were enlarged. His smear is positive. The most probable diagnosis is:
a. Lepromatous leprosy
b. Borderline lepromatous leprosy
c. Borderline tuberculoid leprosy
d. Indeterminate leprosy

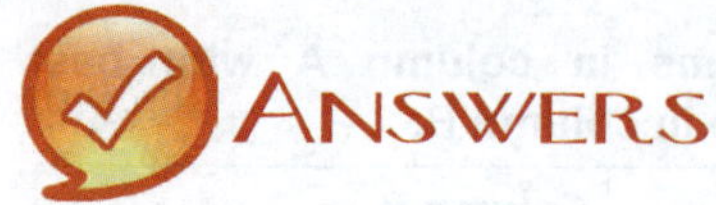

1. **Ans. (a) CNS** *(Ref: IAL Textbook of Leprosy-2nd edn, Page 339)*

CNS is generally regarded as un-involved in leprosy though there have been isolated case reports on cerebral cortex involvement.

2. **Ans. (b) Neuritic** *(Ref: Andrew's textbook, 11th edn, Page 335)*

SSS test involves superficial nicks on skin and it can detect bacilli only if they are >10,000/gm of tissue. Indeterminate, TT, some cases of BT and pure neuritic Hansens have negative SSS. Between neuritic and indeterminate, neuritic would be a better answer as it has pure neural involvement without clinical skin involvement.

3. **Ans. (a) BT** *(Ref: 1. Thangaraj RH, Yawalkars leprosy for Medical Practitioners and Paramedical Workers-8th edn, page 34; 2. IADVL Textbook of dermatology, 3rd edn, Page 2033, 2036; 3. Mani MZ, Mathew M. Leprosy in Punjab - an analysis of 4 years O.P.D. data. Lepr India 1981 Jul;53(3):395-405; 4. Shivaswamy KN et al. Clinico histopathological Correlation in Leprosy. Dermatol Online J. 2012 Sep 15;18(9):2; 5. Singal A et al. Childhood Leprosy in a Tertiary-care Hospital in Delhi, India: a reappraisal in the Post-elimination era. Lepr Rev. 2011 Sep;82(3):259-69)*

Even though Harrison's textbook (19th edn, 18th edn) gives the answer as TT, Indian references and books give the answer as BT.

4. **Ans. (d) Leprosy** (See page 54 for explanation)

5. **Ans. (d) Histiocyte** *(Ref: Levers Histopathology, 10th edn, Page 561)*

6. **Ans. (c) Borderline tuberculoid leprosy** *(Ref: Fitzpatrick's textbook, 8th edn, Page 2255)*

7. **Ans. (c) BB Hansen**

The image is showing an annular, punched out lesion of BB Hansen. Note the prominent elevated edge and central clearing of an annular lesion

8. **Ans. (b) BT** *(Ref: Fitzpatrick's Textbook, 8th edn, Page 2255)*

9. **Ans. (d) Presence of granulomas subdermally** *(Ref: Fitzpatrick's Textbook, 8th edn, Page 2258)*

Tuberculoid granulomas are a feature towards tuberculoid side.

10. **Ans. (d) Borderline lepromatous leprosy**

In questions like these, first decide whether the patient is towards tuberculoid or lepromatous side. Multiple lesions and symmetrical nerves suggests towards lepromatous side. But it cannot be LL as LL does not have hypoesthesia. So, it would be one step before LL, i.e. BL.

11. Ans. (d) Borderline leprosy

In questions like these, first decide whether the patient is towards tuberculoid or lepromatous side. Multiple lesions, hypopigmented lesions and numerous AFB suggests towards lepromatous side. But it cannot be LL as LL does not have hypoesthesia or hypopigmentation. It cannot be indeterminate which would not have hypoesthesia and also not have numerous bacilli. It cannot be tuberculoid which will have a single lesions and is paucibacillary. Hence, best answer is borderline.

12. Ans. (c) Decreased proprioception *(Ref: IAL textbook of leprosy, 2nd edn, Page 324)*

Nerve involvement is leprosy causes motor palsy (hence abnormal EMG). Voluntary muscle testing would detect these motor changes. Decreased sensations are classically seen. Increased tactile response indicates type 1 lepra reaction with hyperesthesia. Proprioception and vibration sense is not impaired in leprosy.

13. Ans. (d) Temperature *(Ref: Andrew's Textbook, 11th edn, Page 338)*

14. Ans. (c) Indeterminate leprosy *(Ref: Andrew's Textbook, 11th edn, Page 336)*

15. Ans. (b) Borderline tuberculoid leprosy *(Ref: Fitzpatrick's Textbook, 8th edn, Page 2255)*

16. Ans. (c) Vesicles

17. Ans. (d) Early nerve involvement *(Ref: IAL Textbook of Leprosy, 2nd edn, Page 324)*

Nerve involvement in LL is typically slow and late. Symmetrical nerve involvement causes glove and stocking anesthesia and mononeuritis multiplex in LL.

18. Ans. (a) BL Hansen

Note the almost symmetrical lesions of BL Hansen. Also note the single annular, punched out lesion on the left side of trunk. Annular lesions can be seen both in BB and BL. The widespread number of lesions would favor BL instead of BB

19. Ans. (c) Monthly rifampicin 450 mg, Clofazimine-150 mg. Daily- Dapsone 50 mg, clofazimine 50 mg

20. Ans. (d) 100%

Even though clinically nerve enlargement is not seen in all leprosy types (indeterminate Hansen's has normal diameter of nerves), nerve is involved in all patients of leprosy subclinically.

21. Ans. (a) Leprosy *(Ref: Andrew's Textbook, 11th edn, Page 339)*

22. Ans. (b) Type 2 lepra reaction

LL patients can show a type 2 lepra reaction after treatment. Fever, painful papules/nodules with lymphadenopathy all suggest ENLs

23. Ans. (d) Tuberculoid *(Ref: IAL Textbook of Leprosy, 2nd edn, Page 143)*

24. Ans. (a) Leonine facies; (b) Saddle nose; (d) Lagophthalmos

Leonine leprosy is nodular LL. Saddle nose is also common in LL due to collapse of bridge of nose. Lagophthalmos is due to facial nerve involvement (When leprosy involves the ophthalmic division of a patient's fifth nerve, cornea becomes anaesthetic. When it involves the zygomatic branch of seventh nerve, orbicularis muscle is paralysed, so that patient cannot shut eyes properly (lagophthalmos). LL usually causes ear lobe infiltration, hence large, pendulous ear lobes called Buddha ears—not small lobes. Microstomia has no relation to LL.

25. Ans. (b) Lepromin test

Multiple hypopigmented lesions suggest BL. Sensory testing would show hypoesthesia. SSS is positive. Biopsy would show few tuberculoid granulomas and plenty of foam cells. Lepromin is a prognostic test, not useful for diagnosis.

26. Ans. (c) and (d) LL; BL *(Ref: Andrew's Textbook, 11th edn, Page 341)*

27. Ans. (c) Tumor necrosis factor–alpha

(Ref: Rook's Textbook of Dermatology, 9th edn, Pg 28.6)

28. Ans. (c) Borderline lepromatous leprosy *(Ref: Fitzpatrick's Textbook, 8th edn, Page 2259)*

(Ref: Mckee's Pathology of skin, 4th edn, Page 827)

Borderline leprosy (BT, BB, BL) have type 1 lepra reaction. Amongst these, BL has the maximum type 1 lepra reaction.

29. Ans. (c) Cyclosporine (See page 56 for explanation)

30. Ans. (a) Steroids *(Ref: IAL Textbook of Leprosy, 2nd edn, Page 469)*

31. Ans. (a) Thalidomide *(Ref: IAL Textbook of Leprosy, 2nd edn, Page 470)*

32. Ans. (d) Corticosteroid

The image is showing type 1 lepra reaction. Note the edematous, erythematous plaque.

33. Ans. (d) Thalidomide *(Ref: IAL Textbook of Leprosy, 2nd edn, Page 466)*

34. Ans. (d) Clofazimine (See page 56 for explanation)

35. Ans. (b) Leprosy (See page 56 for explanation)

36. Ans. (b) 1 year (See page 60 for explanation)

37. Ans. (b) Dapsone, Rifampicin and Clofazimine—6 months

Single dose ROM therapy has been withdrawn from the Indian programme.

38. Ans. (b) MDT + steroid

MDT needs to be continued during reaction. Steroids are the DOC.

39. Ans. (b) Incision and drainage *(Ref: IAL Textbook of Leprosy, 2nd edn, Page 468)*

For a nerve abscess, steroids may not be sufficient. Incision and drainage decompresses the nerve and restores function

40. Ans. (b) Rifampicin *(Ref: Rook's Textbook of Dermatology, 9th edn, Page 28.15)*

Rifampicin is a potent bactericidal. Four days after a single 600 mg dose, bacilli in the patient are no longer viable

41. Ans. (b) Dapsone, Rifampicin, Clofazimine—6 months

42. Ans. (a) Clinical, bacteriological, immunological, histological

(Ref: Andrew's Textbook, 11th edn, Page 335)

Ridley-Jopling does not include indeterminate and pure neural types of Hansen's.

43. Ans. (b) Post-kala-azar dermal leishmaniasis (See page 63 for explanation)

Refer Chart in the Chapter

44. Ans. (b) Indeterminate leprosy (See page 47 for explanation)

Refer Chapter text for chart to differentiate hypopigmented patch on cheek. Bihar is an endemic state for leprosy.

45. Ans. (c) Indeterminate leprosy (See page 47 for explanation)

Refer Chapter text for chart to differentiate hypopigmented patch on cheek.

46. Ans. (a) Ulnar

Ulnar is the commonest peripheral nerve involved in leprosy.

Most books as quoted below give evidence on ulnar as commonest. Harrison 19th edn (pages 1024, 1125), Harrison-18th edn, the Classical Dharmendra Textbook of Leprosy Vol. 1 (page 101, 209), IAL Textbook, 2nd edn page 252, Yawalkar book page 30, 33, 88, all give ulnar conclusively. 2 cohort studies (1999, 2000) say posterior tibial as the commonest involved nerve. Take it as ulnar > posterior tibial.

47. Ans. (c) Uterus *(Ref: Andrew's Textbook, 11th edn, Page 339)*
(Ref: IAL Textbook of Leprosy, 2nd edn, Page 334)
(Ref: Blaustein's Pathology of the Female Genital Tract, 4rth edn, Page 602)

GIT, Brain, lungs, heart, prostrate and female reproductive system is thought to be spared in leprosy, though case reports have described involvement. Between ovary and uterus, uterus should be chosen for this question.

48. Ans. (a) Non-caseating granuloma in skin
(Ref: Mckee's Pathology of Skin, 4th edn, Page 829)
(Ref: IADVL Textbook of Dermatology, 3rd edn, Page 2017)

49. Ans. (d) All of the above (See page 47 for explanation)

50. Ans. (c) LL (See page 46 for explanation)

51. Ans. (c) Prognosis (See page 59 for explanation)

52. Ans. (a) Lepromin test (See page 59 for explanation)

53. Ans. (a) It is diagnostic (See page 59 for explanation)

Lepromin is used for prognosis and not diagnosis since it is a marker of immunity. Early infancy has a poor immune system and will have lepromin negativity. BCG vaccine would also convert it to positive.

54. Ans. (a) Stop anti-leprosy drug

The patient has type 1 lepra reaction with nerve inflammation. Steroids, splinting of limb and analgesics help. Anti-leprosy drugs should not be stopped.

55. Ans. (d) Corticosteroid

Steroid is the DOC for type 1 lepra reaction. The image is showing neuritis with ulceration. Dapsone as a part of MDT should be continued during treatment for reaction. Incision and drainage is done for nerve abscess as a consequence of severe neuritis.

56. Ans. (a) and (d) Pancreatitis; Arthritis (See page 56 for explanation)

ENL causes fever, red tender skin nodules, hepatitis, arthralgia (not arthritis)

57. Ans. (c) Thalidomide

Thalidomide may cause peripheral neuropathy which would then lead to numbness of hands and feet. The image is showing ENLs on arms.

58. Ans. (c) Cyclosporine (See page 56 for explanation)

59. Ans. (a) Rifampicin

60. Ans. (a) Clofazimine

The dark brown hyperpigmentation seen on the face is likely due to clofazimine given in MB-MDT for LL. Ceroid-lipofuscin pigment is deposited inside macrophages of affected patients which contributes to this skin color.

61. Ans. (b) Clofazimine

62. Ans. (b) Ofloxacin

63. Ans. (d) HIV associated neuropathy

Thalidomide itself causes peripheral neuropathy is about 20% patients within 1 year.

64. Ans. (d) Immunoprophylaxis have no role in leprosy

Vaccines have variable efficacy for leprosy prevention. BCG, BCG+ Killed M. leprae, Mycobacterium vaccae and ICRC vaccine have all been tried.

65. Ans. (a) Skin biopsy (See page 47 for explanation)

66. Ans. (c) He should be given Dapsone, Rifampicin, Clofazimine for a period of 6 months

Refer chapter text ROM therapy is now outdated. Blindness, testicular atrophy are features of LL. Serology is not helpful in diagnosis.

67. Ans. (b) Steroids + Clofazimine *(Ref: IAL textbook of leprosy, 2nd edn, Page 473)*

68. Ans. (b) Insect bite *(Ref: IAL textbook of leprosy, 2nd edn, Page 40)*

69. Ans. (d) Pityriasis alba (See page 47 for explanation)

Refer to the chart in chapter

70. Ans. (b) Inverted saucer lesions (See page 49 for explanation)

Inverted saucer is classical of BB. Extensive glove and stocking, ENL and facial lesions-LL.

71. Ans. (c) Membrano proliferative glomerulonephritis

(Ref: IAL Textbook of Leprosy, 2nd edn, Page 126)

Mesangioproliferative glomerulonephritis > MPGN > MPN.

New Answers

72. Ans. a-True; b-True; c-True; d-False; e-True

73. Case 1: Ans. (f) Borderline Hansen

In the options given, hypopigmented lesions are seen in pityriasis versicolor, PKDL, pityriasis alba and Hansen's disease. Pityriasis versicolor will have scaling and Wood's lamp positivity. Pityriasis alba will be on face with scaling, usually in a child. PKDL will usually a past history of fever. Hansen's disease appears to be the best option.

Case 2: Ans. (h) Pityriasis alba

Pityriasis alba typically being a minor sign of atopy has scaly patches on face. Asthmatic episodes are s/o atopy.

74. Ans. (a) Both Assertion and Reason are true and Reason is correct explanation of Assertion

75. Ans. (a) Both Assertion and Reason are true and Reason is correct explanation of Assertion

76. Ans. (1) If a, b, d are correct

77. Ans. 1-d; 2-a; 3-f; 4-c

78. Ans. (b) 2 and 3 are correct

79. Ans. (b) Borderline lepromatous leprosy

The answer would be borderline lepromatous leprosy as the question mentions hypoaesthetic lesions. First try to decide the side of leprosy we are dealing with here. Multiple lesions and multiple nerves go in favour of the lepromatous side. So it would be either LL or BL. Since LL will not have sensory loss, we will go in favour of BL.

Explanation for other incorrect answers:

- Option A: LL will have diffuse, normal sensation areas all over the body with peripheral glove and stocking anesthesia.
- Option C: BT will have satellite lesions (not multiple lesions) and multiple thickened nerves would not be present
- Option D: Indeterminate leprosy will have faint hyperpigmented patches on the cheeks in children with normal sensation and normal sweating. No thick nerves.

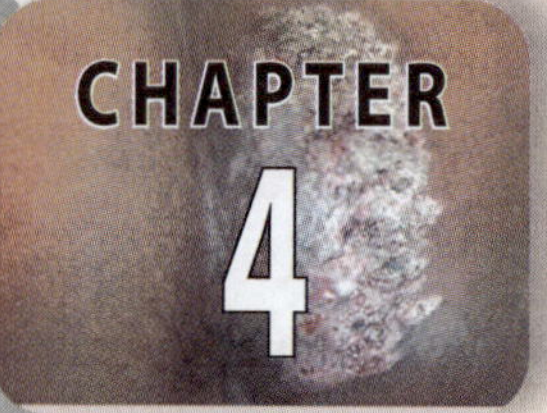

Tuberculosis and Other Bacterial Infections

CLASSIFICATION OF CUTANEOUS TUBERCULOSIS (TB)

The classification of cutaneous TB is done taking into account the mode of acquisition.

Inoculation from an exogenous source	Tuberculous chancre
	Tuberculosis verrucosa cutis (TBVC)
	Lupus vulgaris-**m/c form in India (adults)**(MCQ)
Endogenous	Scrofuloderma-**m/c form in India (children)**(MCQ)
	Periorificial tuberculosis
Tuberculids	Micropapular (Lichen scrofulosorum)(MCQ)
	Papular (Papulonecrotic tuberculid)
	Nodular-Erythema induratum [Bazin disease](MCQ)

* If adult or child not mentioned in MCQ—mark lupus vulgaris as m/c type in India.

Exogenous Variety

Tuberculous chancre (primary tuberculosis complex)

- Inoculation of TB bacilli into skin of a person with **no previous exposure to TB** (TB-naïve). Hence, poor immunity towards bacilli and MT negative
- Presents as an ulcer (**Chancre = ulcer**) with an **undermined edge**(MCQ) (Figs. 1A and B)

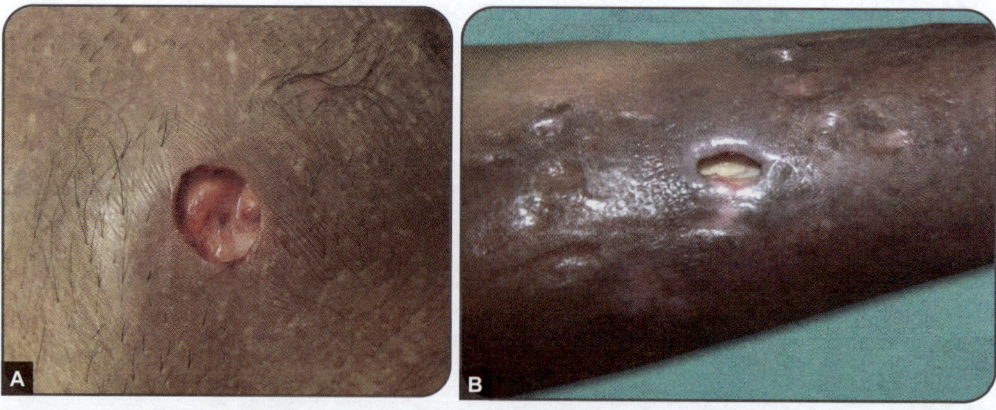

Figs. 1A and B: (A) Undermined ulcer; (B) Note the undermined edge of the ulcer in TB chancre

- **Primary skin TB**(MCQ)
- Since the immunity is low-bacilli proliferate freely (multi-bacillary disease). Hence, bacteria easy to demonstrate.

Tuberculosis verrucosa cutis (TBVC, Warty TB)

- Inoculation of TB bacilli into skin of a person who is **already sensitized** by a previous exposure to TB. Hence, **strong immunity towards bacilli** and MT strongly positive
- Hypertrophic, wart-like, cauliflower-like masses (verrucosa = verruca-like)
- Dorsa of fingers, buttocks and feet (Figs. 2 and 3)
- Since the immunity is good—bacilli are less (**pauci-bacillary disease**). Hence, bacteria difficult to demonstrate
- **Anatomist's wart/Pathologist's wart**—Misnomer and are not types of warts but TBVC in anatomists or pathologists due to accidental inoculation **onto fingers** from cadavers.

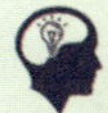

Aid to Remember

- Tuberculosis verrucosa cutis = TB + verrucosa (like verruca, meaning cauliflower-like masses) + cutis (skin)

High Yield Points

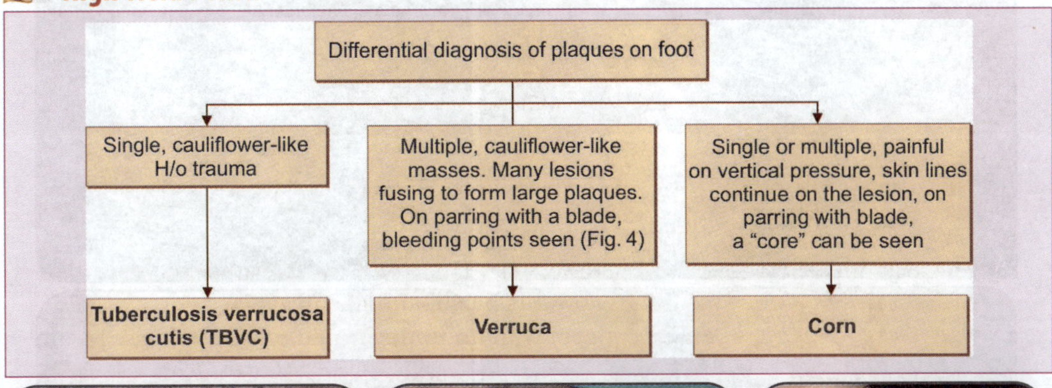

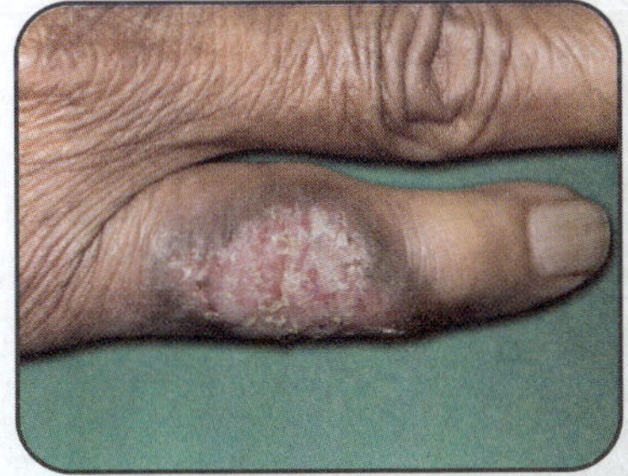

Fig. 2: Verrucous mass on finger—TBVC

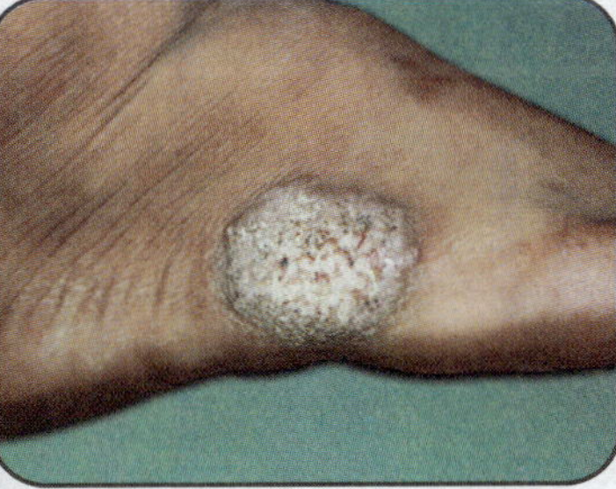

Fig. 3: Verrucous mass on foot—TBVC

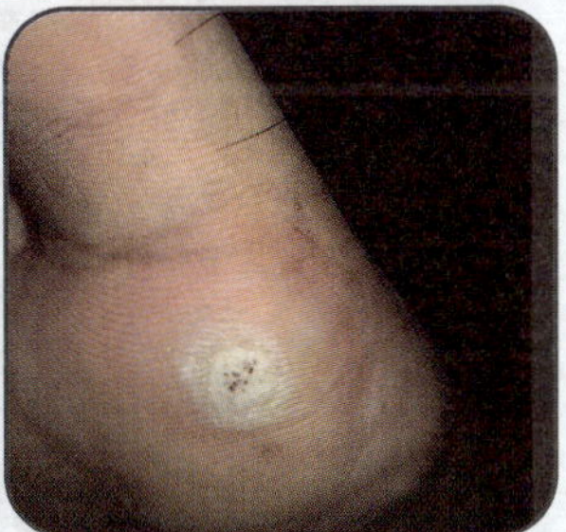

Fig 4: Verruca (wart)- Note the lesion on sole which has been parred horizontally with a blade revealing black/red dots (bleeding points and thrombosed vessels)

Lupus vulgaris

- Typically presents as a single plaque of grouped red-brown papules which **heal at one end and progress at the other end**(MCQ)
- **Healing leaves central scars**(MCQ) (Figs. 5A to C)
- **Face and buttocks**(MCQ) are common sites.
- Since the immunity is good-bacilli are less (pauci-bacillary disease). Hence, bacteria difficult to demonstrate
- Diagnosis of lupus vulgaris:
  - Diascopy: When lesions of lupus vulgaris are pressed by a glass slide, pale brownish yellow **"apple-jelly"**(MCQ) color nodules are seen (Fig. 5D)
  - Skin biopsy: **Tuberculoid granulomas (scanty or absent caseation)**. AFB is seen rarely on smear (PCR may help)
  - Culture is only positive in half the cases.

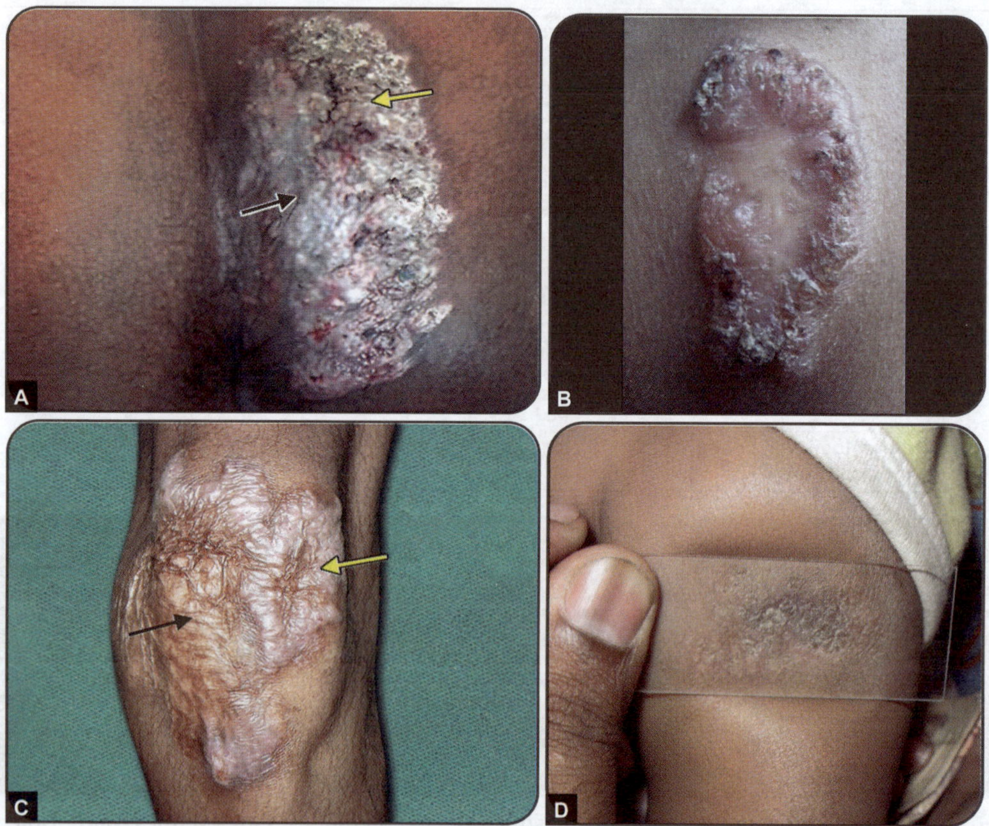

Figs. 5A to D: (A) Plaque on buttock with peripheral extension (yellow arrow) and scarring on old areas (black arrow); (B) Classical lesion with central scarring and peripheral extension; (C) Central scarring (black arrow) and peripheral extension (yellow arrow); (D) Diascopy-pressing with the glass slide shows "apple-jelly" nodules

High Yield Points

Pick-up words in MCQs on lupus vulgaris
- Central scarring
- Healing in the center, extending on periphery
- Buttocks or face

High Yield Points

Central clearing = Tinea(MCQ)
Central crusting = Leishmaniasis(MCQ)
Central scarring = Lupus vulgaris(MCQ)

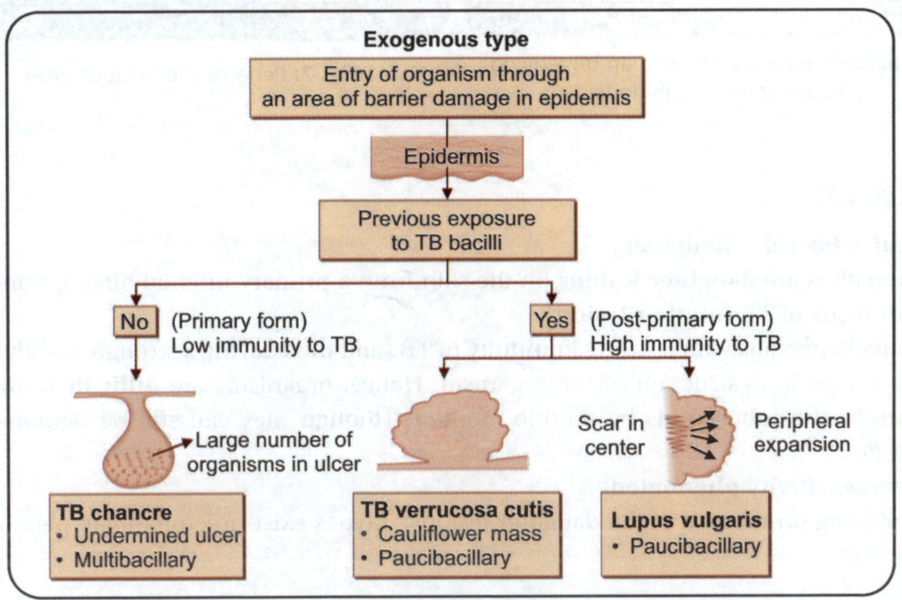

Endogenous Variety (Spread to Skin by Direct Extension)

Scrofuloderma

- Direct extension from an underlying focus of infection, e.g. over infected cervical lymph nodes, over bone or around joints. Begins as nodules which suppurates (**cold abscess**), drains, and forms **nonhealing sinuses** (Fig. 6).(MCQ) Bacteria easy to demonstrate.

Periorificial TB

- Skin TB **around orifices** from spread of internal progressive TB (Fig. 7). Hence, at **mucocutaneous borders** of the nose, mouth (local spread from laryngeal TB, pulmonary TB), anus (local spread from rectal TB), urinary meatus, and vagina
- Since the immunity is low-bacilli proliferate freely (multi-bacillary disease hence bacteria easy to demonstrate). MT negative

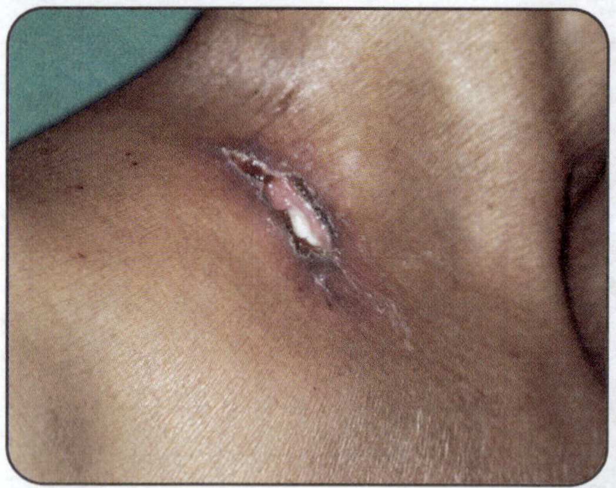

Fig. 6: Undermined ulcer with an underlying tuberculous lymph node

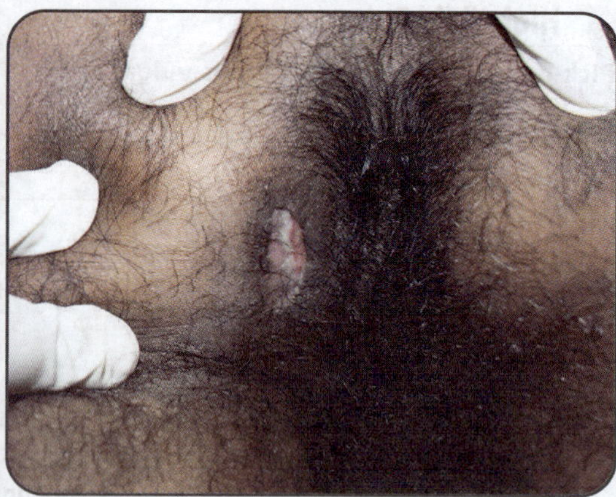

Fig. 7: Perianal tuberculous ulcer

Tuberculids

Tubercul + ids (id = daughter)

- Tuberculids are **daughter lesions** on the skin from a primary internal often ignored and silent focus of TB (**mother lesion**)
- Occurs in persons with a strong immunity to TB (and thus having a strongly positive MT). This results in destruction of the organism. Hence, organisms are **difficult to demonstrate in the tuberculids** by routine methods (though they can still be demonstrated with PCR)
- **Hypersensitivity phenomenon**
- Depending on the size of the daughter lesions, 3 types exist- micropapular, papular and nodular.

Micropapular tuberculid (lichen scrofulosorum)	Papulonecrotic tuberculid (papules + necrosis)	Nodular tuberculid (Bazin disease, Erythema induratum)
Micropapules in groups on trunk (Fig. 8A)	An asymptomatic, chronic disorder with repeated crops of papulonecrotic lesions symmetrically on extensor parts of extremities (elbows, knees, hands and feet)	**Tender dusky nodules on calf in women of middle age which often ulcerates** (Fig. 8B)

High Yield Points

Pick up word in MCQs on tuberculids:
- "Perifollicular tuberculoid granulomas"—suggests lichen scrofulosorum
- "Tender nodules on calf which ulcerate" in an MCQ–suggests nodular tuberculid

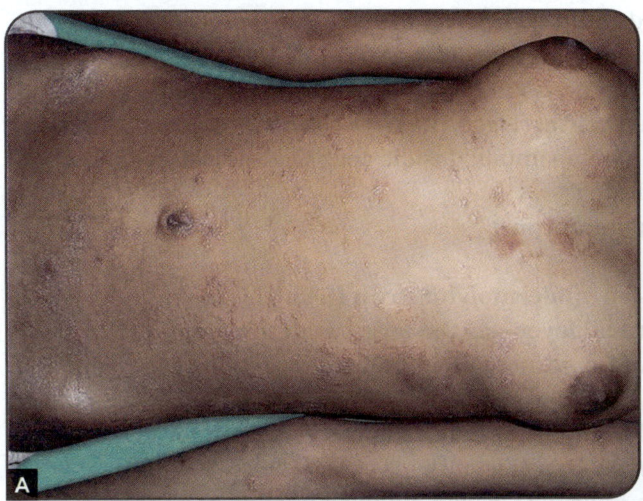

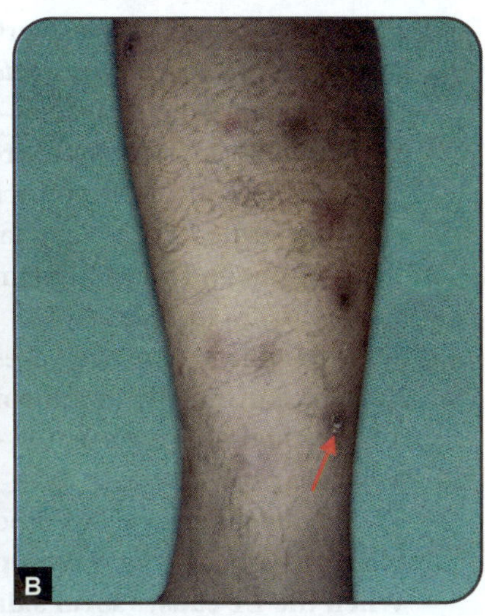

Figs. 8A and B: (A) Grouped micropapules on trunk; (B) Nodules on calf, one lesion ulcerating topped by a crust (red arrow).

ATYPICAL MYCOBACTERIAL INFECTIONS

1. **Mycobacterium ulcerans**-causes **Buruli ulcer**
2. **Swimming pool granuloma/Fish-tank granuloma**[PGI Nov 17]
   - **Fish handlers or swimmers affected**
   - Due to *Mycobacterium marinum* in aquariums or swimming pools (resides in fresh/salt water)
   - Nodules and discharging sinuses along lymphatics, **resembles sporotrichosis**
   - **Minocycline is the drug of choice**. Azithromycin is also effective.

High Yield Points

Pick-up word in MCQ—would be a swimmer or fish-handler,[MCQ] not a farmer or gardener as in sporotrichosis.

IMPETIGO

Two Types Occur—Non-bullous (Impetigo Contagiosa) and Bullous Impetigo

1. **Non-bullous impetigo (Impetigo contagiosa)**
   - Staphylococcal, streptococcal, or combined infection
   - Commonest skin infection in children. More on exposed parts of the body in children—**face is a common site**
   - Contagious—hence called impetigo **contagiosa**

- Etiology—Overall in the world, ***Staphylococcus aureus* > *Streptococcus pyogenes*, *but in warmer climates in developing countries—Streptococcus* > *Staphylococcus***
- Starts as very flaccid blisters—rupture soon to create an erosion covered classically by **golden-colored/honey-colored crusts** (Fig. 9A)
- Treatment: Topical—mupirocin, retapamulin, fusidic acid, Oral—dicloxacillin, amoxicillin + clavulanic acid, cephalexin

2. **Bullous impetigo (pemphigus neonatorum)**
   - **Caused by *S. aureus***
   - *S. aureus* phage type 2 releases an **epidermolytic Toxin (ET)**. This toxin ruptures desmosomes **primarily in subcorneal layer—as the target is desmoglein-1** (Note—It is a toxin-mediated destruction of Dsg-1, not autoimmune destruction as in pemphigus foliaceus)
   - The organism can be cultured from blister fluid. The pus settles on lower end of the blister as it is heavier—**Hypopyon sign** (Fig. 9B)[(MCQ)]
   - **When the ET causes local skin infection—called bullous impetigo and when it disseminates hematogenously—called Staphylococcus Scalded Skin Syndrome (SSSS)**
   - **Histopathology**—Blister below stratum corneum (within or below the granular layer) with plenty of neutrophils

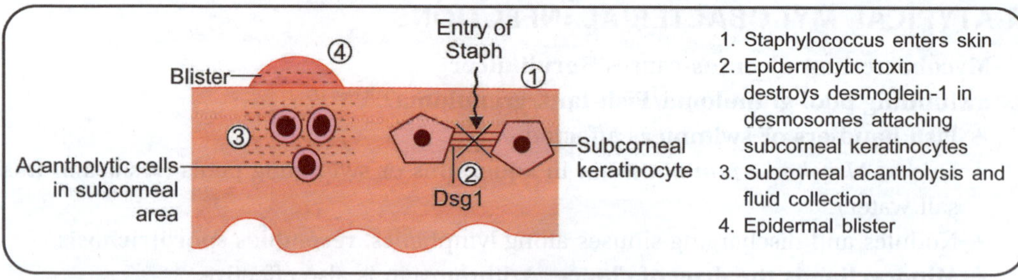

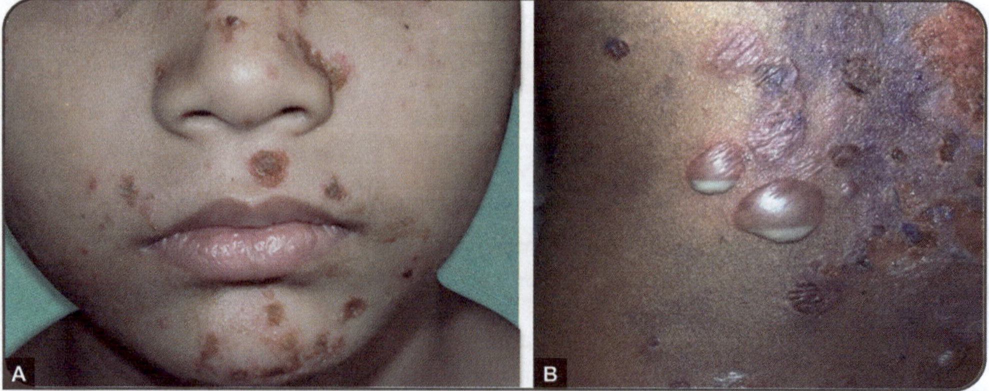

Figs. 9A and B: (A) Typical honey-colored crusts in non-bullous impetigo; (B) Hypopyon sign in bullous impetigo

3. **SSSS/Ritter's disease**
   - Generalized, superficially blistering disease in neonates and young children <5 years
   - There is a focus **of staphylococcal infection** (e.g. otitis media or a furuncle from where the ET spreads hematogenously). Fever is usual.
   - Presents typically as **perioral scaling and crusting, superficial erosions and absence of mucosal involvement** (Dsg target, mucous membrane is not involved since Dsg-1 is absent in mucous membrane) (Figs. 10A and D).
   - The blister ruptures and leads to widespread sheet-like separation of skin (Fig. 10C). Skin surface is fragile and it shears off easily with finger leaving erosions—**Positive Nikolsky sign** (Fig. 10B)(MCQ)
   - **Histopathology**—Similar to bullous impetigo

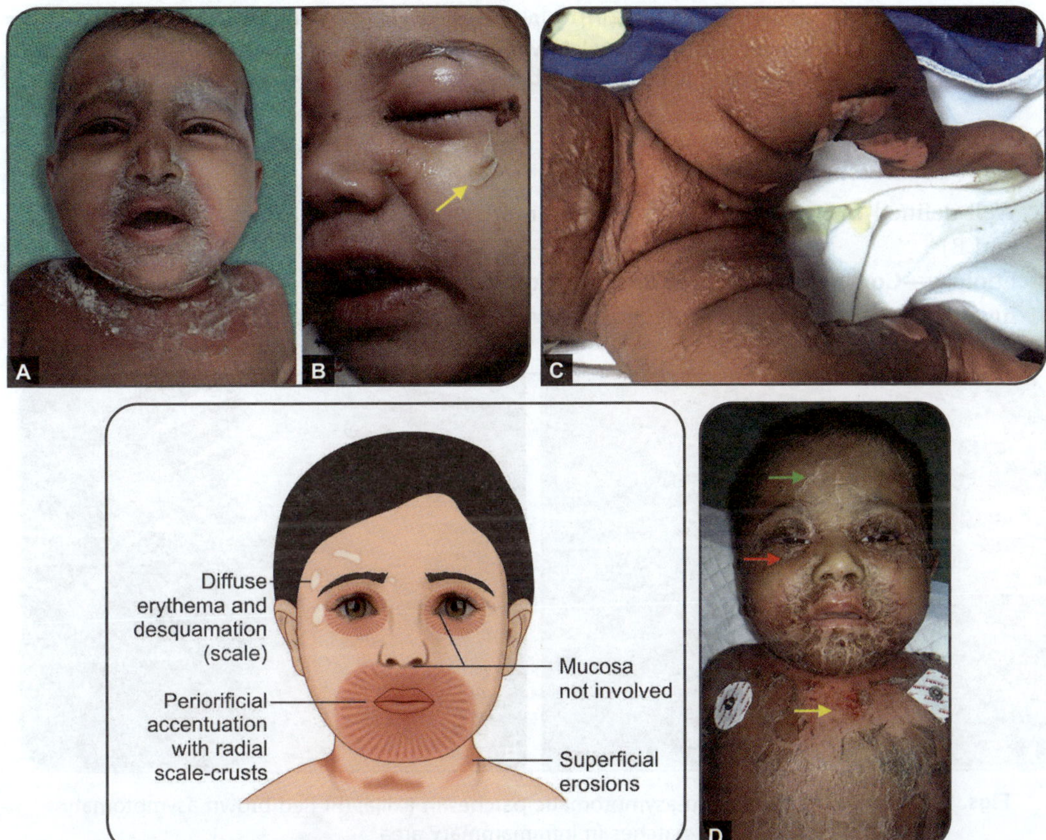

Figs. 10A to D: (A) Note perioral/nasolabial fold scaling and crusting, absent eye involvement and superficial erosions on chest; (B) Nikolsky sign positivity in SSSS—Note the peeling of skin on upper cheek after an attempt was made to pull down the eyelid for examination with finger (yellow arrow). (C) Flaccid blisters, superficial erosions; (D) SSSS— Perioral and periocular scaling (red arrow), Exfoliation (green arrow), Superficial erosions (yellow arrow)

How to Differentiate SSSS, Pemphigus Vulgaris and Toxic Epidermal Necrolysis (TEN)/Stevens-Johnson Syndrome (SJS) in an MCQ?

	SSSS	Pemphigus vulgaris (more details in Chapter 9)	TEN/SJS (more details in Chapter 14)
Age	Infants, children	Adults	Adults
Mucosal involvement	No	Yes	Yes
Targetoid lesions	No	No	Yes
Nikolsky sign	Yes	Yes	Pseudo – Nikolsky sign
Perioral scaling—crusting	Yes	No	No (Hemorrhagic crusting on lips +)
Histopathology	Acantholytic cells with subcorneal (midgranular or subgranular) blister	Acantholytic cells with suprabasal blister	• Intrabasal split or subepidermal blistering. • Necrotic keratinocytes

ERYTHRASMA

- Well-defined **brown-red patches** in the intertriginous areas (axillae, groins) (Figs. 11A and B)
- Etiology—**Corynebacterium minutissimum**(MCQ)
- Investigation—Wood's light is diagnostic—**coral red fluorescence**

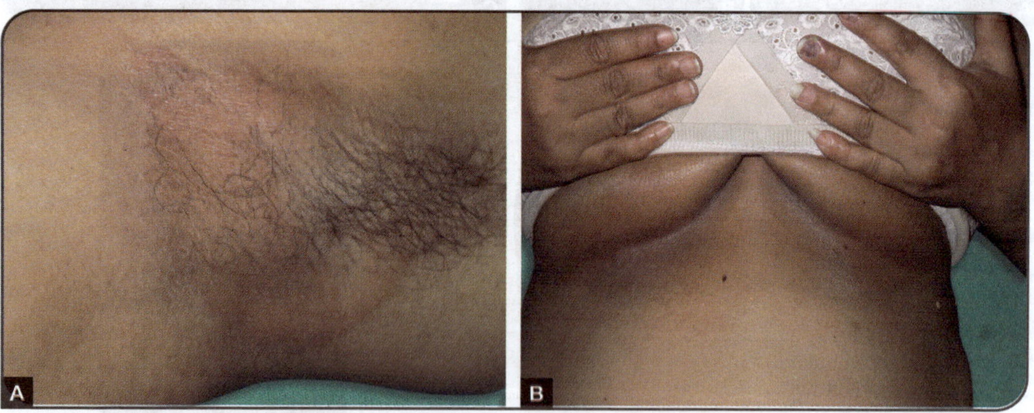

Figs. 11A and B: (A) Red-brown asymptomatic patches in axilla; (B) Red-brown asymptomatic patches in inframammary area

MENINGOCOCCEMIA

- Meningococcal septicemia presents as fever, meningitis
- Skin lesions—**Petechiae** on the trunk and lower extremities, and bullous hemorrhagic lesions. **Angular cutaneous infarcts are classical** (Fig. 12)

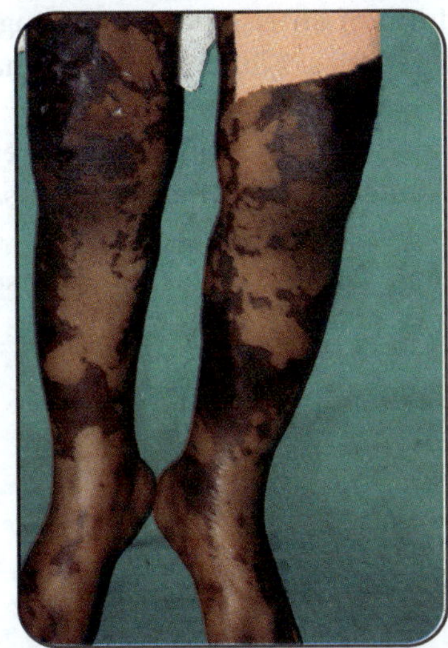

Fig. 12: Meningococcemia—angulated cutaneous infarcts in purpura fulminans caused by meningococcus

SCARLET FEVER

- A generalized erythematous rash often with co-existing streptococcal pharyngitis.
- Primarily in children, who develop the eruption 24–48 h after the onset of pharyngeal symptoms.
- Throat symptoms are in the form of swollen, red tonsils covered with exudate.
- Tongue shows a **white strawberry tongue** (white coating through which reddened, hypertrophied papillae project). Later, the coating disappears and the tongue is bright red (red **strawberry tongue**) (Fig. 13).

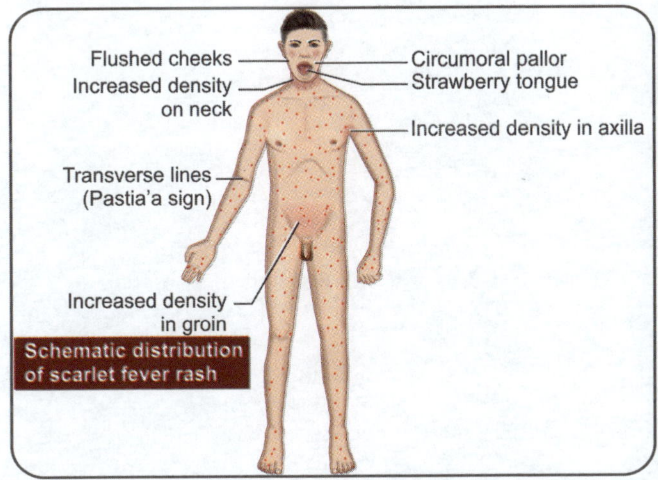

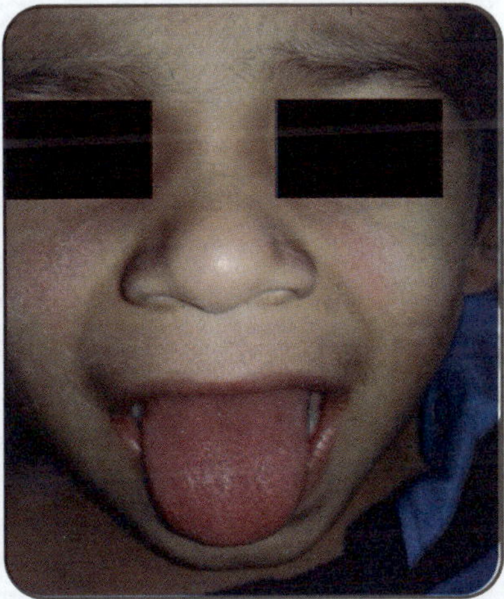

Fig. 13: Facial erythema, red strawberry tongue, circumoral pallor

- Skin involvement is in the form of an eruption beginning on the neck, then spreading to the trunk reaching the extremities. Within the erythema, small papules give the skin a **rough sandpaper quality**.
- Increased erythema over the skinfolds, and **a linear petechial eruption**, **called Pastia lines**, is often present in the antecubital and axillary folds.
- Facial flushing, circumoral pallor.
- A fine exfoliation on palms and soles occurs as the disease subsides.

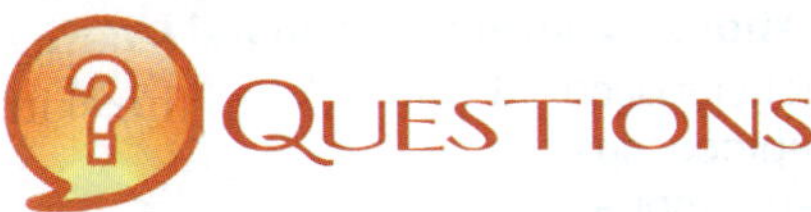

QUESTIONS

1. Most common type of cutaneous TB is:
a. Lupus vulgaris
b. Scrofuloderma
c. Tuberculosis verrucosa cutis
d. Erythema induratum

2. Tuberculosis of skin is called as:
a. Lupus vulgaris b. Lupus pernio
c. Lupus profundus d. Scrofuloderma

3. Forms of skin tuberculosis include all *except*:
a. Lupus vulgaris
b. Scrofuloderma
c. Erythema nodosum
d. Erythema annulare centrifugum

4. Apple-jelly nodules are seen in:
a. Lupus vulgaris
b. Discoid lupus erythematosus
c. Lichen planus
d. Psoriasis

5. A young patient presents with fever with rash as shown. The diagnosis would be: *(AIIMS Nov 18)*

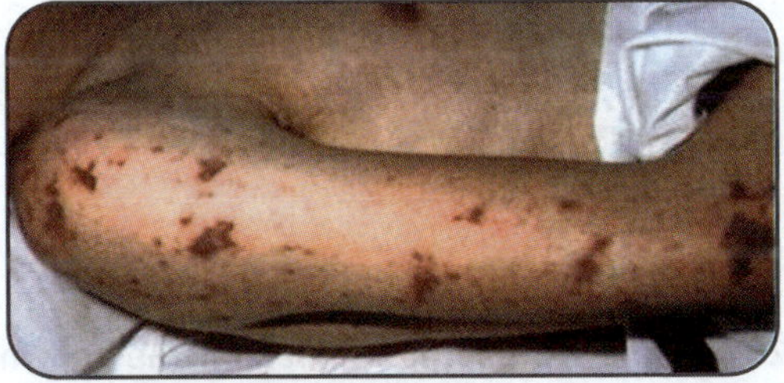

a. Dengue hemorrhagic fever
b. Meningococcemia
c. Leptospirosis
d. Scrub typhus

6. Skin TB which involves skin after involving lymph nodes: *(AIIMS)*
a. Scrofuloderma
b. Lupus vulgaris
c. Lupus erythematosus
d. Lupus pernio

7. Cutaneous tuberculosis secondary to underlying tissue is called as: *(AI)*
a. Lupus vulgaris
b. Scrofuloderma
c. TB chancre
d. Tuberculous verrucosa cutis

8. Tuberculid is:
a. Lupus vulgaris
b. Scrofuloderma
c. Lichen scrofulosorum
d. Erythema nodosum

9. Which of the following is a tuberculid?
a. Lichen scrofulosorum
b. Lichen nitidus
c. Lichen aureus
d. Erythema nodosum

10. Which of the following is characterized by involvement of sweat glands and hair follicles with non-caseating epithelioid granuloma?
a. Lichen scrofulosorum
b. Miliary tuberculosis
c. Papulonecrotic type
d. Lupus vulgaris

11. A 12-year-old boy had a gradually progressive plaque on a buttock for the last 3 years. The plaque was 15 cm in diameter, annular in shape, with scarring in the center. The most likely diagnosis is:
a. Tinea corporis
b. Granuloma annulare
c. Lupus vulgaris
d. Borderline leprosy

12. A young boy presented with lesion over his right buttock which had peripheral extension and central scarring. The investigation of choice would be: *(AIIMS)*
a. Tzanck smear
b. KOH preparation
c. Biopsy
d. Sabouraud dextrose agar

13. Tuberculosis verrucosa cutis is a form of:

a. Tuberculid
b. Primary tuberculosis
c. Post primary tuberculosis with good resistance
d. Post primary tuberculosis with poor resistance

14. A farmer has a single warty lesion on leg. Which of the following could be the most likely lesion?

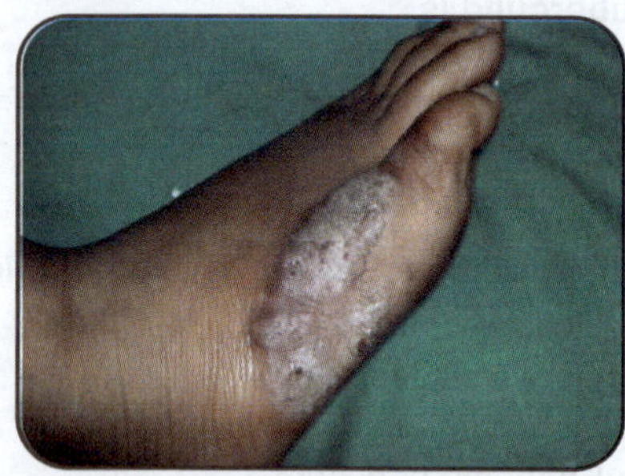

a. Verruca vulgaris
b. Tuberculosis verrucosa cutis
c. Mycetoma
d. Lichen planus hypertrophicus

15. Mycobacterium causing skin ulcer:

a. M. smegmatis b. M. scrofulaceum
c. M. ulcerans d. M. fortuitum

16. Skin hazards of swimming are:

a. Verrucae
b. Pyoderma gangrenosum
c. M. marinum infection
d. M. ulcerans infection

17. A 12-year-old boy presented with a gradually progressive annular plaque on buttock. Likely diagnosis is:

a. Granuloma annulare *(AIIMS Nov 16)*
b. Lupus vulgaris
c. Tinea cruris
d. Annular psoriasis

18. Most common form of cutaneous tuberculosis is: *(MHCET 09)*

a. Scrofuloderma
b. Lupus vulgaris
c. Primary cutaneous tuberculosis
d. Tuberculosis verrucosa cutis

19. Toxic shock syndrome is caused by:

a. Staphylococcal infection
b. Streptococcus
c. Pseudomonas
d. Escherichia coli

20. False statement about impetigo:

a. Mostly caused by Staphylococcus or Streptococcus or both
b. It predisposes to glomerulonephritis
c. Produces scar on healing
d. Erythromycin is drug of choice
e. It is an infectious lesion

21. Commonest skin infection in children is:

a. Scabies
b. Impetigo contagiosa
c. Molluscum contagiosa
d. Warts

22. A patient presents with the following lesions. Investigations shows cocci in long chains. The diagnosis is:

(Recent NEET pattern)

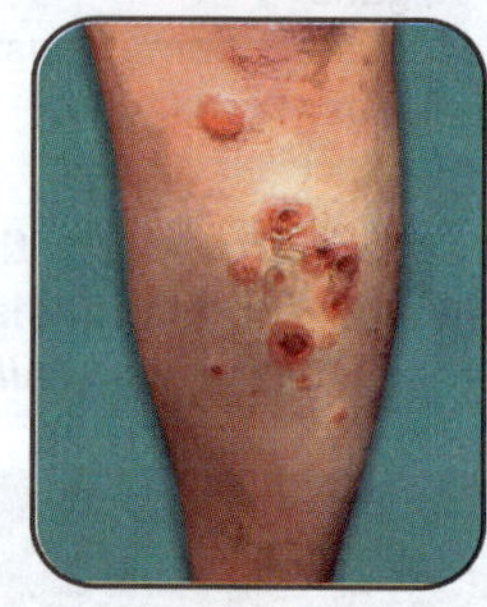

a. Bullous impetigo
b. Impetigo contagiosa
c. Furuncle
d. Cellulitis

23. A patient presents with lesions as shown. The likely diagnosis is:

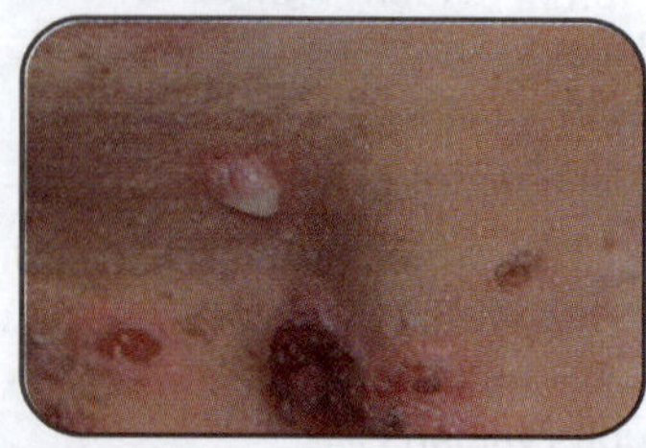

a. Folliculitis b. Bullous impetigo
c. Abscess d. Furuncle

24. True about Impetigo is: *(PGI June 08)*
a. Contagious
b. Bacterial infection
c. Noncontagious
d. Honey coloured crusts
e. Viral infection

25. A 6-month-old male infant developed otitis media. A few days later, he developed extensive peeling of the skin. There were no mucosal lesions. The most likely diagnosis is:

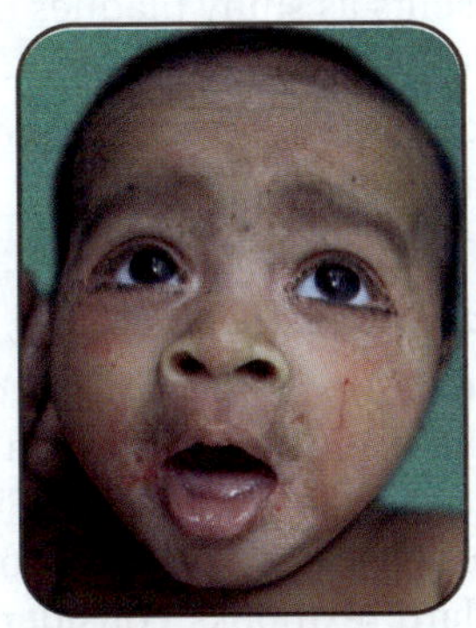

a. Toxic epidermal necrolysis
b. Staphylococcal scalded skin syndrome
c. Stevens-Johnson syndrome
d. Infantile pemphigus

26. Coral red color on Wood's lamp is seen in:
a. Pityriasis versicolor *(DNBCET 2013)*
b. Amyloidosis
c. Melasma
d. Erythrasma

27. Pemphigus neonatorum is: *(MHCET 2015)*
a. Bullous impetigo
b. Epidermolysis bullosa
c. Congenital syphilis
d. Pemphigus

28. Ecthyma gangrenosum is typically due to: *(COMEDK 2011, TNPG 2012)*
a. Escherichia coli
b. Pseudomonas aeruginosa
c. Staphylococcus aureus
d. Candida albicans

29. The causative organism of erythrasma is: *(MHCET 2015)*
a. Corynebacterium b. Staphylococcus
c. Streptococcus d. Pseudomonas

30. Botryomycosis is caused by: *(TNPG 2002)*
a. Bacteria b. Fungus
c. Virus d. Protozoa

31. Which amongst these is a tuberculid?
a. Lichen scrofulosorum *(Recent Nov 17)*
b. Scrofulderma
c. Lupus vulgaris
d. Erythema nodosum

32. Sporotrichoid pattern of lesion is seen in: *(PGI Nov 17)*
a. Lupus vulgaris b. Sporothrix
c. Lichen nitidus d. Fish tank granuloma
e. Impetigo

New Questions

33. The following statements are true/false regarding types of cutaneous TB:
a. Lupus pernio
b. Lupus vulgaris
c. Lichen nitidus
d. Lupus erythematosus
e. Lichen scrofulosorum

34. Assertion: TB chancre is a Paucibacillary TB
Reason: TB chancre is an exogenous TB due to inoculation of TB organisms in patients with good immunity
a. Both Assertion and Reason are true and Reason is correct explanation of Assertion
b. Both Assertion and Reason are true but Reason is not correct explanation of Assertion
c. Assertion is true and Reason is false
d. Assertion is false and Reason is true
e. Both Assertion and Reason are false

35. The diseases caused by staphylococcus are:
a. Non bullous impetigo
b. Pemphigus neonatorum
c. Erysipelas
d. Ritter's disease
1. If a, b, d are correct
2. If a and b are correct
3. If b and d are correct
4. If all four (a, b, c, & d) are correct

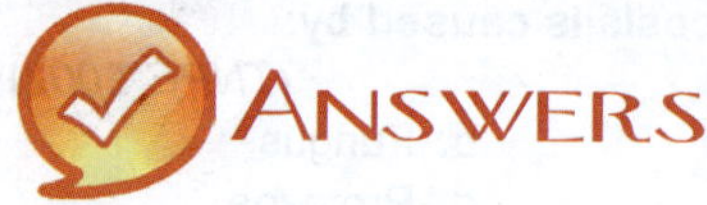

1. **Ans. (a) Lupus vulgaris** *(Ref: Rook's Textbook of Dermatology, 9th edn, Page 27.21)*

In India, lupus vulgaris is the commonest cutaneous TB in adults. In children, the commonest form is scofuloderma.

2. **Ans. (a) Lupus vulgaris** (See page 77 for explanation)

Why not:

- Lupus pernio is a skin lesion in sarcoidosis. It presents as shiny plaques on the nose and may disfigure it. Most cases have underlying respiratory involvement.
- Lupus profundus is also called as lupus panniculitis and is an inflammation of subcutaneous fat in chronic cutaneous lupus erythematosus.

3. **Ans. (d) Erythema annulare centrifugum**

(Ref: Fitzpatrick's Textbook, 8th edn, Page 2233)

Erythema annulare centrifugum is an annular erythema (explained in the chapter on parasitic diseases) and is not related to TB. Lupus vulgaris and scrofuloderma are typical forms of cutaneous TB. Erythema nodosum is not a classical form of TB but Fitzpatrick's textbook includes it in the category of "facultative tuberculids", i.e. TB is only one of the many causes of erythema nodosum. Other standard textbooks consider Erythema nodosum separately and not as tuberculids.

4. **Ans. (a) Lupus vulgaris** *(Ref: Andrew's textbook, 11th edn, Page 325)*

Apple-jelly nodules are also seen in cutaneous leishmaniasis and in sarcoidosis.

5. **Ans. (b) Meningococcemia**

Angular infarcts of skin as shown are classical of meningococcus

6. **Ans. (a) Scrofuloderma** (See page 81 for explanation)
7. **Ans. (b) Scrofuloderma** (See page 81 for explanation)
8. **Ans. (c) Lichen scrofulosorum** (See page 81 for explanation)

Lichen scrofulosorum is a micropapular tuberculid and underlying tuberculosis can be found in majority of patients. Erythema nodosum has many causes, one amongst them is TB. Hence, it is not a classical tuberculid. Also see explanation for question number 3.

9. **Ans. (a) Lichen scrofulosorum** (See page 81 for explanation)

Why not:

- Lichen nitidus is a chronic inflammatory disease characterized by pin-point, shiny, flat topped on dorsum of hands and penis. Etiology is unknown.
- Lichen aureus (aureus = gold). It is due to stasis of circulation in legs due to inadequate venous return causing leakage of hemosiderin from engorged vessels. This group of disorders is called pigmented purpuric dermatosis (PPD). Lichen aureus is a type of PPD. Presents as golden or rust-colored macules on legs.

10. **Ans. (a) Lichen scrofulosorum** *(Ref: McKee's Pathology of Skin, 4th edn, Page 819)*

11. Ans. (c) Lupus vulgaris (See page 79-80 for explanation)

All the 3 pointer words- Progressive, buttocks, central scarring suggests lupus vulgaris

12. Ans. (c) Biopsy (See page 79-80 for explanation)

Buttock involvement and central scarring indicates lupus vulgaris. Skin biopsy classically shows non-caseating tuberculoid granulomas.

13. Ans. (c) Post primary tuberculosis with good resistance

(Ref: Andrew's textbook, 11th edn, Page 324)

14. Ans. (b) Tuberculosis verrucosa cutis (See page 78 for explanation)

Why not:

- Verruca vulgaris—Usually plantar verruca will be multiple lesions and tends to fuse
- Mycetoma will have a big swollen edematous foot with discharging sinuses (see the triad of mycetoma from the chapter on fungal infections)
- Lichen planus hypertrophicus has lesions of lichen planus on lower legs with itching.

15. Ans. (c) M. ulcerans (See page 82 for explanation)

16. Ans. (c) M. marinum infection (See page 82 for explanation)

17. Ans. (b) Lupus vulgaris (See page 79-80 for explanation)

18. Ans. (b) Lupus vulgaris (See page 77 for explanation)

19. Ans. (a) Staphylococcal infection *(Ref: Fitzpatrick's Textbook, 8th edn, Page 2154)*

20. Ans. (c) and (d) Produces scar on healing; Erythromycin is drug of choice

(Ref: Andrew's Textbook, 11th edn, Page 251-252)

21. Ans. (b) Impetigo contagiosa *(Ref: Fitzpatrick's Textbook, 8th edn, Page 2130)*

22. Ans. (b) Impetigo contagiosa

Investigation showing long chains indicates Streptococcus. Impetigo contagiosa is caused by Streptococcus. The image is showing honey colored crust.

23. Ans. (b) Bullous impetigo

Note the hypopyon sign

24. Ans. (a, b, d) Contagious; Bacterial infection; Honey coloured crusts

25. Ans. (b) Staphylococcal scalded skin syndrome (See page 83–84 for explanation)

A focus of infection (otitis media) is present in the question. Extensive peeling and toxicity in the baby without mucosal involvement also points to SSSS. Toxic epidermal necrolysis and Stevens-Johnson syndrome will have mucosal involvement.

26. Ans. (d) Erythrasma (See page 86 for explanation)

27. Ans. (a) Bullous impetigo *(Ref: Fitzpatrick's Textbook, 8th edn, Page 1697)*

28. Ans. (b) Pseudomonas aeruginosa *(Ref: Fitzpatrick's Textbook, 8th edn, Page 2186)*

29. Ans. (a) Corynebacterium *(Ref. Andrew's Textbook, 11th edn, Page 261)*

30. Ans. (a) Bacteria *(Ref: Fitzpatrick's Textbook, 8th edn, Page 2136)*

31. Ans. (a) Lichen scrofulosorum

32. Ans. (a, b, d) Lupus vulgaris; Sporothrix; Fish tank granuloma

New Answers

33. Ans. a-False; b-True; c-False; d-False; e-True

34. Ans. (e) Both Assertion and Reason are false

TB chancre is multibacillary and in patients with poor immunity to TB bacilli.

35. Ans. (1) If a, b, d are correct

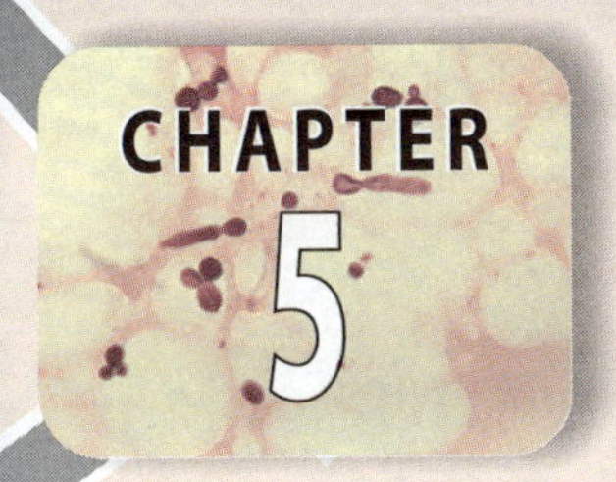

Fungal Infections

FUNGAL INFECTIONS (MYCOSES)

SUPERFICIAL MYCOSES (INFECTION RESTS IN THE EPIDERMIS)

PITYRIASIS VERSICOLOR (TINEA VERSICOLOR)

Etiology

- Caused by **Malassezia yeasts.**[MCQ]
- Malassezia species **normally inhabit** human skin,[MCQ] especially in **seborrheic areas (lipophilic fungus)**.[MCQ] Since, maximum sebum is around the hair follicle; it normally colonizes **perifollicular areas.**[MCQ]
- A shift in the balance between the host and normal flora allows fungus to proliferate
- Most authors have found **Malassezia globosa** as most frequently associated; some have however found **M. sympodialis and M. furfur** as the commonest.[MCQ]

Clinical Features

- Infects only the **top of the corneum** (superficial mycosis) (Figs. 1A and B)
- Presents as discrete initially, then **confluent, scaly, variously colored lesions**, mainly on oily areas which are also sweaty like the **upper trunk -m/c site** (Fig. 2A).[MCQ] Other sites are arms, neck and abdomen.
- The scale **is fine, powdery, and branny**[MCQ]
- Since, the fungus is very superficial in the top part of corneum; the antigen may not be picked by the immune system. Hence, **itching is unusual.**
  The usual presentation in Indian skin is **hypopigmented macules and patches.** The lesions may have other colors like pink (Fig. 3B), brown (Fig. 3C), ochre, etc.[MCQ]
- Since the distribution of the fungus is **perifollicular**, the initial hypopigmentation is often **perifollicular** (Fig. 2B)[MCQ]

Scratch sign (coup d'ongle sign, Besnier's sign, stroke of the nail sign)—Since scaling is minimal; it may be emphasized by **firmly** scratching the skin (Figs. 3A and D).[MCQ]

Aid to Remember

- "Versi-color" (versi = various, meaning variously colored referring to the various colors like brown, white, ochre, pink)
- The literal meaning of the word "pityriasis" is "powdery" or "branny". Hence, powdery, branny scales are seen.

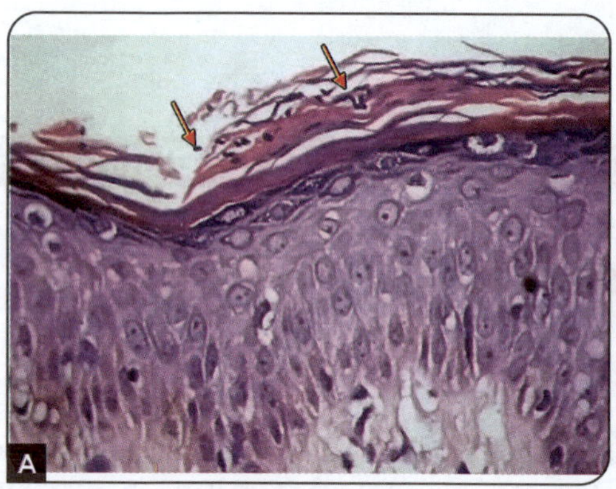

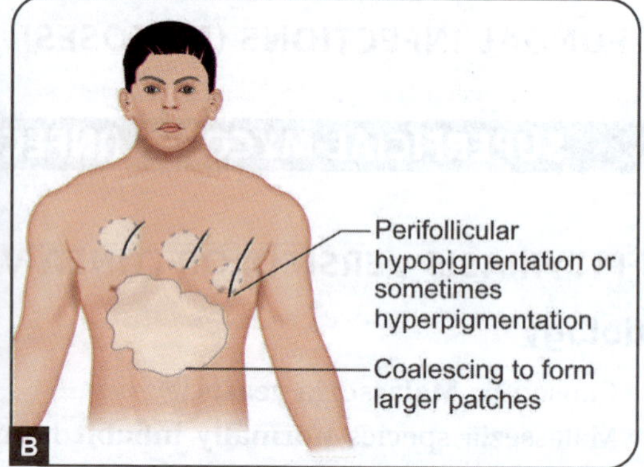

Figs. 1A and B: Histopathology in pityriasis versicolor- note the superficial budding yeasts and short septate hyphae in corneum (A). Schematic representation of the clinical features (B)

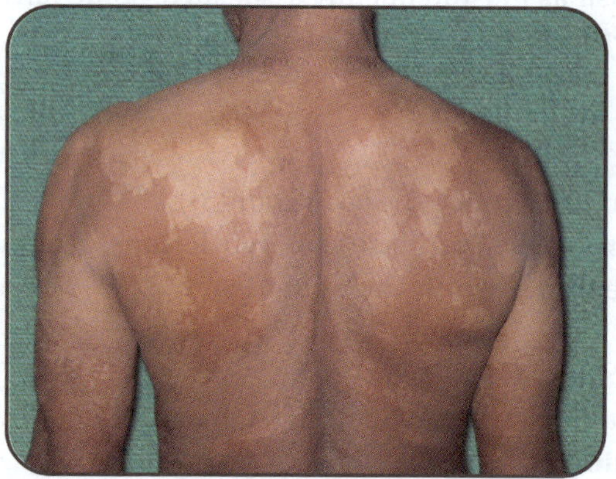

Fig. 2A: Pityriasis versicolor—Hypopigmented macules and patches on back

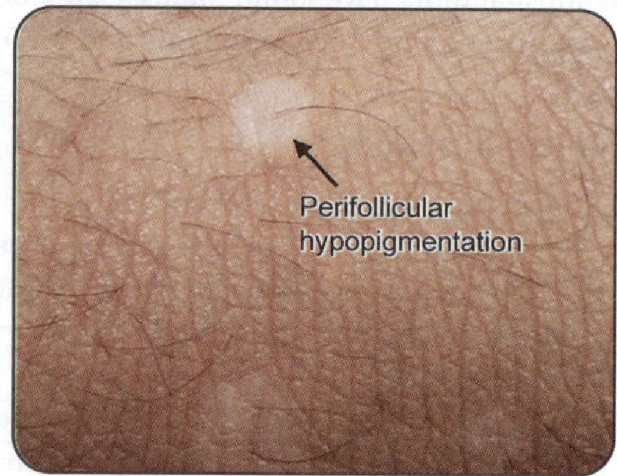

Fig. 2B: Pityriasis versicolor—Perifollicular hypopigmentation

Reasons for Color Change

- **Hypopigmentation**
  - Due to production of **azelaic acid** by Malassezia species which inhibits tyrosinase in the melanin production pathway(MCQ)
- **Hyperpigmentation** (seen more in fairer skin) is due to abnormally large melanosomes in hyperpigmented lesions (Fig. 3C).

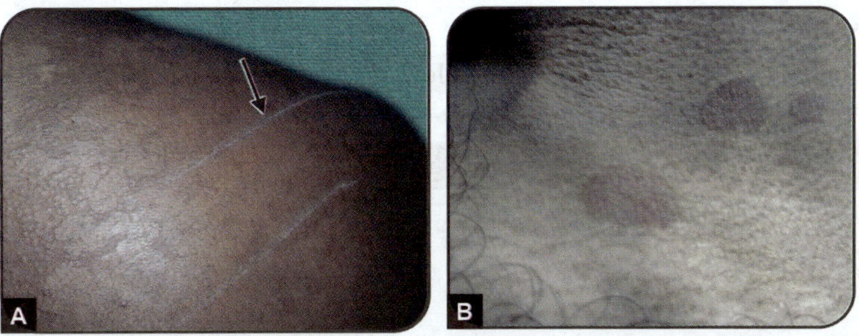

Figs. 3A and B: (A) Pityriasis versicolor—Scratch sign positive; (B) Erythematous variant of pityriasis versicolor

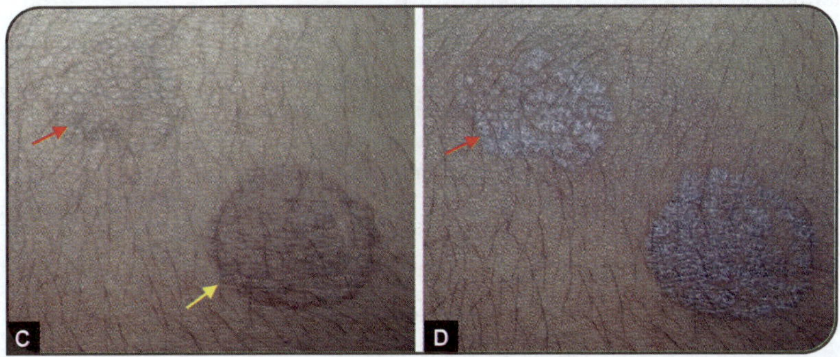

Figs. 3C and D: (C) 2 Hyperpigmented lesions in pityriasis versicolor (red and yellow arrows)—upper lesion depicted by the red arrow only faintly visible; (D) Prominent scales after scratching making even previously unremarkable lesion prominent (red arrow)

Investigations

1. **Wood's lamp**: The scaly lesions show **pale yellow fluorescence**(MCQ) (yellow-green sometimes). (See Figure 22B in Chapter 2 for image).
2. **KOH**: Microscopically, there are short, thick fungal hyphae (like "spaghetti" or "banana") and large numbers of variously sized spores (like "meatballs" or "grapes"), referred to as **"spaghetti and meatballs" ("Banana and grapes") appearance** (Fig. 4).(MCQ)
3. Malassezia fungal culture is of **no help** as the organism is a part **of normal skin flora**.

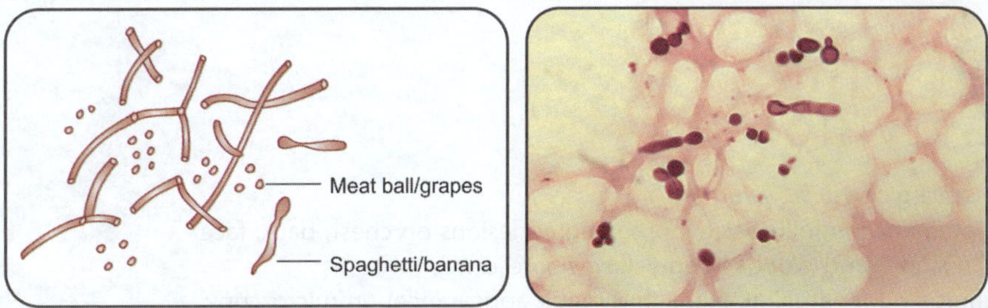

Fig. 4: Thick-walled spores in grape-like/meat ball-like clumps along with short stubby hyphae (spaghetti shaped/banana shaped)

Treatment

It may take several months for the skin color to become normal, even after anti-fungals removes the fungus.

First line	Second line
Topical azoles- **DOC** (Clotrimazole/Econazole/ Miconazole/Sertoconazole/ketoconazole, etc.)(MCQ)	Oral Itraconazole
Topical Terbinafine	Oral Fluconazole
Topical Selenium sulphide(MCQ)	Oral ketoconazole(MCQ) (not preferred now as it is hepatotoxic)

* Oral terbinafine and oral griseofulvin do not work(MCQ)

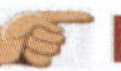

High Yield Points

Pick up these "pointer" words in MCQs on pityriasis versicolor

1. Hypopigmented small macules coalescing to form patches on chest, back, face
2. Fine scaling on lesions becoming prominent on scratching
3. Perifollicular distribution

High Yield Points

Chart on to differentiate from other hypopigmented diseases in MCQs?

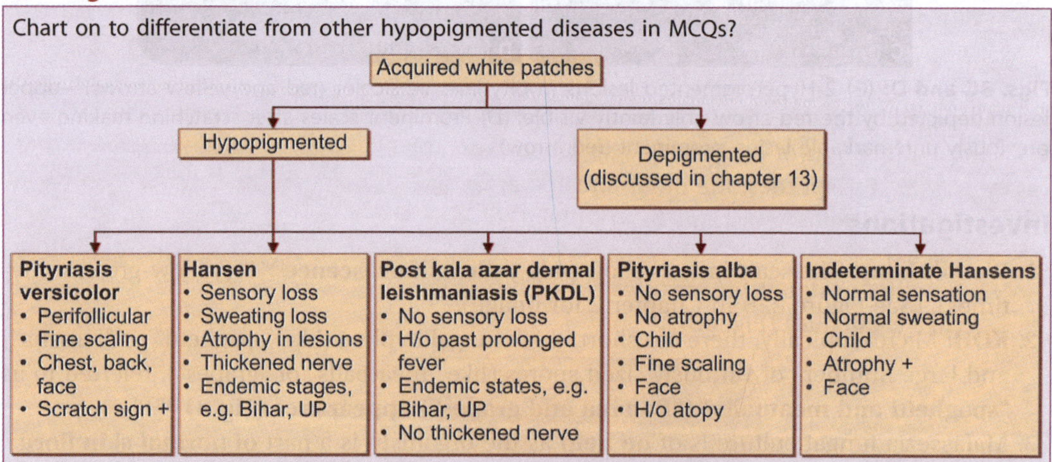

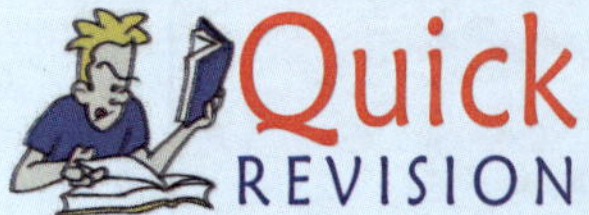

- Malassezia globosa > *M. furfur*
- Asymptomatic perifollicular hypopigmented lesions on chest, back, face
- Scratch sign + and Woods lamp-yellow fluorescence
- Spaghetti and meatball (Banana and grape appearance) on microscopy
- Azoles, selenium sulphide help. Griseofulvin does not work

CANDIDIASIS (MONILIASIS, THRUSH)

C. albicans is a **commensal flora** of skin. Under favorable conditions, it becomes a pathogen **(opportunistic pathogen).**

Predisposing Factors

- In normal adults and children—it may be due to antibiotic therapy which eliminates competing commensal bacteria allowing the commensal candida to grow (called **"antibiotic mouth"**).
- Moisture favors the disease. Hence, folds (called **intertriginous areas**)(MCQ) are frequently involved
- HIV-Immunosuppression helps the fungus grow
- **Diabetes**
- Ill-fitting dentures-causing candida to grow in between spaces (called **"denture mouth"**).

Types of Candidiasis

- Oropharyngeal candidiasis (OPC)
  Often the first presentation of AIDS, it is the **commonest fungal infection in HIV**(MCQ)
  Grayish-white creamy or curdy(AI 10) plaques are found on the surface of the mucous membrane of tongue, buccal mucosa. Since, these **can be scrapped-off by spatula**, these are **pseudomembranes**(MCQ) (Leucoplakia, which is premalignant cannot be scrapped off has a true membrane) (Fig. 5).
- **Candidal intertrigo (Intertriginous literally means "in between folds")**(Recent NEET pattern)
  - Inflammation of body folds, e.g. diaper area, inframammary area, between toes and finger (Except toes, the other affected areas are red and moist)
  - Erythematous, moist patches (groin) (Fig. 6A) and whitish macerated moist patches (webs)
  - **Satellite or daughter pustules**(MCQ)—Tiny white pustules at the periphery of the lesion (like a satellite) (Fig. 6B)

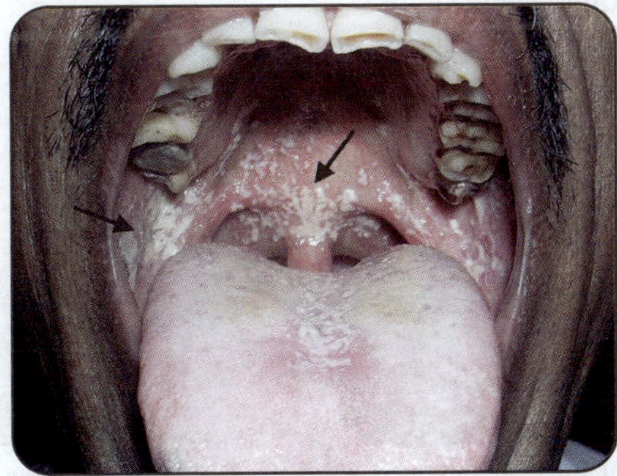

Fig. 5: Oral pseudomembranous candidiasis—White curdy creamy plaques

***Another cause of satellite lesion is borderline tuberculoid (BT) Hansen's disease.**(MCQ) For image of satellite lesion in BT, see Figure 3 in Chapter 3.

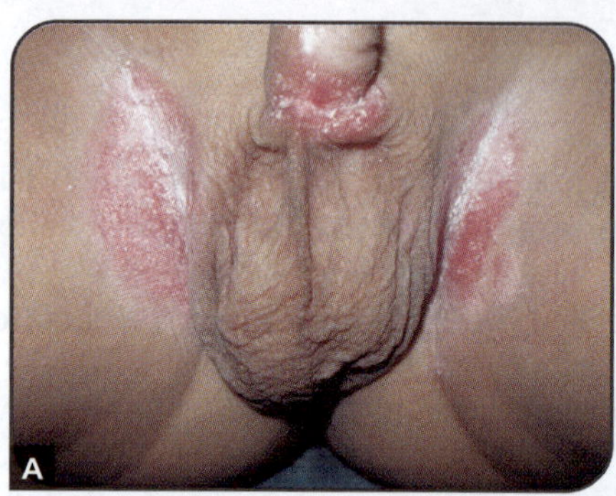
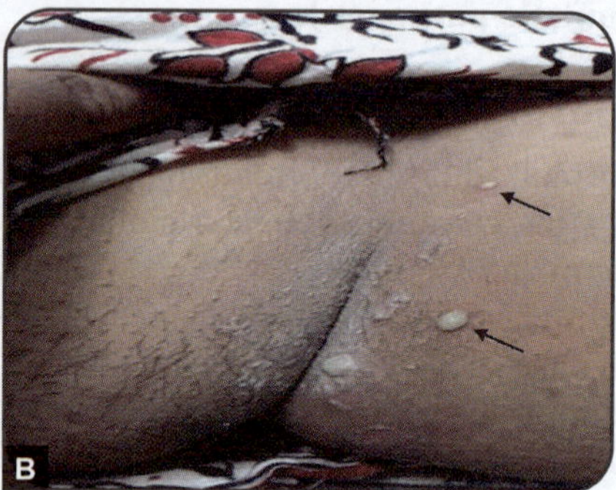

Figs. 6A and B: (A) Candidal intertrigo—Erythematous shiny moist plaques in groins; (B) Satellite pustules in axilla

Aid to Remember

- Candida albicans shows budding—satellites are like buds to a planet (satellite lesions in candida)
- Candida grows in moist environment—causes moist lesions in folds

- **Perlèche**: When the angles of the mouth are involved
- **Vulvovaginitis:**
  - Candidal vaginitis is **2nd most common** cause of vaginal discharge overall **(In diabetic females, it is the commonest)**,(MCQ) **most common overall being bacterial vaginosis**(MCQ)
  - Severe pruritus, burning, and **white curdy discharge** (Figs. 7A and B) (trichomonal vaginitis in contrast causes profuse, **greenish-brown** frothy discharge)
  - Most forms of candida are non-sexual (due to diabetes, pregnancy, broad spectrum antibiotics, OCPs, Intrauterine devices). **Hence, sexual partner treatment is not done in candidal infection**(MCQ) **(Partner treatment is also not done in bacterial vaginosis and herpes genitalis)**(MCQ)

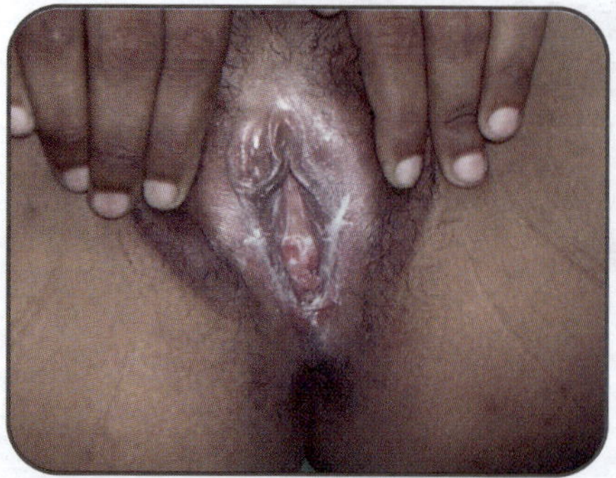

Fig. 7A: Candidal vulvovaginitis—White, scanty curdy discharge

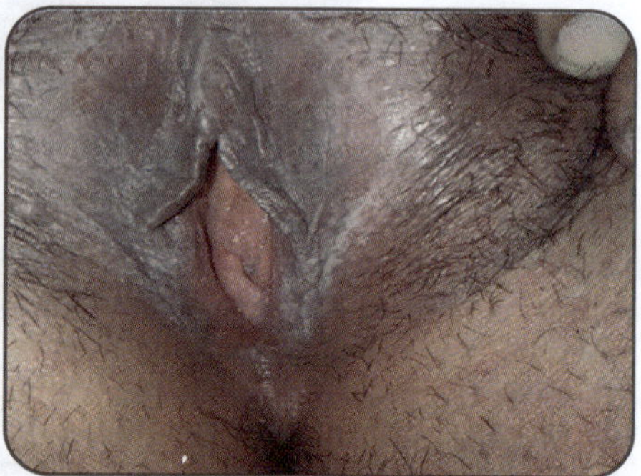

Fig. 7B: Candidal vulvitis—Whitish macerated area on labia

High Yield Points

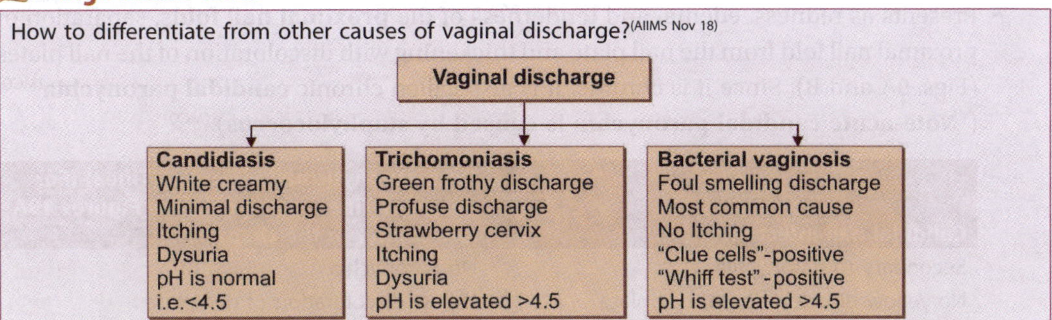

Aid to Remember

Mnemonic to remember Vaginal discharge

- **Candidal vaginitis**: alba = white discharge. **2 C**-Candida, Curdy
- **Trichomoniasis**- 5 Fs- Flagella, Frothy, Fornication (meaning STD), Fruit (strawberry cervix), Flagyl (metronidazole for treatment)
- **Bacterial vaginosis**- take a "whiff" and smell the "clue". Whiff test, presence of clue cells and foul smell are features of this disease.

Treatment

- A single tablet of fluconazole (150 mg) is usually enough(MCQ)
- Itraconazole 200 mg/day for 5–10 days may be needed.
- Topical antifungals are equally effective.
- **Griseofulvin does not work** in candidal infections

- **Candidal balanitis**
  - In mild cases—transient tiny papules or pustules develop on the glans penis a few hours after intercourse. In more severe and chronic cases—inflammatory erosions develop over glans (Fig. 8A)
  - If the prepuce is also involved, it is called a **balanoposthitis** and often presents with **fissures** on prepuce with phimosis (Fig. 8B). **If recurrent candidal balanoposthitis occurs, underlying diabetes should be suspected.**(MCQ)

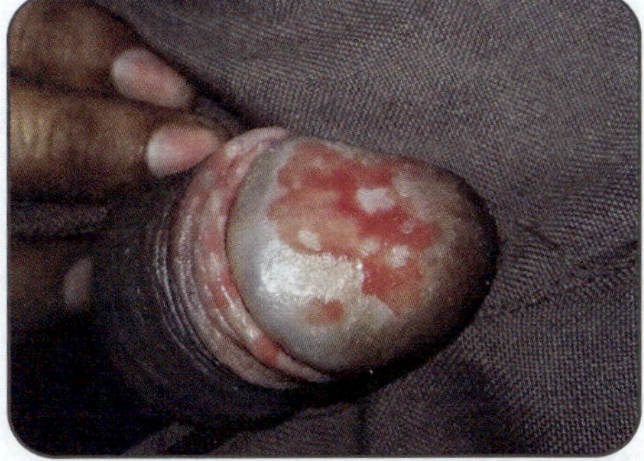

Fig. 8A: Candidal balanitis—Itchy, erythematous, macerated lesions on glans

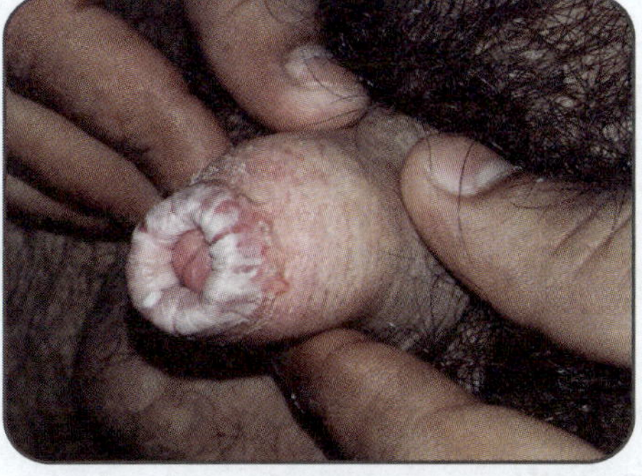

Fig. 8B: Candidal balanoposthitis—Fissured whitish plaques with phimosis

- **Candidal paronychia**
  - Presents as redness, edema, and tenderness of the **proximal nail folds**, separation of proximal nail fold from the nail plate and thickening with discoloration of the nail plates (Figs. 9A and B). Since it is chronic, it is also called chronic **candidal paronychia**(MCQ) (***Note-acute candidal paronychia is caused by staphylococcus**).(MCQ)

Candidal nail infection	Dermatophytic nail infection (Tinea) (For image of Tinea of the nail, see Figures 19A and D later in the chapter)
Secondary to paronychia	No paronychia
No yellow discoloration of nail plate	Yellow discoloration of nail plate
No subungual hyperkeratosis	Subungual hyperkeratosis
Loss of nail cuticle	Nail cuticle intact
Usually h/o wet water work like washing and cleaning, underlying diabetes, atopy	No such factors

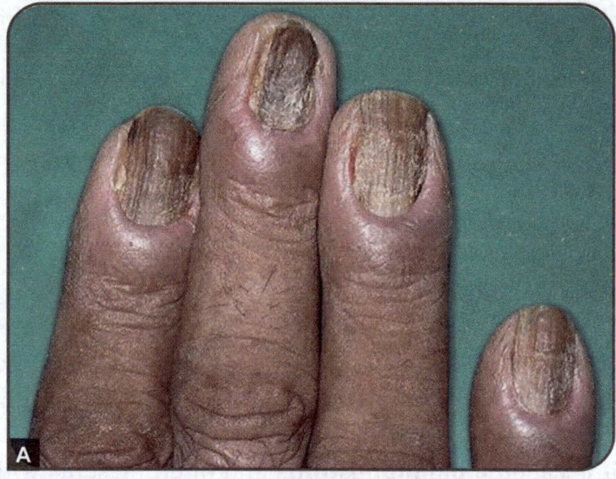

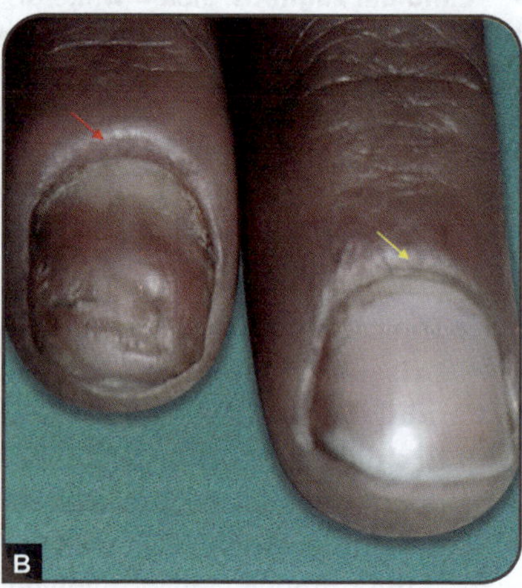

Figs. 9A and B: (A) Candidal paronychia—Swollen nail folds with secondary nail plate abnormalities; (B) Swollen nail fold (red arrow) with secondary nail change- left nail and normal nail (yellow arrow) - right nail

Aid to Remember

- Par = around, onychia = nail (Inflammation of the skin around the nail)
- Candida in all folds, e.g. nail folds, skin folds, etc., tinea in the nail plate
- Candida likes moisture-hence in people doing wet work

Investigations in Candidiasis

- KOH preparation—Spores and pseudohyphae(MCQ)
- Gram stain—gram positive, ovoid bodies(MCQ)

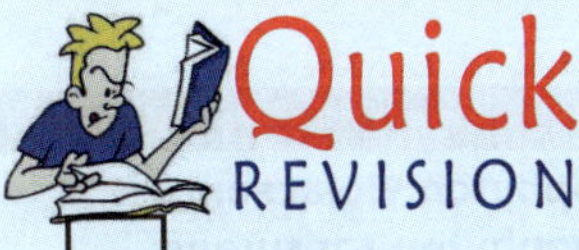

- Candida is an opportunistic pathogen
- Causes oropharyngeal candidiasis (pseudomembranous type-m/c fungal infection in HIV), intertrigo, balanitis, balanoposthitis (indicator of DM), chronic paronychia, vaginitis (white curdy itchy discharge)
- Candidal intertrigo—Satellite pustules
- KOH shows spores and pseudohyphae

DERMATOPHYTOSIS (RING WORM, TINEA)

Three genera of dermatophytes infect skin, hair and nails—**Microsporum (does not infect nail), Epidermophyton (does not infect hair) and Trichophyton (infects all 3 areas)**.

Aid to Remember

- In the English alphabet—M and N are close (microsporum does not infect nail, E and H are also close—Epidermophyton does not infect hair)

The fungi persist in the corneum mainly as it is a **keratinophilic fungus.** Typically, it causes **annular lesions**(MCQ) (ring lesions) with peripheral scaling which spreads outwards (**"central clearing"** indicates annular lesions in MCQs) (Fig. 10).

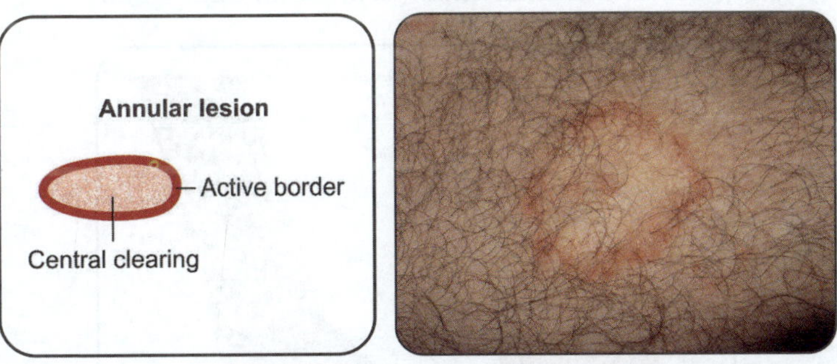

Fig. 10: Tinea—Annular lesion

High Yield Points

Central clearing = Tinea(MCQ)
Central crusting = Leishmaniasis(MCQ)
Central scarring = Lupus vulgaris(MCQ)

Most Common Organisms(MCQ)

All tineas (apart from Tinea capitis)	Tinea capitis
M/c organism is **Trichophyton mentagrophytes**	In India—m/c **Trichophyton violaceum** In US/UK—m/c **Trichophyton tonsurans** In Europe—m/c **Microsporum canis**

*m/c Tinea in India- Tinea corporis(MCQ)
*m/c Tinea in the world- Tinea pedis(MCQ)

Tinea Capitis

- Invasion of scalp hair shaft

Clinical Features

- Disease of children. Rare in adults
- Patchy alopecia occurs
- Either inflames the scalp (inflammatory T. capitis) or does not inflame (non-inflammatory T. capitis)

High Yield Points

- All MCQs on T. capitis will have a **child** in the question
- Pick up phrase in the MCQ—**"Easy pluckability of hair", "broken hairs"**

Classification of T. Capitis

- Endothrix-Fungal spores inside hair shaft (Endo = in, thrix = hair)
- Ectothrix-Fungal spores outside hair shaft (Ecto = out, thrix = hair)

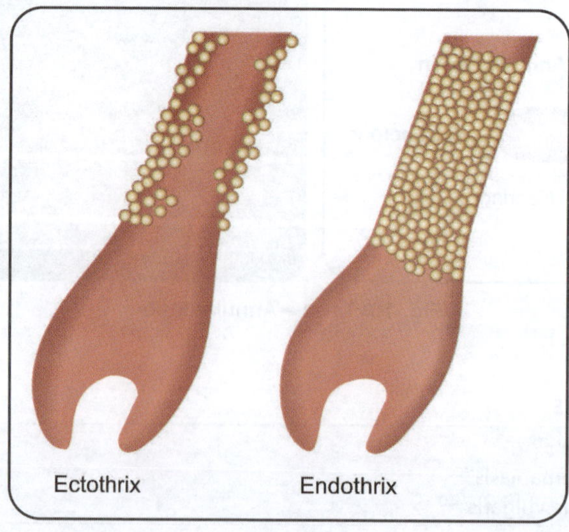

Non-inflammatory type (causing non-scarring alopecia)	Inflammatory type (causing scarring alopecia)
1. Black dot (Endothrix) Organism: *Trichophyton violaceum* : *Trichophyton tonsurans* 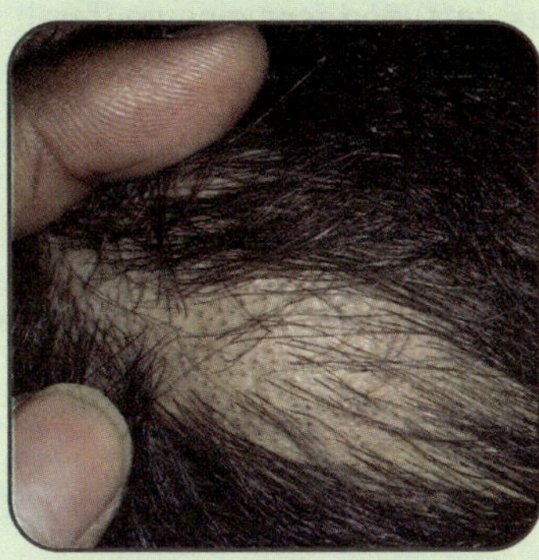 **Fig. 11:** Tinea capitis (Black dot)-multiple black dots (hair broken at scalp surface) seen with non-scarring hair loss Clinical: Due to fungal spores inside the hair in this endothrix variety, hair becomes weak and breaks right at the surface of scalp as they grow up. These broken tips are seen as black dots (Fig. 11).	**1. Kerion (either ectothrix or endothrix)** Organism: *Trichophyton mentagrophytes* : *Trichophyton verrucosum* : *Microsporum canis* 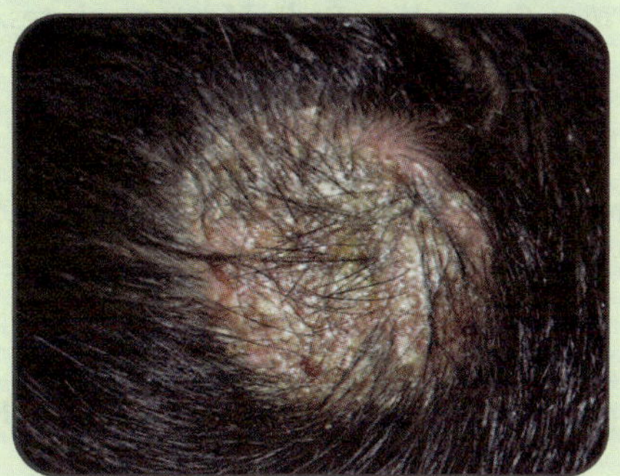 **Fig. 12:** Tinea capitis (kerion)–Boggy swelling with pus discharge and matted hairs Clinical: Painful, inflammatory **boggy swelling**, with pus and sinus formation (Fig. 12)
2. Gray patch (Ectothrix) Organism: *M. ferrugineum, Microsporum canis, Microsporum audouinii* *Fluoresces under Wood's lamp (green) (Fig. 13) 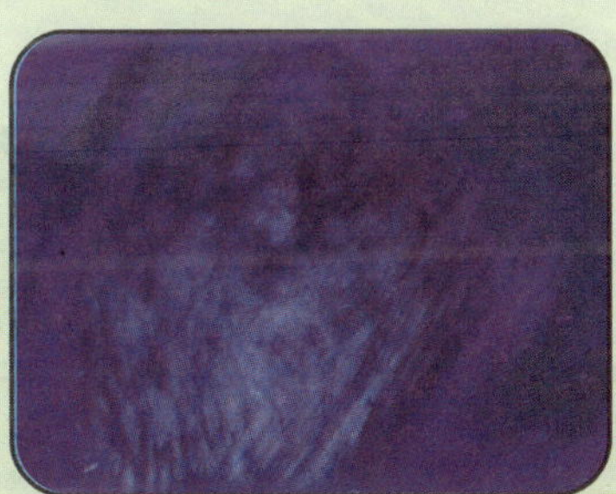 **Fig. 13:** Tinea capitis (woods lamp of gray patch)- greenish fluorescence Clinical: gray colored areas of alopecia with scales, hence called gray patch. Broken hairs (breaking 3–4 mm above scalp surface)	**2. Favus (endothrix with air spaces inside hair)** Organism: *Trichophyton schoenleinii* Clinical: Concave **yellow cup-shaped crust called scutula** form on scalp (Fig. 14). The fungus is inside the hair and forms **air spaces**. 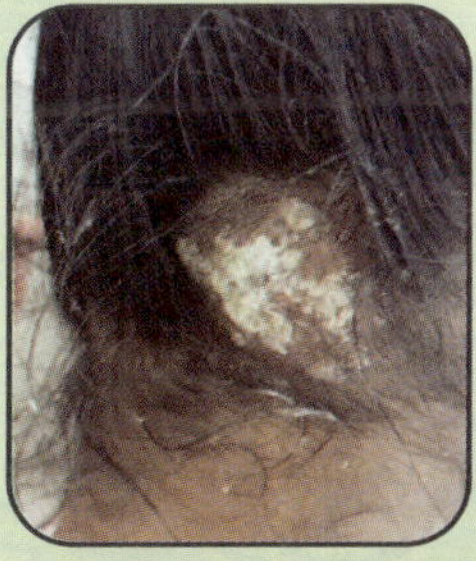 **Fig. 14:** Favus- Note yellow colored cup shaped scutulum with scarring alopecia

Aid to Remember

- Organisms causing endothrix- "**TV** is seen **in the house**" (**T**-Trichophyton tonsurans, **V**-violaceum **in** endothrix = **in the house**)
- Black dot- Black means dark, i.e. no fluorescence
- **Gray Cats** are **fer**als- **Gray** patch dot is caused by canis (= **cats**) and **fer**rugineum (**fer**al) species
- "**Men Can** be **Very Red**"- **Men**tagrophytes, **Can**is, **Ver**rucosum cause **Red** inflamed lesions (kerion)

Treatment(MCQ)

Microsporum species (grey patch and some types of kerion)	**Trichophyton species** (e.g. black dot, favus and some types of kerion)
Oral griseofulvin is the DOC(MCQ)	Oral terbinafine is the DOC

***If species not mentioned in,**(MCQ) **mark oral griseofulvin as DOC**

Tinea Barbae

- Ringworm of the beard.

Tinea Faciei

- Ringworm of the facial skin (Fig. 15B).

Tinea Manuum

- Ringworm of the hands (Fig. 15A).

Tinea Corporis (Tinea Circinata- "Circinata" = Rings, T. Glabrosa)

- Ringworm of skin other than scalp, beard, face, hands, feet, and groin (Figs. 16, 18A).

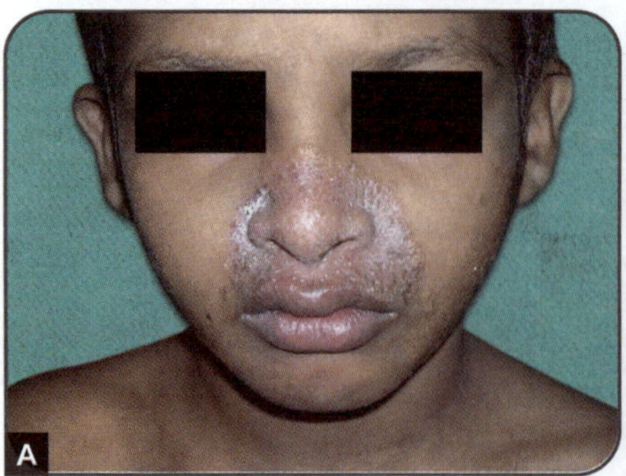

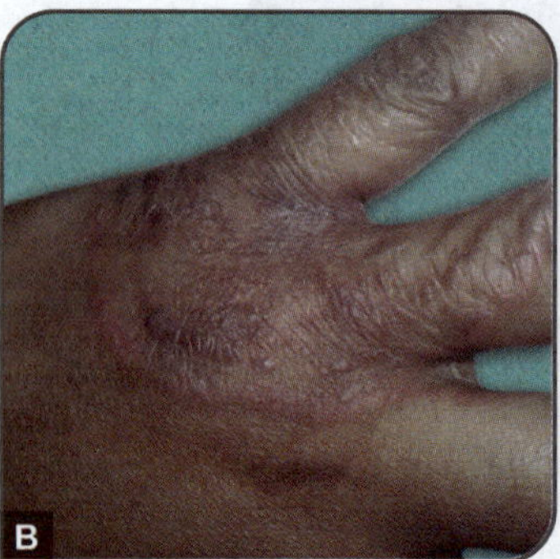

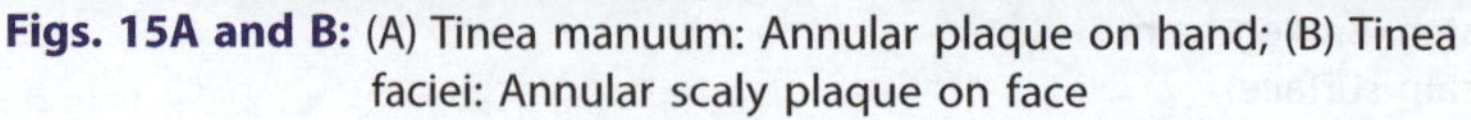

Figs. 15A and B: (A) Tinea manuum: Annular plaque on hand; (B) Tinea faciei: Annular scaly plaque on face

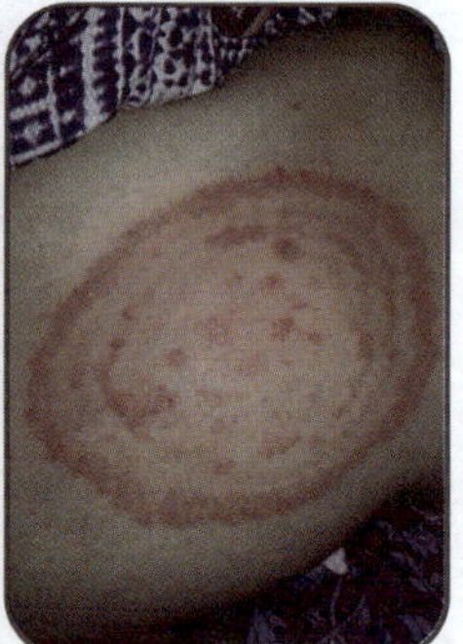

Fig. 16: Tinea corporis—Annular ring lesion on abdomen

Tinea Pedis (Athlete's Foot)[(MCQ)]

Tinea pedis is associated with increased **sweat** on feet and increased use of **closed footwear**. It is of two types:

1. **Interdigital**: Scaling and itching in between toes, especially last web (Fig. 17A). The sweat between the toes has a high pH, and damp keratin is a good culture medium for the fungi.
2. **Moccasin foot**[(MCQ)] —Chronic plantar scaling type (Fig. 17B)

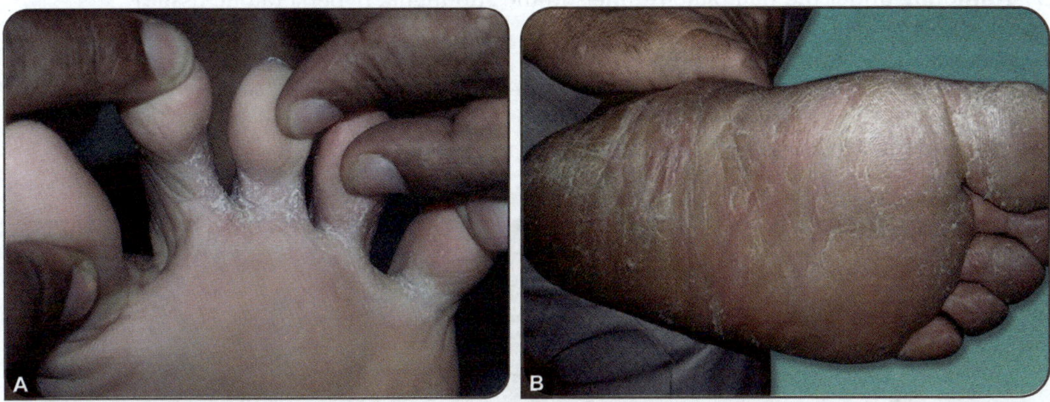

Figs. 17A and B: (A) Tinea pedis (Interdigital)—Scaly plaque between toes: Note the first web (most open and ventilated, hence dry) is yet to get involved; (B) Moccasin foot—Diffuse plantar scaling

Tinea Cruris (Jock Itch, Crotch Itch, Dhobi Itch)

- Ringworm in groin **(m/c site in males)** (Figs. 18A and B)

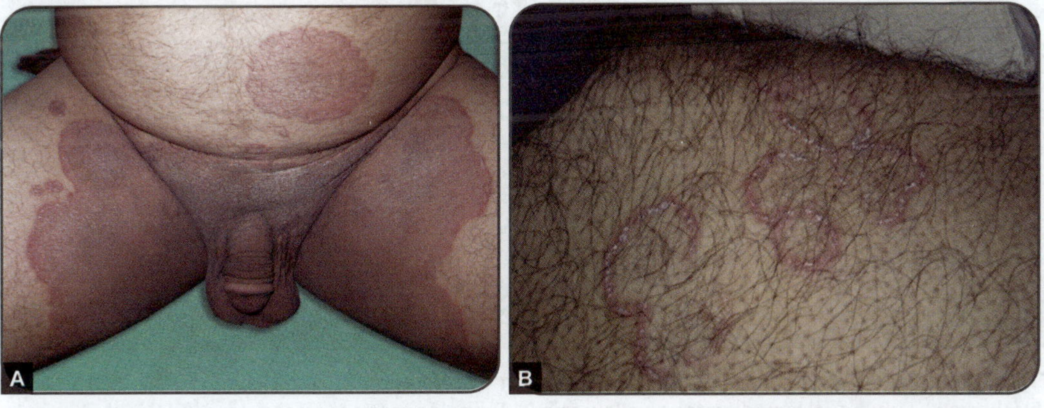

Figs. 18A and B: (A) Tinea cruris with corporis—Erythematous scaly annular plaques in groin and abdomen; (B) Tinea cruris—Annular lesions with peripheral scaling on inner thigh and groin

Onychomycosis (Tinea Unguium)

- Ringworm of the nail

Clinical Features

- **Yellow discoloration** of nail (Figs. 19A and D)(MCQ)
- **Thickened nail plate** (Fig. 19B)
- Subungual hyperkeratosis (Figs. 19B and C)(MCQ)
- **Tunneling** under the nail plate (tunnels in the subungual hyperkeratotic tissue)(MCQ)

Type

Distal and lateral subungual onychomycosis (DLSO) m/c type. Distal + lateral nail plate and nail bed involved (Fig. 19A)(MCQ)

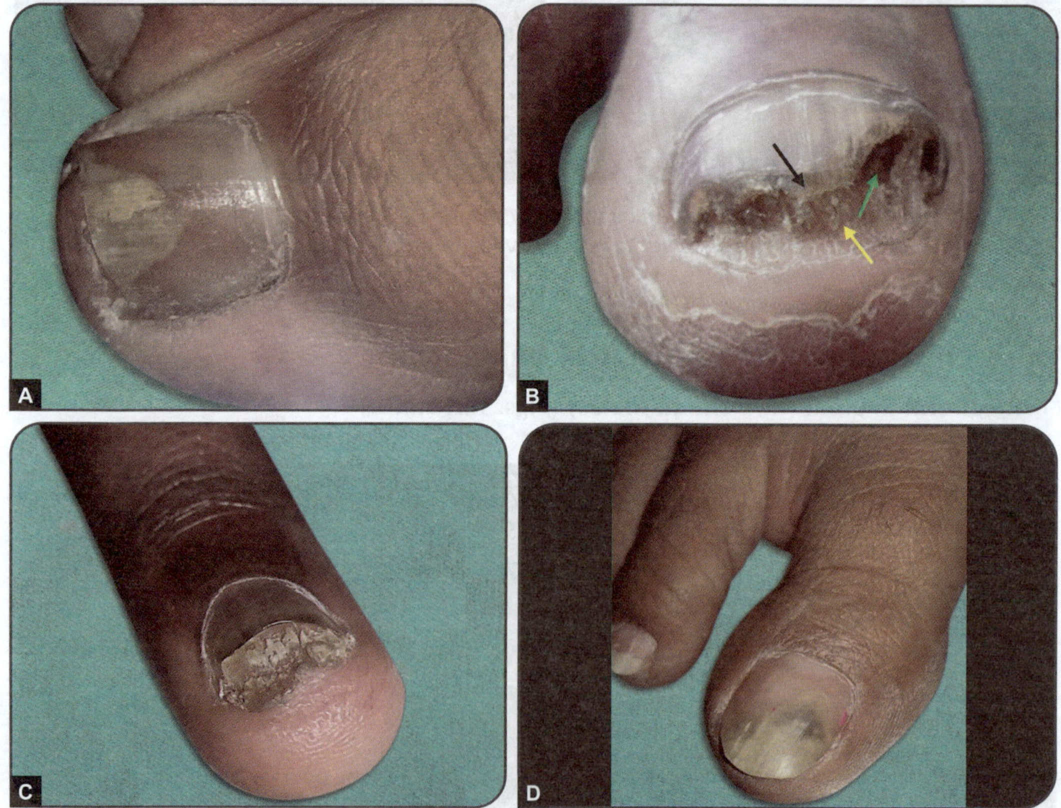

Figs. 19A to D: (A) Onychomycosis (DLSO)—yellowish discoloration of distal edge of nail; (B) Thick nail (black arrow), Subungual hyperkeratosis (yellow arrow), Tunnel formation (green arrow); (C) Onychomycosis-Note the friable subungual hyperkeratosis, onycholysis and yellow nail plate; (D) DLSO-Note the yellow discoloration of nail plate

Treatment

Fingernails	Toenails
• Oral terbinafine (250 mg/day for 6 weeks) • Oral itraconazole (pulsed dosing-400 mg per day for 1 week of each month, for 2 months)	• Oral terbinafine (250 mg/day for 12 weeks) • Oral itraconazole (pulsed dosing-400 mg per day for 1 week of each month, for 3 months)

*Topical treatment with amorolfine or ciclopirox olamine(MCQ) can be used in mild nail infections.

Tinea Incognito ("Incognito" = No Cognition, i.e. not be Able to Diagnose Easily)(MCQ)

A term applied to **atypical clinical lesions** of tinea, usually produced by incorrect treatment with a **topical corticosteroid**. Since steroids suppress inflammation without treatment of fungus, the lesions may be **asymptomatic and extensive, and may even lack scaling**. Often long term steroid application create hypopigmentation and striae (Figs. 20A and B).

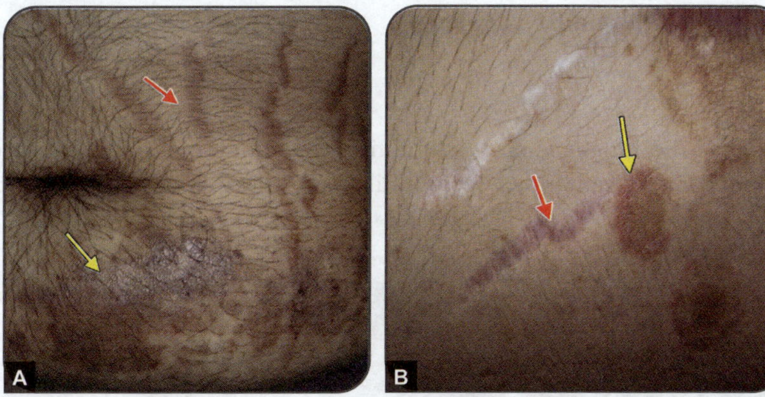

Figs. 20A and B: Tinea incognito— Note the tinea (yellow arrow) and striae (red arrow) due to steroid abuse. This was a case of tinea corporis incorrectly treated with topical steroids

Investigations in Tinea

- KOH smear(MCQ)–from scales, nail plate or tissue under nail, loose hairs
- Fungal culture on Sabouraud's dextrose agar

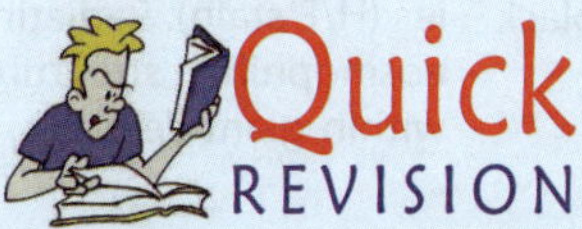

- Caused by Microsporum (does not infect nail), Epidermophyton (does not infect hair) and Trichophyton (infects all 3 areas)
- Annular lesions with central clearing
- M/c cause of all tineas (except T. capitis) = T. rubrum. For T. capitis = T. violaceum (In India)
- T. capitis—Easy pluckable hairs in children causing patchy alopecia and broken hairs
- Gray patch and Favus fluoresces on Wood's lamp. Black dot, Kerion
- Terbinafine is the DOC for all tineas. For T. capitis—Griseofulvin is the DOC

SUBCUTANEOUS MYCOSES

The infections rests in the dermis or subcutaneous tissue:

- Sporotrichosis
- Mycetoma
- Chromoblastomycosis

SPOROTRICHOSIS

- Caused by the dimorphic fungus *Sporothrix schenckii,* which as a saprophyte lives on grass and other plants **(hence, occupations like florists, gardeners, farmers are prone when they get thorn pricks)**.
- Most common cutaneous presentation-**"lymphatic type"**- organism progresses along lymphatics to create **a linear chain of ulcerating nodules and sinuses along these lymphatics** (Figs. 21A and B).

Investigation

On histopathology, the fungus is seen in the tissue as **small cigar-shaped or oval yeasts**, or be surrounded by a radiating, eosinophilic substance **(called as asteroid bodies)** (Fig. 22).(MCQ)

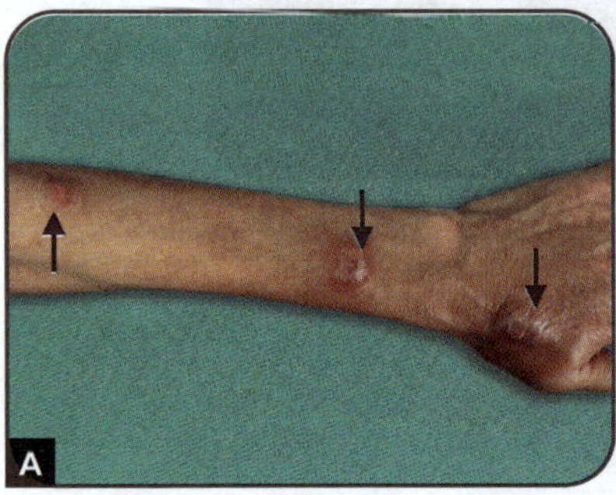

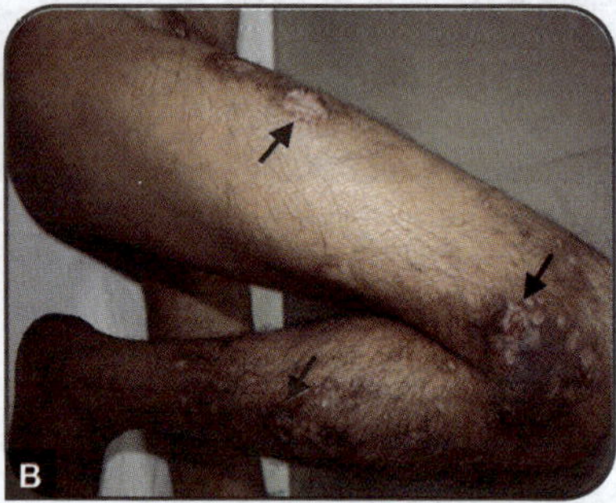

Figs. 21A and B: (A) Sporotrichosis—Linear nodules with sinus discharge on upper limbs in a gardener; (B) Linear discharging sinuses on lower limb (black arrows)

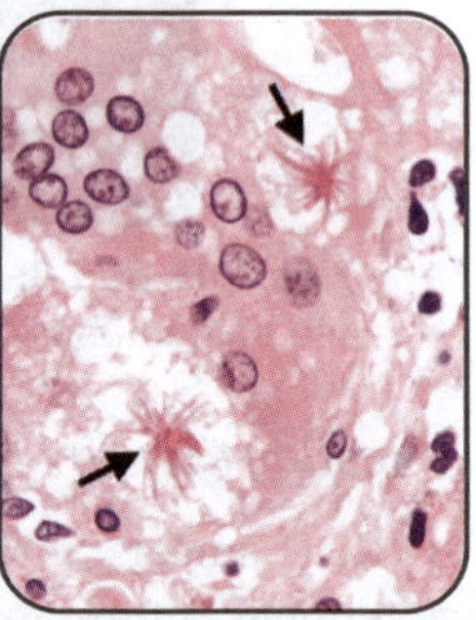

Fig. 22: Asteroid bodies (H/E stain). Radiating eosinophilic structures within giant cells

High Yield Points

- The mycobacterial infection caused by *Mycobacterium marinum* (fish-tank granuloma) closely resembles sporotrichosis
- Pointer word in MCQs would be a **"swimmer"** or **"fish-handler"** for Fish-tank granuloma [MCQ] and a **"farmer"** or **"gardener"** in sporotrichosis.

Treatment

First line	Second line
Itraconazole 100–200 mg/day until clinical recovery (at least 3 months) *Or* Terbinafine 250 mg/day until clinical recovery (at least 3 months)	Potassium iodide

MYCETOMA (MADURA FOOT, MADURAMYCOSIS)

- Caused either by filamentous bacteria **(actinomycetoma)** or true fungi **(eumycetoma)**, both being saprophytes in soil
- Causes severe destruction of dermis, subcutaneous tissue and even underlying bone
- **Triad of mycetoma:**

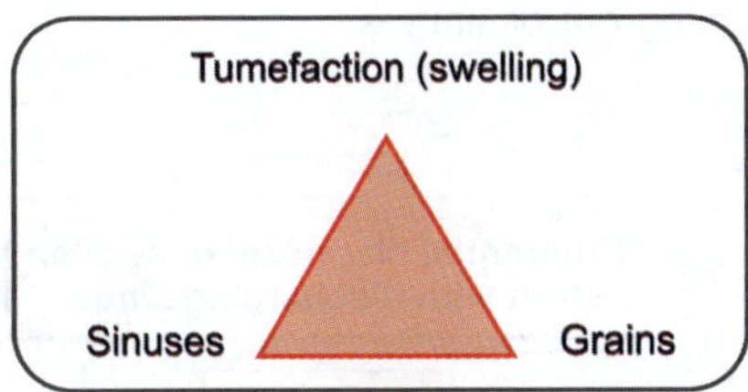

Organisms

Eumycetoma (produce dark colored grains) (Figs. 23A and B)	**Actinomycetoma** (produce white, pale colored grains)
Caused by madurella species	Caused by Nocardia species, Actinomadura species, Streptomyces species

Aid to Remember

- **NASA** has a **white** logo—"**N**ocardia", "**A**ctinomadura", "**S**treptomyces"- cause "**A**ctinomycetoma" with **white** grains
- **MAD**—**M**adurella causes **d**ark grains

Clinical Features

- Entry of organisms is by a **thorn prick on the foot**
- Painless nodule develops which then breaks down to form **draining sinuses** (Fig. 23A)
- The whole foot becomes hard and swollen, without pain.
- Hence, the **triad of mycetoma** (see above) forms.
- Extension to underlying bones and joints can occur giving rise to periostitis, osteomyelitis and arthritis. **Lymphatic involvement is rare (contrast to sporotrichosis).**

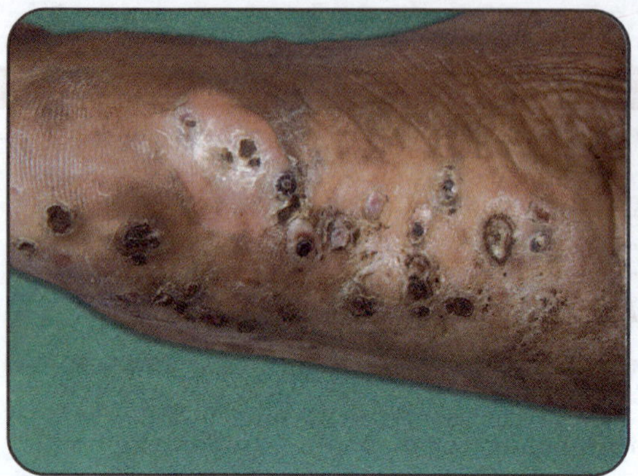

Fig. 23A: Eumycetoma—Swollen foot with discharging sinuses and dark grains coming out of sinuses

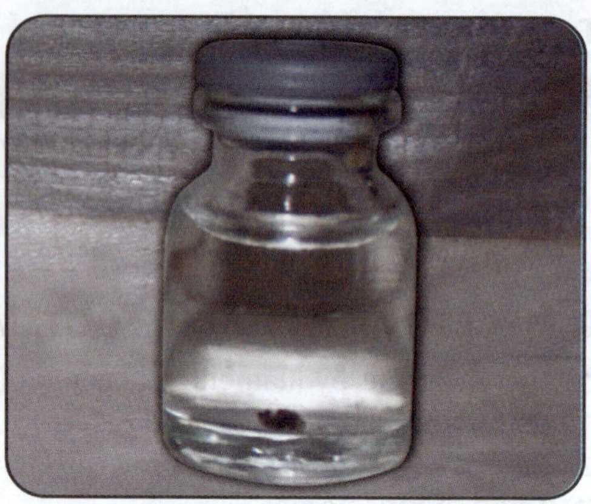

Fig. 23B: Black grains in eumycetoma

High Yield Points

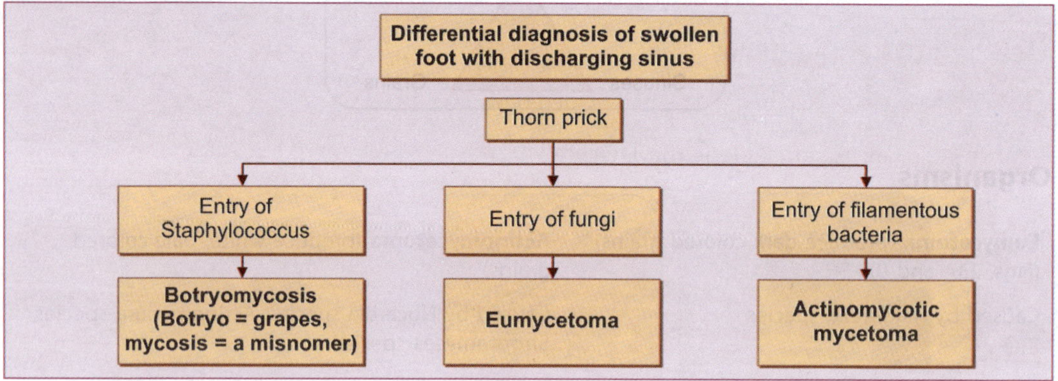

Investigations

- **KOH smear**—from grains in pus (fungal grains will show broader while actinomycotic grains show finer filaments)
- **Skin biopsy** is the **best method**—Chronic inflammatory reaction leading to abscess formation. Grains are found in the center of the inflammatory response while club formation in the periphery of a grain is seen.
- **Fungal culture**—Grains are cultured—For eumycetoma (On sabouraud dextrose agar) while for actinomycetes grains (brain-heart infusion agar)

Treatment

Actinomycotic mycetoma	Eumycetoma
* **Welsh regimen**(MCQ)—Amikacin + Cotrimoxazole	Itraconazole
* **Modified Welsh regimen**(MCQ)—Same as Welsh regimen but with added Rifampicin	Potassium Iodide
	Amputation

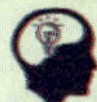

Aid to Remember

- "**Walsh** (the cricketer Courtney Walsh) was an **Ami**cable and a **Co**urteous guy"—**Welsh** regimen- **Ami**kacin + **Co**trimoxazole

CHROMOBLASTOMYCOSIS

- Chronic infection caused by **pigmented fungi**(MCQ) (Phialophora and Fonsecaea species)
- Inoculation of the organism through a thorn prick

Clinical: Warty, cauliflower-like growth on the foot or lower leg at the site of prick(AIIMS Nov 17) (Fig. 24A).

Histology: A foreign-body granuloma forms. Groups of fungal cells may be seen within giant cells. These fungal cells are **golden brown in color (sclerotic, copper penny, medlar or muriform bodies) (Fig. 24B)**.(MCQ) (AIIMS NOV 17)

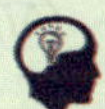

Aid to Remember

- "Chromo"= color- coloured pigmented golden-brown fungi

Treatment: Oral Itraconazole is the DOC(MCQ)

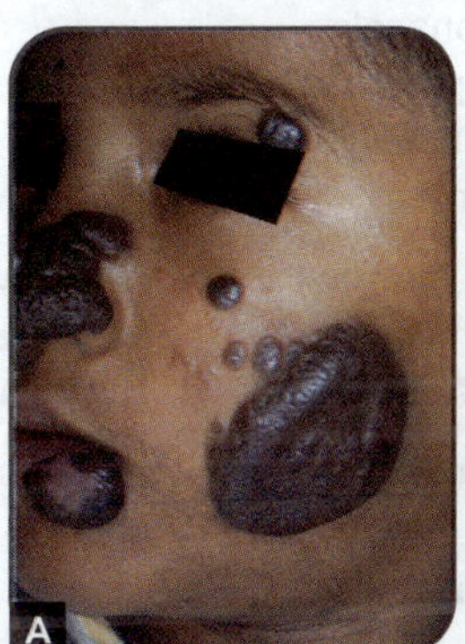

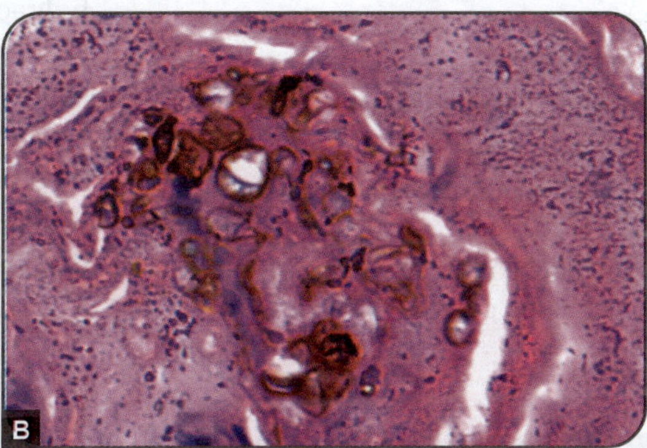

Figs. 24A and B: (A) Verrucous mass on face after thorn prick (even though this lesion is of the face, the most common site is the foot); (B) Thick-walled golden brown sclerotic bodies in dermis

(*Ref:* Department of Pathology, Calicut Medical College, https://commons.wikimedia.org/wiki/File: Chromoblastomycosis_40x.jpg), crop by saurabh, https://creativecommons.org/licenses/by-sa/4.0/legalcode)

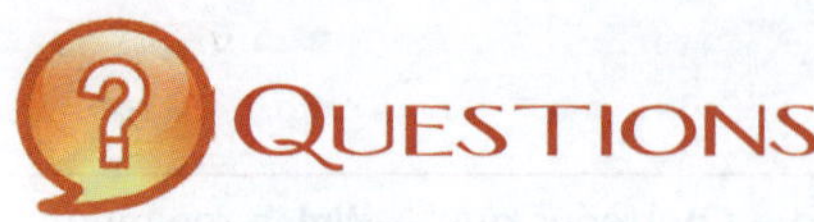

1. **Which of the following are used to diagnose fungal infections?** *(AI 10)*
   a. PAS b. Alizarin red
   c. Von Kossa d. Masson's trichrome
2. **Dermatophytes primarily involves:**
   a. Stratum corneum *(AIIMS)*
   b. Stratum granulosum
   c. Stratum basale
   d. Stratum spinosum
3. **Which species does not cause tinea capitis?** *(AIIMS)*
   a. Epidermophyton floccosum
   b. Microsporum canis
   c. Trichophyton violaceum
   d. Trichophyton tonsurans
4. **Most common species causing tinea capitis:**
   a. Trichophyton violaceum
   b. Candida albicans
   c. Epidermophyton
   d. Trichophyton mentagrophyte
5. **A child presents with scalp lesions with pain and suppuration. The likely diagnosis is:** *(AIIMS)*
   a. Black dot tinea capitis
   b. Grey patch tinea capitis
   c. Kerion
   d. Favus
6. **Black dot tinea is caused by:** *(AIIMS)*
   a. Trichophyton b. Microsporum
   c. Epidermophyton d. Candida
7. **An 8-year-old child presents with localized non-scarring alopecia over scalp with itching and scales. The diagnosis is:** *(AIIMS)*
   a. Alopecia areata b. Tinea barbae
   c. Tinea capitis d. Lichen planus
8. **A 10-year-old boy presented with painful boggy swelling of scalp, multiple sinuses with purulent discharge, easily pluckable hair and enlarged lymph nodes in occipital region. Which one of the following would be most helpful for diagnosis?** *(AIIMS May 13, 09, AI 01)*
   a. KOH mount b. Biopsy and culture
   c. Bacterial culture d. Patch test
9. **An 11-year-old is having tinea capitis. The most appropriate line of therapy is:**
   a. Oral griseofulvin
   b. Topical griseofulvin
   c. Selenium sulphide shampoo
   d. Shaving of hair
10. **Tinea unguium affects:** *(AI)*
    a. Nail fold b. Nail plate
    c. Interdigital space d. Joints
11. **Drug/s for tinea unguium:**
    a. Fluticasone
    b. Itraconazole
    c. Ciclopirox olamine
    d. Terbinafine
    e. Neomycin
12. **Drug of choice for tinea unguium is:**
    a. Amphoterecin B b. Miconazole
    c. Oral terbinafine d. Nystatin
13. **Griseofulvin is effective in all *except:*** *(AIIMS)*
    a. Tinea capitis b. Tinea versicolor
    c. Tinea corporis d. Tinea unguium
14. **Regarding athelete's foot, true is:** *(PGI)*
    a. 4th web is commonly involved
    b. Severe itching
    c. Caused by Trichophyton rubrum
    d. Hyperhidrosis present
    e. All of the above
15. **Dhobi's itch is:** *(DNB)*
    a. Tinea corporis
    b. Tinea cruris
    c. Tinea barbae
    d. Tinea capitis

16. A patient comes with itching in the groin since 2 months. All can cause this, *except*: *(AIIMS Nov 18)*

a. Aspergillus b. Trichophyton
c. Microsporum d. Epidermophyton

17. A 22-year-old male presents with complaints of severe itching and scaly lesions in groin for the past month. Which of the following is the most likely causative agent? *(AIIMS Nov 03, JIPMER 05)*

a. Trichophyton rubrum
b. Candida albicans
c. Malassezia furfur
d. Candida glabrata

18. A 36-year-old factory worker developed itchy annular scaly plaques in groin. Application of steroid ointment gives temporary relief but the plaques continued to grow at periphery. The most likely diagnosis is:

a. Erythema annulare centrifugum
b. Granuloma annulare
c. Tinea incognito
d. Annular lichen planus

19. The test likely to help in the diagnosis of itchy annular plaques on the face is:

a. Gram stain
b. Potassium hydroxide mount
c. Tissue smear
d. Wood's lamp

20. Which of the following is not an antifungal?

a. Capsofungin b. Ciclopirox
c. Clofazimine d. Undecylenic acid

21. An otherwise healthy male presents with a creamy curd like white patch on the tongue. The probable diagnosis is:

a. Candidiasis b. Histoplasmosis
c. Lichen planus d. Aspergillosis

22. Commonest fungal infection on the genitalia in a female diabetic patient is:

a. Candidal vulvovaginitis
b. Aspergillosis
c. Maduramycosis
d. Cryptococcus

23. A child presents with lesions in groin as shown. The likely diagnosis is:

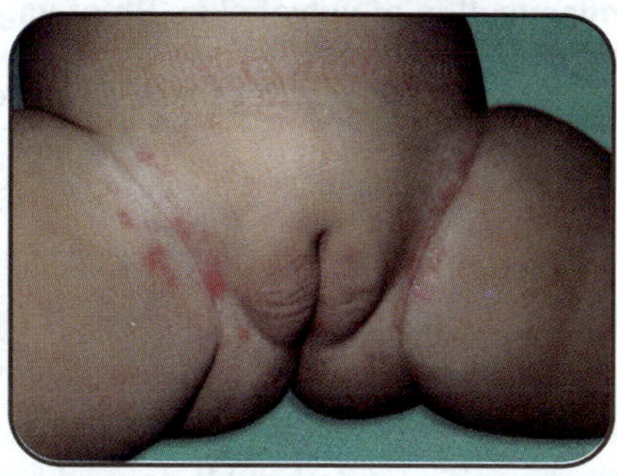

a. Psoriasis
b. Tinea unguium
c. Candidiasis
d. Pseudomonas

24. About dermatophytes all are true, *except:* *(AIIMS)*

a. *Candida albicans* usually causes systemic infection in immunocompetent people
b. Dermatophytes primarily involve stratum corneum
c. Microsporum does not involve nail
d. Epidermophyton does not involve hair

25. A patient presents with lesions as shown. The next step would be: *(AIMS Nov 18)*

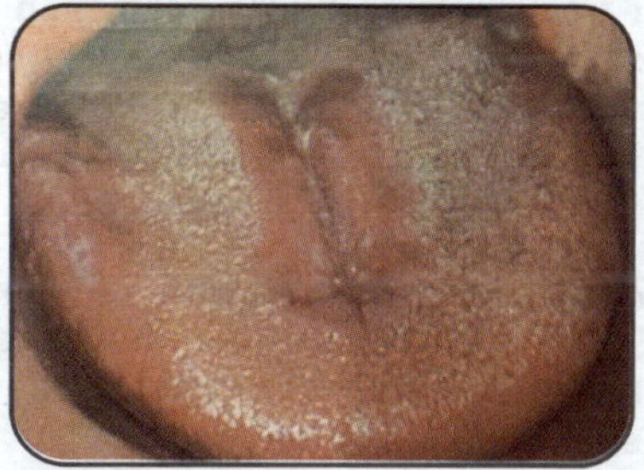

a. Give antifungal
b. Send blood for Vitamin B_{12} and folic acid levels
c. Give dapsone and topical steroids
d. Ask to stop smoking and ask to get tested for malignancy

26. Linear nodules are seen in:

a. Lichen planus b. Psoriasis
c. Pemphigus d. Sporotrichosis

27. A female patient presents with green frothy, itchy vaginal discharge with inflammation of vulval skin. Ph of vagina is 5.4. The diagnosis is: *(Recent NEET pattern)*

a. Candidal infection
b. Trichomonas infection
c. Bacterial vaginosis
d. Mixed infection

28. Ringworm affects:

a. Dermis b. Papillary layer
c. Stratum corneum d. Prickle layer

29. Tinea capitis (endothrix) is caused by:

a. Epidermophyton
b. Trichophyton tonsurans
c. Trichophyton rubrum
d. Trichophyton violaceum
e. Microsporum

30. A 60-year-old male presents with discolouration, thickening and tunneling of 2 fingernails and one toe nail. Which of the following will clinch the diagnosis at the earliest?

a. Wood's lamp b. Gram stain
c. Slit skin smear d. KOH mount

31. Tinea incognito is seen with:

a. Steroids b. Antibiotics
c. 5% permethrin d. Antifungals

32. For treating tinea cruris, for which drug, widespread resistance is developing in last 2 yrs? *(AIIMS May 18)*

a. Itraconazole b. Griseofulvin
c. Terbinafine d. Voriconazole

33. A 25-year-old presents with itchy lesions on glans as shown. He often washes his genitalia for hygiene purposes. The diagnosis will be made by doing:

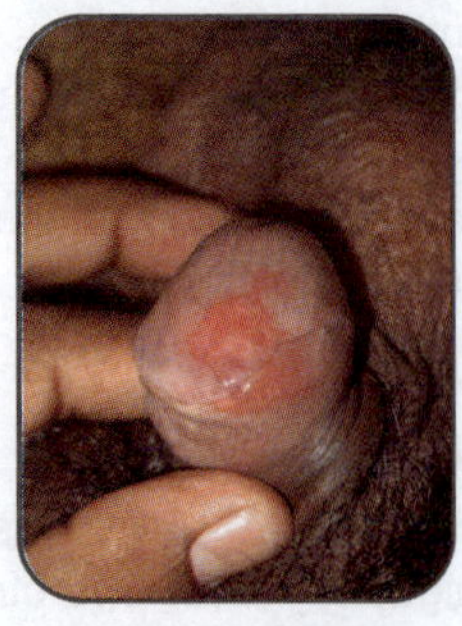

a. Tzanck smear b. KOH smear
c. Giemsa stain d. Biopsy

34. A 24-year-old male had multiple small hypopigmented macules on the upper chest and back for the last three months. The macules were circular, arranged around follicles and many had coalesced to form large sheets. The surface showed fine scaling. He had similar lesions one year ago which subsided with treatment. The most appropriate investigation to confirm the diagnosis is: *(AIIMS May 12, Nov 13)*

a. Potassium hydroxide mount
b. Slit skin smear
c. Skin biopsy
d. Tzanck smear

35. Potassium iodide is used in the treatment of:

a. Sporotrichosis
b. Impetigo
c. Dermatitis herpetiformis
d. Warts

36. A child presents with image as shown. The diagnosis is: *(Recent NEET pattern)*

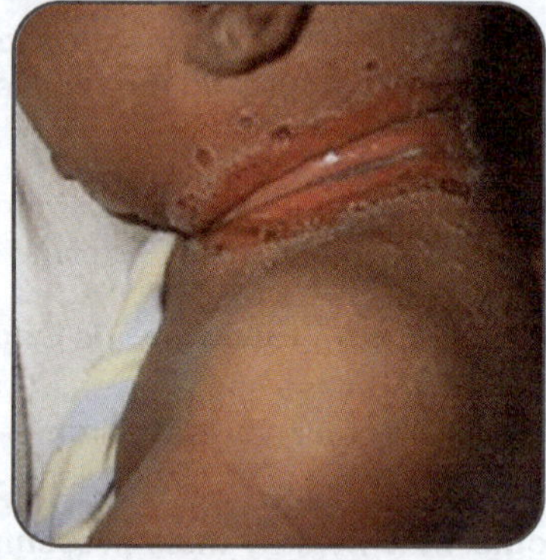

a. Bullous impetigo
b. Staphylococal scalded skin syndrome
c. Candidal intertrigo
d. Scrofuloderma

37. A child comes with a circular 3 cm x 3 cm scaly patchy hair loss with itching in the lesions. The investigation of choice is: *(AIIMS May 17)*

a. Slit skin smear b. KOH
c. Gram stain d. Tzanck smear

38. A patient from Himachal Pradesh gets a thorn prick and subsequently presents with a verrucous lesion (an image of a cauliflower-like lesion on feet and microscopy stain image of copper penny bodies was shown). The diagnosis is: *(AIIMS Nov 17)*

a. Sporothrix
b. Chromoblastomycosis
c. Eumycetoma
d. Verruca

New Questions

39. The following statements are true/false regarding pityriasis versicolor:

a. Oral terbinafine is the drug of choice
b. Spaghetti and meatball appearance on KOH mount
c. Pteridine is the reason for the fluorescence on woods lamp
d. Collarette scales are seen
e. Dermatophytic infection

40. Assertion: Partner treatment is not done for male partner of females with vulvovaginal candidiasis

Reason: Candida is usually non sexual in its transmission

a. Both Assertion and Reason are true and Reason is correct explanation of Assertion
b. Both Assertion and Reason are true but Reason is not correct explanation of Assertion
c. Assertion is true and Reason is false
d. Assertion is false and Reason is true
e. Both Assertion and Reason are false

41. Regarding dermatophytic infections mark the correct options:

a. Central clearing
b. Involve the dermis and subcutaneous tissue primarily
c. Keratophilic fungi
d. Red discoloration is the classical pattern of nail involvement

1. If a, b, d are correct
2. If a and b are correct
3. If a and c are correct
4. If all four (a, b, c, & d) are correct

42. Match items in column A with best alternative in column B

Column A	Column B
1. Sporotrichosis	a. Immunosuppression may be the cause
2. Chromoblastomycosis	b. Welsh regimen
3. Mycetoma	c. Sclerotic bodies
4. Oral candidiasis	d. Asteroid bodies
	e. Kligman regimen
	f. Woods lamp positive

43. A young man presents with linear lesions as shown. All the following can cause this spread along lymphatics *except*: *(INICET Nov 22)*

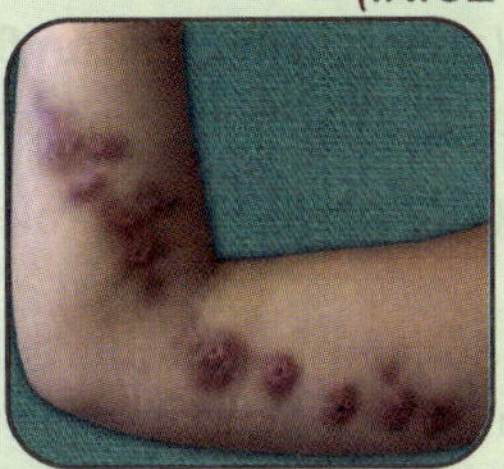

a. Sporothrix
b. Nocardia
c. *Staphylococcal aureus*
d. Mycobacterial marinum

44. A forest worker has a history of warty/cauliflower lesion on foot. His histology is as shown. The histology image is of:

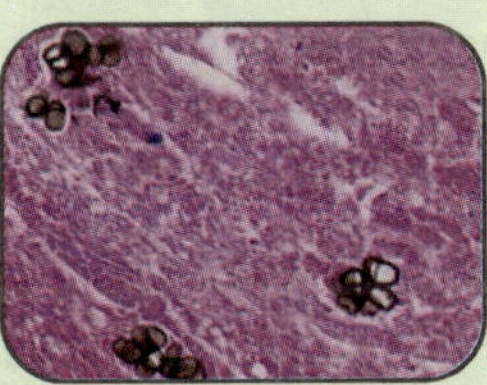

a. Broad base non-capsulated
b. Splendore–Hoeppli phenomenon
c. Encapsulated budding yeast
d. Sclerotic body

45. A patient has central clearing and peripheral redness as shown. The morphology would be: *(INICET May 22)*

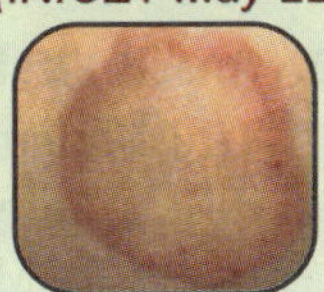

a. Targetoid
b. Discoid
c. Nummular
d. Annular

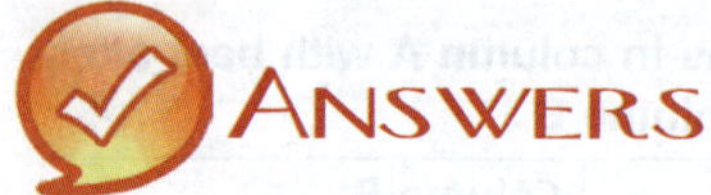

1. **Ans. (a) PAS** *(Ref: Fitzpatrick's Textbook, 8th edn, Page 2281)*
Lab methods used for fungal infections are KOH smear, fungal culture on sabouraud's dextrose agar. Special stains staining the fungal cell wall like PAS stains (pink) and Grocott-Gomori's methenamine silver (black) are also used. Von Kossa and alizarin red is used to stain calcium while masson's trichrome is used to stain collagen, muscle, keratin and nerve.

2. **Ans. (a) Stratum corneum** *(Ref: Habif's Clinical Dermatology, 5th edn, Page 491)*
Dermatophytes have the ability to infect and survive only on dead keratin layer (stratum corneum), the hair, and the nails.

3. **Ans. (a) Epidermophyton floccosum** *(Ref: Andrew's textbook, 11th edn, Page 228)*
Epidermophyton floccosum and trichophyton concentricum do not cause tinea capitis.

4. **Ans. (a) Trichophyton violaceum** *(Ref: Andrew's textbook, 11th edn, Page 289, IADVL textbbook of dermatology 3rd edn, Page 254)*
Trichophyton tonsurans is the commonest cause of tinea capitis in US while in Europe it is microsporum canis. In South-east Asia including India, the predominant species is trichophyton violaceum.

5. **Ans. (c) Kerion**

6. **Ans. (a) Trichophyton** (See page 109 for explanation)

7. **Ans. (c) Tinea capitis** (See page 108 for explanation)
Alopecia areata and tinea capitis both cause non-scarring localized patchy hair loss. Itching and scaling favors the diagnosis of tinea capitis (alopecia areata will have a "smooth surfaced" patch of asymptomatic hair loss). Lichen planus causes patchy scarring alopecia.

8. **Ans. (a) KOH mount** (See page 109 for explanation)
Easily pluckable hairs, sinuses and painful boggy swelling point to a diagnosis of kerion. KOH smear on the loose hairs plucked from scalp will show either endothrix or ectothrix hair infection.

9. **Ans. (a) Oral griseofulvin** *(Ref: Rook's Textbook of Dermatology, 9th edn, Page 32.40)*
Oral griseofulvin (it is not available in topical form) is useful for tinea capitis caused by microsporum species, while oral terbinafine is more suitable for trichophyton infections of scalp. Selenium sulphide only has a supportive role.

10. **Ans. (b) Nail plate** *(Ref: Rook's Textbook of Dermatology, 9th edn, Page 32.47)*
Tinea unguium (onychomycosis) is defined as invasion of the nail plates by species of dermatophytes. Nail fold involvement is classical of candidal infection (paronychia) and not tinea. Most common organism causing tinea unguium is trichophyton rubrum.

11. Ans. (b), (c), (d) Itraconazole; Ciclopirox olamine; Terbinafine
(Ref: Rook's Textbook of Dermatology, 9th edn, Page 32.49)

First line therapy for tinea unguium is oral terbinafine or oral itraconazole. Topical amorolfine and topical ciclopirox are useful for mild infections of nail.

12. Ans. (c) Oral terbinafine *(Ref: Rook's Textbook of Dermatology, 9th edn, Page 32.49)*

13. Ans. (b) Tinea versicolor *(Ref: Rook's Textbook of Dermatology, 9th edn, Page 32.13, Fitzpatrick Textbook, 8th edn, Page 2311)*

Oral griseofulvin and oral terbinafine do not work in tinea versicolor.

14. Ans. (e) All of the above (See page 111 for explanation)

15. Ans. (b) Tinea cruris (See page 112 for explanation)

16. Ans (a) Aspergillus

17. Ans. (a) Trichophyton rubrum *(Ref: Rook's Textbook of Dermatology, 9th edn, Page 32.46)*

The MCQ indicates tinea cruris. All tineas (except tinea capitis) are most commonly caused by trichophyton rubrum.

18. Ans. (c) Tinea incognito (See page 113 for explanation)

All the above are annular lesions. Tinea incognito is steroid-modified tinea cruris here.

Why not other options?

Erythema annulare centrifugum is annular (erythema = red, annulare = annular, centrifugum = spreads centrifugally) but is not necessarily in groins, Granuloma annulare is also annular but classically non-scaly, Annular lichen planus is classically on mucosal areas and not groins.

19. Ans. (b) Potassium hydroxide mount (See page 114 for explanation)

Tinea faciei is diagnosed by KOH smears.

20. Ans. (c) Clofazimine

Capsofungin is an intravenous antifungal useful for aspergillosis and candida. Undecylenic acid is a topical antifungal though not in use now.

21. Ans. (a) Candidiasis (See page 103 for explanation)

"Creamy" or "curdy" white points to a diagnosis of candidiasis. Oral candidiasis can occur in an apparently healthy patient (for example with undiagnosed diabetes).

22. Ans. (a) Candidal vulvovaginitis *(Ref: Fitzpatrick's Textbook, 8th edn, Page 2300)*

23. Ans. (c) Candidiasis (See page 104 for explanation)

The lesions are erythematous macules with few satellite lesions in the groin which suggests candidal intertrigo

24. Ans. (a) *Candida albicans* usually causes systemic infection in immunocompetent people (See page 103 for explanation)

Candida is an opportunistic pathogens causing invasive candidiasis in immunocompromised patients not in immunocompetent patients (Esophageal candidiasis is a marker of AIDS).

25. Ans. (a) Give antifungal

The image shows acute erythematous candidiasis in an HIV patient.

26. Ans. (d) Sporotrichosis *(Ref: Fitzpatrick's Textbook, 8th edn, Page 2313)*

Linear nodules and discharging sinuses are classical of lymphangitic sporotrichosis. Lichen planus will have the "5P" words (purple, polygonal, plane topped, pruritic, papules). Pemphigus creates blisters. Psoriasis presents as scaly silvery plaques.

27. Ans (b) Trichomonas infection

28. Ans. (c) Stratum corneum (See page 107 for explanation)

29. Ans. (b) and (d) Trichophyton tonsurans; Trichophyton violaceum *(Ref: Rook's Textbook of Dermatology, 9th edn, Page 32.38)*

30. Ans. (d) KOH mount *(Ref: Rook's Textbook of Dermatology, 9th edn, Page 32.48)*

The MCQ points to a diagnosis of onychomycosis. Pointers in the MCQ are thickened nails, discoloration of nail. Tunneling indicates tunnel-like gaps under nail plate by the invading fungus.

31. Ans. (a) Steroids (See page 113 for explanation)

32. Ans. (b) Griseofulvin

33. Ans. (b) KOH smear

The image is of candidal balanitis for which a KOH mount would help.

34. Ans. (a) Potassium hydroxide mount (See page 100 for explanation)

Diagnosis is pityriasis versicolor. Pointers in the MCQ are "circular around hair follicles", "hypopigmented macules", "fine scaling" and location on chest.

35. Ans. (a) Sporotrichosis *(Ref: Rook's Textbook of Dermatology, 9th edn, Page 32.73)*

For treatment of sporotrichosis, oral itraconazole is the drug of choice. Potassium iodide is cheap and effective, though with more side-effects (dry mouth, taste alteration, nausea). Potassium iodide worsens dermatitis herpetiformis.

36. Ans. (c) Candidal intertrigo

The image shows erythematous erosions on flexure with satellite lesions- classical of candida.

Why not:

a: Will have blister with hypopyon sign

b: Will have scaling, face, trunk involvement, fever, Nikolsky positive

d: Will have lymphadenitis with sinus on neck/axillae

37. Ans. (b) KOH

Scaly, itchy, localized patchy hair loss in a child is tinea capitis. KOH smear is done from loose hairs. SSS is for leprosy and leishmaniasis. Tzanck smear is for herpes, pemphigus, etc.

38. Ans. (b) Chromoblastomycosis

New Answers

39. Ans. a-False; b-True; c-True; d-False; e-False

40. Ans. (a) Both Assertion and Reason are true and Reason is correct explanation of Assertion

41. Ans. (3) If a and c are correct

42. Ans. 1-d; 2-c; 3-b; 4-a

43. Ans. (c) Staphylococcal aureus

44. Ans. (d) Sclerotic body

The diagnosis is chromoblastomycosis

45. Ans. (d) Annular

CHAPTER 6

Viral Infections

HERPES GROUP

- Herpes simplex virus (HSV) 1 and 2
- Human herpes virus 3 (Varicella zoster virus—VZV)
- Human herpes virus 4 (Epstein-Barr virus—EBV)
- Human herpes virus 5 (Cytomegalovirus—CMV)
- Human herpes viruses (HHV) 6, 7
- Human herpes virus 8

Herpes Simplex Virus (HSV)

- HSV1—Orolabial herpes.(MCQ) HSV2—Genital herpes(MCQ)
- Virus remains **latent in sensory ganglia** after primary episode from where it periodically **reactivates**
- Histologically, HSV causes edema of the keratinocytes **(ballooning degeneration)**. Adjacent keratinocytes fuse and appear large and multinucleate. These ballooned cells rupture **(reticular degeneration)** to create an intraepidermal blister
- The most common test used to diagnose is the **Tzanck smear which shows multinucleated giant cells**(MCQ) (For image of multinucleate giant cells, see topic discussion of acantholytic cell in Chapter 1).

High Yield Points

- Tzanck smear **does not differentiate between HSV and VZV infections**MCQ (multinucleate epidermal giant cells are seen in both).

Infections Caused by HSV

1. **Orolabial herpes (fever blister, cold sore)**(MCQ)
   Etiology: Virtually always caused by HSV1
   Triggers: Fever,(MCQ) Ultraviolet (UVB) exposure, surgical and dental procedures of the lips
   Clinical:
   - Present as **grouped vesicles**(MCQ) which rupture to create **grouped erosions** in the mouth and on lips.
   - Initial episodes are **severe and painful** (Fig. 1). After the primary episode, the virus migrates to the cervical dorsal root ganglia and remains latent. It reactivates after fever, menstruation, dental procedures, etc. to cause repeated episodes. Recurrences

which occur with fever **(hence called fever blisters)** are milder and milder as time progresses (Fig. 2).

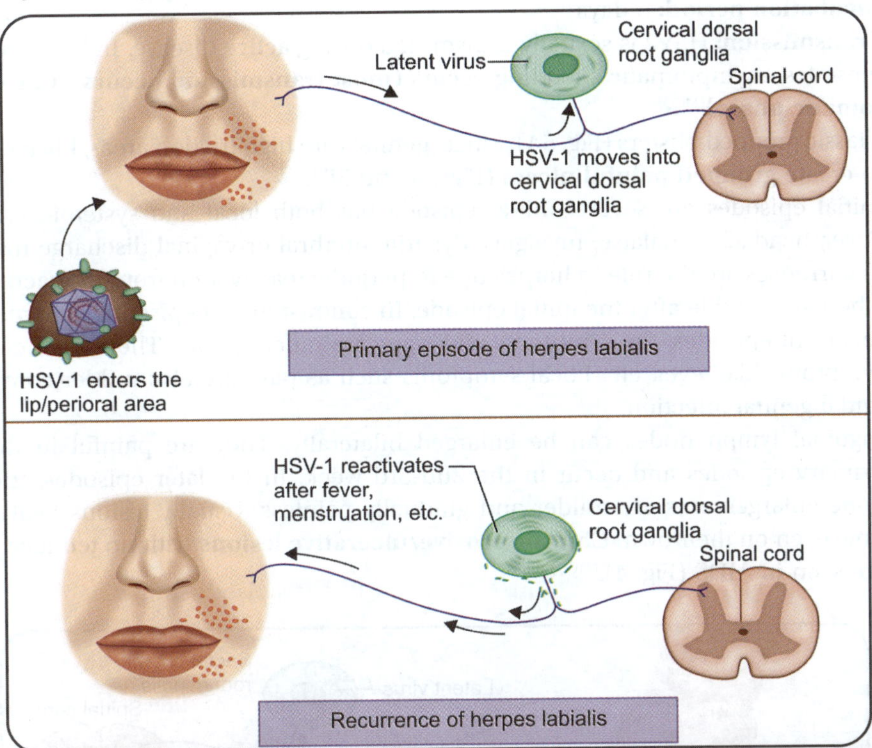

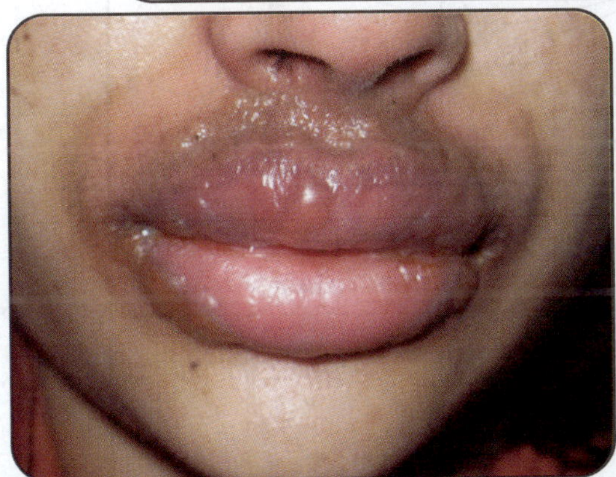

Fig. 1: Herpes labialis (Primary episode): Grouped vesicles and bullae with severe inflammatory edemaon lips

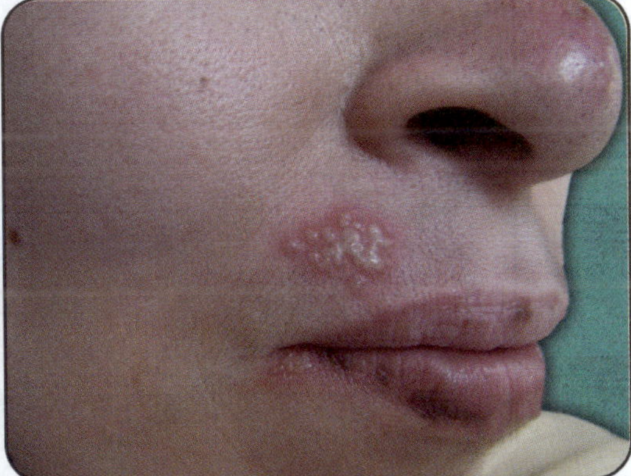

Fig. 2: Herpes labialis (Recurrence): Grouped vesicles with less inflammation

Treatment: Antivirals like acyclovir, famciclovir, valaciclovir are given during clinical episodes.

High Yield Points

- Pick-up words in an MCQ—**Grouped blisters** and **recurrence** point to a diagnosis of herpes.

2. **Genital herpes (m/c STD in the world)**(MCQ)
   - Mainly HSV2, sometimes HSV1. Many HSV infections are subclinical
   - **Incubation period:** 5 days
   - **Transmission:** HSV2 is sexually transmitted during active disease. In between clinical episodes, asymptomatic shedding occurs **(most transmission occurs in this asymptomatic phase)**(MCQ)
   - Classic grouped blisters (Fig. 5A). Since, genitals are high friction areas, blisters rupture to create **grouped painful ulcers** (Figs. 3 and 5B).
   - Initial episodes are severe. Initial episode has both local and systemic symptoms. Fever, headache, malaise, myalgias, dysuria, urethral or vaginal discharge may occur. Recurrences are the rule in herpes due to periodic reactivation from the sacral ganglia where they reside after the initial episode. In contrast to first episodes of herpes, in the recurrent episodes, the symptoms and signs are much milder. There are no systemic symptoms like fever, etc. Local symptoms such as pain are also milder compared to initial genital infection.
   - Inguinal lymph nodes can be enlarged bilaterally. They are painful in the initial primary episodes and occur in the 2nd-3rd week. In the later episodes, the lymph node enlargements are milder and gradually painless. Usually lesions heal in some time even on their own. **Chronic erosive/ulcerative lesions** with no tendency to heal are seen in AIDS (Fig. 4).(MCQ)

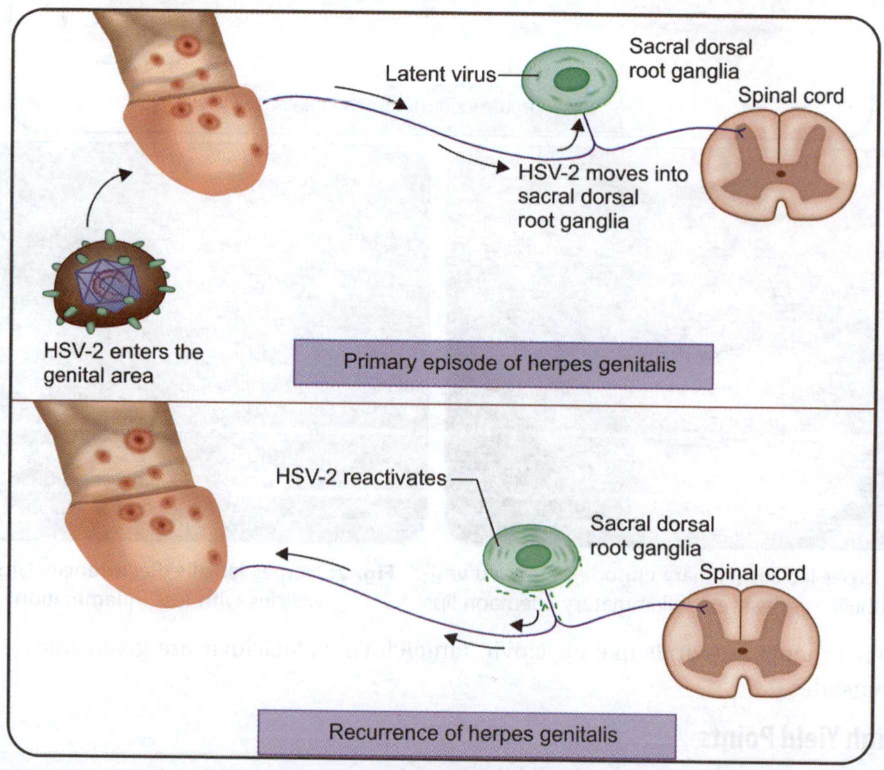

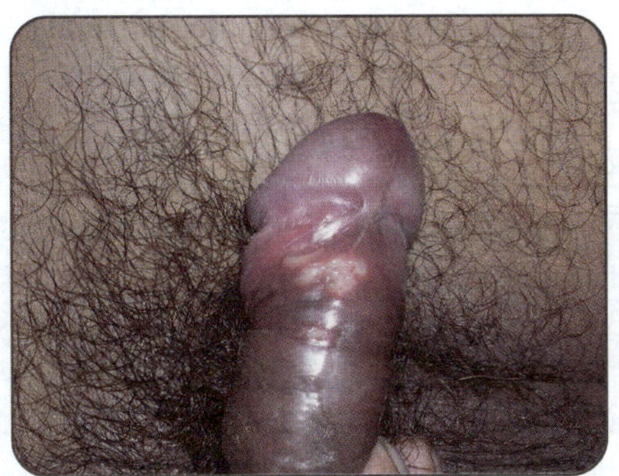

Fig. 3: Herpes genitalis: Grouped tender erosions (after rupture of grouped blisters)

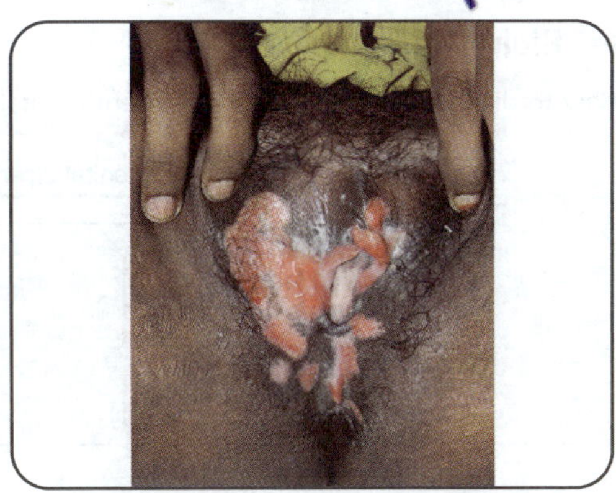

Fig. 4: Herpes genitalis (chronic erosive type): Severe chronic ulceration (lasting more than 1 month) in AIDS

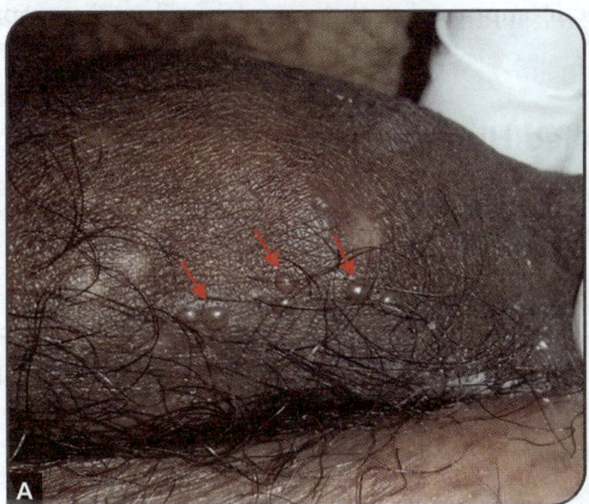

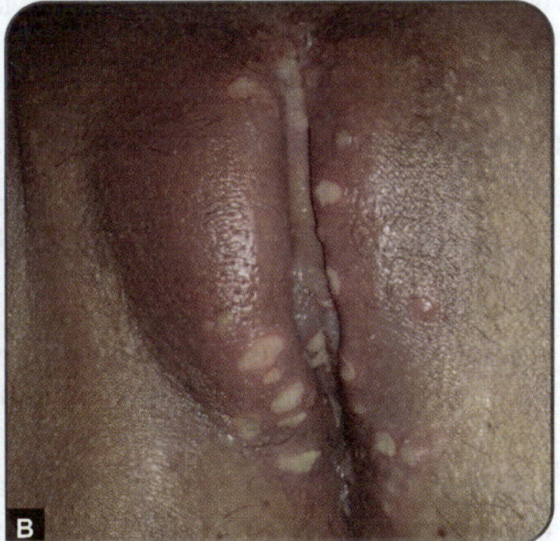

Figs. 5A and B: (A) Grouped blisters (red arrows); (B) Superficial painful erosions

High Yield Points

How to diagnose genital herpes in an MCQ? *(PGI Nov 2017)*

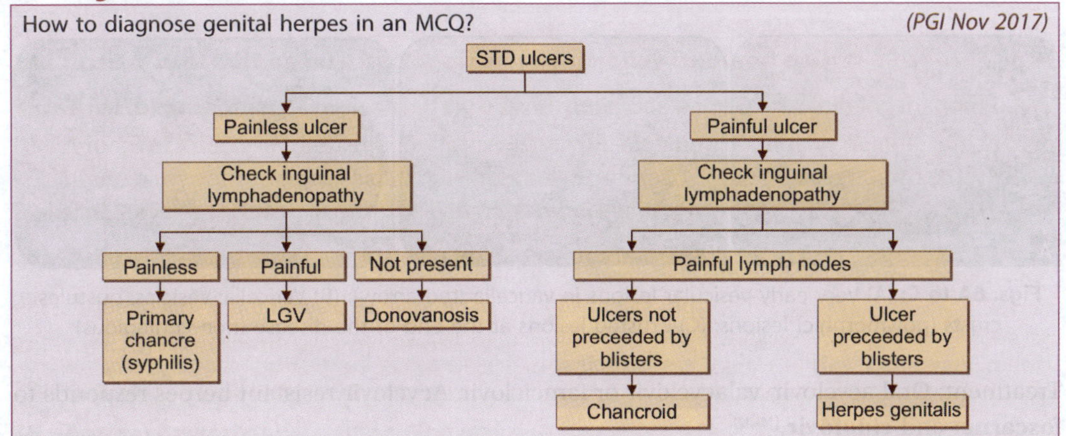

High Yield Points

How to diagnose in an MCQ on recurrent genital ulcers/blisters?

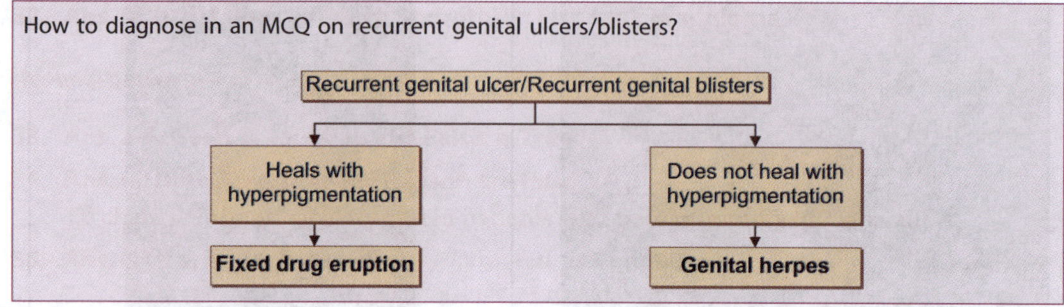

Treatment: Antivirals like acyclovir, famciclovir, valaciclovir are given during clinical episodes. For those having more than 6–12 episodes a year—continuous antiviral prophylaxis is recommended (continuous prophylactic suppressive therapy also reduces asymptomatic shedding).[MCQ]

Varicella Zoster Virus (VZV-also Called Human Herpes Virus-3)

- Primary VZV (HHV-3) infection—**Varicella**
- Reactivation of VZV due to immunosuppression—**Herpes zoster**.

1. **Varicella**[DNB 89]

   Pathology: VZV causes **ballooning degeneration**[MCQ] of keratinocytes due to intracellular edema creating **Tzanck cells** with multiple nuclei inside. Blisters form in the epidermis.

   Clinical: After a day or two of fever, papules → vesicles → red halo at base **("dewdrop on rose petal" appearance)** → pustule → crust.

   - Polymorphic lesions (lesions in various stages of development) (Figs. 6A to C)
   - Centripetal distribution
   - Crust formation indicates patient **is not contagious** to other people.[MCQ]

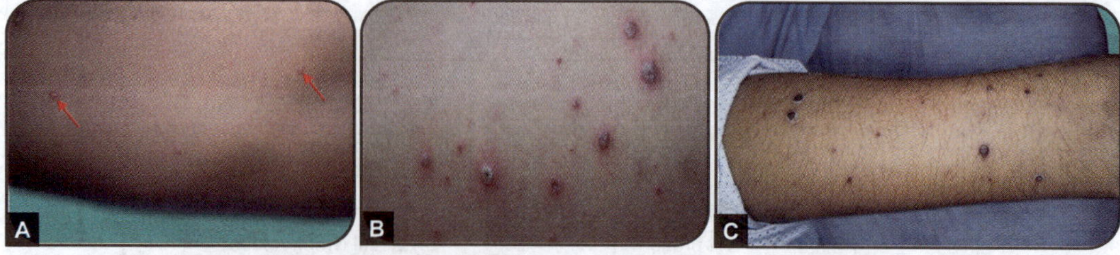

Figs. 6A to C: (A) Very early vesicular lesions in varicella (red arrow); (B) Varicella: Vesicles, pustules, crusts (polymorphic) lesions; (C) Crusted lesions at the end of the disease (non-contagious)

Treatment: Oral acyclovir, valacyclovir or famciclovir. Acyclovir resistant herpes responds to **foscarnet** and **cidofovir**.[MCQ]

Varicella in pregnancy(MCQ)

- If infection occurs **within 20 weeks of gestation** (most risk is between 13–20 weeks), there is a 2% risk of fetal damage (congenital varicella syndrome—limb hypoplasia, cutaneous scars, ocular and neurological defects). Treatment is with oral acyclovir.
- Maternal primary infection in perinatal period (5 days before till 2 days after delivery) spreads to the immunologically unprotected neonate rapidly causing a very severe neonatal varicella (mortality of 30%). In such cases VZIG to baby and intravenous acyclovir therapy intravenously to mother is given.(MCQ)
- If mother has been exposed to a varicella case, VZIG alone should be given to mother within 72–96 hrs of exposure to prevent maternal varicella.

2. **Herpes Zoster (Shingles)**

After varicella subsides, VZV stays latent in the dorsal root ganglia. Reactivation of this VZV occurs in immunosuppression (e.g. HIV, old people) and creates **vesicles on an erythematous base occurs along unilateral dermatomes** (lines along nerves) and is then called herpes zoster (Fig. 7A). Commonest dermatome involved is **thoracic**(MCQ) while commonest cranial nerve involved is **trigeminal**. Treatment is with oral acyclovir, valacyclovir or famciclovir.(MCQ) The commonest complication of herpes zoster is **post herpetic neuralgia (PHN)**(MCQ) (defined as pain even **after 3 months** of herpes zoster but some also consider it at **4 weeks** after herpes zoster).(AIIMS Nov 16)

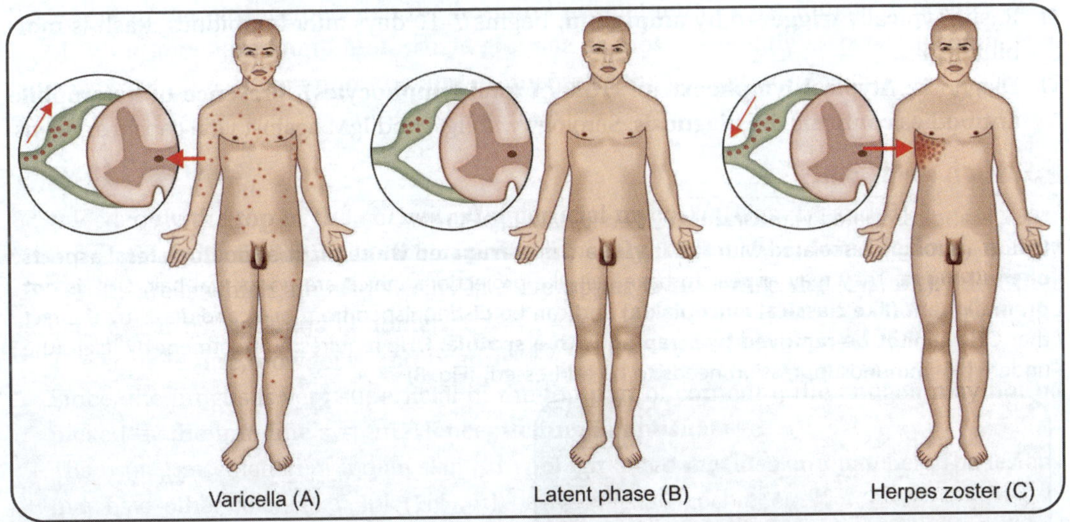

(A) Varicella (centripetal lesions). VZV then enters spinal/cranial ganglia; (B) Latent phase. VZV remains latent in ganglia; (C) Herpes Zoster—Reactivation of VZV occurs with immunosuppression and occurs along dermatomes (a truncal dermatome is shown here)

- **Hutchinson's sign**(MCQ): The sign states that, if vesicles are seen on the side of the nose in ophthalmic nerve zoster, the eye is usually affected (Fig. 7B).
- **Ramsay Hunt syndrome**(MCQ): Facial paralysis in some cases of herpes zoster oticus.

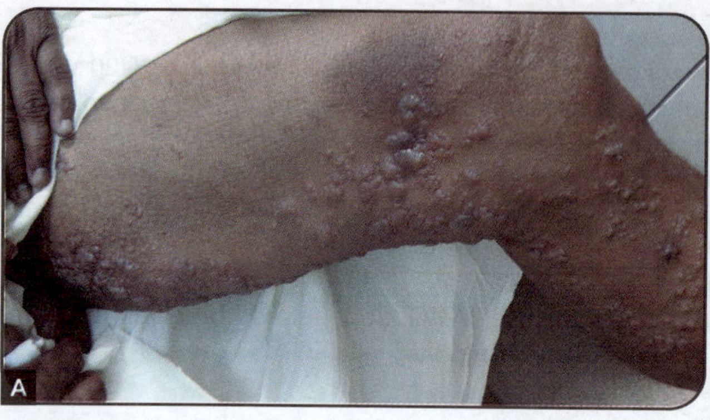

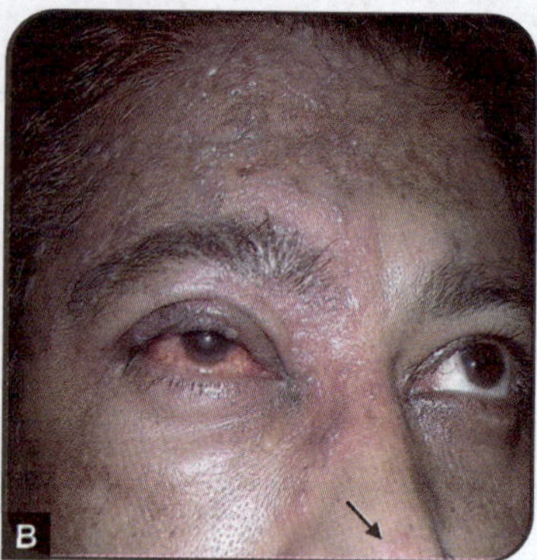

Figs. 7A and B: (A) Herpes zoster: Dermatomal distribution of vesicles and bullae on thigh; (B) Hutchinson's sign in herpes zoster ophthalmicus- Note the nasal vesicles (black arrow) and ipsilateral eye involvement. Explanation in the box before

HH4 (EBV)—Causes Infectious Mononucleosis (Glandular Fever, Kissing Disease)

- **Classic triad is fever, posterior cervical lymphadenopathy, and pharyngitis.** Petechiae at the junction of the hard and soft palate are a classical feature of the disease and usually appear on the **second or third day** of fever
- Rash: Typically **triggered by ampicillin,** begins 7–10 days after antibiotics. Rash is morbilliform
- Diagnosis: **Atypical lymphocytes (>10% of total lymphocytes), presence of heterophile antibodies confirms the diagnosis,** Serology with IgG and IgM against viral capsid antigens.

High Yield Points

*EBV is also associated with **Oral Hairy Leucoplakia (OHL)**(AIIMS)

OHL is a strongly associated with HIV. It appears as **corrugated white plaques on the lateral aspects of the tongue**. They may appear to have hair-like projections which are not actual hair. OHL is **not premalignant (like classical leucoplakia)** and can be distinguished from oral candidiasis by the fact that OHL **cannot be removed by scraping with a spatula**. OHL requires no treatment by itself (the underlying immunosuppression needs to be addressed) (Fig. 8)

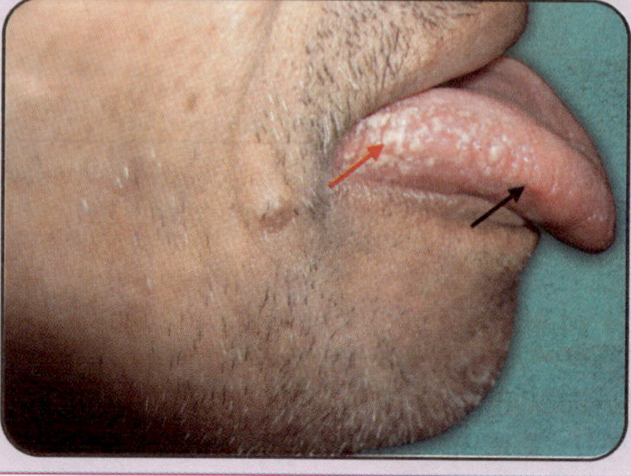

Fig. 8: OHL: Note the corrugated vertical furrows (black arrow); Coexisting white plaques of oral candidiasis can also be seen (red arrow)—both being signs of HIV disease here

Oral premalignant lesions and 10 years risk of malignant conversion		
Very high-risk (70–85%)	*High-risk (10–30%)*	*Low risk (1–5%)*
Erythroplakia(MCQ) (erythroplasia)	Leukoplakia(MCQ) (non homogenous)	Leukoplakia (homogenous)(MCQ)
	Actinic cheilitis (Actinic = sun, cheilitis = inflammation of lip)	Oral lichen planus(MCQ) (mainly ulcerative/erosive type)
	Submucous fibrosis(MCQ)	

*** Leukoplakia is the most common premalignant lesion in the oral cavity(MCQ)**

Pityriasis Rosea (PR)(MCQ)

Pityriasis = powdery scale, rosea = pink

Etiology: HHV-7 > HHV-6.(MCQ)

Clinical:

- Common acute disease typically beginning as a single oval scaly plaque on the trunk **("herald patch" or "mother patch")**.(MCQ)
- The initial lesion is followed later by the appearance of numerous similar-appearing smaller lesions located **along the lines of cleavage (along the ribs). This is called *Christmas tree or fir-tree* pattern.**(MCQ) The lines have also been called Langer's lines (Figs. 9A, 9C to E).
- Typically, the periphery of the lesions have a **collarette scale** ("collar"= something on periphery, "ette"= small) (Fig. 9B).
- The collarette scales are **attached on outer border and free on inner border of the lesions.**(MCQ) When stretched across the long axis, the scales tend to fold across the lines of stretch, called the **"hanging curtain" sign.**(MCQ)

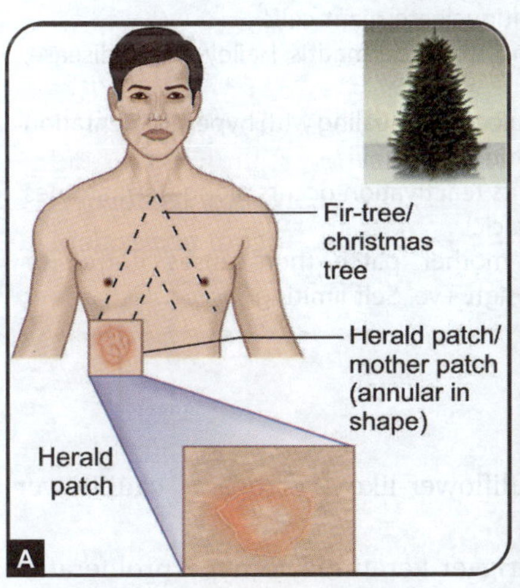

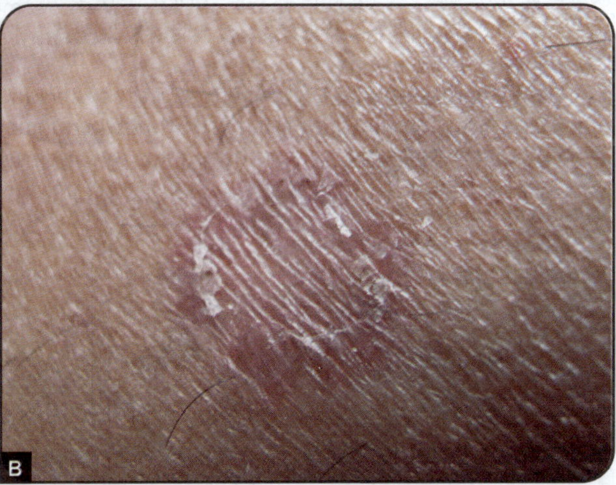

Figs. 9A and B: Pityriasis Rosea: (A) Schematic representation of lesions; (B) Collarette scales: Note attachment of scales on outer border and free on inner border

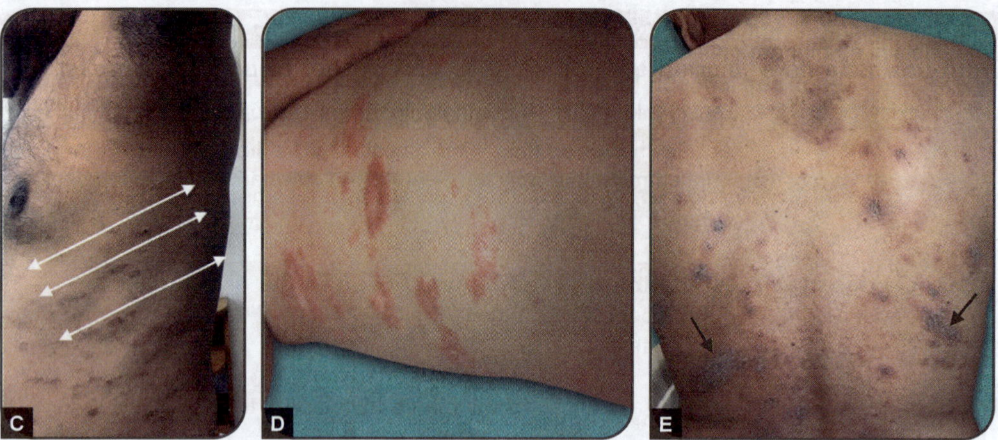

Figs. 9C to E: (C) Lesions along ribs (Langer's lines); (D) Multiple annular plaques in a child on the trunk in a fir-tree pattern; (E) Note the direction of lesions on back oriented towards central (black arrow)

- Treatment: Always **self resolving** in 4–10 weeks and most patients **do not require treatment.**(MCQ) Oral erythromycin (erythromycin has an anti-inflammatory role), high dose acyclovir, mid-potency topical steroids and UVB therapy help in faster resolution.

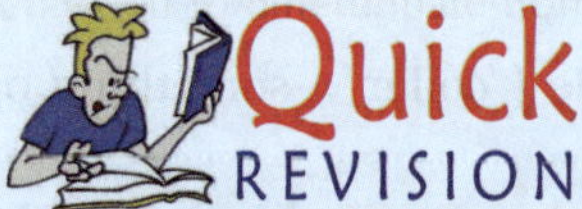

- HSV1—Orolabial herpes (fever blisters). HSV2—Genital herpes
- Severe initial episode and milder recurrences
- Ballooning degeneration, reticular degeneration occurs pathologically in keratinocytes
- Tzanck smear used for diagnosis of HSV, VZV shows multinucleate giant cells
- Eczema herpeticum—Disseminated HSV-1 with underlying atopic dermatitis, Hailey-Hailey disease, pemphigus foliaceous
- Genital herpes—m/c STD. Grouped recurrent blisters and ulcers not healing with hyperpigmentation (Fixed drug eruption is similar, heals with hyperpigmentation)
- VZV causes Varicella (polymorphic centripetal rash,) and its reactivation occurs along dermatomes is called Herpes Zoster (m/c dermatome involved—thoracic)
- Pityriasis rosea (HHV 7 > HHV 6) starts as "herald" or "mother" patch, then causes "fir-tree" or "Christmas-tree" rash, Collarette scales. Hanging curtain sign +ve. Self limiting.

HUMAN PAPILLOMA VIRUS (HPV)

- Causes warts. Presents as warty, verrucous, cauliflower-like (verruca = cauliflower) masses on skin
- HPV enters the epidermis through trauma. They trigger keratinocyte hyperproliferation and consequently are seen as elevated keratotic lesions on skin (see Figures 10A and B)
- Typically HPV can be **subclinical (70% of genital HPV infections are subclinical)**

- Warts are more extensive in immunosuppression
- Typically on removing the top layer with a scalpel, **thrombosed black vessels** are seen as black dots on the surface and is a useful diagnostic sign (Fig. 12B).

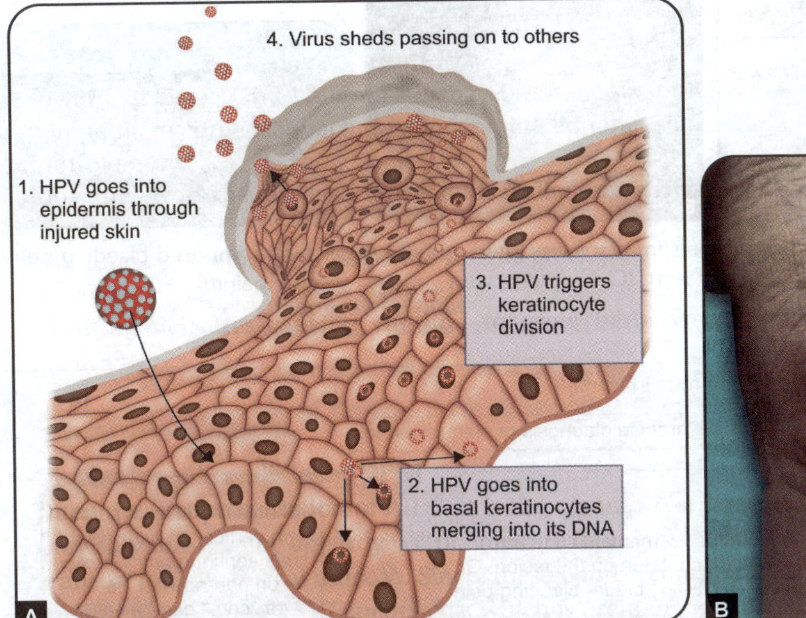

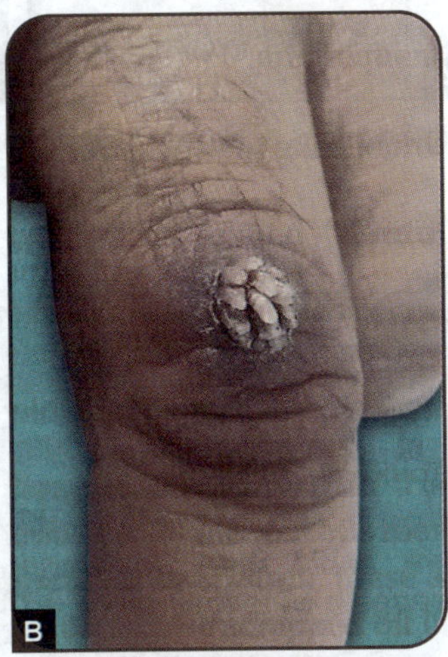

Figs. 10A and B: (A) Schematic representation of pathogenesis in warts; (B) Cauliflower-like, warty growths with finger-like projections

Types of Warts

1. **Common warts (verruca vulgaris)**—most common type (**vulgaris = common**)
   Mainly caused by HPV-2 (Figs. 11A and B)

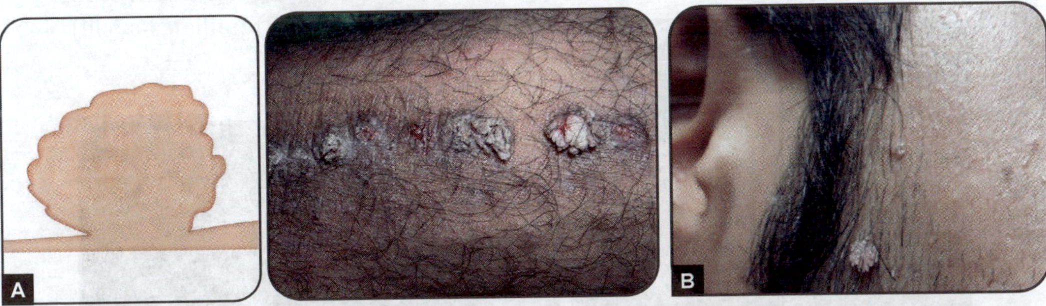

Figs. 11A and B: Verruca vulgaris: Cauliflower masses with pseudo-Koebner's phenomenon due to scratching; (B) Verruca vulgaris: cauliflower mass (beard area is commonly involved)

2. **Plantar warts (Figs. 12A to C):**
   - Superficial warts (**Mosaic warts**)—Painless superficial warts caused by HPV-2
   - Deep warts (**Myrmecia warts**)—Painful deep warts caused by HPV-1 (Fig. 12C)

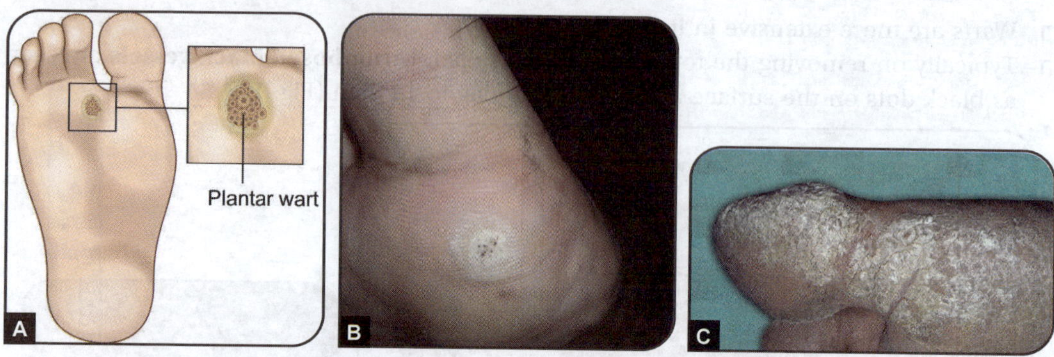

Figs. 12A to C: (A) Schematic representation of plantar wart; (B) Note the thrombosed bleeding points on parring of wart; (C) Myrmecia wart which would be painful

High Yield Points

How to differentiate plaques on foot in an MCQ?

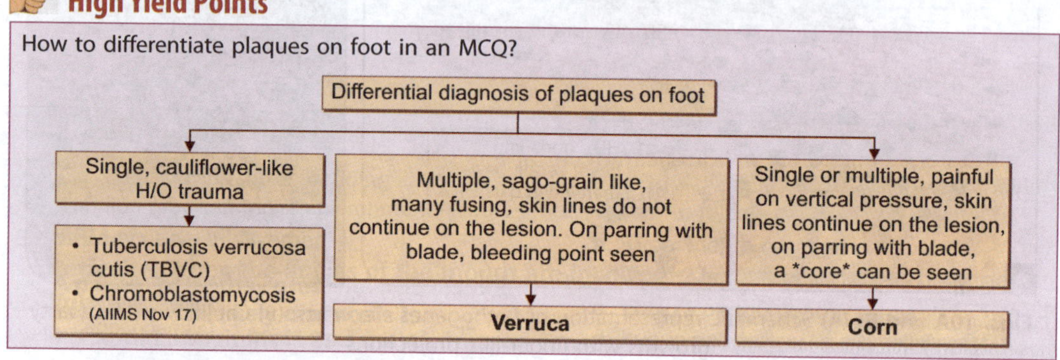

3. **Verruca plana (Plane warts)**
   - Presents as flatter (plana = flat) lesions (Figs. 13A and B)
   - Mainly due to HPV-3 and HPV-10
   - Most likely to increase by Koebner's (more accurately called pseudo-Koebner's) phenomenon.

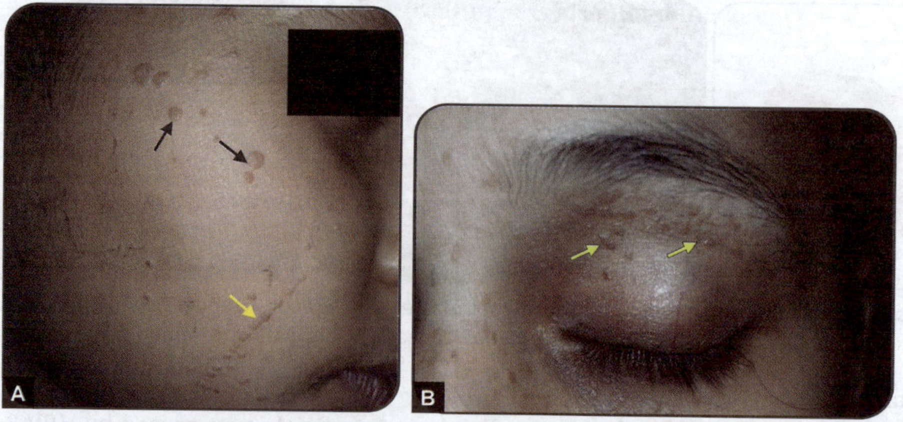

Figs. 13A and B: (A) Verruca plana: multiple lesions (black arrow) and pseudo-Koebner's phenomenon (yellow arrrow); (B) Verruca plana-multiple lesions on eyebrow area after parlor threading (yellow arrows)

Histopathology of Verruca

- Characteristic feature of **koilocytosis** of upper keratinocytes (spinous and granular layer), along with papillomatosis (elevation of dermal papilla) (Fig. 14).

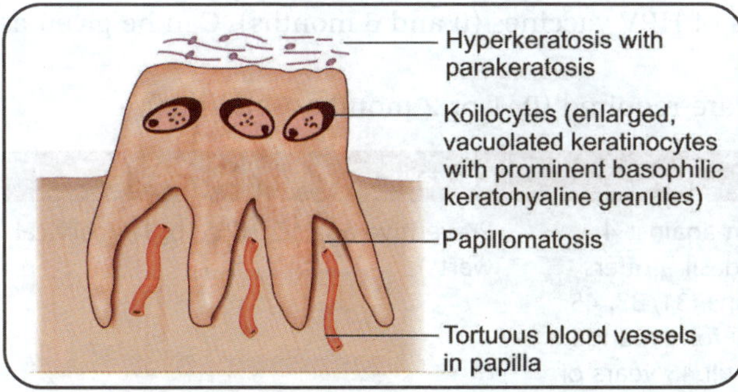

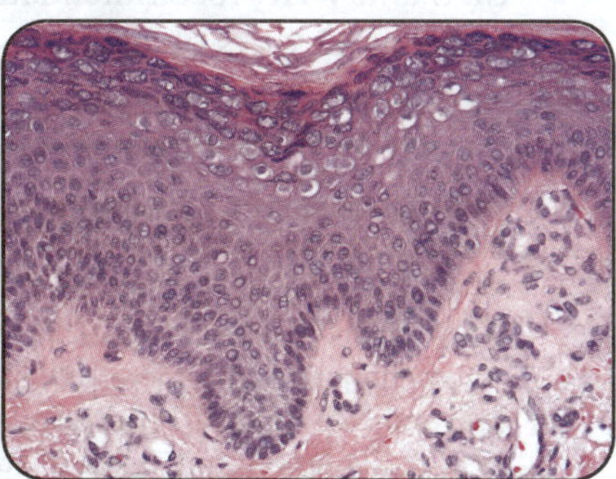

Fig. 14: Koilocytes with enlarged cells, pyknotic nucleus and clear cytoplasm (high power view)

Treatment for Common Warts, Plantar Warts and Plane Warts

- Spontaneous clearance of warts can occur at any time
- For cutaneous warts, destruction of infected area is commonly done.

First line (Self-applied by patient)	Second line (done by physician)
• **Salicylic acid**—Works as a keratolytic—**DOC** for common and plantar warts • Trichloroacetic acid, Glutaraldehyde, Formalin, 5- fluorouracil—all used topically	• Cryotherapy—cold liquid nitrogen is applied (Figs. 15A and B) • Electrocautery (Figs. 16A and B)

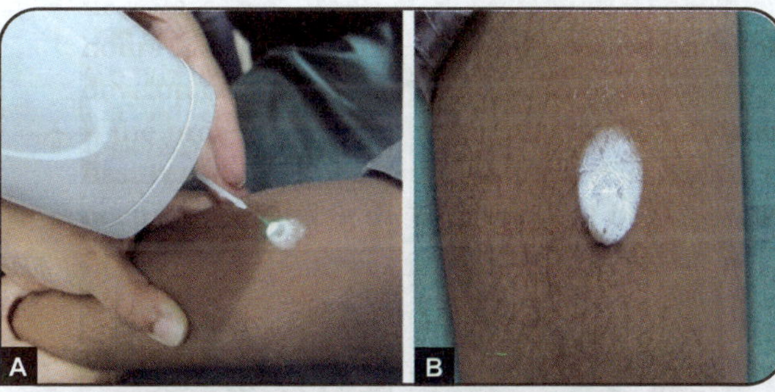

Figs. 15A and B: Cryotherapy with liquid nitrogen spray (A) being done; (B) Immediately afterwards

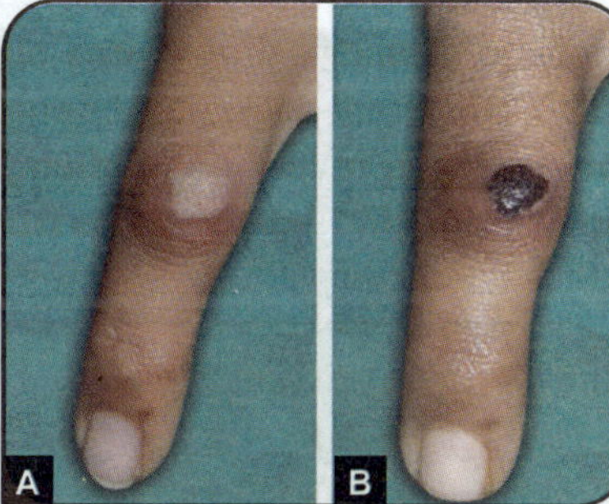

Figs. 16A and B: Electrocautery done for verruca (A) before; (B) Immediately afterwards

4. **Ano-genital warts (condyloma acuminata, external genital warts)**
   - Transmission is usually by sexual route
   - HPV 6 > HPV 11[(MCQ)]
   - **Pointed masses on genitalia** (Figs. 17A and B)

- Application of **acetic acid** to genital warts enhances visualization of the lesions by making them white (**aceto-whitening**)
- Prevention of genital wart is only by Gardasil HPV vaccine, not by Cervarix vaccine.
- CDC and WHO recommendations for HPV vaccines:
  - Below 15 years of age: 2 doses of HPV vaccines (0 and 6 months). Can be given as early as 9 years of age.
  - After 15 years of age: 3 doses are required (0, 1 or 2 months, 6 months).

Gardasil vaccine	Cervarix vaccine
Gardasil originally offered protection against 4 HPV strains (6, 11, 16, 18). Now Gardasil 9 offers protection against 5 more HPV strains (31, 33, 45, 52, and 58). FDA has given approval for expanded use of Gardasil from 9 years of age till 45 years of age for both males and females	Preventive against HPV 16, 18 (cervical warts)

- Low risk vs high risk HPVs

Low-risk HPV types	High-risk types
HPV 6,11—causes external genital warts	HPV-16, -18, 45, -31, -33, -52 and -58 causes cervical warts
Viral genomes replicate as extra chromosomal episomes	Viral DNA is integrated into the cellular chromosomes * In high-risk genital HPV types, *E6* and *E7* gene products bind and inactivate p53 (tumor suppressor gene) and retinoblastoma protein (pRb), respectively causing carcinogenesis.

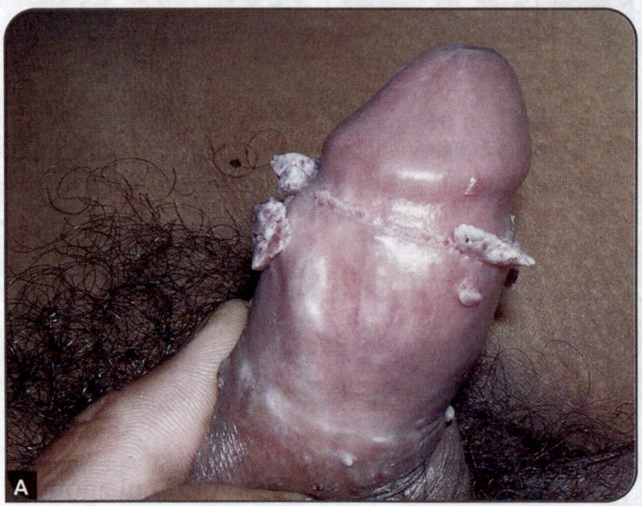

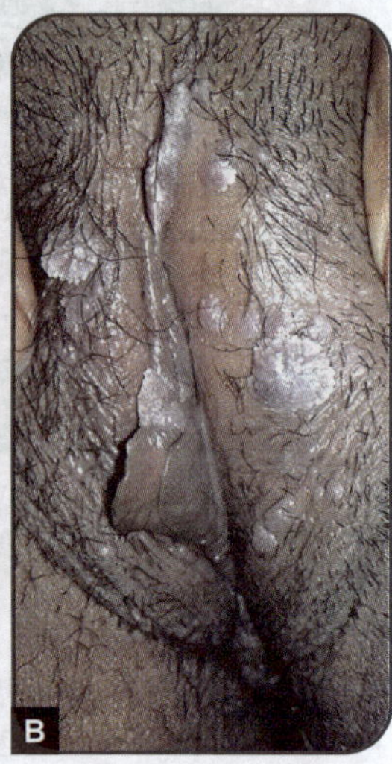

Figs. 17A and B: (A) Condyloma acuminata: Pointed (acuminate) masses on penile area; (B) Condyloma acuminata: Pointed (acuminate) masses on labia

Aid to Remember

"Acuminata" means pointed. Hence, pointed, finger-like masses seen in genital warts.

⅄ Treatment:

First line	Second line	Third line
Imiquimod—DOC[MCQ] * Imiquimod acts by stimulating Toll-like receptors (TLR) 7 and 8 and increasing several proinflammatory cytokines. Increased immunosurveillance removes warts (Figs. 18A to D)	**Cryotherapy with liquid nitrogen** (**more effective** than imiquimod and podophyllin but since it has to be administered by the doctor and not by patient, **it is not the therapy of choice**)	Interferon
Podophyllotoxin (purified form of podophyllin) *Act as antimitotics which disrupt the formation of the mitotic spindles	Trichloroacetic acid (80–90%) Surgery if numerous warts. Shave excision (where a superficial area of skin is shaved off with a blade) can also be used.[JIPMER Nov 17]	

Figs. 18A to D: (A) Condyloma acuminata: Pretreatment; (B) Condyloma acuminata: Same patient after imiquimod application; (C) Condyloma—Pretreatment; (D) Same patient after imiquimod application

High Yield Points

- Since podophyllin/podophyllotoxin/Imiquimod is better absorbed from **moist** surfaces, they are first line for genital warts and only third line for drier cutaneous warts.
- Topical 5% imiquimod is **FDA approved for treatment of genital warts, small superficial non-facial basal cell carcinoma and actinic keratosis**[MCQ]
- **Treatment of genital warts in pregnancy: Cryotherapy > Trichloroacetic acid**[MCQ]
  - Podophyllin/Podophyllotoxin is **contraindicated in pregnancy**[MCQ]
  - Routine cesarean section is not recommended for genital warts at labor (only a small risk for laryngeal papillomatosis of the newborn)

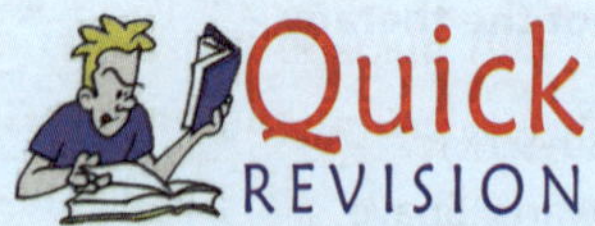

- HPV causes warts. Verruca is the term for non-genital warts and condyloma acuminata for genital warts
- HPV 6 > 11—Genital warts (Low risk types). HPV 16, 18—cervical warts (high risk HPV)
- Verruca vulgaris—HPV 2, Plantar warts- HPV 2 > HPV 1, Flat warts- HPV 3, 10
- Vacuolated keratinocytes (koilocytes) on histopathology
- Salicylic acid—DOC for cutaneous warts, Imiquimod as an immunomodulator—DOC for genital warts (Podophyllotoxin is an alternative for genital warts)
- Cryotherapy > TCA for genital warts in pregnancy
- Gardasil—Tetravalent HPV vaccine—Preventive for genital warts

Other Viral Infections

1. **Measles (Rubeola)**
   - RNA virus
   - Patients are contagious from 1 to 2 days before onset of symptoms to 4 days after the rash
   - Clinical—First prodrome occurs for up to 4 days (fever, palpebral conjunctivitis, coryza and cough). **Koplik spots** (pathognomonic- red macules with a blue-white speck within them) are seen on the **buccal mucosa near the lower second molars**(MCQ) 1–2 days before and 2 days after the rash. Exanthem is red, non-itchy, **begins on forehead,**(MCQ) behind the ear and quickly progresses to neck, abdomen and limbs. Rash disappears by 5 days.
2. **Rubella (German measles, 3-day measles)**
   - Mild, short prodrome with low grade fever, headache, conjunctivitis, rhinitis, cough, sore throat, and **lymphadenopathy (prominently suboccipital)**
   - As prodrome subsides, rash occurs beginning on the face quickly progressing to trunk and extremities. Petechiae confined to the soft palate (Forchheimer sign) are seen during the prodromal period or on the first day of the rash.
   - Rashes subside in 2- to 3-day duration (**faster than measles**)
3. **Erythema infectiosum (fifth disease)**(PGI Nov 15)
   - Caused by Parvovirus B19

- The classical rash begins with confluent, erythematous plaques on cheeks **("slapped cheeks")**(MCQ) soon followed by an erythematous, lacy rash on the trunk and extremities.

4. **Roseola infantum (exanthema subitum, sixth disease)**(MCQ)
   Etiology: Caused by HHV 6 > HHV 7
   Clinical: Typically starts with fever and on the fourth day as the fever drops, morbilliform rose-coloured macules appear on the neck, trunk, and buttocks (hence called roseola).
5. **Molluscum contagiosum**(MCQ) (AIIMS May 16, Nov 15)
   - Common in children (usually MCQs mention the child age-group)
   - Type 1 molluscum contagiosum virus (MCV-1) causes majority of infections
   - **Clinical**: Shiny, pearly white, umbilicated papules are classically seen (Figs. 20A and B). Pseudo-Koebner's phenomenon causes increase of lesions with scratching and trauma.

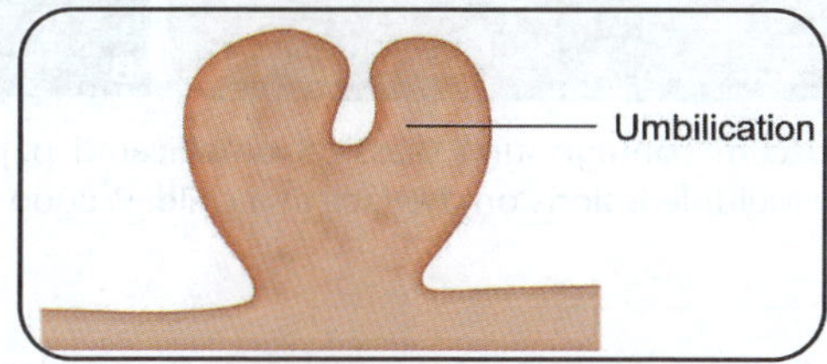

   - **Pathology:** MCV enters the basal epidermis causing it to increase division. This cellular proliferation produces epidermal growths which are seen as papules clinically. Infected keratinocytes show **hyaline bodies (molluscum bodies, Henderson-Paterson bodies)**(MCQ) (AIIMS May 2016) (Figs. 19A and B).

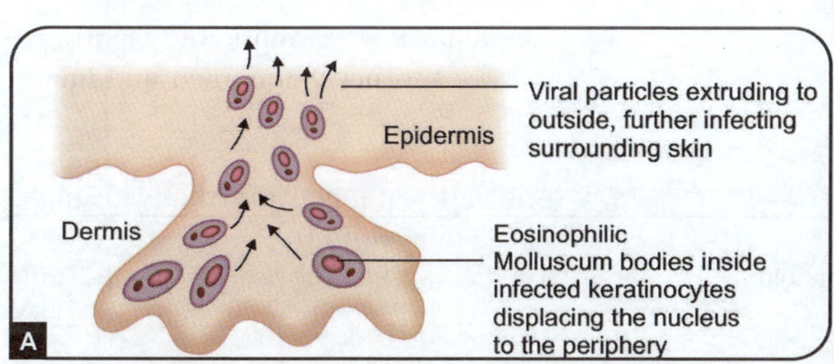

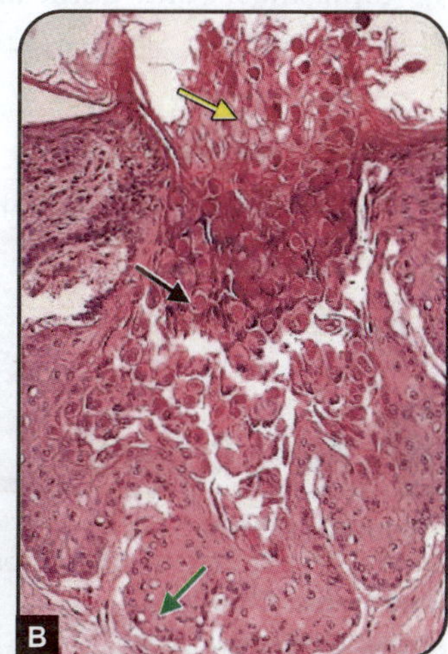

Figs. 19A and B: (A) Schematic representation of molluscum exiting the epidermis; (B) Compare this actual histopathology to the schematic 19A image. Note the basal epidermis first (green arrow). Also note the molluscum bodies (black arrow). These molluscum bodies are extruding to the outside from the top and will then infect the surrounding skin (yellow arrow)

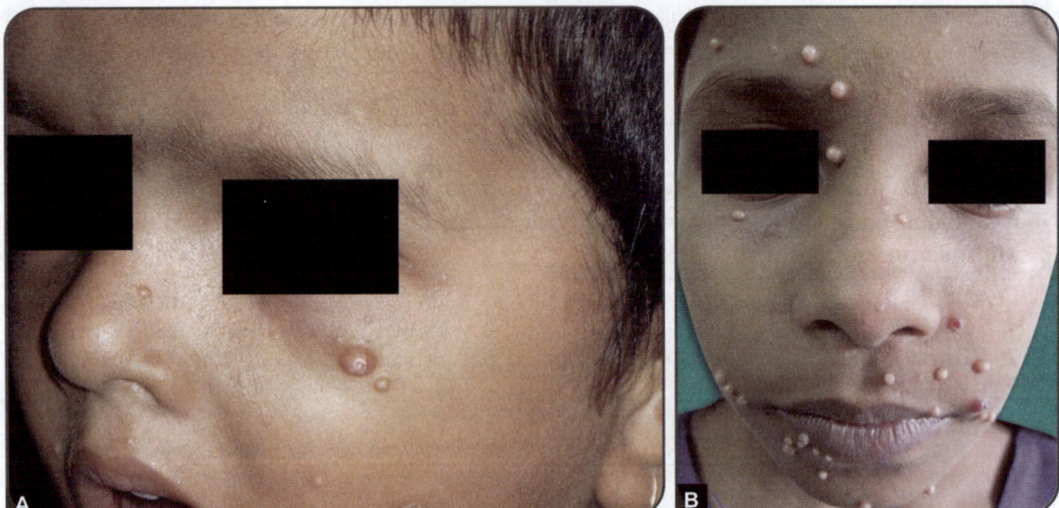

Figs. 20A and B: (A) Molluscum contagiosum: Classical umbilicated papules on the face in a child; (B) Molluscum contagiosum: Multiple lesions on the face in a child. Pseudo-Koebner's phenomenon seen near right angle of mouth

- **Treatment:** Most cases are self-limiting within 6–9 months.
- 1st line: Trichloroacetic acid, salicylic acid, KOH, Topical retinoids
  2nd line: Needle removal, cryotherapy

- Molluscum-like lesions also occur in cryptococcosis-associated with meningitis, histoplasmosis and penicilliosis-associated with lung manifestation (all AIDS defining illnesses)

 **High Yield Points**

- Pick-up word in MCQs—Pearly papule, face, child, umbilication

6. Kawasaki disease

Aid to Remember

Diagnostic criteria
5 = Fever > **5** days, Child < **5** years old
Mnemonic: CHILD
Conjunctivitis (bilateral)
Hyperthermia (fever) > 5 days
Idiopathic polymorphic rash
Lymphadenopathy (cervical)
Dryness and redness of (i) lips and tongue, (ii) palms and soles

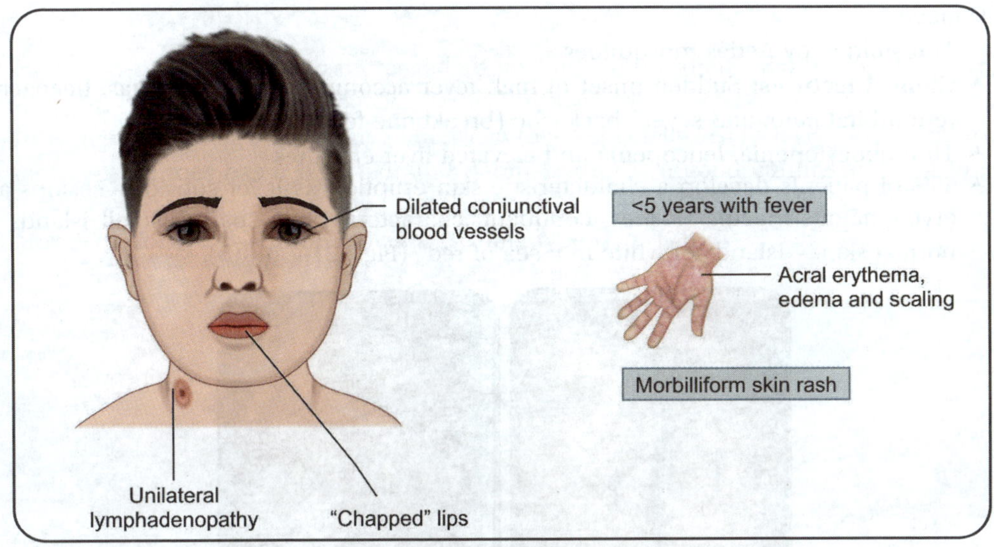

7. Various common skin rashes with fever (exanthems)

Aid to Remember

Mnemonic **"M**any **S**enior **R**esidents **D**o **E**ncounter **E**xanthems"	**Day of appearance of rash after fever** **Mnemonic: "V**ery **S**ick **P**erson **M**ust **T**ake **D**ouble **T**ablets"
Measles (Rubeola)—1st disease **S**carlet fever—2nd disease **R**ubella (German measles)—3rd disease **D**uke's disease—4th disease **E**rythema infectiosum—5th disease **E**xanthem subitum (Roseola)—6th disease	**V**ery (Varicella-day 1) **S**ick (Scarlet fever-day 2) **P**erson (Pox-small pox-day 3) **M**ust—(Measles-day 4) **T**ake—(Typhus-day 5) **D**ouble (Dengue-day 6) **T**ablets—(Typhoid-day 7)

8. Centripetal vs Centrifugal rashes[(AIIMS)]

Primarily central/truncal Mnemonic: "**R**ed **R**ashes **S**care **P**arents **V**ery **M**uch"	Primarily on extremities Mnemonic: You drive **CARS** with your Hands and Feet
Rubella	**CA**—**C**oxsackie **A** virus (Hand, foot, mouth disease)
Roseola	**R**—Rocky mountain spotted fever
Scarlet fever	**S**—Secondary syphilis
Parvovirus B19 (Erythema infectiosum)	
Varicella	
Measles	

9. Dengue
   - Transmitted by Aedes mosquitoes
   - **Clinical features:** Sudden onset of high fever accompanied by myalgias, headache, retroorbital pain, and severe backache (breakbone fever)
   - Thrombocytopenia, leucopenia and elevated liver enzymes
   - 50% of patients develop a characteristic skin eruption as fever subsides–Lesions are erythematous macular rashes, confluent, characteristically sparing small islands of normal skin—"islands of white in a sea of red" (Figs. 21A and B).

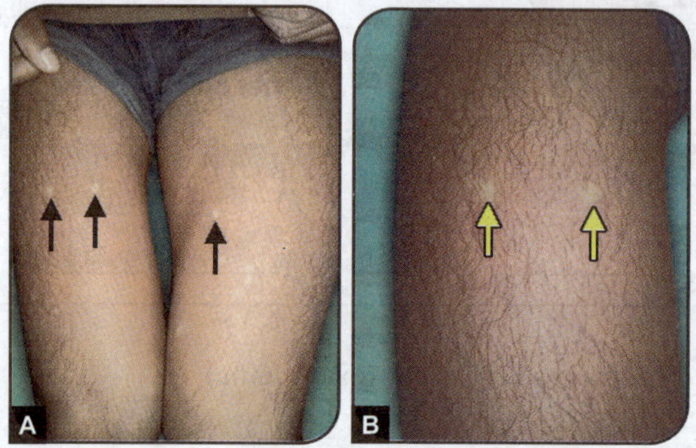

Figs. 21A and B: (A) Dengue rash—"Islands of white in a sea of red" (black arrows); (B) Close up of the rash. Note the spared areas (yellow arrows)

10. Hand, foot and mouth disease (HFMD) (Figs. 22A and B)(PGI Nov 17)
    - Caused by coxsackie virus A in children from 2 to 10
    - Begins with fever, followed by oral lesions (small rapidly ulcerating vesicles surrounded by a red border)
    - Lesions on the hands and feet occur with small vesicles surrounded by a red halo. They are often parallel to the skin lines on the fingers and toes
    - Especially in children who wear diapers, similar lesions occur on buttocks.

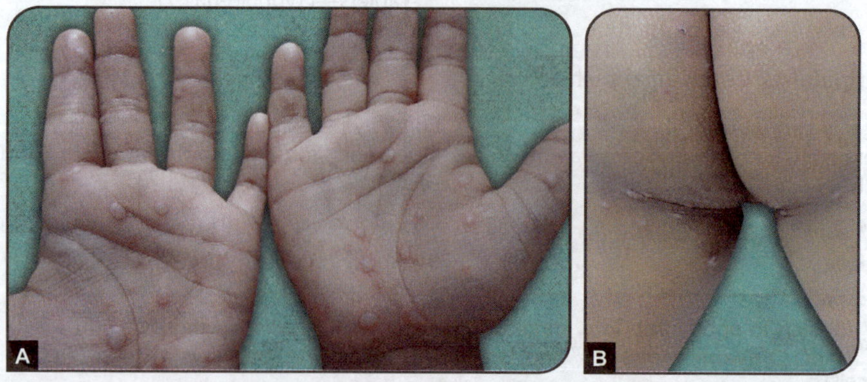

Figs. 22A and B: (A) Vesicles surrounded by a red halo, few along skin creases; (B) Vesicles on buttocks and thigh

QUESTIONS

1. Cervical warts are seen with which HPV?

a. 11, 13 b. 6, 11
c. 16, 18 d. 5, 8

2. Genital warts are most commonly caused by which of the following serotype of HPV?

a. HPV 6 b. HPV 16
c. HPV 18 d. HPV 33

3. Myrmecia wart is:

a. Planar wart
b. Plantar wart
c. Verrucous wart
d. Palmar wart

4. A male patient with flat lesions on face which are increasing gradually. The diagnosis would be:

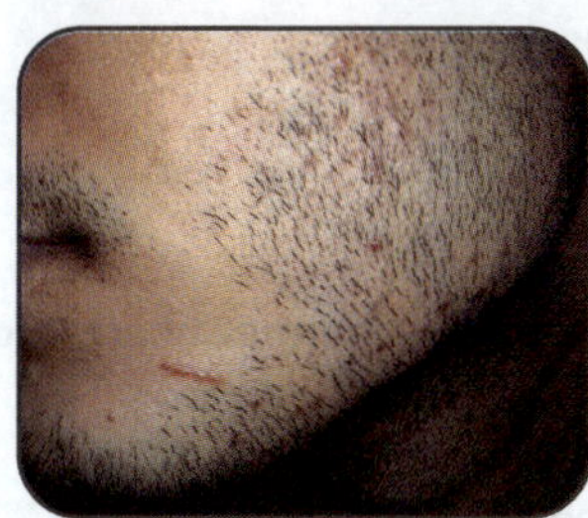

a. Psoriasis
b. Lichen planus
c. Verruca plana
d. Molluscum

5. Verruca vulgaris is caused by:

a. CMV b. EBV
c. HIV d. HPV

6. Type of human Papilloma virus associated with carcinoma cervix:

a. Types 6, 12, 18
b. Types 16, 18, 31
c. Types 6, 8, 11
d. Types 3, 10, 19

7. Low risk HPV: *(DNB June 14)*

a. Type 31 b. Type 6
c. Type 18 d. Type 16

8. Podophyllum resin is indicated in the treatment of:

a. Pemphigus
b. Psoriasis
c. Condyloma lata
d. Condyloma acuminata

9. Topical immunomodulator used for the treatment of genital warts is:

a. Imiquimod
b. Interferon
c. Acyclovir
d. Podophyllin

10. Imiquimod used in treatment of anogenital warts acts mainly as:

a. Antiviral
b. Keratolytic
c. Antifungal
d. Immunostimulator

11. All are true regarding viral warts *except:* *(PGI)*

a. Basophilic stippling
b. Koilocytes are characteristic
c. Spontaneous regression common in children
d. Perinuclear vacuolization
e. Verruca vulgaris is associated with HPV 12

12. Regarding podophyllin resin which of the following statement is true?

a. Derived from plant source
b. Safe in pregnancy
c. Teratogenic
d. High recurrence rate of wart after podophyllin resin treatment
e. Individual variation in response rate

13. Treatment of choice in genital warts in pregnancy:

a. Salicylic acid with lactic acid solution
b. Podophyllin
c. Imiquimod
d. Cryotherapy

14. HPV vaccine is:
a. Monovalent
b. Bivalent
c. Quadrivalent
d. Bivalent and quadrivalent

15. Multiple erythematous annular lesions with peripheral collarette of scales arranged predominantly on trunk are seen in:
a. Pityriasis rosea
b. Pityriasis versicolor
c. Pityriasis rubra pilaris
d. Pityriasis lichenoides chronica

16. Christmas tree arrangement of skin lesion is seen in:
a. Pityriasis versicolor
b. Pityrosporum folliculitis
c. Pityriasis rosea
d. Tinea corporis

17. Herald patch is seen in:
a. Pityriasis rosea
b. Discoid lupus erythematosus
c. Lichen planus
d. Lichen nitidus

18. Types of scale observed in pityriasis rosea is:
a. Mica like b. Silvery
c. Powdery d. Collarette-like

19. Slapped cheek appearance is caused by:
a. Parvovirus b. Rubella
c. Measles d. HHV-6

20. A lady presents with pearly white papule on forehead with central umbilication. Which of the following will most probably be the causative organism?
a. Pox b. Coxsackie
c. Herpes d. HHV-6

21. Pearly umbilicated lesions on face are seen in:
a. Molluscum contagiosum
b. Impetigo
c. Congenital syphilis
d. Norwegian scabies

22. A patient presents with the following lesions. The diagnosis is: *(Recent NEET pattern)*

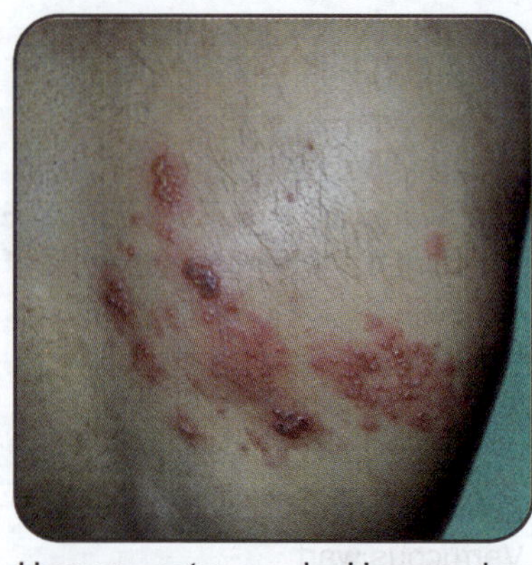

a. Herpes zoster b. Herpes simplex
c. Insect bites d. Pemphigus

23. A 3-year-old female child develops umbilicated papule over face. Probable diagnosis is: *(AIIMS)*
a. Lichen planus
b. Chickenpox
c. Molluscum contagiosum
d. Scabies

24. Treatment of genital wart include all, *except*:
a. Trichloroacetic acid 10–25%
b. Trichloroacetic acid 30–50%
c. Podophyllin
d. Interferon
e. Salicylic acid

25. A 25-year-old pregnant women presents with a growing vulval warty lesion to you. The best treatment would be:
a. Podophyllum
b. Cryotherapy
c. Trichloroacetic acid
d. Electrosurgery

26. Herpes zoster is commonly seen in:
a. Cervical region b. Thoracic region
c. Lumbar region d. Genital region

27. Ballooning is a classical feature of:
a. Herpes zoster b. Pemphigus
c. Pemphigoid d. Insect bite

28. Most common site of herpes simplex is:

a. Thorax b. Abdomen
c. Extremities d. Face

29. A patient with recurrent raw lesions on the genitals as shown in the image. These lesions healed without hyperpigmentation. The likely diagnosis is:

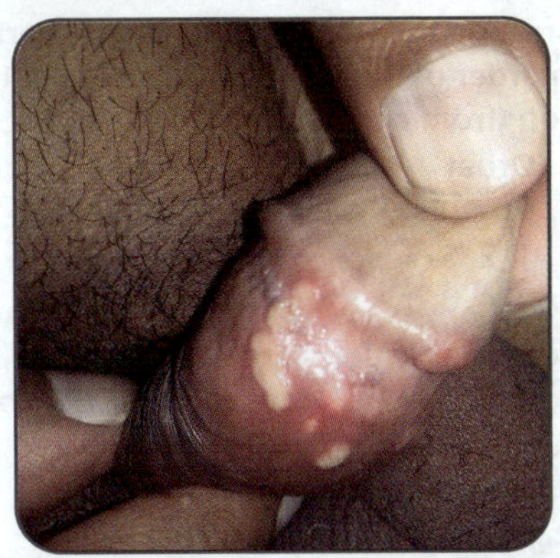

a. Herpes genitalis b. Aphthous ulcer
c. Syphilis d. Chancroid

30. A child presents with dome shaped, pearly lesions on forehead. Mother also similar lesions. The likely diagnosis is:

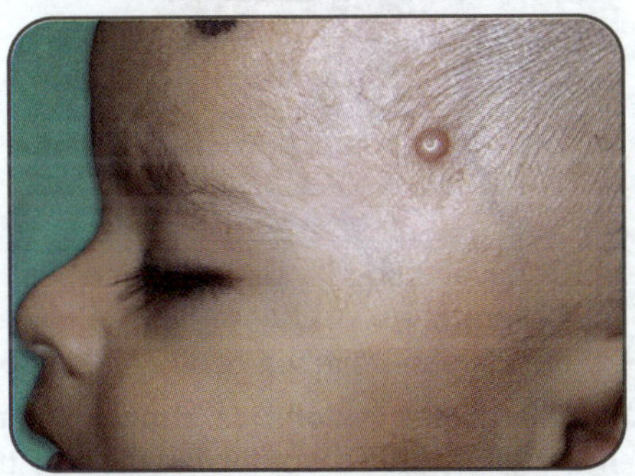

a. Scabies b. Pox
c. Herpes d. Molluscum

31. Herpes resistant to acyclovir is treated by:

a. Foscarnet b. Lamivudine
c. Valacyclovir d. Ganciclovir

32. Imiquimod is approved for use in all *except:*

a. Condyloma acuminata
b. Basal cell carcinoma
c. Squamous cell carcinoma
d. Actinic keratosis

33. A 28-year-old lady has asymptomatic dome shaped small lesions on forehead for last 2 months. She has a 2-year-old daughter with similar lesions. What is the causative agent? *(AIIMS Nov 15)*

a. Papillomavirus b. Poxvirus
c. Herpesvirus d. Coxsackievirus

34. Slapped cheek appearance is seen in:

a. Parvovirus b. EBV
c. HHV 6 d. HHV 4
e. Toxic shock syndrome

35. The rash which is not central in predisposition is:

a. Epidemic typhus
b. Measles
c. Secondary syphilis
d. Typhoid

36. A patient presents with lesions as shown. The likely pathogen is:

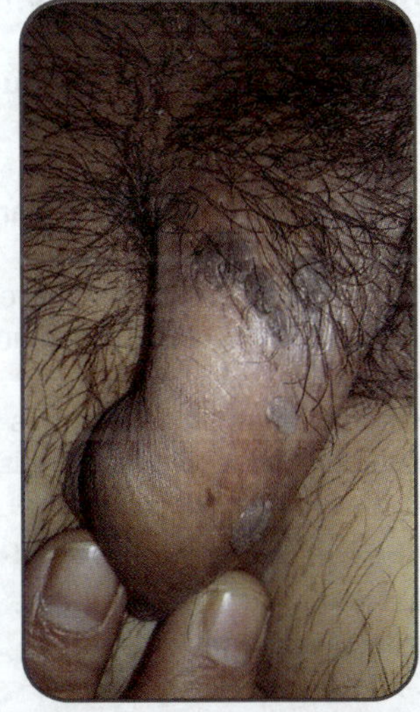

a. HPV 16, 18 b. HPV 6, 11
c. HPV 2, 3 d. HPV 7

37. Postherpetic neuralgia is defined as pain lasting beyond how many weeks?

a. 1 week b. 2 weeks
c. 3 weeks d. 4 weeks

New Questions

38. The following statements are true/false regarding causes of rash on skin which is primarily truncal, relatively sparing the acral areas:

a. Rubella
b. Secondary syphilis
c. Coxsackievirus infection
d. Measles
e. Varicella

39. Assertion: Imiquimod is the drug of choice for genital warts
Reason: Imiquimod is an anti-mitotic

a. Both Assertion and Reason are true and Reason is correct explanation of Assertion
b. Both Assertion and Reason are true but Reason is not correct explanation of Assertion
c. Assertion is true and Reason is false
d. Assertion is false and Reason is true
e. Both Assertion and Reason are false

40. Assertion: HPV 16 and 18 are high risk HPV types
Reason: *E6* and *E7* gene products bind and inactivate *p53* gene

a. Both Assertion and Reason are true and Reason is correct explanation of Assertion
b. Both Assertion and Reason are true but Reason is not correct explanation of Assertion
c. Assertion is true and Reason is false
d. Assertion is false and Reason is true
e. Both Assertion and Reason are false

41. Mark the treatment options for HPV:
a. Interferon
b. Gardasil vaccine
c. Inj. MMR
d. Acitretin

1. If a, c, d are correct
2. If a and b are correct
3. If b and d are correct
4. If all four (a, b, c, & d) are correct

42. Match items in column A with best alternative in column B:

Column A	Column B
1. HHV-1	a Most common STD in the world
2. HHV-4	b Kaposi varicelliform eruption
3. HHV-2	c Atypical lymphocytes on smear
4. HHV-7	d Collarette scales
	e Kaposi sarcoma
	f. Dermatomal distribution classically

43. Arrange the following lesions in varicella in order of their time of onset in the infection (from earliest to last):

1. Crust **2. Vesicle**
3. Pustule **4. Papule**

a. 1, 2, 3, 4 b. 2, 1, 4, 3
c. 2, 4, 3, 1 d. 4, 2, 3, 1

44. Vesicular lesions are seen in: *(INICET Nov 22)*

a. Hand, foot mouth disease
b. Roseola
c. Dengue
d. Measles

45. A child presents with multiple lesions on thigh and genital area. Some lesions have umbilication. Histology is as shown. What is being shown? *(INICET Nov 22)*

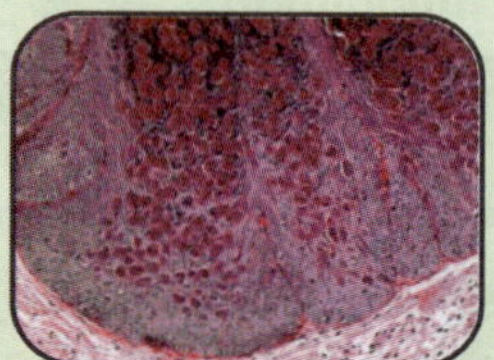

a. Donovan body b. Tzanck cell
c. Koilocyte
d. Henderson-Peterson body

46. A patient has lesions as shown. Patient mentioned that a spider crawled in that area while sleeping. The diagnosis is: *(INICET May 22)*

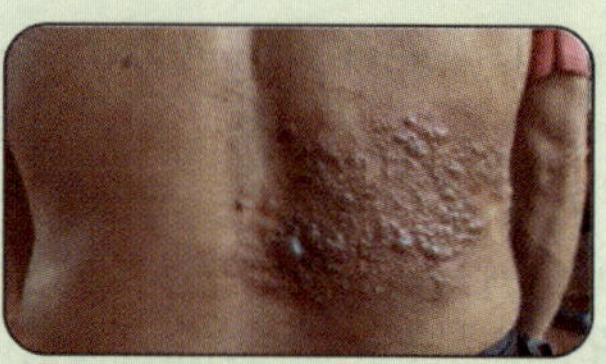

a. Allergic dermatitis b. Irritant dermatitis
c. Herpes zoster d. Chickenpox

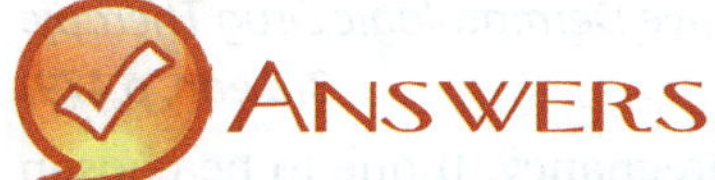

1. **Ans. (c) 16, 18** *(Ref: Rook's Textbook of Dermatology, 9th edn, p 25.29)*

   High-risk HPV (16, 18) is commonly detected in dysplastic cervical lesions and is found in majority of cervical cancers.

2. **Ans. (a) HPV 6** *(Ref: Rook's Textbook of Dermatology, 9th edn, p 25.56)*

   The low-risk HPVs cause most cases of ano-genital warts, most commonly HPV-6 (in 45–90%) or HPV-11.

3. **Ans. (b) Plantar wart** *(Ref: Andrew's Textbook, 11th edn, p 399)*

4. **Ans. (c) Verruca plana**

   The image is showing flat verruca lesions with pseudo-Koebners phenomenon on the chin area

5. **Ans. (d) HPV** (See page 135 for explanation)

6. **Ans. (b) Types 16,18,31** *(Ref: Fitzpatrick's Textbook, 8th edn, p 2422)*

   High-risk HPVs (HPV 16 > 18, 45, 31, 33, 52 and 58) cause cervical warts and hence cervical cancers.

7. **Ans. (b) Type 6** (See page 140 for explanation)

8. **Ans. (d) Condyloma acuminata** *(Ref: Fitzpatrick's Textbook, 8th edn, p 2432)*

9. **Ans. (a) Imiquimod** *(Ref: Andrew's Textbook, 11th edn, p 403)*

   Imiquimod is an immune response modifier that induces local interferon production at the site of application. It is more effective than podophyllotoxin in treating women with genital warts, but equally effective in men.

10. **Ans. (d) Immunostimulator** *(Ref: Andrew's Textbook, 11th edn, p 403)*

11. **Ans. (e) Verruca vulgaris is associated with HPV 12**

    (Ref: McKee's Pathology of Skin, 4th edn, p 763)

    Genital warts in children spontaneously resolve in 75% cases. On histopathology, large cells with prominent vacuolated cytoplasm and a small pyknotic nucleus are seen in the upper layers of the epidermis (koilocytes). A prominent granular cell layer containing large clumps of irregular basophilic keratohyaline is also seen. Verruca vulgaris is associated with HPV-2 and butchers wart with HPV-7.

12. **Ans. (a, c, d, e) Derived from plant source; Teratogenic; High recurrence rate of wart after podophyllin resin treatment; Individual variation in response rates**

    Podophyllin is an extract of cytotoxic material from the May apple plant (either Podophyllum peltatum or Podophyllum emodi). Podophyllotoxin is the active ingredient in podophyllin. Podophyllin is contraindicated in pregnancy as it has mutagenic properties. Response rates vary with podophyllin due to difficulty in standardizing the molecule. Recurrence rates are more than imiquimod.

13. Ans. (d) Cryotherapy *(Ref: Wolverton's Comprehensive Dermatologic Drug Therapy, 3rd edn, p 479)*

Both cryotherapy and trichloroacetic acid are useful in pregnancy. If one to be chosen between them, choose cryotherapy.

14. Ans. (d) Bivalent and quadrivalent (See page 140 for explanation)

15. Ans. (a) Pityriasis rosea *(Ref: Fitzpatrick's Textbook, 8th edn, p 458)*

16. Ans. (c) Pityriasis Rosea *(Ref: Fitzpatrick's Textbook, 8th edn, p 458)*

17. Ans. (a) Pityriasis rosea (See page 134 for explanation)

18. Ans. (d) Collarette-like *(Ref: Fitzpatrick's Textbook, 8th edn, p 458)*

Mica-like scale and silvery scales are seen in psoriasis. Powdery scale are seen in pityriasis versicolor.

19. Ans. (a) Parvovirus *(Ref: Andrew's Textbook, 11th edn, p 393)*

20. Ans. (a) Pox (See page 144 for explanation)

21. Ans. (a) Molluscum contagiosum (See page 144 for explanation)

22. Ans. (a) Herpes Zoster

23. Ans. (c) Molluscum contagiosum (See page 144 for explanation)

In molluscum infection in children, facial involvement is commonly seen.

24. Ans. (a, b) Tricholoroacetic acid 10–25%; Tricholoroacetic acid 30–50%

Tricholoroacetic acid is used in concentration of 80-90% in external genital warts.

25. Ans. (b) Cryotherapy

26. Ans. (b) Thoracic region *(Ref: Andrew's Textbook, 11th edn, p 372)*

Thoracic involvement is most commonly seen (55%) followed by cranial (20%, with the trigeminal nerve being the most common single nerve involved), lumbar (15%), and sacral (5%).

27. Ans. (a) Herpes zoster *(Ref: Mckee's Pathology of Skin, 4th edn, p 774)*

28. Ans. (d) Face (See page 126 for explanation)

29. Ans. (a) Herpes genitalis (See page 128 for explanation)

30. Ans. (d) Molluscum

31. Ans. (a) Foscarnet *(Ref: Fitzpatrick's Textbook, 8th edn, p 2793)*

Thymidine kinase is important for action of acyclovir on HSV. In resistant herpes strains, there is mutation in thymidine kinase. Foscarnet does not utilize thymidine kinase but acts on viral DNA polymerases. Hence, it is effective on resistant strains.

32. Ans. (c) Squamous cell carcinoma

(Ref: Wolverton's Comprehensive Dermatologic Drug Therapy, 3rd edn, p 476)

Imiquimod is FDA approved for the treatment of genital warts, Actinic keratosis and small (<2 cm) non-facial superficial BCC, if surgery is inappropriate.

33. Ans. (b) Poxvirus (See page 144 for explanation)
Dome shaped lesions are seen in molluscum.

34. Ans. (a) Parvovirus (See page 144 for explanation)

35. Ans. (c) Secondary syphilis (See page 146 for explanation)

36. Ans. (b) HPV 6,11 (See page 140 for explanation)

37. Ans. (d) 4 weeks (See page 132 for explanation)

New Answers

38. Ans. a-True; b-False; c-False; d-True; e-True

39. Ans. (c) Assertion is true and Reason is false

40. Ans. (a) Both Assertion and Reason are true and Reason is correct explanation of Assertion

41. Ans. (1) If a, c, d are correct
Gardasil is a preventive vaccine and not for treatment of HPV

42. Ans. 1-b; 2-c; 3-a; 4-d

43. Ans. (d) 4, 2, 3, 1

44. Ans. (a) Hand, foot mouth disease

45. Ans. (d) Henderson-Peterson body

46. Ans. (c) Herpes zoster

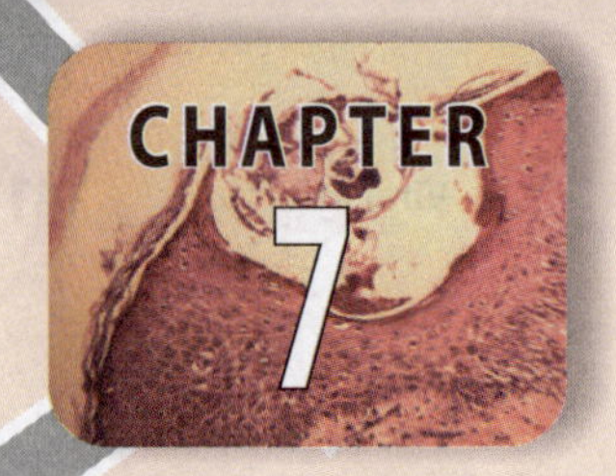

Protozoal, Arthropods and Parasitic Infections

SCABIES

- Highly contagious disease caused by the mite Sarcoptes scabiei var. hominis
- Transmitted by intimate personal contact, sharing of inanimate objects, and fomite
- **Genital scabies is an STD**(MCQ)

Mite Anatomy and Life Cycle

- The adult female mite is 0.4 × 0.3 mm in size while male is 0.2 mm × 0.15 mm with a flattened, oval body and eight legs (Fig. 1).
- Fertilized female mite penetrates the corneum (creating a **burrow**(MCQ) at the entry point in the stratum corneum) and as it advances lays **3 eggs a day**.
- The larvae hatch from these eggs and mature in 14 to 17 days.
- Itching starts **after 3–4 weeks of infestation.**
- Reinfection of a previously cured individual, however, may provoke immediate symptoms **within 2 days.**(MCQ)

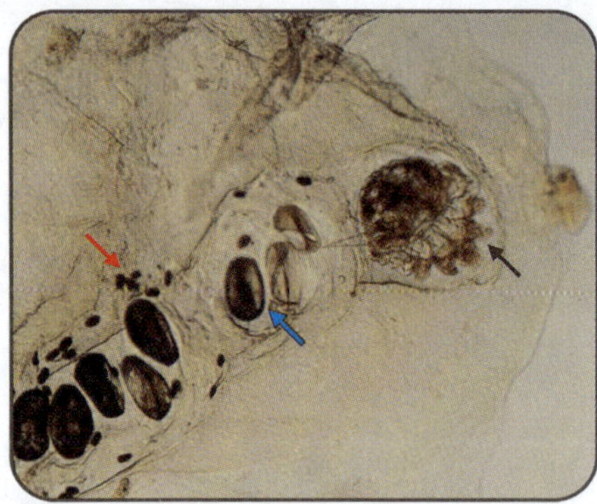

Fig. 1: Sarcoptes scabiei mite (black arrow), Eggs (blue arrow) and fecal pellets (red arrow)

Clinical

- Burrow is the **pathognomonic lesion**(MCQ) of scabies. It is linear, curved, or **S-shaped.**(MCQ) The mite is seen at the advancing edge of the burrow. Burrows are seen in finger webs, wrists, penis, buttocks, scrotum, and the palms and soles of infants (Figs. 2A and B).

***Burrows are absent in animal scabies**(MCQ)

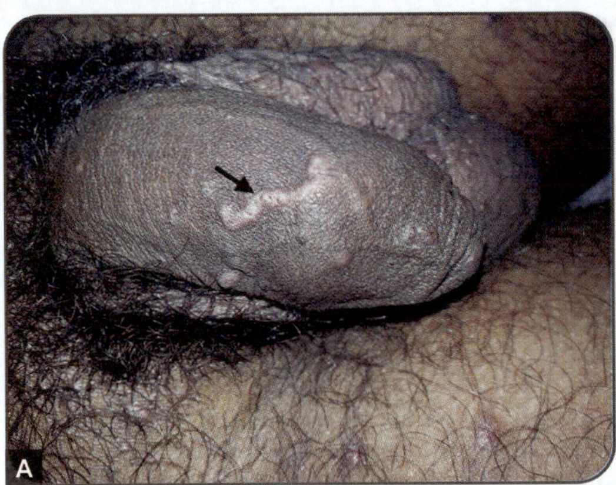

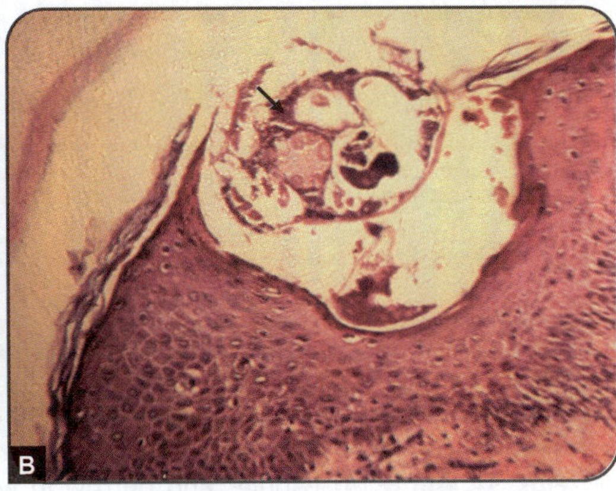

Figs. 2A and B: (A) Classical S-shaped burrow on genitals; (B) Histopathology in scabies- Note the scabies mite (black arrow) in the superficial epidermis

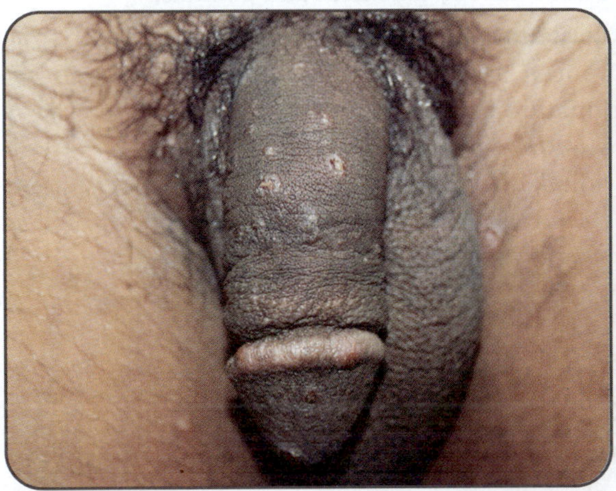

Fig. 3: Excoriated papules on genitals and scrotum

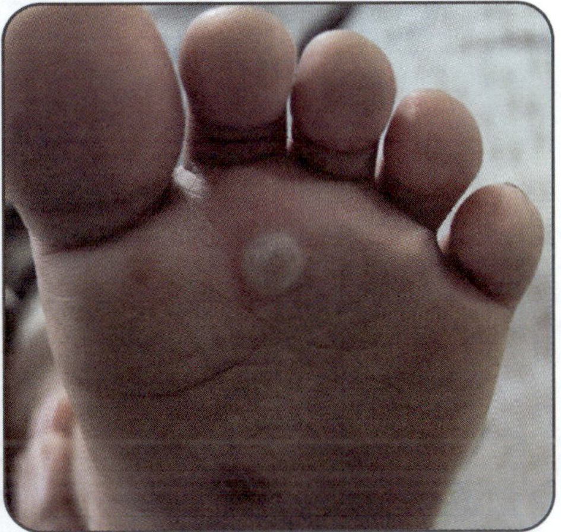

Fig. 4: Vesicles on soles in infants

- **After about a month**, itching starts making the patient scratch (Fig. 3). As the mite is superficial, they are dislodged by nails. This helps control the mite population. Hence, average number of mites on skin is less- **12 (range 5–15)**(MCQ)
- The number of burrows in skin **doesn't correlate with the number of mites on skin**
- **Nocturnal pruritus**(NEET)(MCQ) is highly characteristic of scabies.
- The classical lesion in an adult is an **itchy papule** (Fig. 5A) (papules are due to hypersensitivity and **rarely harbor mites**). Pustules are due to scratching and are a sign of secondary infection (Fig. 5B).

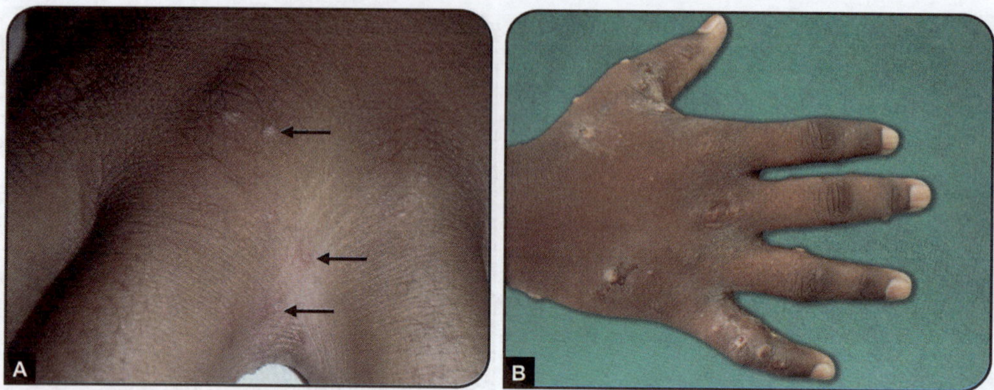

Figs. 5A and B: (A) Papules and burrow in webs (black arrows); (B) Papules with pustules due to secondary infection

- **Circle of Hebra**: An imaginary circle connecting the main sites of involvement—starting from finger webs, wrists, elbow flexures, axillae, areola, umbilicus and genitals.

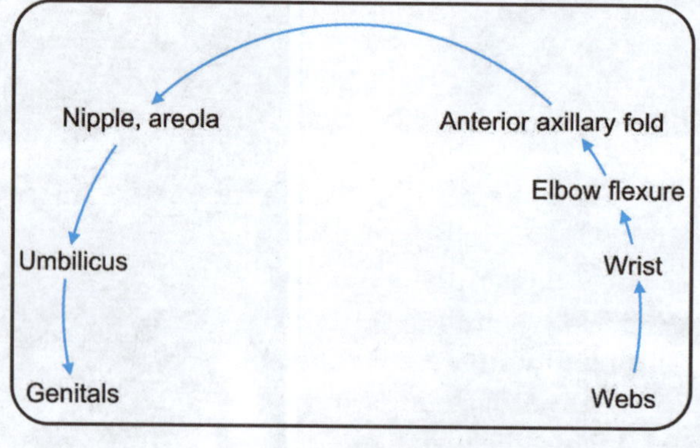

Circle of hebra

High Yield Points

Adult scabies	Infant scabies[MCQ]
Papules	Papules + vesicles (Fig. 4)[MCQ]
Face not involved (sebum protection)[MCQ]	Face involved (no sebum protection)[MCQ]
Palms and soles not involved[MCQ]	Palms and soles involved (classical feature) (Figs. 4 and 6)[MCQ]

High Yield Points

- **Pick up these phrases in MCQs on infantile scabies**—Papulovesicles on palms and soles, face involvement

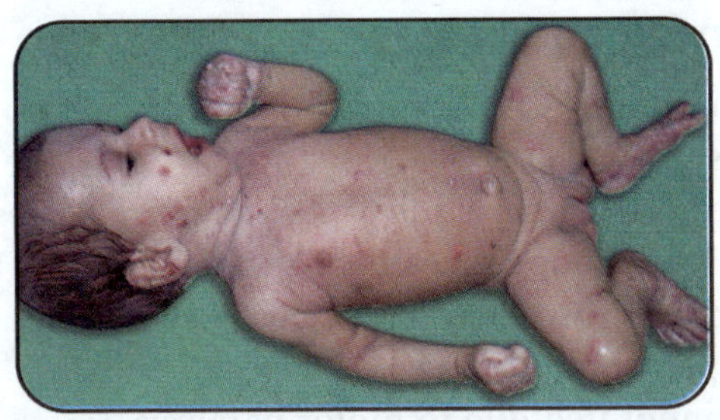

Fig. 6: Infantile scabies: Note the involvement of the face, palms and soles

Diagnosis

- **KOH or mineral oil mount** of scrapings demonstrate the mites, eggs, fecal pellets (scybala) (Fig. 1)
- **Fountain pen ink** when applied on burrows will remain inside the burrow and make them more visible
- **Wood's lamp**: Fluorescent substance like tetracycline paste is applied on burrow. Tetracycline will fluoresce under Wood's lamp.

Treatment

- **Five percent permethrin (single overnight application—neck to toe in adults, head to toe in infants) is the DOC**[MCQ] in **all ages including infants above 2 years of age and pregnant women**. It paralyzes the nerves not allowing the mite to breathe. Permethrin kills both the scabies mite and eggs. Hence, a single application is sufficient.
- **Oral ivermectin**[MCQ]: As ivermectin **does not kill eggs**[MCQ] a repeat dose is given after 1–2 weeks **(200 mcg/kg)**[MCQ] when the eggs become the second wave of adults. It acts on nerve synapses utilizing **glutamate.**[MCQ] It is not recommended for use in children less than 15 kg or in pregnant or lactating women
- Topical sulfur is safe for infants less than 2 months old and pregnant and nursing women but is messy, has an unpleasant odor and stains clothes and is **not preferred**
- **Gamma benzene hexachloride, lindane, benzoyl benzoate, crotamiton** are other agents used[MCQ]
- Itching continues for a week or two even after the mite has been killed. Both sexual and close personal contacts who have had direct prolonged skin-to-skin contact with an infected person within the preceding month should also be treated.
- **Clothing needs disinfection**[MCQ] (hot launder of clothes used in past 72 hours). If not possible, they must be kept in a plastic bag for up to 72 hrs as mites automatically die after this time.[MCQ]

Nodular Scabies[AIIMS 97]

- **Hypersensitivity** response to the mite (Fig. 7)
- Seen as nodules on genitals[MCQ] with severe itching
- Needs anti-scabetics along with intralesional steroids

Crusted Scabies (Norwegian Scabies)

- Classically in this form, there is **no scratching and hence no dislodgement of mites**. Scratching is absent as:
  - **Itching is absent** (e.g. HIV where due to lack of immune response there is no itch)
  - Due to neuropathy which impairs transmission of itch (e.g. Hansen's disease)
  - Mental and neurological disorders (e.g. Down's syndrome, dementia where there is inadequate central perception of itch)
  - When the patient cannot itch due to motor paralysis
- Due to absent scratching and no self-dislodgment of the mites, **large number of mites** are retained in the epidermis
- Thousands of mites routinely survive in skin and **easy to demonstrate by scrapping**. Presents as **scaly-crusted, hyperkeratotic papules** (hence the name crusted scabies, **keratotic scabies**) (Fig. 8)

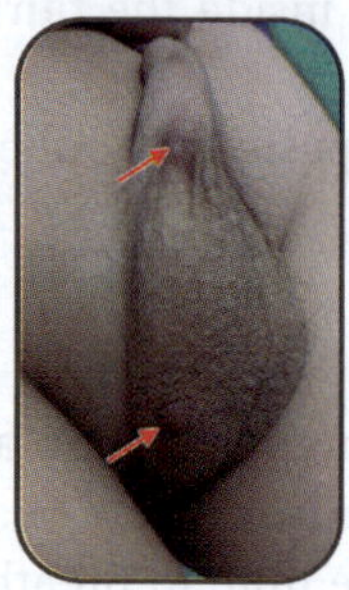

Fig. 7: Nodules on scrotum (red arrows)

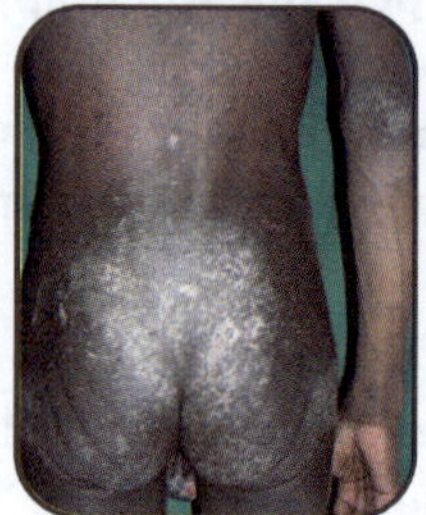

Fig. 8: Norwegian scabies—Hyperkeratotic plaques full of mites in an HIV positive patient

- Treatment[MCQ]: **Ivermectin + topical permethrin**. Repeated courses may be required. Salicylic acid would reduce the hyperkeratosis.

"Scabies incognito" ("incognito" = not to know)

If topical steroids are used on scabies lesions, it modifies the clinical picture to mimic other dermatoses and is called scabies incognito.

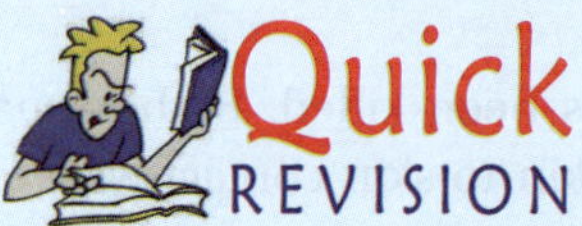

- Caused by the mite Sarcoptes scabiei var. hominis
- S-shaped burrows in webs and genitals—pathognomic. Average no. of mites on skin = 12
- Incubation period- 1st episode- 3–4 weeks, next episode- 2 days
- Nocturnal pruritic papules sparing the face in adults, but in infants causing papulovesicular lesions on face, palms and soles
- Circle of Hebra—describes distribution of lesions in scabies
- Variants—Nodular (hypersensitivity to mite causing nodules on scrotum), Norwegian scabies (in HIV patients present with hyperkeratosis without itching)
- Five percent permethrin is the DOC for adults, infants and pregnancy. Oral ivermectin + permethrin is given in Norwegian scabies.

PEDICULOSIS

- Caused by lice
- 3 louse species exists—**Pediculus humanus capitis (the head louse), P. humanus corporis (the body louse)**, and **Phthirus pubis (the pubic or crab louse)**.
- Head louse and body louse are similar looking while pubic louse is short and stocky.

Pediculosis capitis	Pediculosis corporis ("Vagabonds' disease") (MCQ)	Pediculosis pubis
• Caused by **head louse** (Fig. 9A) • **Children** present with intense scalp itching and often have posterior cervical lymphadenopathy. **Posterior cervical adenopathy without obvious scalp disease is characteristic**(MCQ) • **Nits (egg-cases)** are seen on hair. Nits need to be differentiated from dandruff scales (seborrheic dermatitis). **Scales can easily be flicked off the hair while nits cannot be** (Figs. 9B and C). • **Treatment** – **1% permethrin** (or topical malathion in permethrin-resistant cases) – 5% Permethrin – Oral/Topical ivermectin – Shaving of hair helps – Trimethoprim—sulfamethoxazole works by killing essential bacteria in the louse's gut (which usually help the louse to digest human blood)	• Caused by **body louse** (Fig. 9D) • Disease of poor, homeless and neglected people (vagabonds). Lice is seen on the **seams of clothing only (NOT on body).**(MCQ) Itching on skin is due to salivary antigens of the louse bites • Transmission is mainly by direct close body contact or by sharing infested clothing. • **Treatment** is not for skin but clothing (laundering)(MCQ) ***Body lice are vectors for relapsing fever, trench fever, and epidemic typhus**	• Caused by **pubic/crab louse (Phthirus pubis)** (Fig. 9E) • This louse infests hair in pubic region **(commonest site)**, legs, arms, abdomen, chest, axillae and eyelashes. **Scalp hair is not involved as it is too dense for colonization** • The lice spread through close physical contact, and is often transmitted sexually • **Blue or slate-colored macules (maculae ceruleae)** (Fig. 9F) are located on the sides of the trunk and on the inner aspects of the thighs and are caused by altered blood pigments. • Treatment is 1% permethrin, 5% permethrin, oral/topical ivermectin and shaving of hair

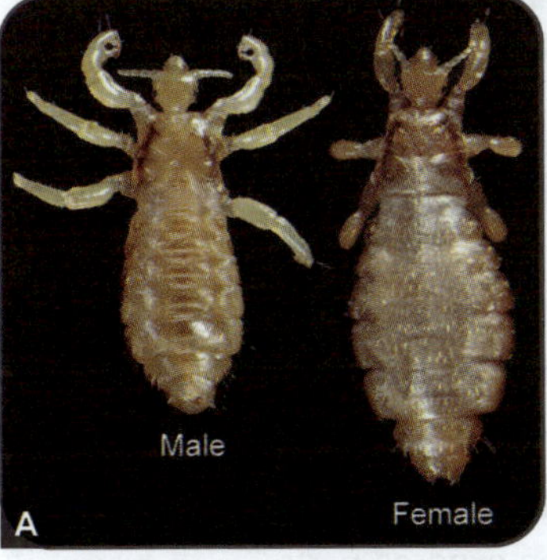

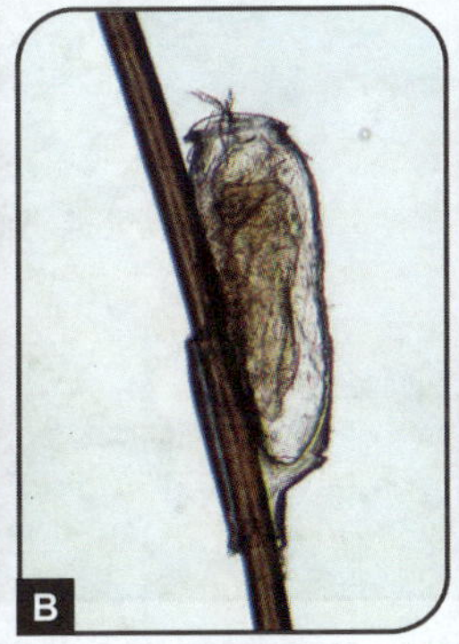

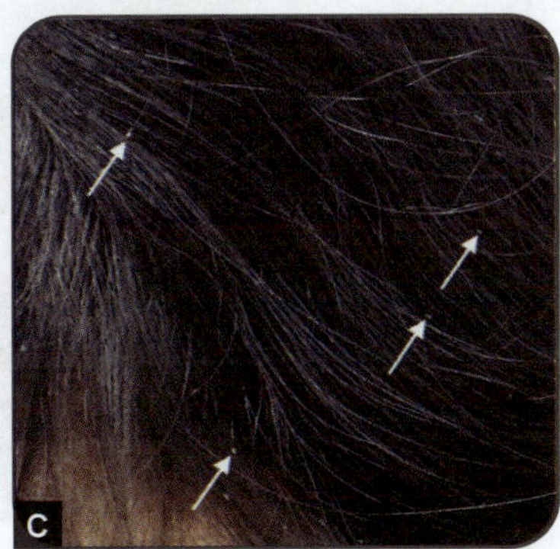

Figs. 9A to C:

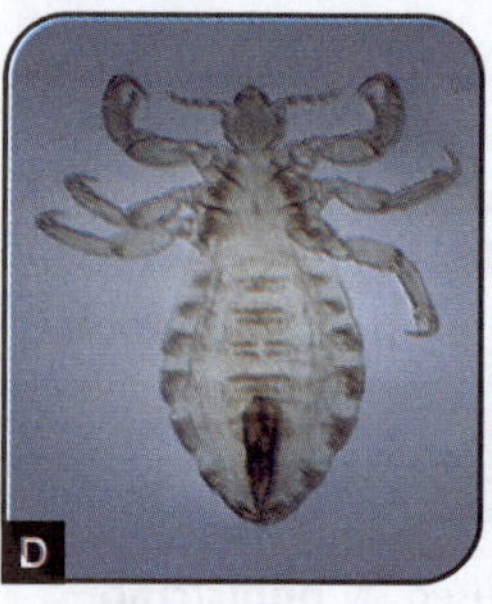

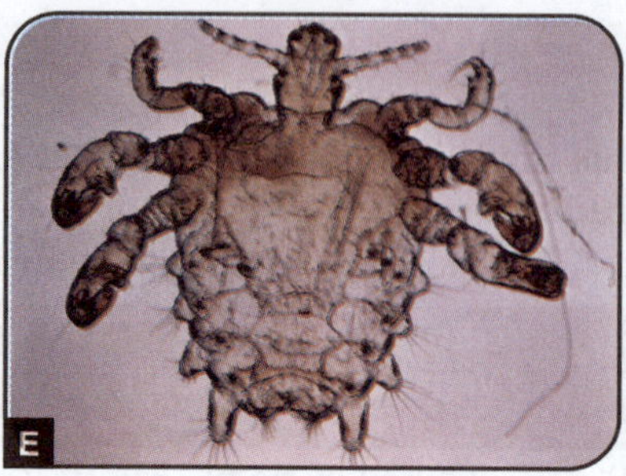

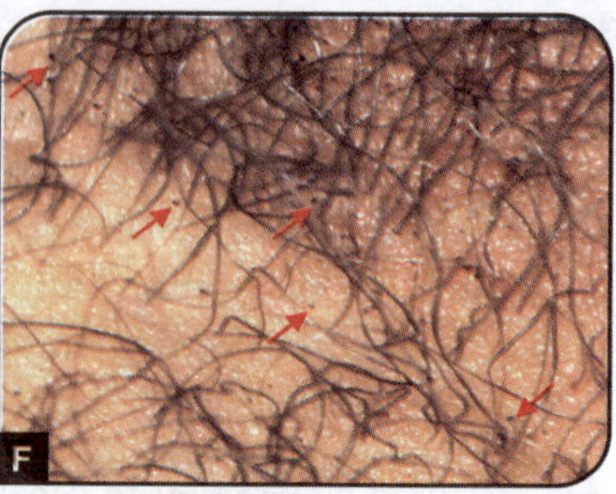

Figs. 9A to F: (A) Head louse (male and female); (B) Nit (egg) of head louse attached to hair; (C) Unflickable nits on occipital area; (D) Body louse; (E) Pubic (Crab) louse; (F) Nits and pigment seen on pubic area (red arrows)

INSECT BITE HYPERSENSITIVITY (PAPULAR URTICARIA)(MCQ)

- **Recurrent pruritic papules** occurring on exposed skin areas due to mosquito, fleas bites, etc.
- **Hypersensitivity reaction** to insect bites especially in children.
- Atopy is an association
- They are seen on **exposed body parts**(MCQ) mainly in **rainy season** (Fig. 10)(MCQ)
- Conservative topical therapy with corticosteroids and antipruritics, along with oral antihistamines.

High Yield Points

- **Pick up phrases in MCQs on insect bite hypersensitivity:**
  - Lesions on exposed sites
  - Lesions increasing in rainy season

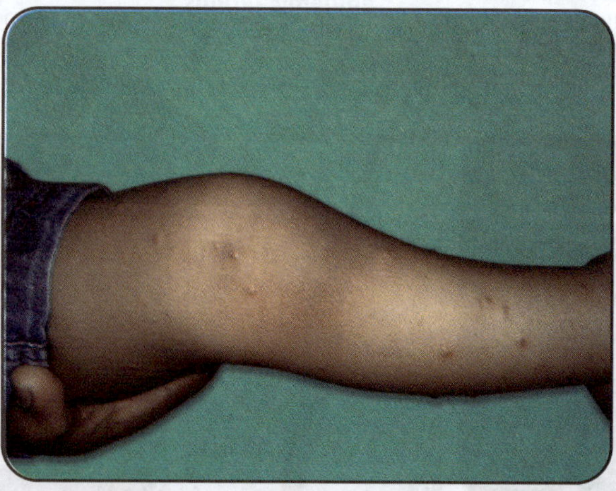

Fig. 10: Recurrent itchy excoriated papules on exposed parts

POST-KALA-AZAR DERMAL LEISHMANIASIS (PKDL)(MCQ)

- In India, PKDL is the **most common skin** manifestation of leishmaniasis
- Develops after 1–2 years of recovery from visceral leishmaniasis
- **This condition closely resembles Hansen's disease**(MCQ)
- There are **two presentations**:
  - Macular, hypopigmented eruption found mainly on the face, arms, and upper part of the trunk (Figs. 11A and B)(MCQ)
  - Papular and nodular eruptions
- Detection of organisms in skin lesions is not always possible as parasite level is low. PCR can detect Leishmania parasites.
- Treatment: Oral miltefosine

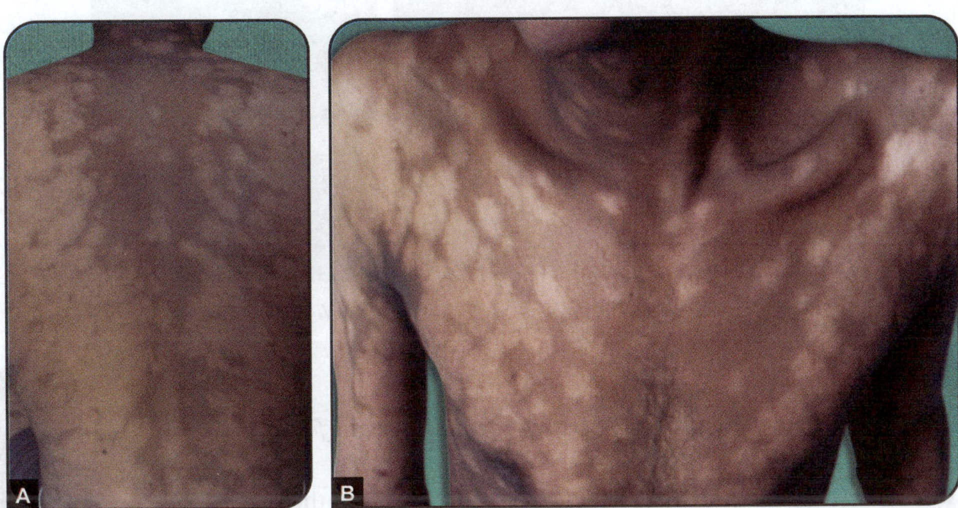

Figs. 11A and B: PKDL—Hypopigmented form (resembling Hansen's disease)

High Yield Points

How to differentiate Leprosy, Pityriasis versicolor and PKDL in an MCQ?
All may cause hypopigmentation on trunk.

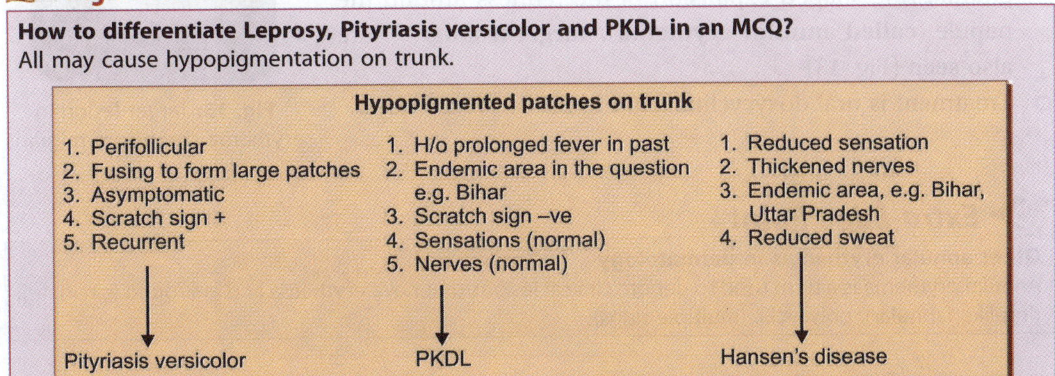

CUTANEOUS LARVA MIGRANS (CREEPING ERUPTION)

- Twisting, creeping, winding linear skin lesions produced by the movement of cat and dog hookworm larvae (ancyclostoma braziliense) (Figs. 12A and B)
- Migration is at the rate of 2 cm/day
- Ivermectin and albendazole are effective treatment.

*Larva currens is caused by strongyloides stercoralis. The name "currens" means "running" or "racing" indicating the fast spread (10 cm/day).

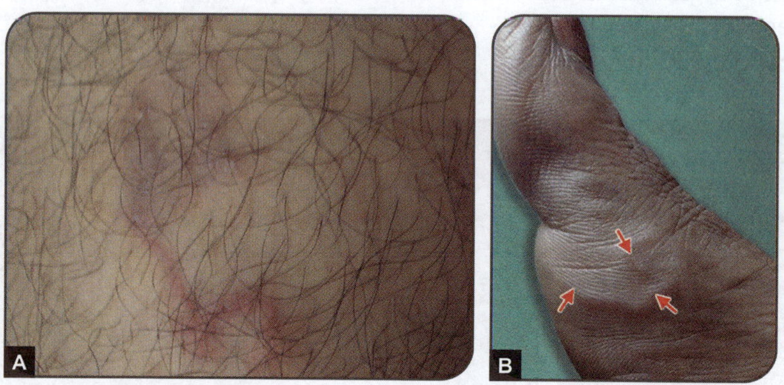

Figs. 12A and B: Cutaneous larva migrans—Wavy, twisting eruptions

ERYTHEMA CHRONICUM MIGRANS(MCQ)

- Skin sign of **Lyme disease** (caused by *Borrelia burgdorferi* sensu lato species)
- **Hard tick** (Ixodidae) bite transmits the spirochetes into the skin
- Starts as a small red macule or papule at the site of the bite, e.g. legs, trunk. Seven days after the bite, there is a gradual ring shaped expansion of the redness around the papule (**called annular erythema**). **Target lesions**(MCQ) are also seen (Fig. 13)
- Treatment is oral doxycycline 100 mg BD for 10–30 days.

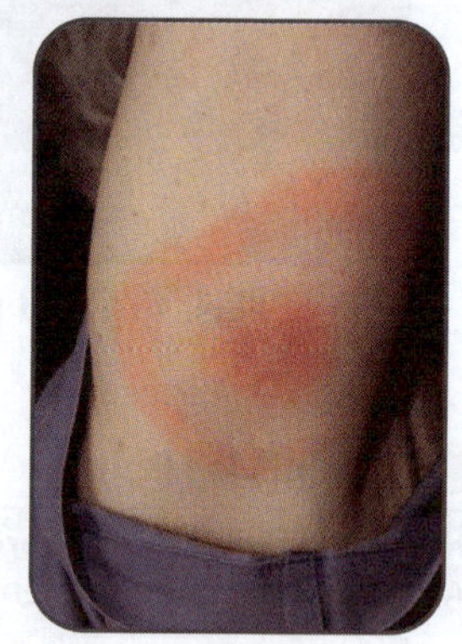

Fig. 13: Target lesion in erythema chronicum migrans

Extra-Edge Point

Other annular erythemas in dermatology

Annular erythema is a term used to denote clinical lesions that have erythema and are round (circinate), ring-like (annular), polycyclic (multiple rings).

QUESTIONS

1. The burrows in scabies is in the:

a. Stratum basale b. Stratum corneum
c. Stratum granulosum
d. Dermis

2. Characteristic lesion of scabies is: *(NEET pattern)*

a. Burrow b. Vesicle
c. Fissure d. Papule

3. Incubation period of scabies is: *(WBPG)*

a. 7 days b. 4 weeks
c. 2 weeks d. 2–3 days

4. Adult scabies is characterized by:

a. Involvement of palms and soles
b. Involvement of anterior abdomen
c. Involvement of face
d. Involvement of genitalia
e. Involvement of web space

5. Scabies in children differs from that in adults in that it affects:

a. Webspace b. Genitalia
c. Axilla d. Face

6. Erythema chronicum migrans is a feature of: *(Recent-May 2017)*

a. Lyme disease
b. Rheumatic fever
c. Tinea
d. Hookworm disease

7. Circle of Hebra is associated with:

a. Syphilis b. Leprosy
c. Scabies d. Lichen planus

8. Not a feature of scabies: *(NEET pattern)*

a. Burrows are seen in stratum corneum
b. Itching is more severe at night
c. Family history is found
d. Fever is a common finding

9. Nodular scabies is found in: *(AIIMS)*

a. Web space of finger
b. Abdomen
c. Axilla
d. Scrotum

10. Treatment of choice of scabies in pregnancy is:

a. Ivermectin b. Permethrin
c. Gamma benzene hexachloride
d. None

11. An 8-month-old child presented with itchy, exudative lesions on the face, palm and soles. The siblings also have similar complaints. The treatment of choice in such patient is:

a. Systemic ampicillin
b. Topical betamethasone
c. Systemic prednisolone
d. Topical permethrin

12. Identify the organism here: *(Recent NEET pattern)*

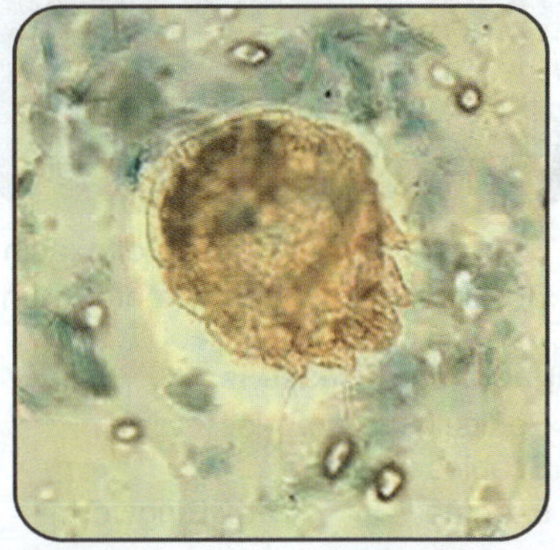

a. Scabies mite b. Demodex mite
c. Louse d. Tick

13. Oral medication used in the treatment of scabies:

a. Albendazole b. Metronidazole
c. Ivermectin d. Ketoconazole

14. Scabies, an infection of the skin caused by sarcoptes scabiei, is an example of:

a. Water-borne disease
b. Water-washed disease
c. Water-based disease
d. Water-related disease

15. **Most severe form of scabies:**
 a. Norwegian scabies
 b. Nodular scabies
 c. Animal scabies
 d. Genital scabies
16. **Drug used in scabies are all *except:***
 a. Crotamiton
 b. Permethrin
 c. Lindane
 d. Gamma benzene hexachloride
 e. Tacrolimus
17. **A patient is suffering from fever from past 1 week along with mild shortness of breath. He is having single painless lesion as shown in the photograph. What is the appropriate treatment?** *(AIIMS May 18)*

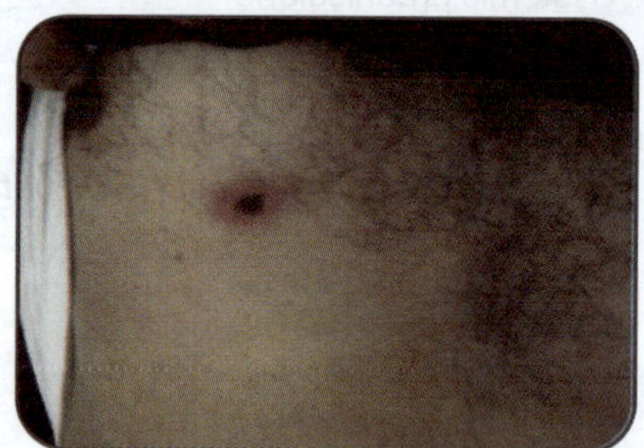

 a. Oseltamivir b. Ciprofloxacin
 c. Doxycycline d. Streptomycin
18. **Vagabond's disease is:**
 a. Pediculosis corporis
 b. Scabies
 c. Eczema d. Ringworm
19. **Maculae ceruleae are seen in:**
 a. Pediculosis corporis *(MHCET 15)*
 b. Pediculosis capitis
 c. Pediculosis pubis
 d. Lupus erythematosus
20. **TOC for pediculosis corporis is:** *(AIIMS)*
 a. 3 application of BHC
 b. 4 application of BHC
 c. Disinfection of all clothes and beddings
 d. DDT application
21. **A patient comes with oval to circular hypopigmented macules on trunk. He reports long standing fever a few years back. His nerves are normal. Which statement is true?**

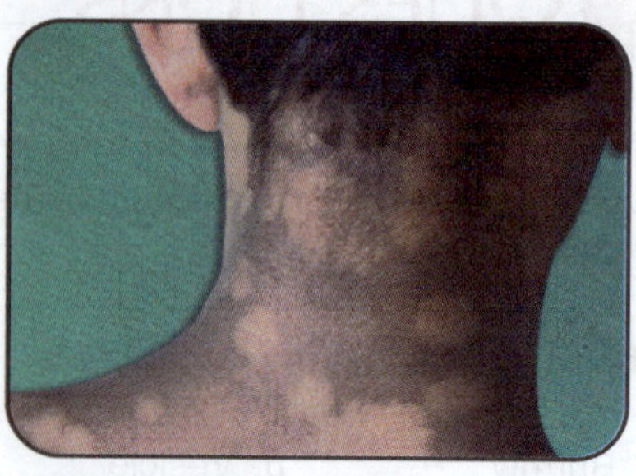

 a. Wood's lamp
 b. Smear for Giemsa stain
 c. KOH mount
 d. Thyroid profile
22. **An infant has papulovesicular lesions on palms, soles and face. The likely diagnosis is:**
 a. Scabies
 b. Atopic dermatitis
 c. Urticaria
 d. Seborrheic dermatitis
23. **A young boy had itchy, excoriated papules on the forehead and the exposed parts of the arms and legs for three years. The disease was most severe in the rainy season and improved completely in winter. The most likely diagnosis is:**

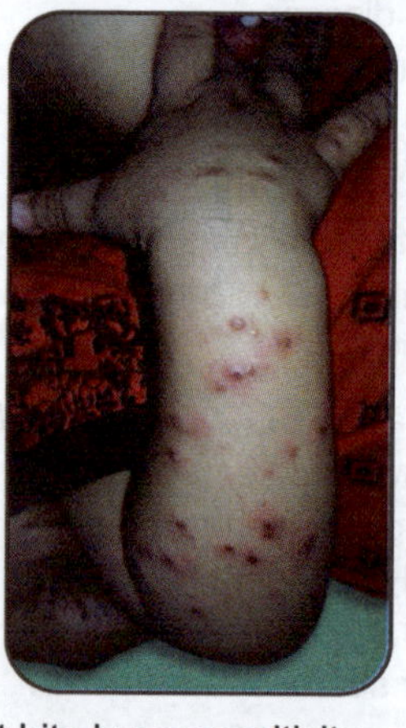

 a. Insect bite hypersensitivity
 b. Scabies
 c. Urticaria
 d. Atopic dermatitis

24. A 20-year-old male from Bihar with erythematous nodule on cheek with central crusting. Likely diagnosis is:

a. SLE
b. Lupus vulgaris
c. Chilblain
d. Cutaneous leishmaniasis

New Questions

25. The following statements are true/false scabies infection:

a. Average number of mites in skin is 12
b. Circle of Willis describes the lesion distribution
c. Vesicle are seen in infantile scabies
d. Nodules are seen in immunosuppressed patients
e. Wood's lamp positive

26. Assertion: Infantile scabies spares the face
Reason: Infants have sebum on face

a. Both Assertion and Reason are true and Reason is correct explanation of Assertion
b. Both Assertion and Reason are true but Reason is not correct explanation of Assertion
c. Assertion is true and Reason is false
d. Assertion is false and Reason is true
e. Both Assertion and Reason are false

27. The treatment options for classical scabies are:

a. Crotamiton
b. Ivermectin
c. Salicylic acid
d. Benzoyl benzoate

1. If a, b, d are correct
2. If a and c are correct
3. If b and d are correct
4. If all four (a, b, c, & d) are correct

28. Match items in column A with best alternative in column B:

Column A	Column B
1. Insect	a. Larva migrans
2. Body louse	b. Vagabond disease
3. Hard tick	c. Papular urticaria
4. Hookworm	d. Larva currens
	e. Erythema chronicum migrans
	f. Leishmaniasis

29. A patient from Bihar had history of very high grade fever. He later developed symmetrical lesions on his back without any nerve thickening and without any sensation loss. The diagnosis is: ***(INICET Nov 21)***

a. Tuberculoid leprosy
b. Lepromatous leprosy
c. Post-kala-azar dermal leishmaniasis
d. Pityriasis versicolor

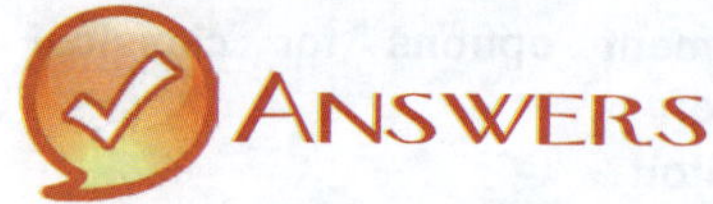

1. **Ans. (b) Stratum corneum** *(Ref: Andrew's Textbook, 11th edn, Page 442)*
2. **Ans. (a) Burrow** *(Ref: Fitzpatrick's Textbook, 8th edn, Page 2570)*

   The pathognomonic lesion is a burrow, which is a thin, thread-like, linear structure 1–10 mm in length.
3. **Ans. (b) 4 weeks** *(Ref: Rook's Textbook of Dermatology, 9th edn, Page 34.40)*
4. **Ans. (b), (d), (e) Involvement of anterior abdomen; Involvement of genitalia; Involvement of web space** *(Ref: Andrew's Textbook, 11th edn, Page 442)*
5. **Ans. (d) Face** *(Ref: Fitzpatrick's Textbook, 8th edn, Page 2580)*
6. **Ans. (a) Lyme disease**
7. **Ans. (c) Scabies** *(Ref: Andrew's Textbook, 11th edn, Page 442)*
8. **Ans. (d) Fever is a common finding** *(Ref: Andrew's Textbook, 11th edn, Page 442)*

   Fever is not a primary finding in scabies. Pustules are seen as a complication and can lead to fever.
9. **Ans. (d) Scrotum** *(Ref: Andrew's Textbook, 11th edn, Page 442)*

   Genitals, particularly scrotum is a common site for nodular scabies. Nodular scabies present as pruritic nodules.
10. **Ans. (b) Permethrin** *(Ref: Habif's Clincial Dermatology, 5th edn, Page 588)*

    Permethrin is pregnancy category B
11. **Ans. (d) Topical permethrin** (See page 157 for explanation)

    Face, palms and sole involvement points to infantile scabies. Exudative lesion suggests a secondary eczematous change which is common in infants. Permethrin is DOC for infantile scabies.
12. **Ans. (a) Scabies mite**
13. **Ans. (c) Ivermectin** (See page 158 for explanation)

    Ivermectin is used in scabies, onchocerciasis and loiasis. Ivermectin is not used in children <15 kg, pregnant and lactating mothers.
14. **Ans. (b) Water-washed disease** (See page 158 for explanation)
15. **Ans. (a) Norwegian scabies** (See page 159 for explanation)
16. **Ans. (e) Tacrolimus** (See page 158 for explanation)

    Tacrolimus is an immunosuppressant used in atopic dermatitis, lichen planus, vitiligo, etc. and not in scabies.
17. **Ans. (c) Doxycycline**

    Characteristic hallmarks of the rickettsial rash: The eschar of the tick bite. In India, the scrub typhus group is more common than the spotted fever group. Scrub typhus is caused by Rickettsia tsutsugamushi. A tick bite with the eschar, petechial rash with predominantly truncal distribution sparing the palms, soles and face (unlike a Rocky mountain spotted fever where these sites are involved) is suggestive of scrub typhus

18. Ans. (a) Pediculosis corporis *(Ref: Andrew's Textbook, 11th edn, Page 437)*

19. Ans. (c) Pediculosis pubis *(Ref: Andrew's Textbook, 11th edn, Page 437)*

20. Ans. (c) Disinfection of all clothes and beddings
(Ref: Fitzpatrick's Textbook, 8th edn, Page 2576)

21. Ans. (b) Smear for giemsa stain (See page 163 for explanation)
Fever points to kala-azar in the past. Hypopigmented macules on trunk indicate PKDL. Smear is done by giemsa stain to look for LD bodies.

22. Ans. (a) Scabies (See page 157 for explanation)
Papulovesicular lesions on palms, soles and face are classical of infantile scabies.

23. Ans. (a) Insect bite hypersensitivity (See page 157 for explanation)
Pointer words in the MCQ- "exposed parts" and "increasing in rainy season".

24. Ans. (d) Cutaneous leishmaniasis (See page 157 for explanation)
Central crusting indicates cutaneous leishmaniasis.

New Answers

25. Ans. a-True; b-False; c-True; d-False; e-True

26. Ans. (e) Both Assertion and Reason are false

27. Ans. (1) If a, b, d are correct

28. Ans. 1-c; 2-b; 3-e; 4-a

29. Ans. (c) Post-kala-azar dermal leishmaniasis

CHAPTER 8

Sexually Transmitted Diseases

Sexually transmitted diseases (STDs) can be divided into three parts:

1. Genital ulcers diseases (GUD)
2. Urethral discharge diseases (UD)
3. Vaginal discharge diseases (VD)

GENITAL ULCER DISEASES

Syphilis

- Caused by **Treponema pallidum. Classical motility**(MCQ)-in the direction of the long axis, a rotation on its long axis, and a **bending corkscrew** twisting from side to side.

I. Primary stage (Hunterian Chancre, Hard chancre)

- Incubation period: **9–90** days (average 3 weeks), then **chancre** (ulcer) develops
- Chancre: **Painless**, **Hard** (cartilage feel, **button-like feel**, **indurated**), **regular edges**, usually **single** (rarely many ulcers) (Figs. 1A and B)

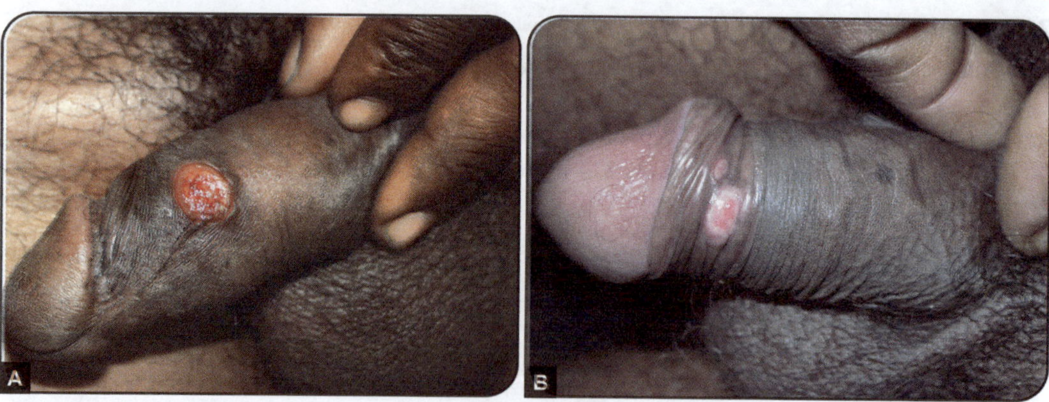

Figs. 1A and B: (A) Single, well defined primary chancre. Notice the clear serum dripping from the ulcer; (B) 2 painless hard ulcers

- Inguinal lymphadenopathy: **Painless**, unilateral or bilateral, shotty and rubbery to feel
- Extra-genital chancre: **m/c site-lip** due to peno-oral contact
- Diagnosis: Smear is taken from ulcer and dark ground illumination **(DGI) test is done (test of choice)**

- **Chancre redux:** If the primary chancre is not treated or treated inadequately, it may subsequently recur, weeks or months later (Fig. 1C). This is called chancre redux ("redux" means recurrence). It is a sign of relapsing syphilis.

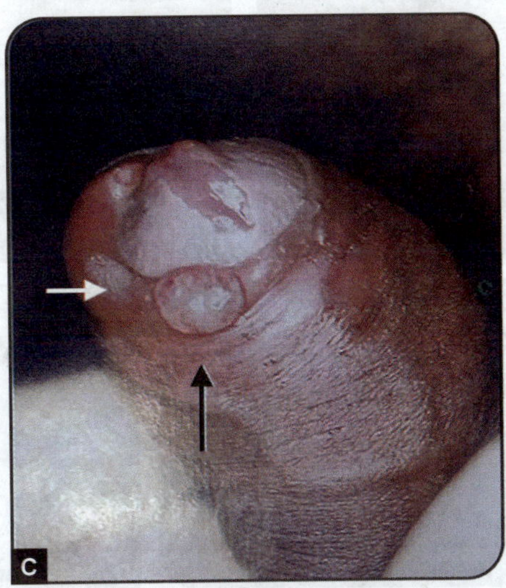

Fig. 1C: New lesion of chancre (black arrow) near the site of a previous healed primary chancre (white arrow)

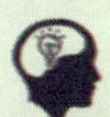

Aid to Remember

- Syphi'LESS'- Pain'LESS' ulcers and Pain'LESS' lymphadenopathy

II. Secondary syphilis (blood dissemination of spirochetes if primary stage is not treated). The main features of this stage are listed in the table below.

Rash	Condyloma lata	Generalized lymphadenopathy	Mucous patches	Moth eaten alopecia
• **Most common feature** • **Non-itchy** • Macules, scaly papules, plaques (Figs. 2A and B) • **Palm, sole** involvement-classical (Fig. 2C) • **No vesicles**	• **Flat cauliflower like masses** on moist skin like anus, groin, etc. (Fig. 3A) • **Moist** in appearance • Very infectious	Diffuse nontender lymphadenopathy	• **Most classical lesion** (Fig. 2D) • **Most infectious lesion** • Full of treponemas • Flat erosions on tongue • These erosions can coalesce to form **snail track ulcers**	• Small areas of hair loss on scalp (Fig. 3B) • Non-scarring type

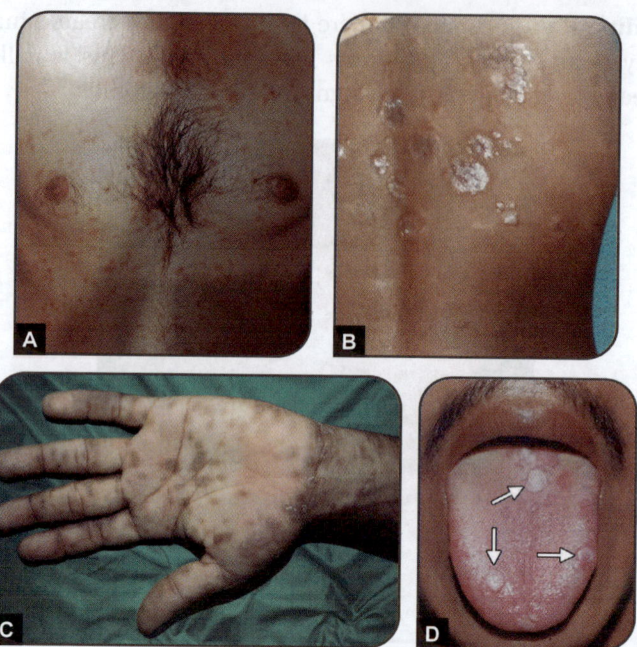

Figs. 2A to D: (A) Secondary syphilis—Multiple, erythematous, mildly scaly papules and plaques on trunk; (B) Secondary syphilis—Multiple, violaceous (purple) plaques; (C) Hyperpigmented and scaly macules, papules on palm (Deep dermal tenderness- DDT +ve); (D) Secondary syphilis—Mucous patches on tongue (white arrows)

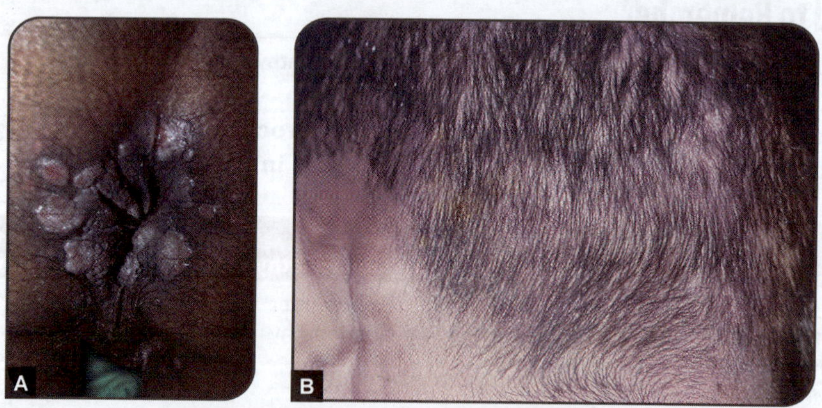

Figs. 3A and B: (A) Condyloma lata (flat, moist plaque teeming with spirochetes); (B) Moth-eaten alopecia

- **Deep dermal tenderness (DDT)/Ollendorff sign in secondary syphilis.** Pressure with a blunt object on the palm and sole lesions elicits severe tenderness
- The **"great imitator"** as it can mimic many other diseases
- Systemic involvement: Acute glomerulonephritis, proteinuria, gastritis, hepatitis, acute meningitis, uveitis, periostitis may all be seen

Aid to Remember

- Nothing bothers the patient much in syphilis—non-painful ulcer, non-painful lymph nodes, non-itchy rash

III. Latent syphilis

- The disease becomes **inactive** automatically after secondary syphilis. Patient is **asymptomatic clinically but has serological evidence of infection**
  - Early latent—First 2 years of infection
  - Late latent—After 2 years of infection

IV. Tertiary syphilis: Tissue invasion (hypersensitivity phenomenon—treponemes difficult to demonstrate)

- **Skin: Gummatous syphilis**—Nodules develop on skin which ulcerates creating deep, punched out ulcers having a **"gum-like" secretion** on floor (Fig. 4A). Mucosal lesions can occur. Gummatous osteitis of the nasal bones, hard palate, and nasal septum can occur causing perforation (Fig. 4B).

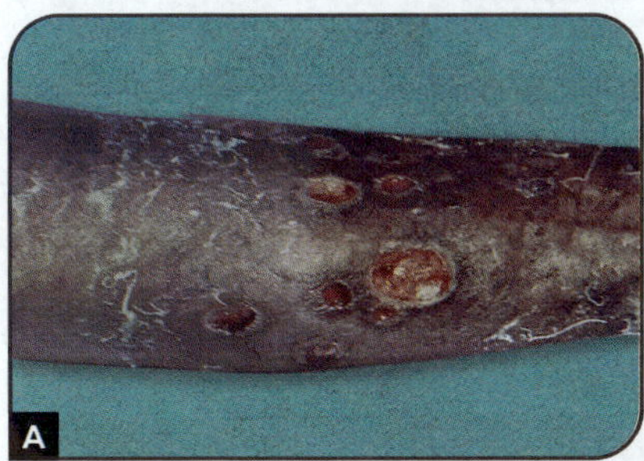

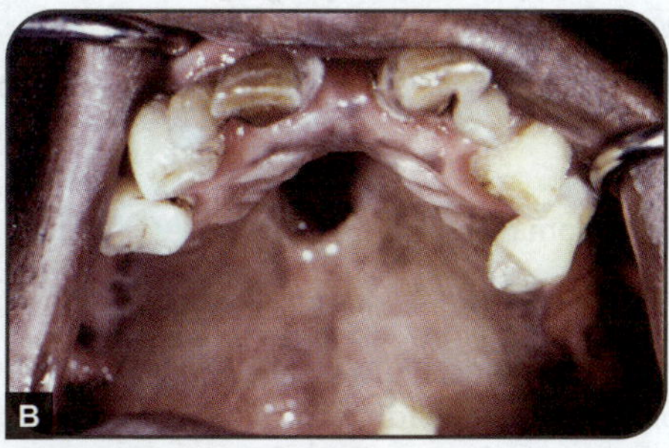

Figs. 4A and B: Gummatous syphilis—Multiple punched out ulcers on extremities; (B) Perforated hard palate in gummatous syphilis

* **Pseudochancre redux** is a gumma occurring at the site of a previous healed chancre

- **CVS: Cardiovascular syphilis—Aortitis of the ascending aorta** leading to ascending aorta aneurysm, coronary disease, aortic aneurysm
- **CNS: Neurosyphilis**—CNS involvement can occur at any stage of syphilis, even in primary syphilis. It may be in the form of asymptomatic state, general paresis of insane or **tabes dorsalis**

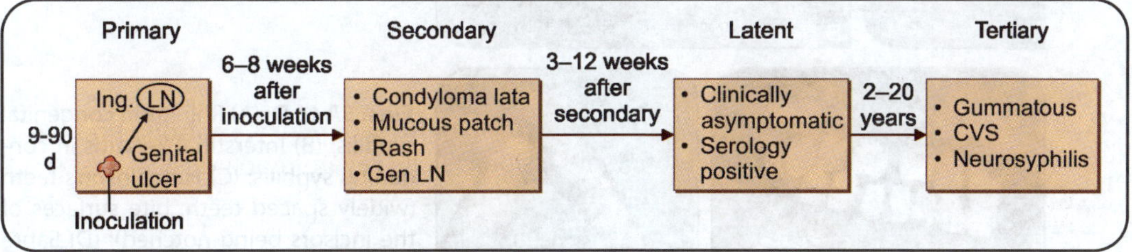

Natural history of untreated syphilis

V. Congenital syphilis

Transmission from mother can occur at any stage of syphilis

- **Early congenital syphilis**: Within the first 2 years of life (Resembles adult secondary syphilis, since the baby is getting infected through mother's blood)
- **Late congenital syphilis**: After 2 years of life (resembles adult tertiary syphilis)
- **Stigmata** (remnants and scars of previous congenital syphilis).

Early congenital	Late congenital	Stigmata
Snuffles (rhinitis): Earliest and the most common sign (Fig. 5A)	**Interstitial keratitis** (Fig. 5B)	**Hutchinson's teeth** (peg shaped upper incisors with a notch)[AI] (Fig. 5D) **Hutchinson's triad**: Hutchinson's tooth + 8th nerve deafness + interstitial keratitis
Bullae (syphilitic pemphigus): Most classical feature	8th nerve deafness	
Mucous patches	**Clutton's joint**: Painless, symmetrical swelling of the knees	
Condyloma lata	Sabre tibia due to periostitis of tibia (Fig. 5C)	
Diaphyseal epiphysitis and osteochondritis: Causes pain on movement, leading to the infant's refusing to move (**Parrot pseudoparalysis**)		
	Saddle nose	

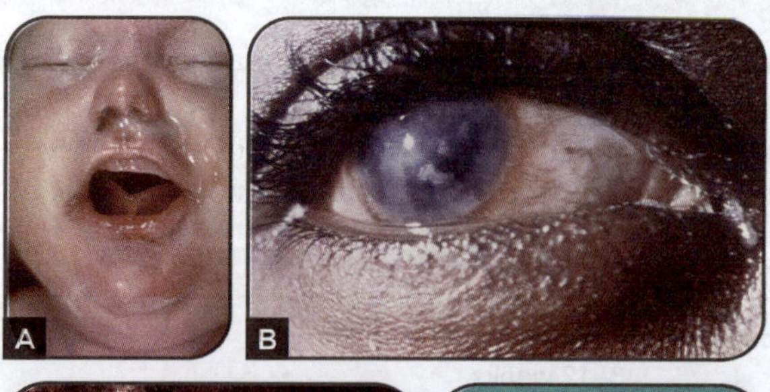
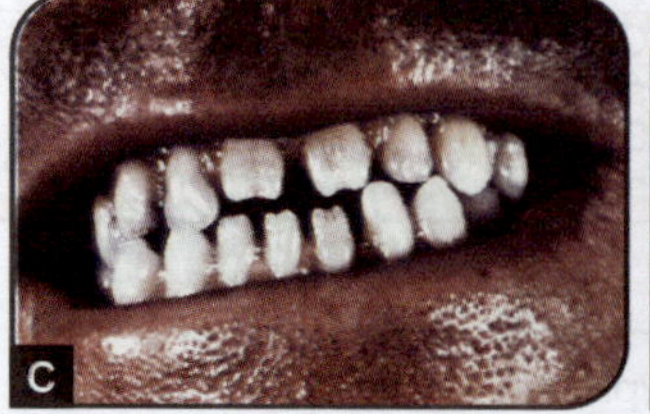
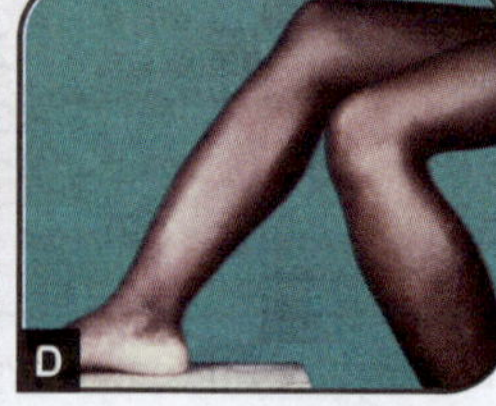

Figs. 5A to D: (A) Rhinitis in congenital syphilis; (B) Interstitial keratitis in congenital syphilis; (C) Hutchinson's teeth (widely spaced teeth, bite surfaces of the incisors being notched); (D) Sabre tibia in congenital syphilis

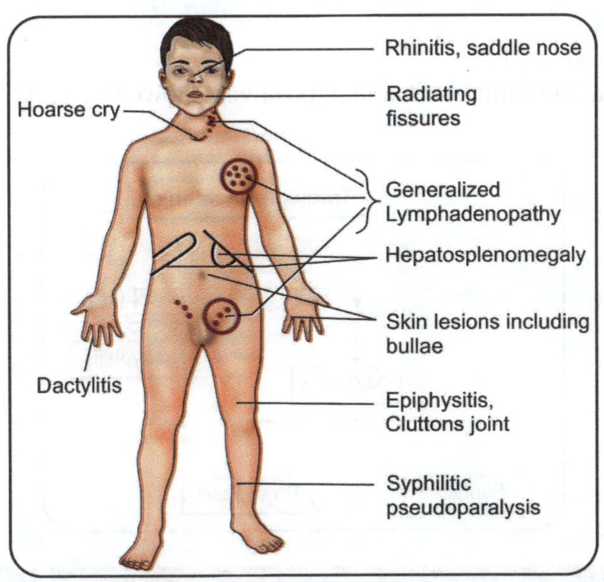

Diagnosis

1. DGI from nasal secretions
2. **VDRL titre of baby 4 times > mother's titre—IOC**

Testing for Syphilis

- Direct visualization of treponema can be done by **dark-ground illumination (DGI)** (Fig. 6)

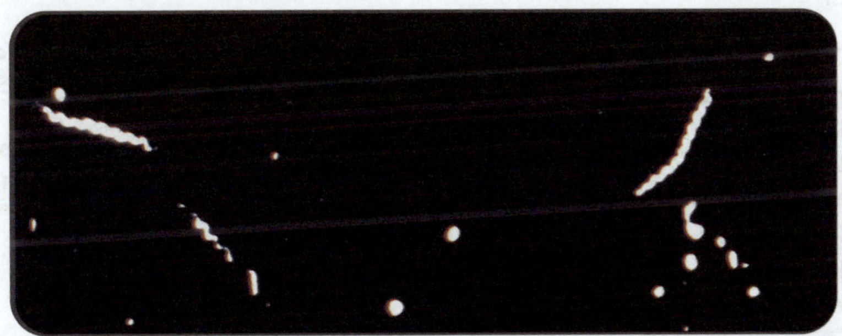

Fig. 6: Treponema pallidum refractile on DGI smear

- Serological tests are of two types:
  1. **Nontreponemal tests**: VDRL/RPR (becomes **negative** after treatment)
  2. **Treponemal tests**: Enzyme immune-assay (EIA)/treponema pallidum haemagglutination (TPHA)/Microhaemagglutination-Treponema pallidum (MHA-TP)/Treponema pallidum particle agglutination (TPPA)/fluorescent treponemal antibody-absorption (FTA-Abs). **Treponemal tests remain positive even after treatment.**

Testing protocol

- Screening test for syphilis
  - **Traditional method:** VDRL and, if positive, followed by TPPA/TPHA for confirmation

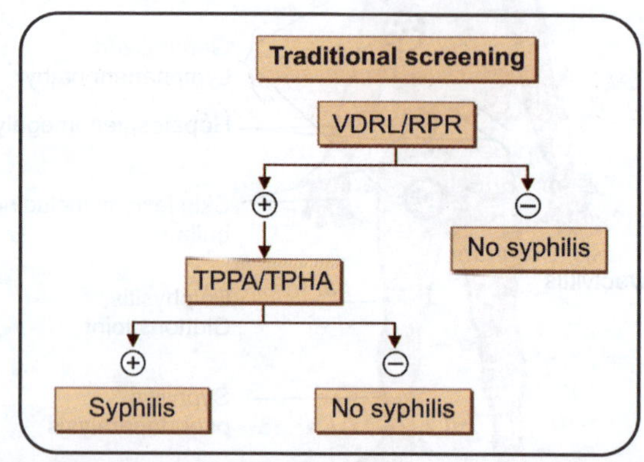

Primary	Secondary	Latent	Tertiary
IOC: DGI on smear from ulcer/lymph node aspirate (**most specific test in primary syphilis**) **The direct fluorescent antibody test** for *T. pallidum* is easier to perform than dark-field microscopy. It detects antigen and, thus, does not require the presence of motile treponemes like DGI	DGI from condyloma lata	Most sensitive EIA > FTA-Abs > TPPA	Most sensitive FTA-Abs > TPPA
If DGI cannot be done then serology **Timings of positive serology after inoculation** 3 weeks—EIA (IgM)* **(screening test of choice)** 3 weeks—FTA-Abs* 4 weeks—VDRL 4–6 weeks—TPHA/TPPA Sensitivity in syphilis EIA > TPPA = FTA-Abs *Between EIA (IgM) and FTA-Abs, since FTA-Abs is outdated now, EIA should be chosen as earliest test to come positive (If not there in the options, choose FTA-Abs)	**IOC-VDRL/RPR**		• **Neurosyphilis** • **CSF-VDRL is the most specific and the IOC**

⅄ **Role of VDRL**

- IOC for **monitoring response to therapy** in syphilis (CDC guideline for effective treatment-titre reduces 4 fold within 6 months in primary and secondary syphilis and 12–24 months of therapy in latent and tertiary syphilis)
- False positive VDRL (titre <1:8).

Acute false positive VDRL	Chronic false positive VDRL
• Malaria, lepromatous leprosy, respiratory tract infection, infectious mononucleosis, active pulmonary tuberculosis, subacute bacterial endocarditis, measles, chickenpox, filariasis, pregnancy • Also positive in non-venereal treponemal infections: Yaws, pinta	Autoimmune diseases (e.g. SLE)

Treatment for Adult Syphilis (WHO 2016)

Classification	Includes	Treatment in adults and in pregnancy	Treatment for penicillin allergic adult patients
Early syphilis (First 2 years of infection)	**Primary, Secondary, Early latent**	Benzathine penicillin G 2.4 million units IM in a single dose	Doxycycline 100 mg twice daily orally for 14 days (preferred) or Ceftriaxone 1 g IM once daily for 10–14 days, or, in special circumstances, azithromycin 2 g once orally
Late syphilis (after 2 years of infection)	**Late latent, Tertiary**	Benzathine penicillin G 2.4 million units IM, 3 doses at weekly intervals (For neurosyphilis- Aqueous crystalline penicillin in the DOC as benzathine penicillin does not cross the blood-brain barrier)	Doxycycline 100 mg BD for 30 days (Penicillin allergy in neurosyphilis—Desensitization)

Chancroid (Soft Chancre)

- Caused by *Haemophilus ducreyi.* Incubation period—3–10 days
- **Multiple, tender, soft ulcers** (Fig. 7A)
- **Irregular edges, undermined ulcers,** bleeds easily
- **Painful, suppurative, unilateral inguinal lymphadenitis (bubo)**—Classical feature (Fig. 7C)
- **Kissing ulcers**—Due to autoinoculation on the genitalia (Fig. 7B)
- Most strongly associated with an increased risk for HIV transmission
- Diagnosis: Gram-stain on smear from the ulcer—**"School of fish"** or **"rail-road track appearance"** (Figs. 7D and E), PCR if facilities available.
- **Treatment (CDC 2015): Tab Azithromycin 1 g single dose or inj. Ceftriaxone 250 mg IM stat.**

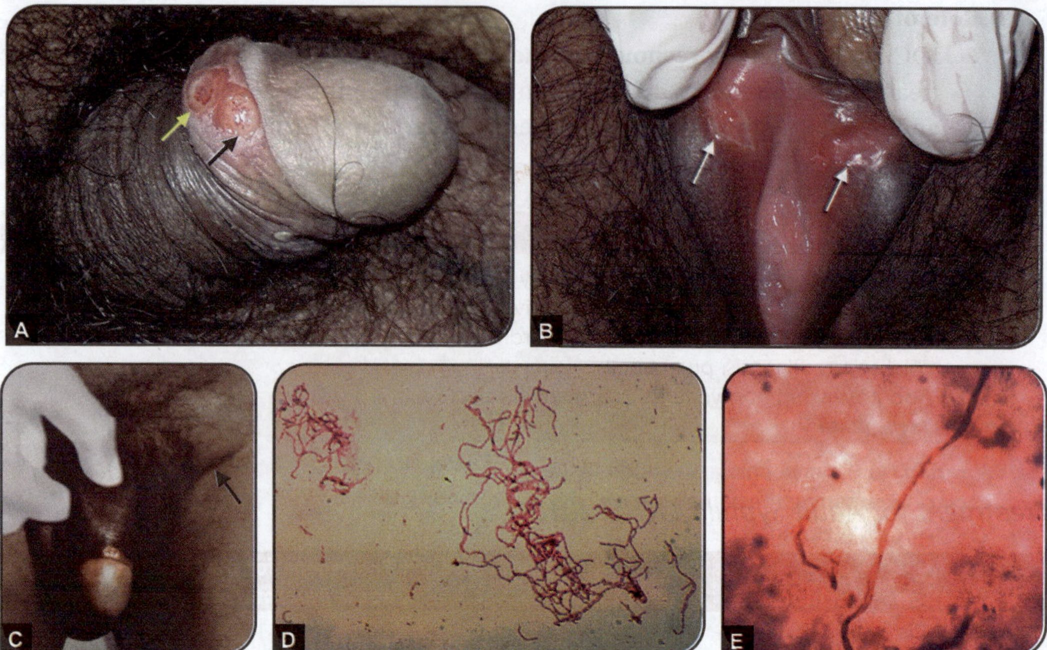

Figs. 7A to E: (A) Two painful soft non-indurated mildly bleeding ulcers; (B) Kissing ulcers due to autoinoculation; (C) Chancroid—Single, irregular penile ulcer with unilateral inflamed bubo; (D) Gram-stain shows pleomorphic. Gram-negative rods that are in short chains, pairs, or schools of fish; (E) Note the "rail road track" arrangement of *haemophilus ducreyi*

Aid to Remember

- du-crey-i: Patients "do" "cry" with this painful ulcer
- Ulcer features are opposite to syphilis

Donovanosis (Granuloma Inguinale)

- Chronic, granulomatous, locally destructive ulceration caused by **Calymmatobacterium granulomatis**
- Painless, foul-smelling ulcers
- **Exuberant vascular granulation tissue on floor** (Fig. 8A)
- **Beefy red appearance**
- **Bleeds readily**
- Regional lymph nodes are **not enlarged.** Granulomatous swellings occur in inguinal area. Since, no lymphadenopathy occurs, these are called as **pseudo-buboes**
- Squamous cell carcinoma can be a late complication
- Investigations: **Crushed smear** of fresh biopsy material stained with **Wright or Giemsa stain shows parasitized histiocytes containing Donovan bodies (showing closed safety pin appearance: prominent staining at the poles)** (Fig. 8B)

- **Treatment-Azithromycin 1 g orally once per week or 500 mg daily for at least 3 weeks and until all lesions have completely healed** (Preferred regimen).

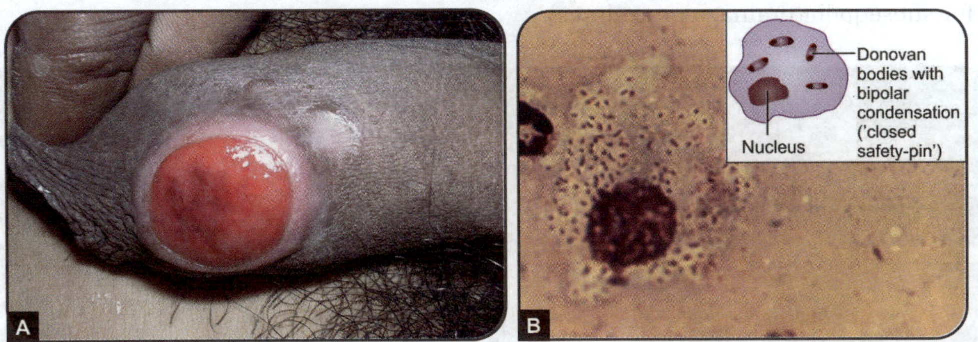

Figs. 8A and B: (A) Hypertrophic granulation tissue on ulcer floor (painless) which bleeds on touch; (B) A white blood cell containing the pathognomonic finding of Donovan bodies (encapsulated, Gram-negative rods). Schematic diagram (inset)

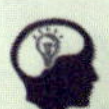

Aid to Remember

- Remember NO in doNOvanosis. "No" lymphadenopathy, "No" pain in ulcer, "No"—Not seen in India commonly.
- **'Gra'**nuloma inguinale—**'gra'**nuloma in the inguinal area, **'gra'**nulation tissue on ulcer floor

Lymphogranuloma Venereum (LGV)

- Caused by **Chlamydia trachomatis** L1, L2, L3
- **Primary genital stage—Transient superficial painless erosion** which often goes unnoticed by the patient
- **Secondary inguinal stage—Painful unilateral or bilateral inguinal lymph nodes (bubo)** (Fig. 9A)
- Swollen buboes above and below inguinal ligament are seen. The inguinal ligament then looks like a groove (**Groove sign-pathognomonic**) (Fig. 9B)
- Not only inguinal, but para-rectal lymph nodes are also enlarged. **Rectal inflammation causes strictures, fissures**
- **Tertiary stage**: Fibrosis of lymph nodes causes obstruction in lymph drainage, lymphedema and **genital elephantiasis. Lymphangiectasias** (bubbles of lymph) form on surface of genitals due to pressure of lymph under skin. These then rupture to cause **lymphorrhea (oozing of lymph)** (Figs. 9C and D)
- **Diagnosis:**
  - **Nucleic acid amplification tests (NAAT)**—test of choice
  - Complement fixation test (CFT) detects antibodies—most commonly done

- **Treatment (CDC 2015): Doxycycline 100 mg BD for 21 days.** For inguinal buboes—Needle aspiration or incision and drainage (although needle aspiration of buboes is a simpler procedure, incision and drainage might be preferred because of reduced need for subsequent drainage procedures).

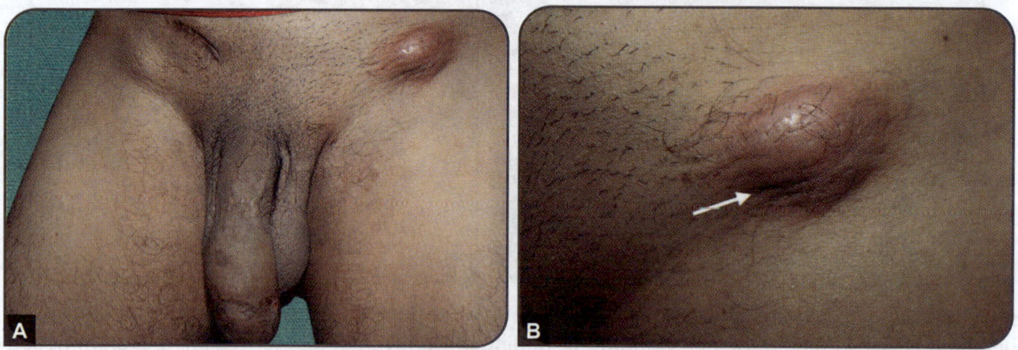

Figs. 9A and B: (A) Bilateral inflamed inguinal buboes; (B) Inguinal bubo. An early "groove" sign is seen developing on medial side

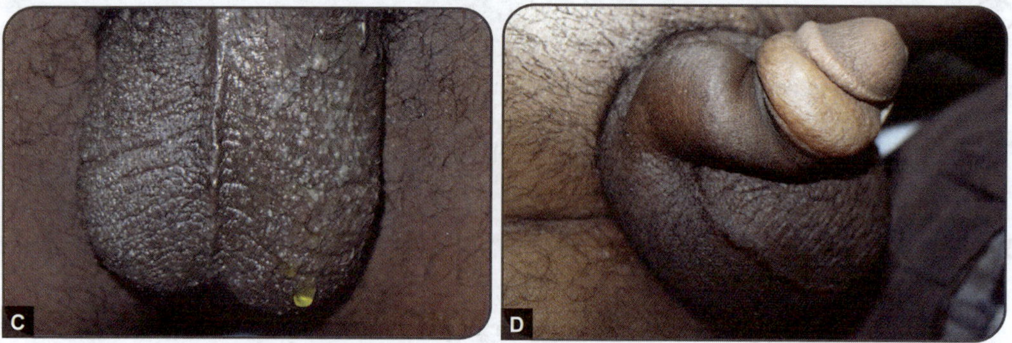

Figs. 9C and D: (C) Oozing of lymph (lymphorrhea) after bursting of lymphangiectasia with scrotal lymphedema; (D) Saxophone penis

Pick up words in MCQs on LGV

- "Transient"
- "Ulcer never seen by the patient"

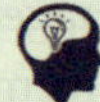

Aid to Remember

- **LGV-L** = **L**ymph nodes painful, **L**ymph oozes out of genitals (**L**ymphorrhea), **G** = **G**roove sign, **V** = **V**ery transient genital ulcers
- Painful ulcer + painful lymph node—Chancroid (All pain)
- Painless ulcer + painless lymph node—Syphilis (All pain'LESS'-Syphi'LESS')
- Painless ulcer + painful lymph node—LGV (having both)

Herpes Genitalis

- For theory, read the topic in Chapter 6. Images of herpes genitalis are shown in Figures 10A and B.

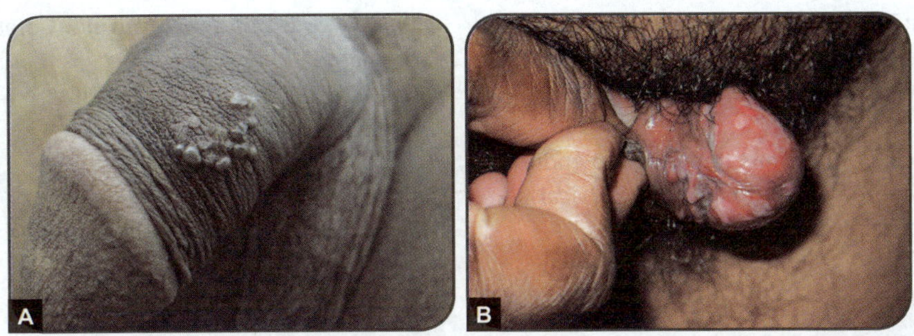

Figs. 10A and B: (A) Grouped vesicles; (B) Grouped erosions

Aid to Remember

- Diseases causing genital ulcers—**CHISEL**: **C**—Chancroid, **H**—herpes, **I**—inguinale (granuloma inguinale), **S**—syphilis, **L**—LGV

High Yield Points

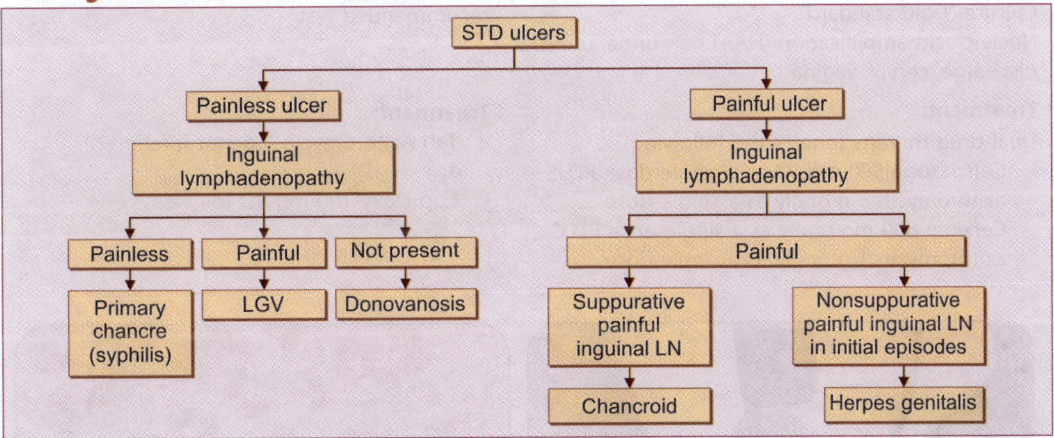

URETHRAL DISCHARGE DISEASES (DUE TO URETHRITIS)

Gonococcal	Non-gonococcal
Caused by N. gonorrhea. It is the second most common bacterial STI in the world (WHO 2016) Treatment for gonococcus is complicated by emerging serious drug resistance[INICET 24]	Caused by **Chlamydia-m/c** Others organisms are ureaplasma (20%) and mycoplasma genitalium (10–20%), rarely trichomonas. It is the most common bacterial STI in the world (WHO 2016)

Contd...

Contd...

Gonococcal	Non-gonococcal
Incubation period: 2–8 days	Incubation period: 1–3 weeks
In males: Thick, **profuse**, **purulent** urethral discharge. Others have prostatitis, epididymo-orchitis (Fig. 11A) *Testis is not involved **In females:** Primary infection is in the endocervix, often asymptomatic but can cause cervical discharge, salpingitis, PID **Asymptomatic infection** in urethra, endocervix, rectum, pharynx **Symptomatic infection and complications** 1. Urethritis 2. Cervicitis 3. Proctitis 4. Bartholin abscess 5. Conjunctivitis 6. Salpingitis 7. Epididymitis	**Watery or a thin muco-purulent** urethral discharge Can also cause epididymitis, PID
Diagnosis: Gram-stain microscopy for gram –ve diplococci (IOC) (Fig. 11B) Culture-"Gold standard" Nucleic-acid amplification (NAAT) on urine, urethral discharge, cervix, vagina	**Diagnosis:** NAAT done on urethral swab or first void urine is the most sensitive and the only recommended test
Treatment: Dual drug therapy (one of the following) • Ceftriaxone 500 mg IM as a single dose PLUS azithromycin 1 g orally as a single dose • Cefxime 800 mg orally as a single dose PLUS azithromycin 1 g orally as a single dose	**Treatment:** • Tab Azithromycin 1 g stat (preferred) or • Cap Doxy 100 mg BD for 7 days

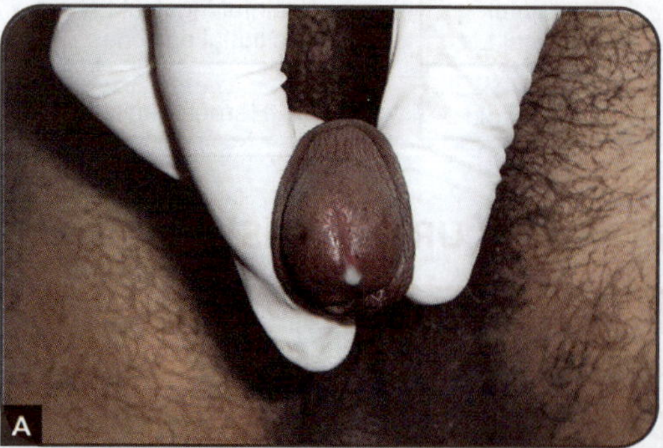

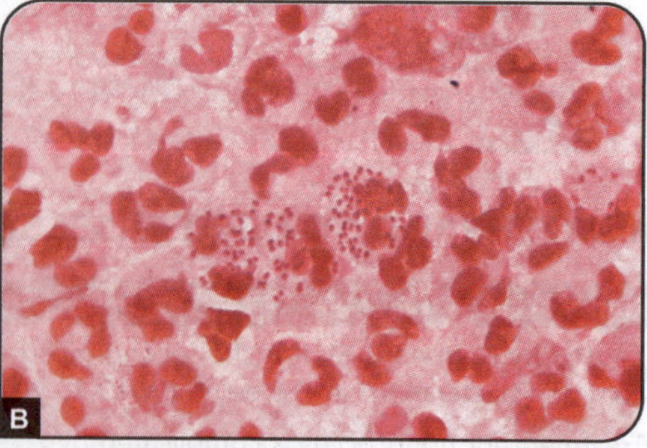

Figs. 11A and B: (A) Gonorrhea—thick purulent urethral discharge; (B) Gram-stain of urethral discharge showing gram-negative diplococci

VAGINAL DISCHARGE

Vulvo-vaginal candidiasis	Trichomoniasis	Bacterial vaginosis
Caused by *Candida albicans*	Caused by *Trichomonas vaginalis*	• **Not sexually transmitted** but due to local factors like douching or use of bidet toilets • **M/c cause of vaginal discharge** • **Pathogenesis:** Due to an imbalance of the bacterial flora normally present in the vagina. Normally, hydrogen peroxide-producing lactobacilli predominate in vagina and other commensals like **Gardnerella vaginalis, mycoplasma hominis, anaerobic bacteria (e.g. Prevotella, bacteroides, fusobacterium) and ureaplasma.** Due to douching, lactobacilli are killed and these other commensals proliferate causing discharge
Thick, curdy, minimal, white vaginal discharge (Fig. 12A)	**Yellow-green, copious** discharge	**Homogenous, thin** vaginal discharge
Vulvar itching Swelling Redness	Itching Dysuria **Strawberry cervix** (punctuate hemorrhages on cervix)–Specific feature	**Fishy odor** **No inflammation** (Hence, the name bacterial "vaginosis" not bacterial "vaginitis") **No itching**
Wet mount (with saline, KOH), gram-stain-shows budding yeasts, hyphae and pseudohyphae (Fig. 12B) pH is <4.5 (normal)	Diagnosis: Wet mount, (Fig. 12C) culture, NAAT pH is >4.5 (elevated)	Clinical criteria- (Amsel criteria-3 out of 4) • Homogenous, thin white discharge • **Clue cells** (vaginal epithelial cells coated with organisms) (Fig. 12D) • **Fishy amine odor after adding KOH (Whiff test)** • Vaginal pH >4.5
Treatment Topical-Azole creams or suppository Oral-tab fluconazole 150 mg stat	**Treatment** DOC-Tab Metronidazole 2 g stat or Tab Tinidazole 2 g stat or Tab Secnidazole 2 g stat	**Treatment** DOC- Tab Metronidazole 500 mg BD for 7 days Or Tab Tinidazole 2 g OD for 1–2 days Or Tab Secnidazole 2 g stat Or Cap Clindamycin 300 mg BD for 7 days Or Metronidazole gel 0.75% intravaginally, once a day for 5 days Or Clindamycin cream 2% intravaginally at bedtime for 7 days

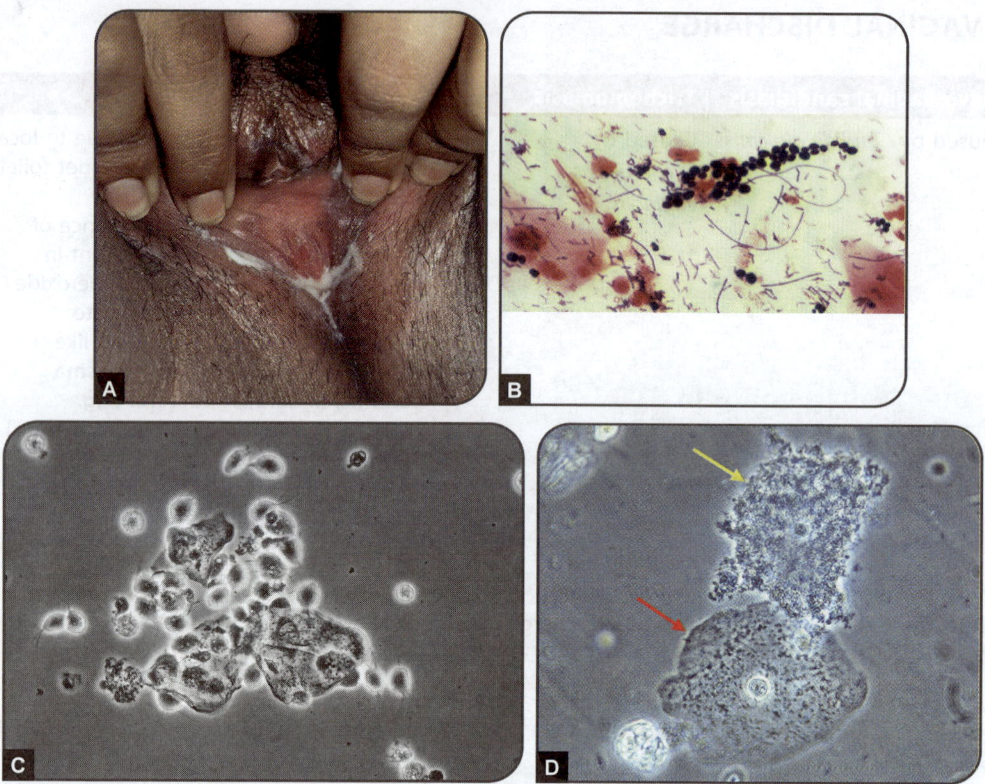

Figs. 12A to D: (A) Vaginal candidiasis—Thick, curdy-white, scanty discharge; (B) Vaginal candidiasis—Gram-stain showing Gram-positive budding yeasts; (C) Wet mount of Trichomoniasis—Plenty of trichomonas on smear; (D) Bacterial vaginosis—Depicts a normal vaginal epithelial cell (red arrow) and an epithelial cell with its exterior covered by bacteria giving the cell a roughened, stippled appearance known as a "clue cell" (yellow arrow)

Aid to Remember

- **Candidal vaginitis** Caused by Candida albicans. Alba = White. Hence, white discharge. **2C**: **C**andida, **C**urdy
- **Trichomoniasis**: **5Fs**—**F**lagella, **F**rothy, **F**ornication (meaning STD), **F**ruit (strawberry cervix), **F**lagyl (metronidazole for treatment)
- **Bacterial vaginosis**: take a "whiff" and smell the "clue". Whiff test, presence of clue cells and foul smell are features of this disease. "vaginosis" not "vaginitis"—no inflammation

ANOGENITAL WARTS

- For theory, read the topic in Chapter 6. Image of condyloma acuminata caused by HPV 6, HPV 11 is shown in Figures 13A and B.

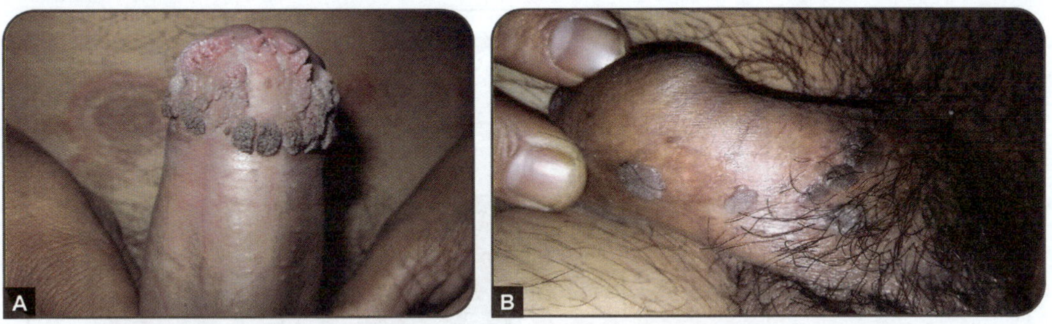

Figs. 13A and B: (A) Condyloma acuminata—Finger-like masses; (B) Condyloma acuminata—Flatter masses

Partner Management in STD

- Usually in all STD prophylactic partner management is done. But for 3 organisms, it is not done-viz **Gardnerella, Candida, herpes.**

Syndromic Approach of STDs

STDs are often treated in the field set up with lack of facilities for accurate diagnosis. In this situation, "syndromic approach" helps where all the possible causes causing a particular presentation are treated.

STI/RTI pre-packed colored kits (Kit 1-Kit 7) are provided to the patient (Fig. 14).

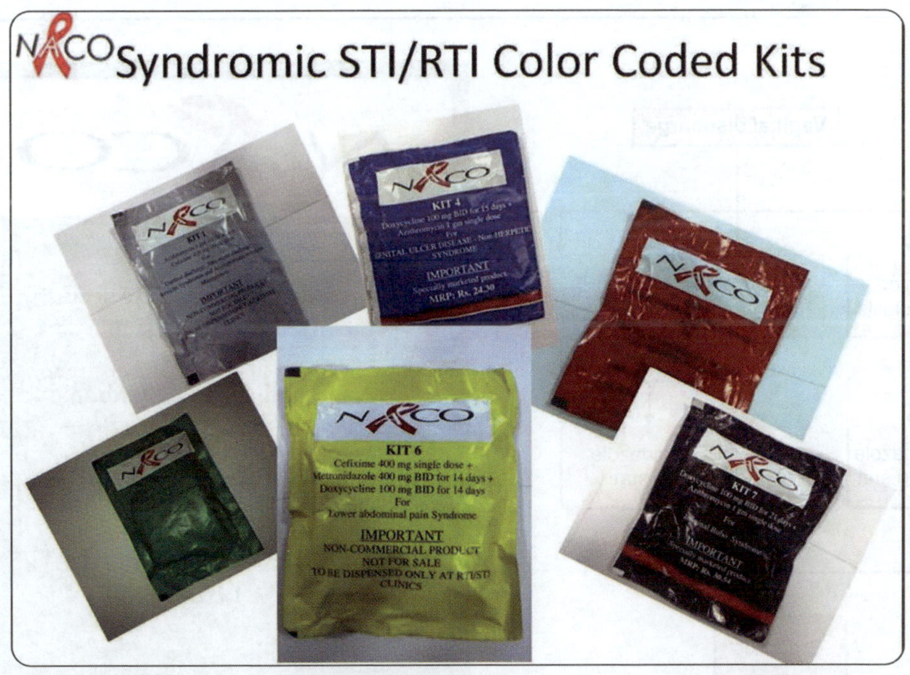

Fig. 14: Syndromic STD packets.

Urethral discharge/cervical discharge
Cover gonorrhea
Cover chlamydia
Tab cefixime single dose
+
Tab azithromycin single dose
(Gray kit)
NACO
KIT 1
Azithromycin 1 gm single dose +
Cefixime 400 mg single dose
For
Urethral discharge, Ano-rectal discharge,
Cervicits Syndromes and Asymptomatic infection
Management
IMPORTANT
NON-COMMERCIAL PRODUCT
NOT FOR SALE
TO BE DISPENSED ONLY AT RTI/STI
CLINICS

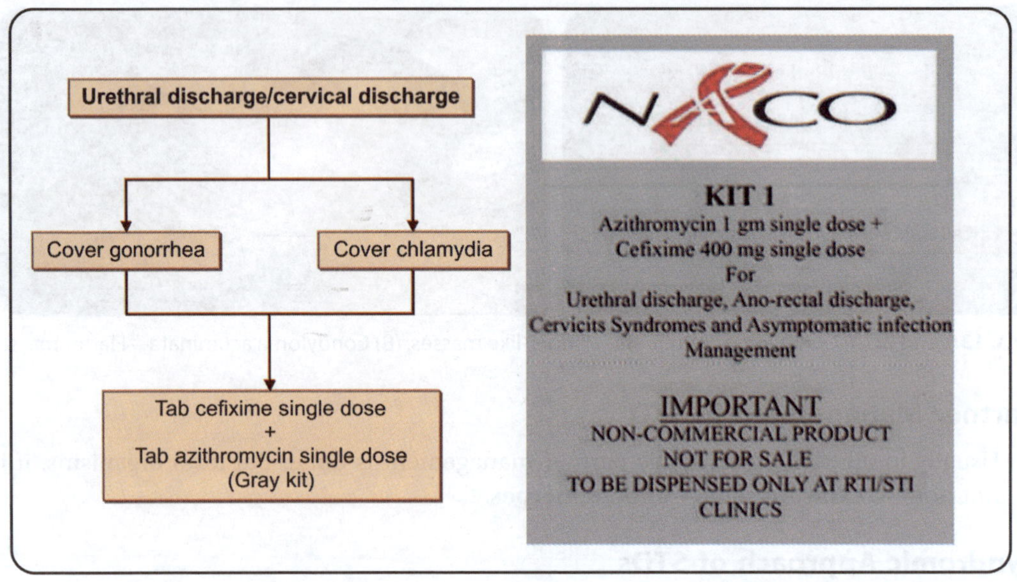

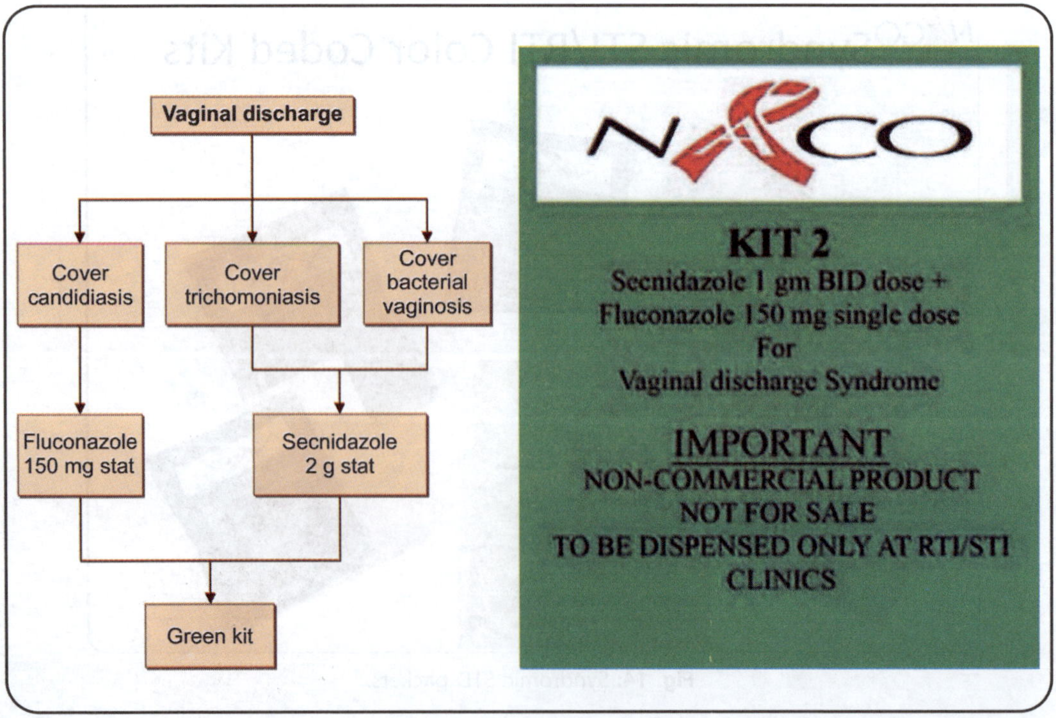

Vaginal discharge
Cover candidiasis
Cover trichomoniasis
Cover bacterial vaginosis
Fluconazole 150 mg stat
Secnidazole 2 g stat
Green kit
NACO
KIT 2
Secnidazole 1 gm BID dose +
Fluconazole 150 mg single dose
For
Vaginal discharge Syndrome
IMPORTANT
NON-COMMERCIAL PRODUCT
NOT FOR SALE
TO BE DISPENSED ONLY AT RTI/STI
CLINICS

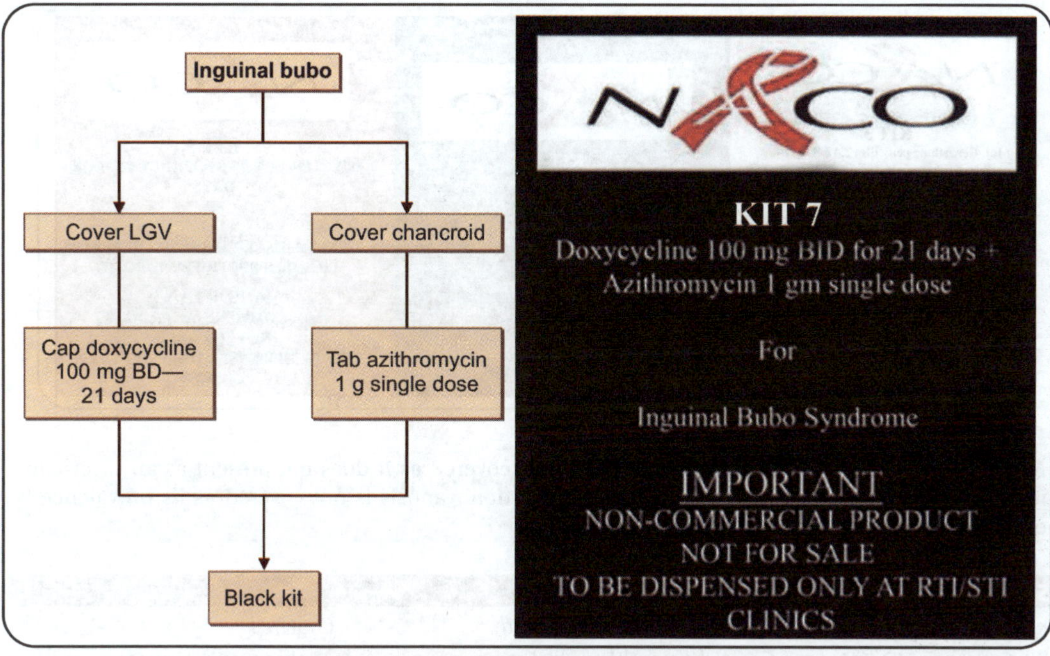

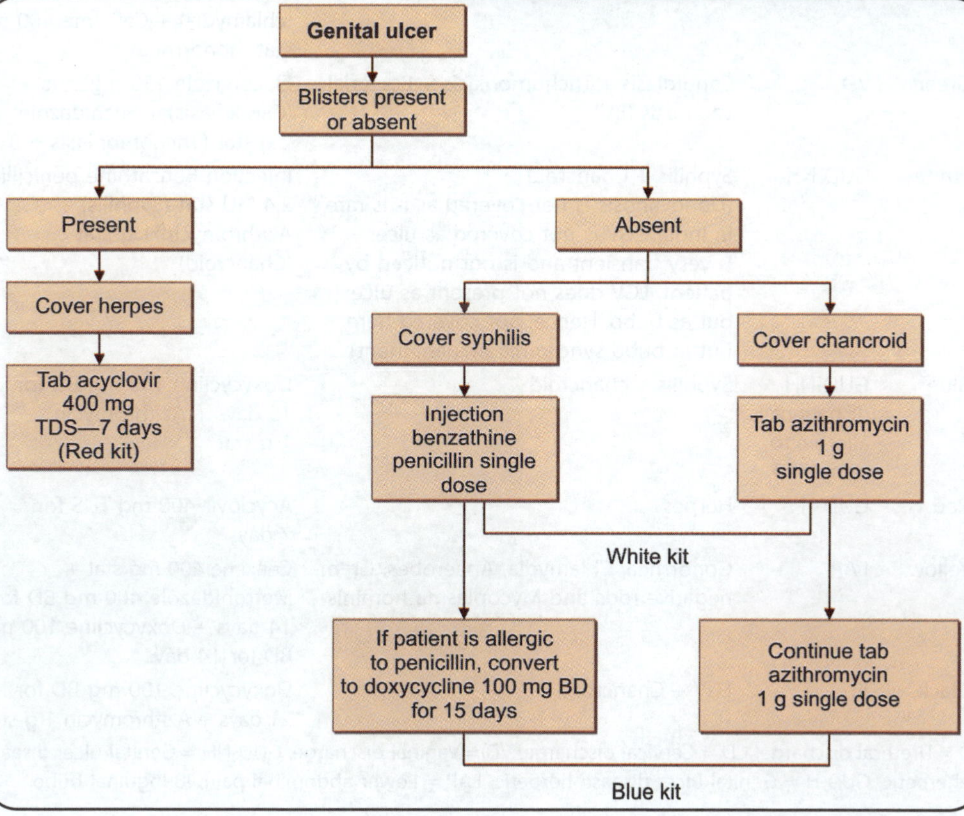

Genital ulcer

Blisters present or absent

- Present → Cover herpes → Tab acyclovir 400 mg TDS—7 days (Red kit)
- Absent
  - Cover syphilis → Injection benzathine penicillin single dose → If patient is allergic to penicillin, convert to doxycycline 100 mg BD for 15 days
  - Cover chancroid → Tab azithromycin 1 g single dose → Continue tab azithromycin 1 g single dose

White kit

Blue kit

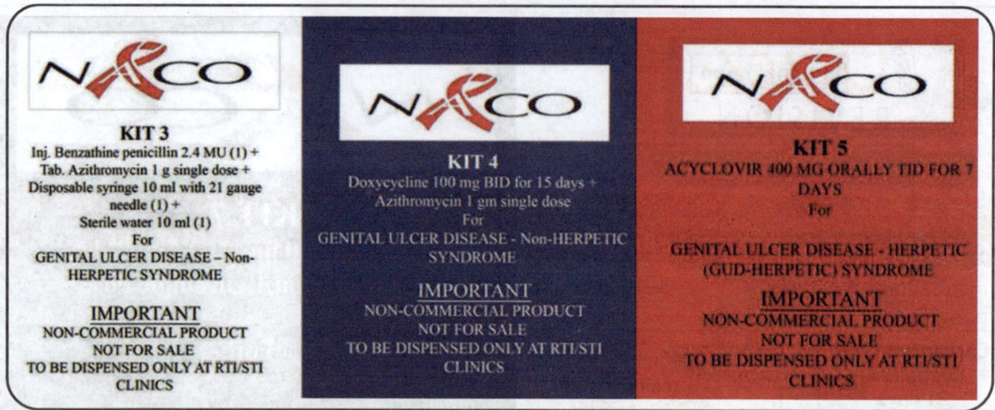

Note: In GUD syndromic management, LGV is not covered as it does not present as an ulcer clinically (more common presentation is a bubo) and donovanosis is not covered as its prevalence is extremely low in India now.

Syndromic management of STIs

Kit color	*Syndrome**	*Organisms/Diseases covered*	*Contents*
Kit Gray	UD, CD	Gonorrhea + chlamydia	Azithromycin 1 g stat (chlamydia) + Cefixime 400 mg stat (gonorrhea)
Kit Green	VD	Candidiasis + Trichomoniasis + Bacterial vaginosis (BV)	Fluconazole 150 mg stat (Candidiasis) + Secnidazole 2 g stat (Trichomoniasis + BV)
Kit White	GUD-NH	Syphilis + Chancroid (Donovanosis is not covered as it is rare in India. LGV is not covered as ulcer is very transient and is not noticed by patient. LGV does not present as ulcer but as bubo. Hence, not covered here but in bubo syndromic management)	Injection Benzathine penicillin 2.4 MU stat (Syphilis) + Azithromycin 1 g stat (Chancroid)
Kit Blue	GUD-NH (If patient is allergic to penicillin)	Syphilis + chancroid	Doxycycline 100 mg BD for 15 days + Azithromycin 1 g stat
Kit Red	GUD-H	Herpes	Acyclovir 400 mg TDS for 7 days
Kit Yellow	LAP	Gonorrhea, Chlamydia, Anaerobes, Gram-negative rods and Mycoplasma hominis	Cefixime 400 mg stat + Metronidazole 400 mg BD for 14 days + Doxycycline 100 mg BD for 14 days
Kit Black	IB	LGV + Chancroid	Doxycycline 100 mg BD for 21 days + Azithromycin 1 g stat

* UD = Urethral discharge, CD = Cervical discharge, VD = Vaginal discharge, GUD-NH = Genital ulcer disease-non-herpetic, GUD-H = Genital ulcer disease-herpetic, LAP = Lower abdominal pain, IB-Inguinal bubo

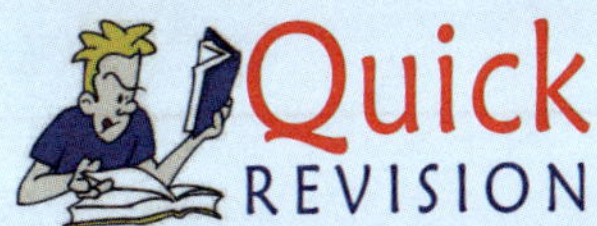

Genital ulcer diseases

Features	Chancre	Chancroid	Herpes genitalis	LGV	Donovanosis
Incubation period	9–90 day	3–10 days	2–20 day	10–30 days	8–80 day
Ulcer features	Single, well-demarcated, round ulcer with firm-indurated base	• Multiple • Soft, painful, tender • Ragged, undermined edges	Grouped vesicles which on rupturing produce grouped erosions	Transient ulcers not noticed by the patient	• Hypertrophic granulation tissue on ulcer floor • Beefy-red • Bleeds easily • Painless
Ulcer features	• Cartilaginous feel, Button-like • Non-tender • Extragenital on lip	• Bleed easily • Auto-inoculation (kissing ulcers)	Recurrent		
Inguinal area	Bilateral, non-tender, shotty, and non-suppurative	• Painful and tender lymph nodes (bubo) • Unilateral, often suppurates	Bilateral-Tender in initial primary episodes	Painful and tender lymph nodes (bubo), "Sign of groove" +	Granulomatous nodules in inguinal area forming "pseudobuboes", not true lymphadenopathy

- Gonococcal urethritis presents with thick, purulent urethral discharge. DOC is Injection Ceftriaxone + Tab azithromycin
- Nongonococcal urethritis caused by Chlamydia presents with mucopurulent thinner urethral discharge. DOC: Tab Azithromycin
- Vaginal discharge: Candidiasis: White, curdy, scanty discharge. Trichomoniasis—Green, frothy, profuse discharge, strawberry cervix. Bacterial vaginosis—Foul smelling, due to Gardnerella. Homogenous thin discharge. Clue cells, Whiff test+
- Herpes genitalis: M/c STD in the world. m/c bacterial STD—Chlamydia
- Gardnerella, Candida, Herpes: No partner management
- Syndromic management: Ulcer: Blue, White, red kits (syphilis+ chancroid+ herpes), Bubo—Black kit (Chancroid + LGV), urethral discharge, cervical discharge—Gray kit (gonococcus + chlamydia), vaginal discharge-green kit (Candida+ trichomonas + bacterial vaginosis)

QUESTIONS

1. **A 23-year-old male had unprotected sexual intercourse with a commercial sex worker. Two weeks later, he developed a painless, indurated ulcer on the glans which exuded clear serum on pressure. Inguinal lymph nodes in both groins were enlarged and not tender. The most appropriate diagnostic test is:**

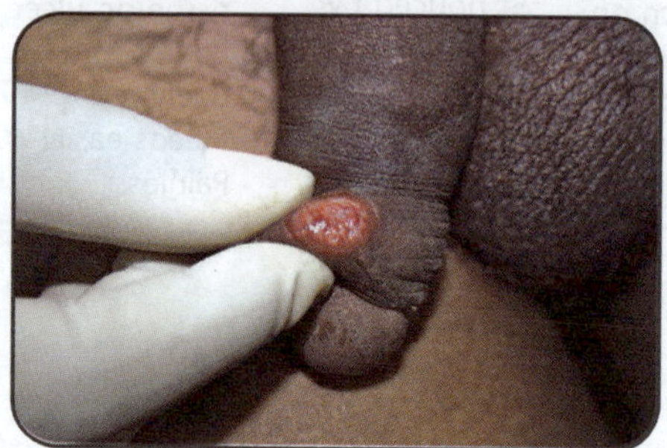

   a. Gram-stain of ulcer discharge
   b. Dark field microscopy of ulcer discharge
   c. Giemsa stain of lymph mode aspirate
   d. ELISA for HIV infection

2. **A 20-year-old male develops ulcers over prepuce and glans which are painful along with suppurative lymphadenopathy 5 days after having sexual intercourse with a sex worker. Most probable diagnosis is:**

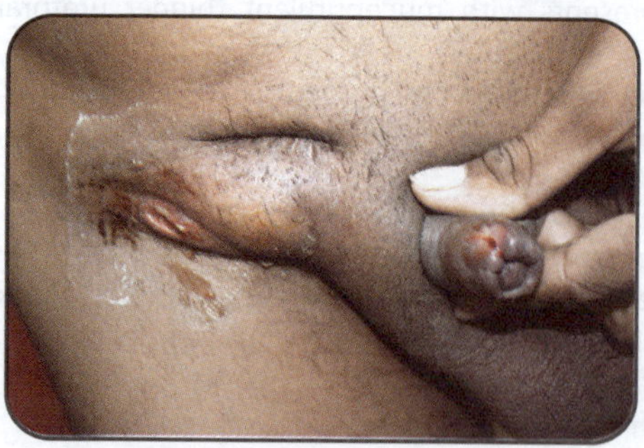

   a. Herpes simplex
   b. Molluscum contagiosum
   c. Syphilis
   d. Chancroid

3. **A man having multiple, painful, non-indurated, undermined, irregular edged ulcers on glans which occurred 5 days after exposure; most likely diagnosis is:**

   a. Chancroid b. Primary chancre
   c. Herpes genitalis d. LGV

4. **A 19 years male develops painless penile ulcers 9 days after sexual intercourse with a professional sex worker. Likely diagnosis is:**

   a. Chancroid b. Herpes
   c. Chancre d. Traumatic ulcer

5. **Multiple painful ulcers over glans without induration is suggestive of:**

   a. LGV
   b. Granuloma inguinale
   c. Chancroid
   d. Syphilis

6. **A 30-year-old male patient has a large, foul-smelling, spreading exuberant ulcer with bright red granulation tissue over the glans penis. There was no lymphadenopathy. The most likely causative organism is:**

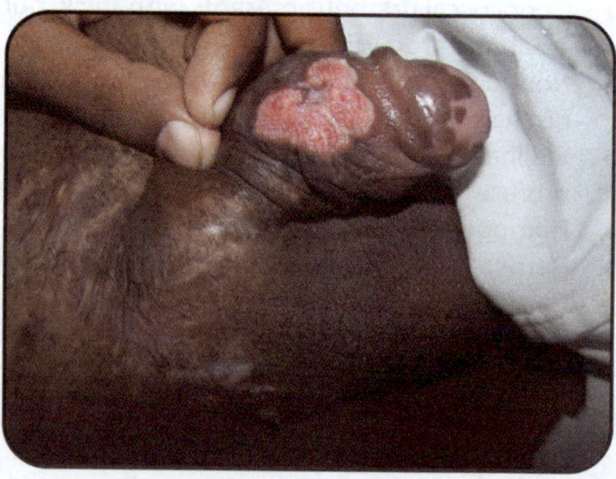

   a. Treponema pallidum
   b. Herpes simplex virus type 1
   c. Herpes simplex virus type 2
   d. Calymmatobacterium granulomatis

7. A 24-year-old male presents to a STD clinic with a single painless ulcer on external genitalia. The choice of laboratory test to look for the etiological agent would be:

a. Scrappings from ulcer for culture on chocolate agar with antibiotic supplement
b. Serology for detection of specific IgM antibodies
c. Scrappings from ulcer for dark field microscopy
d. Scrappings from ulcer for tissue culture

8. Painful ulcers over genitalia are caused by:

a. Primary syphilis
b. Granuloma inguinale
c. Chancroid
d. LGV

9. Ulcer on penis which bleeds on touch, best fits the description of which of the following?

a. Donovanosis
b. Syphilis
c. Herpes genitalis
d. LGV

10. Beefy red genital ulcer with a bleeding ulcer on touch is seen in:

a. LGV
b. Chancroid
c. Primary syphilis
d. Donovanosis

11. A homosexual man presents with pain on defecation. On examination, he has clustered ulcers extending into anal canal. The likely diagnosis is:

a. CMV
b. Gonorrhea
c. Herpes genitalis
d. HIV

12. Genital ulcer is seen in A/E:

a. Granuloma inguinale
b. Syphilis
c. LGV
d. Donovanosis

13. The most frequent cause of recurrent genital ulceration in a sexually active male is:

a. Herpes genitalis
b. Aphthous ulcer
c. Syphilis
d. Chancroid

14. All of the following are sexually transmitted, *except*:

a. Candida albicans
b. Echinococcus
c. Molluscum contagiosum
d. Group B streptococcus

15. Kit 1 used for cervical discharge, urethral discharge and inguino scrotal swelling have which components?

a. Azithromycin b. Cefixime
c. Ciprofloxacin d. Azithromycin
e. Doxycycline

16. Which of the following is an example of a non-venereal disease?

a. Endemic syphilis
b. Gonorrhea
c. Chancroid
d. LGV

17. A female patient presents with green frothy, itchy vaginal discharge with inflammation of vulval skin. Ph of vagina is 5.4. The diagnosis is:

(Recent NEET pattern)

a. Candidal infection
b. Trichomonas infection
c. Bacterial vaginosis
d. Mixed infection

18. Secondary syphilis is manifested by:

a. Painless lymphadenopathy
b. Pruritic rash
c. Mucosal erosion
d. Rash
e. Moist lesions

19. In secondary syphilis all are seen *except*:

a. Condyloma lata b. Interstitial Keratitis
c. Arthritis d. Proteinuria

20. The skin lesions of secondary syphilis include all of the following *except*:

a. Macules
b. Vesicles and Bullae
c. Nodules
d. Papulosquamous lesions

21. In secondary syphilis, true about rash is:
a. Pruritic b. Vesicular
c. Asymptomatic d. Painful

22. Hutchinson's triad in congenital syphilis consists of:
a. Hutchinson teeth, interstitial keratitis, eighth nerve deafness
b. Interstitial keratitis, eighth nerve deafness, mulberry teeth
c. Interstitial keratitis, eighth nerve deafness, strawberry tongue
d. Keratoconjunctivitis sicca, eighth nerve deafness, eighth nerve deafness

23. The lesion characteristic of secondary syphilis:
a. Ulcer
b. Condyloma acuminata
c. Condyloma lata
d. Gumma

24. Which stage of syphilis is most contagious from mother to baby?
a. Primary b. Secondary
c. Early latent d. Later latent

25. A young man presents with a rash which was prominent acrally as shown. He also reports hair loss in patches on scalp and some perianal lesions. The likely etiological agent is:

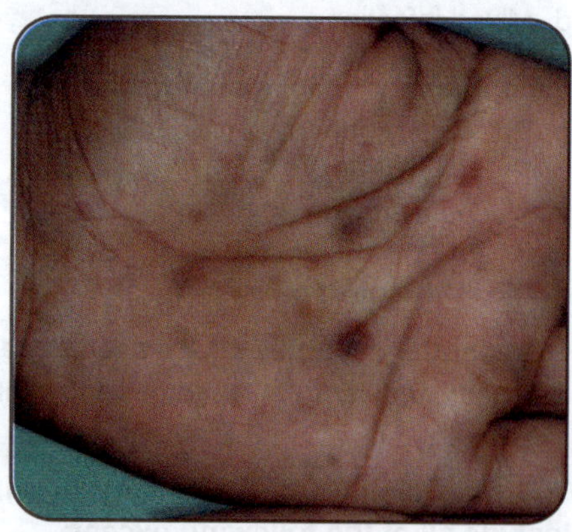

a. Treponema pallidum
b. Treponema pertenue
c. Chlamydia trachomatis
d. Calymmatobacterium

26. Soft sore is caused by: ***(NEET Pattern)***
a. Hemophilus ducreyi
b. Calymmatobacterium granulomatis
c. Chlamydia trachomatis
d. Treponema pallidum

27. "Chancre redux" is a clinical feature of:
a. Early relapsing syphilis
b. Late syphilis
c. Chancroid
d. Recurrent herpes simplex infection

28. Genital elephantiasis is caused by:
a. Donovanosis
b. Congenital syphilis
c. Herpes genitalis
d. Lymphogranuloma venereum

29. Painful lymphadenopathy is seen in:
a. Donovanosis
b. Syphilis
c. Chancroid
d. Herpes simplex
e. Gonorrhea

30. Pseudobubo is seen in: ***(NEET Pattern)***
a. Donovanosis b. LGV
c. Chancroid d. Syphilis

31. Lymphadenopathy is seen in all *except*:
a. Primary syphilis
b. Donovanosis
c. LGV
d. Chancroid

32. Incubation period of Lymphogranuloma venereum is:
a. 1–5 days
b. 5–7 days
c. 60–90 days
d. 10–30 days

33. Treatment of both partners is recommended in all *except*:
a. Candida infection
b. Gardnerella
c. Herpes
d. Trichomonas vaginalis
e. Syphilis

34. Cervical warts are seen with which HPV?
a. 11,13 b. 6,11
c. 16,18 d. 5,8

35. Genital warts are most commonly caused by which of the following serotypes of HPV?

a. HPV 6 b. HPV 16
c. HPV 18 d. HPV 33

36. Condyloma acuminata is caused by:

a. HPV b. HSV
c. HIV d. All

37. The treatment of late stage of cardiovascular syphilis would be:

a. Inj. Benzathine Penicillin 2.4 million units single dose
b. Oral Tetracycline 2 gm/day for 14 days
c. Inj. Benzathine Penicillin 12 to 24 million units/day for 21 days
d. Inj. Benzathine Penicillin 7.2 million units in 3 divided doses weekly

38. Low risk type of HPV:

a. Type-16 b. Type-6
c. Type-18 d. Type-31

39. Podophyllum resin is indicated in the treatment of:

a. Psoriasis
b. Pemphigus
c. Condylomata acuminata
d. Condylomata lata

40. Topical immunomodulator used for the treatment of genital warts is:

a. Imiquimod b. Podophyllin
c. Interferon d. Acyclovir

41. Imiquimod used in treatment of anogenital warts acts manly as:

a. Antifungal
b. Antiviral
c. Immunostimulator
d. Keratolytic

42. The syndromic management of urethral discharge includes treatment of:

a. Neisseria gonorrhoeae and herpes genitalis
b. Chlamydia trachomatis and herpes genitalis
c. Neisseria gonorrhoeae and Chlamydia trachomatis
d. Syphilis and chancroid

43. The syndromic management of genital ulcer syndrome in India includes which of the following disease?

a. Chancroid and primary chancre
b. Chancroid and herpes simplex
c. Chancroid, primary chancre and herpes simplex
d. Herpes simplex and primary chancre

44. A 32-year-old pregnant woman is asymptomatic and has a history of syphilis 7 years back. Her VDRL is negative and TPPA is positive. Which statement is correct?

a. Significant risk for congenital syphilis
b. CSF examination needs to be done for mother
c. Mother has active syphilis
d. No management required

45. A 27 years old sexually active wife of a long distance truck driver presents with copious vaginal discharge of 2 days duration. According to syndromal management of vaginal discharge, which of the following can be given?

a. Azithromycin + metronidazole + fluconazole
b. Azithromycin
c. Metronidazole + fluconazole
d. Fluconazole

46. Olympian brow and rhagades are seen in:

a. CMV inclusion disease
b. Ectodermal dysplasia
c. Congenital syphilis
d. Hyper IgE syndrome

47. A young man presents with asymptomatic macules on trunk and painless lesion on glans penis with generalized lymphadenopathy. The treatment of choice is:

a. Ceftriaxone
b. Benzathine penicillin
c. Acyclovir
d. Fluconazole

48. After giving treatment for syphilis, the response is best assessed by:

a. FTA-Abs b. VDRL
c. TPHA d. Immobilization test

49. Painful genital ulcers are/is seen in:
a. Herpes b. Chancroid
c. Donovanosis d. LGV
e. Syphilis

50. Test used to screen syphilis in pregnant females? *(PGI Nov 18)*
a. TPPA
b. TPHA
c. VDRL
d. RPR
e. Dark ground microscopy

51. Treatment of choice for genital warts in pregnancy is:
a. Salicylic acid b. Podophyllin
c. Imiquimod d. Cryotherapy

52. The best single drug for combined gonococcal and non-gonococcal infections in cervix is:
a. Azithromycin 2 g stat
b. Ceftriaxone 250 mg stat
c. Cefixime 400 mg stat
d. Ciprofloxacin 500 mg stat

53. Drug of choice in syphilis in a pregnant woman is:
a. Azithromycin b. Penicillin
c. Tetracycline d. Ceftriaxone

54. All is/are true about syphilis *except*:
a. Seropositive infant not treated at birth if mother was treated in last trimester
b. For neurosyphilis, CSF-FTA-Abs is sensitive, VDRL is diagnostic but CSF pleocytosis is best treatment response guide
c. HIV patients are less likely to become VDRL nonreactive after treatment
d. EIA +, RPR + indicates past or current treatment
e. Sulphonamides and quinolones are 2nd line

55. A parous woman has nontender indurated ulcer on genitals with no inguinal lymphadenopathy. The diagnosis is:
a. Syphilis b. LGV
c. Herpes d. Chancroid

56. A female comes with frothy, green vaginal discharge of 5 days duration. There was a strawberry cervix on examination. The drug of choice is:
a. Metronidazole b. Tetracycline
c. Fluconazole d. Ciprofloxacin

57. Groove sign is seen in:
a. Chancroid b. Syphilis
c. LGV d. Psoriasis

58. Moth eaten alopecia is seen in:
a. Black dot tinea
b. Telogen effluvium
c. Alopecia areata
d. Secondary syphilis

59. Regarding Donovanosis true is/are:
a. Caused by leishmania species
b. Caused by Calymmatobacterium granulomatis
c. Treated by miltefosine
d. Treated by amphotericin B
e. Pseudobubo

60. A patient presents with multiple penile ulcers with inguinal bubo. Which statement is/are true?
a. Will find school of fish on gram-stain
b. Donovan bodies from scrapings collected from swollen lymph nodes
c. Incision and drainage to be done for fluctuant lymph node swelling
d. Painful genital ulcers
e. Azithromycin in the treatment

61. A woman presents with heavy foul smelling discharge with sharply demarcated ulcers without induration on the perineum and the labia majora. Inguinal lymphadenopathy is also present. What is the most probable diagnosis?
a. Gonorrhea b. Tuberculosis
c. Chancroid d. Trichomoniasis

62. Which of the following tests is NOT used for diagnosing syphilis?
a. Frei test
b. Direct fluorescent antibody test
c. FTA – ABS test
d. TPHA

63. Which of the following cause/causes bacterial vaginosis?

1. Gardnerella
2. Mycoplasma
3. Ureaplasma urealyticum

Select the correct answer using the code given above:

a. 1 only b. 2 and 3 only
c. 1 and 3 only d. 1, 2 and 3

64. Which of the following is correctly matched?

a. Syphilis—painless ulcer and suppurative lymphadenopathy
b. Herpes – painful small vesicles and painful lymphadenopathy
c. LGV - painful vesicle and suppurative lymphadenopathy
d. Chancroid – painful ulcer and painless lymphadenopathy

New Questions

65. A female comes with profuse vaginal itchy discharge. She has strawberry cervix on examination. The treatment is:

(INI CET Nov 21)

a. Metronidazole b. Tetracycline
c. Aciclovir d. Azithromycin

66. Match the entries in the columns:

(INICET July 21)

STD	Kit
1. Green	a. Lower abdominal pain
2. Grey	b. Vaginal discharge
3. Yellow	c. Urethral discharge
4. White	d. Bubo
	e. Genital ulcer—Herpes
	f. Genital ulcer—Non herpes

A. 1-a, 2-b, 3-e, 4-d B. 1-b, 2-d, 3-f, 4-c
C. 1-d, 2-f, 3-a, 4-c D. 1-b, 2-c, 3-a, 4-f

67. A patient presents with painful ulcers at glans penis. Which all options are correct? *(INICET Nov 2020)*

1. Hemophilus ducreyi
2. Herpes simplex
3. Chlamydia
4. Neisseria

a. 1, 2 are correct
b. 1, 2, 3 are correct
c. 2, 3 are correct
d. 1, 2, 4 are correct

68. What all are seen in chancroid?

(INICET Nov 2020)

1. Bleeding
2. Pain
3. Groove sign
4. School of fish

a. 1, 2 are correct
b. 1, 2, 3 are correct
c. 2, 3 are correct
d. 1, 2, 4 are correct

69. The STD showing the most drug resistance: *(INICET May 24)*

a. Gonorrhea b. Chancroid
c. Syphilis d. Donovanosis

70. The following statements are true/false regarding syphilis:

a. Hunterian chancre is best diagnosed by VDRL
b. Moist lesions are seen in tertiary syphilis
c. Inguinal bubo
d. Secondary syphilis classically has blisters
e. Paired VDRL for diagnosis of congenital syphilis

71. Arrange the features of syphilis in the order of their onset (from earliest to latest):

1. Palm and sole lesions
2. Gumma
3. VDRL positive but clinically asymptomatic
4. Hard chancre

a. 1, 2, 3, 4 b. 2, 1, 4, 3
c. 4, 1, 3, 2 d. 1, 2, 4, 3

72. Assertion: VDRL can be used for monitoring treatment efficacy is syphilis

Reason: VDRL is a screening test for syphilis

a. Both Assertion and Reason are true and Reason is correct explanation of Assertion
b. Both Assertion and Reason are true but Reason is not correct explanation of Assertion
c. Assertion is true and Reason is false
d. Assertion is false and Reason is true
e. Both Assertion and Reason are false

73. Painful genital ulcers:

a. Chancroid **b. Herpes**
c. LGV **d. Donovanosis**

1. If a, b, c are correct
2. If a and b are correct
3. If b and d are correct
4. If all four (a, b, c, & d) are correct

74. Match items in column A with best alternative in column B:

Column A	Column B
1. Herpes genitalis 2. LGV 3. Donovanosis 4. Trichomonas vaginalis	a. Profuse vaginal discharge b. Red beefy ulcer c. Kissing ulcers d. White curdy discharge e. Partner treatment not required f. Lymphatic involvement

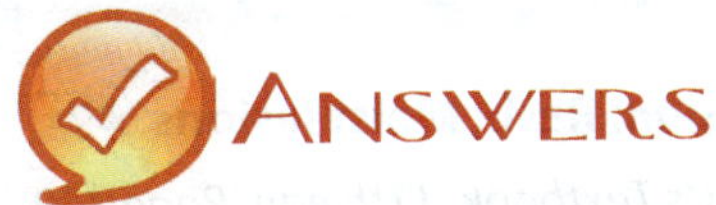

ANSWERS

1. **Ans. (b) Dark field microscopy of ulcer discharge**

   (Ref: Fitzpatrick's Textbook, 8th edn, Page 2486)

   Indurated, painless ulcers with painless lymphadenopathy suggest primary chancre. Incubation period for syphilis is 9–90 days. DGI is the best test here. Gram stain is for chancroid and Giemsa stain is done for donovanosis.

2. **Ans. (d) Chancroid** *(Ref: King K. Holmes and others. Sexually Transmitted Diseases, 4th edn, Page 390-91)*

   Multiple painful ulcers and suppurative lymphadenopathy suggests chancroid. Incubation period for chancroid is 3–10 days which also fits.

3. **Ans. (a) Chancroid** (See page 182 for explanation)

4. **Ans. (c) Chancre** *(Ref: Rook's Textbook of Dermatology, 9th edn, Page 29.8)*

5. **Ans. (c) Chancroid** (See page 182 for explanation)

6. **Ans. (d) Calymmatobacterium granulomatis** *(Ref: Andrew's Textbook, 11th edn, Page 269)*

   Bright red granulation tissue suggests donovanosis. Bubo is not seen (pseudobubo).

7. **Ans. (c) Scrappings from ulcer for dark field microscopy** (See page 164 for explanation)

   DGI is the test of choice for chancre and is the most specific and sensitive test. Serology by EIA (IgM) is a useful screening test but is done only if DGI cannot be done.

8. **Ans. (c) Chancroid** (See page 182 for explanation)

9. **Ans. (a) Donovanosis** (See page 183 for explanation)

10. **Ans. (d) Donovanosis** (See page 183 for explanation)

11. **Ans. (c) Herpes genitalis** (See page 185 for explanation)

    For more details refer to this topic in Chapter 6.

    Grouped blisters and ulcers are classically seen in herpes.

12. **Ans. (c) LGV** *(Ref: Fitzpatrick's Textbook, 8th edn, Page 2506)*

    The primary lesion of LGV is transient, often heals within a few days, and may go unnoticed.

13. **Ans. (a) Herpes genitalis** (See page 185 for explanation)

    For more details refer to this topic in Chapter 6.

    Recurrent ulcers are typical of herpes.

14. **Ans. (b) Echinococcus** *(Ref: Clin Infect Dis. 2004;39:380-388)*

    Group B streptococcus may sometimes be sexually transmitted.

15. **Ans. (a, b) Azithromycin; Cefixime**

16. **Ans. (a) Endemic syphilis** *(Ref: Andrew's Textbook, 11th edn, Page 358)*

    Endemic syphilis (bejel) is a nonvenereal treponematosis occurring in the nomadic tribes. It is caused by *T. pallidum endemicum* and presents with oral ulcers and is transmitted by skin contact or from mouth to mouth by kissing.

17. **Ans. (b) Trichomonas infection**

18. **Ans. (a, c, d, e) Painless lymphadenopathy; Mucosal erosion; Rash; Moist lesions**

19. **Ans. (b) Interstitial Keratitis** *(Ref: Andrew's Textbook, 11th edn, Page 350)*

 Interstitial keratitis is a stigmata of congenital syphilis.

20. **Ans. (b) Vesicles and Bullae** *(Ref: Andrew's Textbook, 11th edn, Page 348)*

21. **Ans. (c) Asymptomatic** (See page 174 for explanation)

22. **Ans. (a) Hutchinson teeth, interstitial keratitis, eighth nerve deafness**

23. **Ans. (c) Condyloma lata** (See page 174 for explanation)

24. **Ans. (b) Secondary** (See page 177 for explanation)

 Secondary syphilis transmits most easily from mother to child through passing of infected blood. Primary stage is most transmissible by the sexual route.

25. **Ans. (a) Treponema Pallidum** (See page 175 for explanation)

 The image is showing a classical palmar lesion of secondary syphilis. The perianal lesions would indicate condyloma lata. Hair loss in patches on scalp would point to moth-eaten alopecia.

26. **Ans. (a) Haemophilus ducreyi** (See page 182 for explanation)

27. **Ans. (a) Early relapsing syphilis** *(Ref: Fitzpatrick's Textbook, 8th edn, Page 2476)*

28. **Ans. (d) Lymphogranuloma venereum** (See page 183 for explanation)

29. **Ans. (c, d) Chancroid; Herpes**

30. **Ans. (a) Donovanosis** (See page 183 for explanation)

31. **Ans. (b) Donovanosis** *(Ref: Fitzpatrick's Textbook, 8th edn, Page 2511)*

32. **Ans. (d) 10–30 days**

33. **Ans. (a, b, c) Candida infection; Gardnerella; Herpes**

 (Ref: 2015 STD Treatment Guidelines, CDC)

 Data from clinical trials indicate that a woman's response to therapy and the likelihood of relapse or recurrence are not affected by treatment of her sex partner(s) as bacterial vaginosis is not a sexually transmitted pathogen. Vulvovaginal candidiasis is usually not sexually acquired, but due to local factors like moisture, DM, antibiotics. Herpes genitalis will continue to be recurrent even if partner management is done as recurrence in herpes is due to reactivation from sacral ganglia and partner treatment is done primarily to prevent recurrence.

34. **Ans. (c) 16, 18**

 For more details refer to this topic in Chapter 6.

35. **Ans. (a) HPV 6** (See page 183 for explanation)

 For more details refer to this topic in Chapter 6.

36. **Ans. (a) HPV** (See page 183 for explanation)

 For more details refer to this topic in Chapter 6.

37. **Ans. (d) Inj. Benzathine Penicillin 7.2 million units in 3 divided doses weekly**

38. Ans. (b) Type-6

For more details refer to this topic in Chapter 6.

39. Ans. (c) Condylomata acuminata

For more details refer to this topic in Chapter 6.

40. Ans. (a) Imiquimod

For more details refer to this topic in Chapter 6.

41. Ans. (c) Immunostimulator

For more details refer to this topic in Chapter 6.

42. Ans. (c) Neisseria gonorrhoeae and Chlamydia trachomatis

(Ref: NACO STD Syndromal Approach Guidelines)

43. Ans. (c) Chancroid, primary chancre and herpes simplex

(Ref: NACO STD Syndromal Approach Guidelines)

44. Ans. (d) No management required

VDRL becomes negative after successful treatment, while treponemal tests remain positive.

45. Ans. (c) Metronidazole + fluconazole *(Ref: NACO STD Syndromal Approach Guidelines)*

46. Ans. (c) Congenital syphilis *(Ref: Fitzpatrick's Textbook, 8th edn, Page 2486)*

47. Ans. (b) Benzathine penicillin

Asymptomatic rash, generalised lymphadenopathy indicates secondary syphilis. Genital ulcer here is an indication of possibly a primary stage ulcer which is yet to heal.

48. Ans. (b) VDRL (See page 180 for explanation)

49. Ans. (a) Herpes; (b) Chancroid

50. Ans. (c, d) VDRL; RPR

51. Ans. (d) Cryotherapy

For more details refer to this topic in Chapter 6.

52. Ans. (a) Azithromycin 2 g stat

Please note that single dose 2 g azithromycin therapy for combined infection is no longer recommended (CDC 2015 guideline) for fear of resistance and azithromycin treatment failures in gonococcal infection. For combined infection the recommendation is injection Ceftriaxone 250 mg/m stat/Cefixime 400 mg stat + Azithromycin 1 g stat. However, since this is not in the options—the best option would still be 2 g azithromycin stat.

53. Ans. (b) Penicillin (See page 181 for explanation)

54. Ans. (a, d, e) Seropositive infant not treated at birth if mother was treated in last trimester; EIA +, RPR + indicates past or current treatment; Sulphonamides and quinolones are 2nd line

Infected infants do need treatment even if mother was treated. HIV patients often remain VDRL positive even after treatment. EIA + RPR + indicates active syphilis, not past syphilis. Doxycycline is the 2nd line.

55. Ans. (a) Syphilis (See page 173 for explanation)

56. Ans. (a) Metronidazole

57. Ans. (c) LGV

58. Ans. (d) Secondary syphilis (See page 174 for explanation)

59. Ans. (b, e) Caused by Calymmatobacterium granulomatis; Pseudobubo

60. Ans. (a, c, d, e) Will find school of fish on gram-stain; Incision and drainage to be done for fluctuant lymph node swelling; Painful genital ulcers; Azithromycin in the treatment

The diagnosis here is chancroid.

61. Ans. (c) Chancroid

Non-indurated ulcer (soft chancre) and inguinal lymphadenopathy suggests chancroid

62. Ans. (a) Frei test

63. Ans. (d) 1, 2 and 3

64. Ans. (b) Herpes – painful small vesicles and painful lymphadenopathy

New Answers

65. Ans. (a) Metronidazole

The diagnosis is trichomoniasis due to profuse itchy discharge with strawberry cervix.

66. Ans. (d) 1-b, 2-c, 3-a, 4-f

67. Ans. (a) 1, 2 are correct

68. Ans. (d) 1, 2, 4 are correct

69. Ans. (a) Gonorrhea

70. Ans. a-False; b-False; c-False; d-False; e-True

Correct answers: a- Best diagnosed by DGI, b- Moist lesions are seen in secondary syphilis, c- Bubo is not seen in syphilis, d- Congenital syphilis has blisters

71. Ans. (c) 4, 1, 3, 2

72. Ans. (b) Both Assertion and Reason are true but Reason is not correct explanation of Assertion

Correct reason: VDRL is used for monitoring as its titre reduces 4 folds within 6 months after successful treatment.

73. Ans. (2) If a and b are correct

74. Ans. 1-e, 2-f, 3-b, 4-a

CHAPTER 9

Blistering (Vesiculobullous) Diseases

BLISTERING DISORDERS

Classification

A. Based on etiology:

- Acquired—Autoimmune mechanism of blister formation
- Congenital—Genetic defects

B. Based on level of blister formation

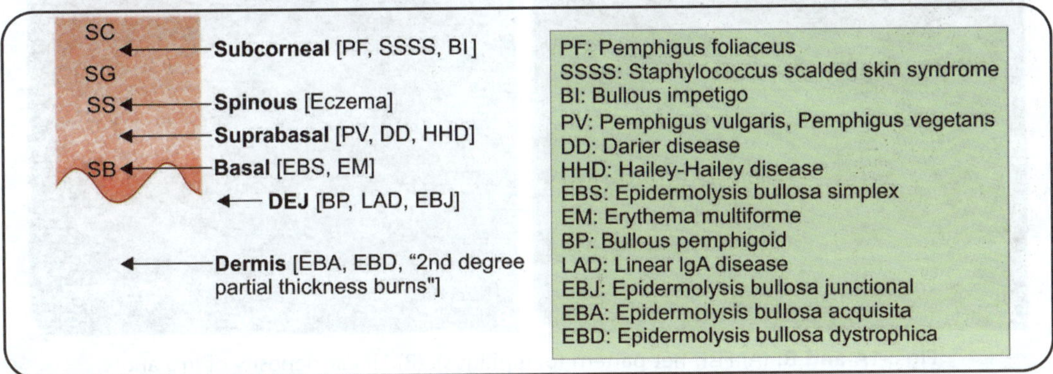

Investigation in Blistering Disorders

- **Direct immunofluorescence (DIF):** DIF is a test which detects the abnormal antibody formation in autoimmune blistering diseases and its position of deposition in skin via tagging with immunofluorescent dyes.
  Site for DIF: Biopsy is taken from **perilesional skin** (normal skin immediately next to the blister). Since it is a test for autoimmune blistering disorders, it will be negative in congenital epidermolysis bullosa, Hailey-Hailey disease, Darier disease.

Disease	Pattern
Pemphigus	**Intercellular** or **fish-net pattern** (**IgG and C3** deposits) (Fig. 1A)
Bullous pemphigoid/Cicatricial pemphigoid/ Epidermolysis bullosa acquisita	**Linear, homogeneous deposits of IgG and C3** at the DEJ (Fig. 1B)
Linear IgA dermatosis	**Linear homogenous deposits of IgA at the DEJ**
Dermatitis herpetiformis	Focal **granular** deposits of **IgA at the papillary tips**

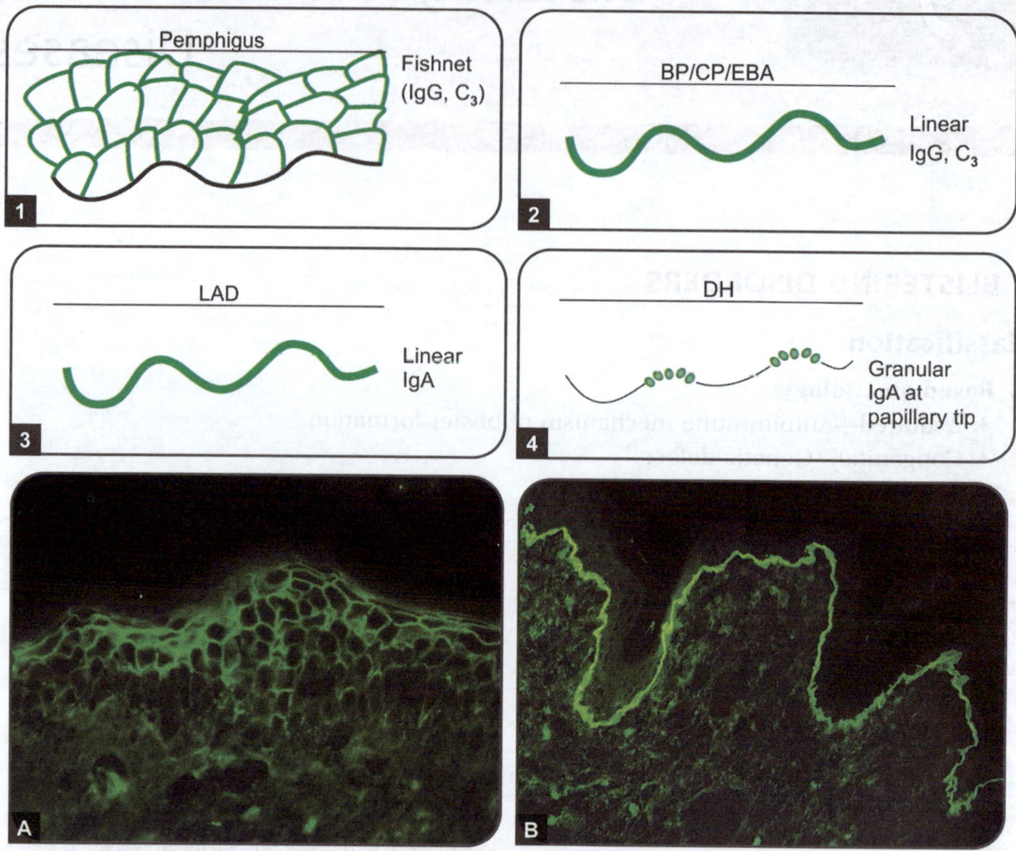

Figs. 1A and B: (A) Fish net pattern (pemphigus); (B) Linear deposits of IgG and C3 along the DEJ (BP/CP/EBA)

ACQUIRED BLISTERING DISORDERS

Pemphigus

- A group of **chronic autoimmune blistering diseases** typically with presence of **antibodies (usually IgG) against desmosomes/intercellular substance** leading to separation of epidermal keratinocytes **(acantholysis)** and epidermal flaccid blisters. (There is a rare type of pemphigus where IgA is deposited in epidermis, called as **IgA pemphigus**).
- The term **"pemphigus"** is derived from the Greek ***pemphix*, meaning blister or bubble**.
- **Pathology**: Desmosomes are intercellular adhesion molecules which keep the keratinocytes glued together in epidermis. Desmoglein (Dsg) is a protein inside desmosomes. Central pathology in pemphigus is the formation of **anti-desmoglein antibodies** causing collapse of the desmosome. As there is no adhesion between keratinocytes now, they separate from each other, become circular (**acantholytic cells**) and accumulate fluid in between them.

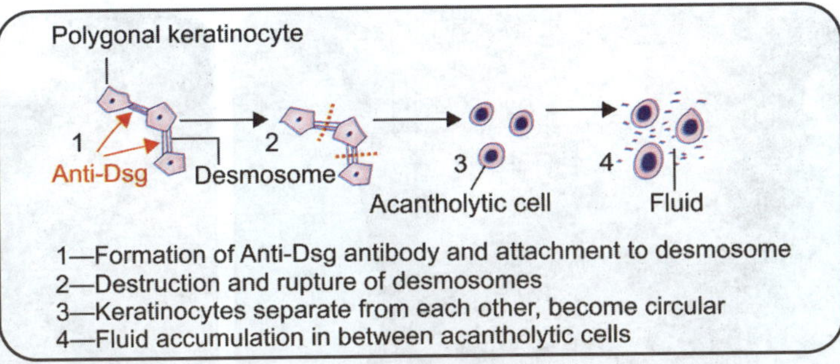

Types of pemphigus

a. Pemphigus vulgaris (PV)

- **Most common type** ("vulgaris" means common)

High Yield Points

Remember that all diseases which have the word "vulgaris" attached are the most common forms of that disease. For example, psoriasis vulgaris is the most common form of psoriasis, lupus vulgaris is the most common type of cutaneous TB, vitiligo vulgaris is the most common form of vitiligo and so on.

- Presents as **flaccid** (as they are epidermal), **easily rupturable bullae** (hence cutaneous erosions are more commonly seen clinically) **with mucosal erosions** (Figs. 2 and 3). Lesions are all over the body and are typically **very slow to heal.**

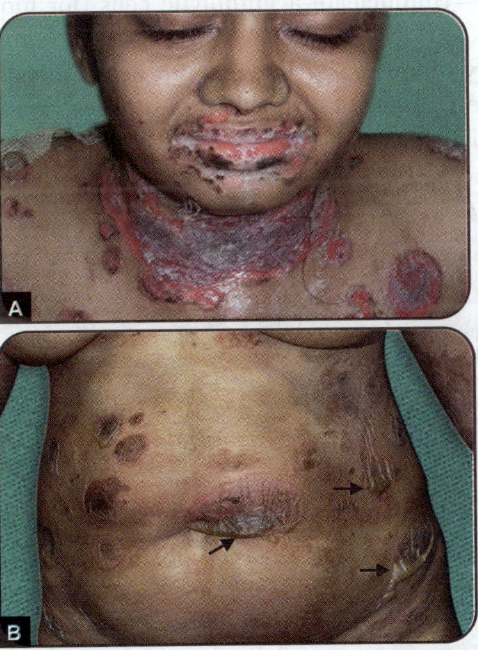

Figs. 2A and B: (A) Pemphigus vulgaris—cutaneous erosions and oral erosions; (B) Pemphigus vulgaris— flaccid blisters

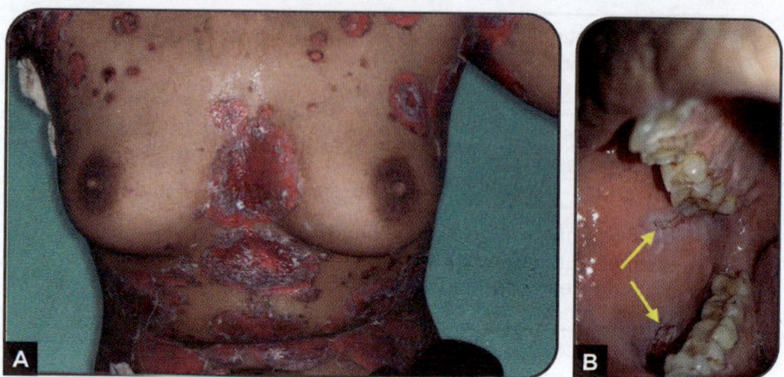

Figs. 3A and B: (A) Pemphigus vulgaris—widespread erosions; (B) Pemphigus vulgaris—angular, irregular oral ulcers (yellow arrows)

- **First site of involvement—mouth**, then skin gets involved after a few months. Mean age of onset—40 years in India.
- **The Nikolsky sign and bulla-spread sign (Asboe-Hansen sign) are positive.** Nikolsky sign refers to erosions extending into visibly normal skin by rubbing at the periphery of active lesions (more on Nikolsky sign and bulla spread sign—see Chapter 2).
- **2 types—Mucosal** (only Anti-Dsg 3 antibodies are present) **and mucocutaneous** (Both anti-Dsg 3 and anti-Dsg 1 antibodies are present).
- **Diagnosis:**
  - **Tzanck smear**—Uninucleate acantholytic cells (for more on Tzanck smear—see Chapter 2)
  - **Histopathology—Suprabasal blister with acantholysis**. The basal cells are still attached to the DEJ and appear like tombstones in a grave (**row of tombstone appearance**) (Fig. 3C).

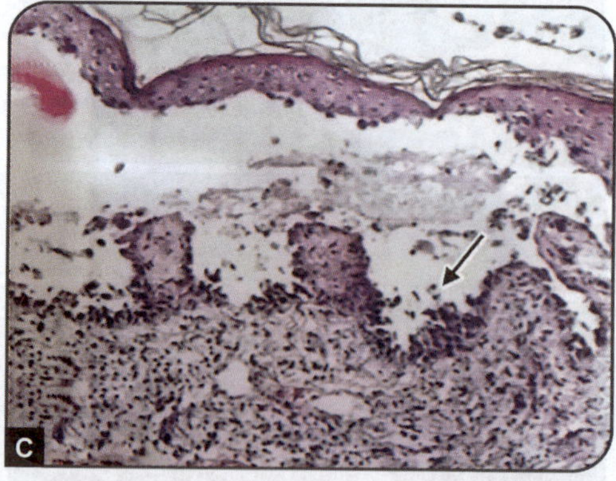

Fig. 3C: Histopathology in PV—Note the suprabasal split and row of tombstone appearance of stratum basale

  - **DIF**—see above
  - **ELISA testing** for Dsg-1 and Dsg-3 autoantibodies.

- **Treatment:**
  - **High-dose Prednisolone (1 mg/kg/day)—DOC**
  - Azathioprine, Mycophenolate mofetil, cyclophosphamide and methotrexate—often added with steroids (all used as steroid-sparing drugs to help reduce dose of steroids)
  - **Rituximab** (anti-CD20 monoclonal antibody) attacks autoimmune B cells and hence reduces anti-Dsg antibody formation—DOC in patients not responding to steroids/mycophenolate/azathioprine
  - Intravenous immunoglobulin (IVIG), Plasmapheresis (dilutional effect on pathogenic autoantibodies)
  - **Pulse therapy**—Intravenous pulse therapy with megadose corticosteroids (methylprednisolone, dexamethasone), often combined with cyclophosphamide called DC pulse (D-dexamethasone, C-cyclophosphamide) at monthly intervals are often given to avoid side effects of daily steroids.

b. Pemphigus vegetans

- Flaccid blisters, erosions, **vegetating masses** (cauliflower-like vegetations) in flexural areas. **Hence the name pemphigus "vegetans"—Vegetans = vegetable-like, i.e., cauliflower-like** (Fig. 4)
- A variant of pemphigus vulgaris (**rare type** of pemphigus)

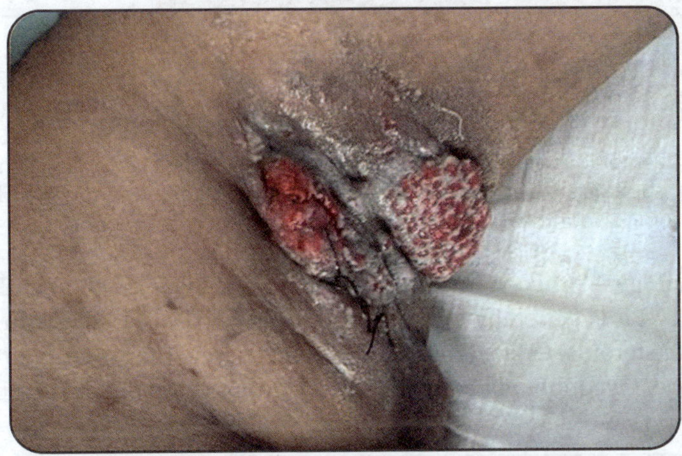

Fig. 4: Vegetating, cauliflower-like masses in flexure

c. Pemphigus foliaceus (PF)

- **Flaccid bullae** (so flaccid and superficial that intact blisters are **not seen; instead scales and crusts are seen**). Lesions are not widespread like in PV but **in seborrheic distribution**, including the face, scalp, and upper trunk. **Mucosa is not involved (contrast to pemphigus vulgaris)** (Figs. 5 and 6)
- Antibodies target **only Dsg 1.**
- **Nikolsky sign is positive. Bulla spread sign is however negative** as the blisters are too fragile to be pushed in bulla spread sign (more information and image of bulla spread sign in the topic of pemphigoid next)

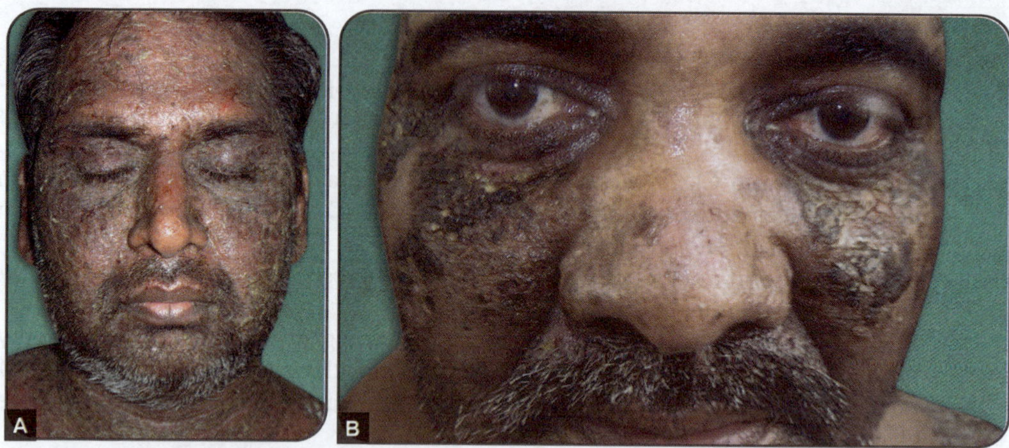

Figs. 5A and B: (A) Pemphigus foliaceus—Scales on face (seborrheic area); (B) Pemphigus foliaceous—Scales—crusts on cheeks. Note the absent mucosal involvement

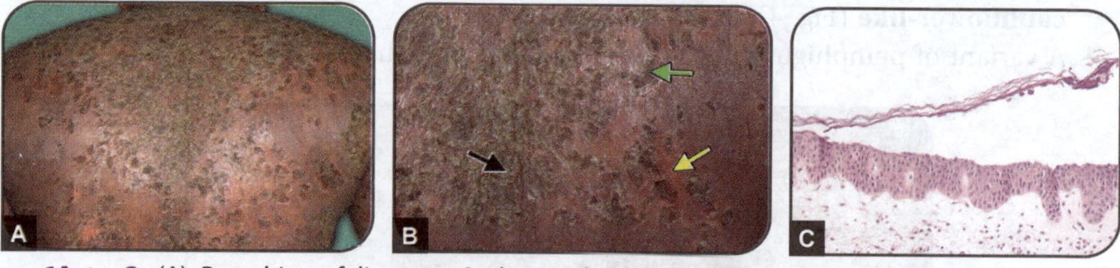

Figs. 6A to C: (A) Pemphigus foliaceus—Scales on back (seborrheic area); (B) Pemphigus foliaceus-Close-up showing superficial erosions (yellow arrow), crusts (green arrow), scales (black arrow); (C) Histopathology of PF. Note the subcorneal split

- **Histopathology—Subcorneal blister (in granular layer) with acantholysis** (Fig. 6C)
- **Treatment**—PF is generally less severe than PV and mild cases can only be treated with topical steroids. Oral steroids and steroid sparers (dapsone, hydroxychloroquine, azathioprine, mycophenolate mofetil, or cyclophosphamide) are given in more severe cases.

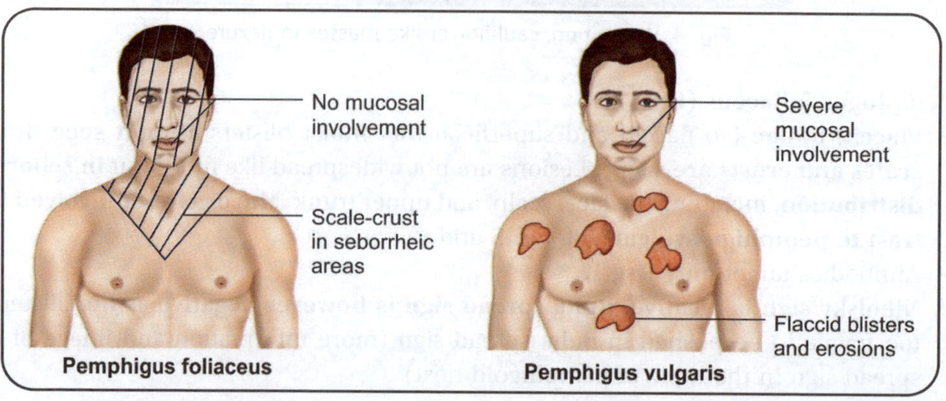

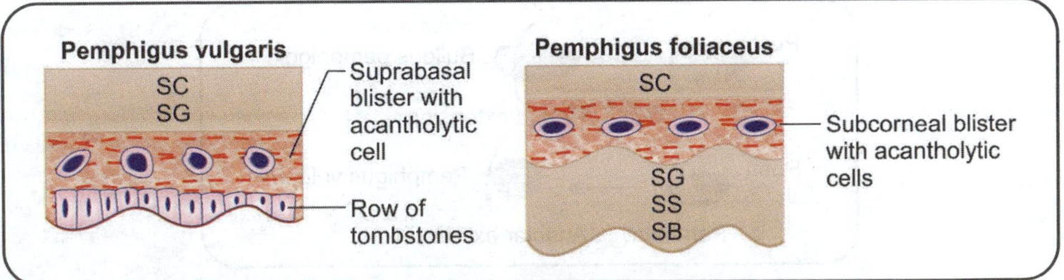

Pemphigoid (Bullous Pemphigoid—BP)

- **Tense itchy blisters** (since it is subepidermal) on the **trunk**, **thigh**, groin, axillae, limb
- The blisters tend to **heal fast** (contrast to PV)
- Blisters often come on a **background of urticarial wheals and redness** (contrast to PV which comes on normal skin). **Blisters heal with hypopigmentation** (Figs. 7A to D)

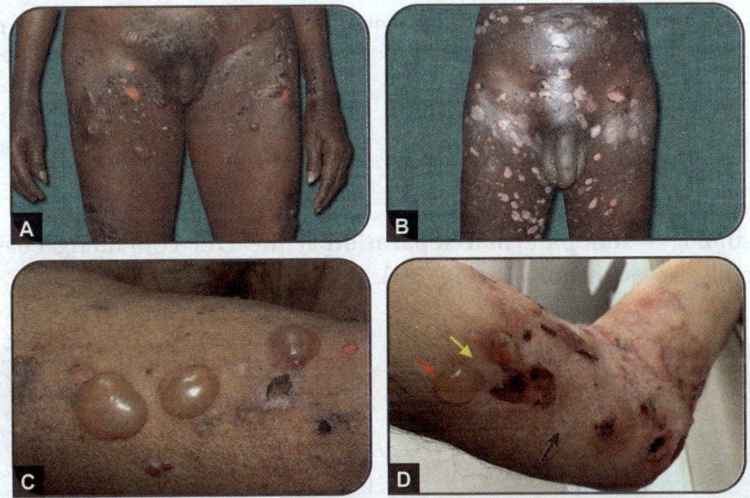

Figs. 7A to D: (A) Bullous pemphigoid—tense blisters on red skin, few have ruptured; (B) Bullous pemphigoid—after treatment—healing with hypopigmentation; (C) Bullous pemphigoid—Tense blisters on upper limb; (D) Bullous pemphigoid—tense blister (red arrow) with mild erythema around it (yellow arrow), few healed areas with hypopigmentation (black arrow)

- Age group—Classically **elderly** population (65–75 years—contrast to PV)
- **Anti-BP 1 (BP 230) and Anti-BP 2 (BP 180)** antibodies are pathogenic (BP-2 > BP-1)
- **Nikolsky sign—negative, bulla spread sign (Asboe-Hansen sign)—positive**
- Bulla spread sign involves making a pen mark at one edge of the blister and pushing it from the other side to extend it beyond the pen mark. It extends in both PV and BP (Figs. 8A and B) but their patterns of extension are different (oval extension in BP and pointed extension in PV, as shown next).

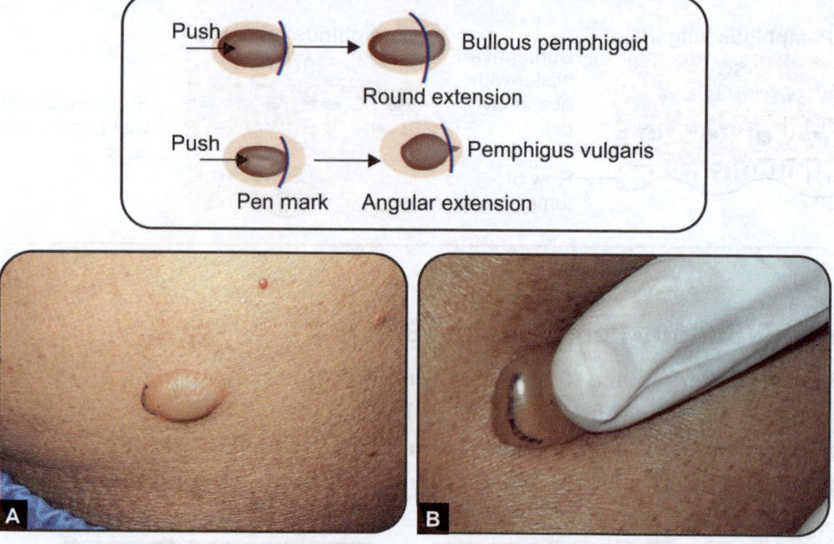

Figs. 8A and B: (A) Bulla spread sign—one edge of blister is marked with a pen; (B) Rounded extension of blister beyond the pen mark—bullous pemphigoid

- **Diagnosis**:
  - Tzanck smear—negative
  - DIF—See Figures 1B and 8C
  - Histopathology—**subepidermal separation** at the DEJ containing **eosinophils** and neutrophils. **No acantholysis (Fig. 8D)**.

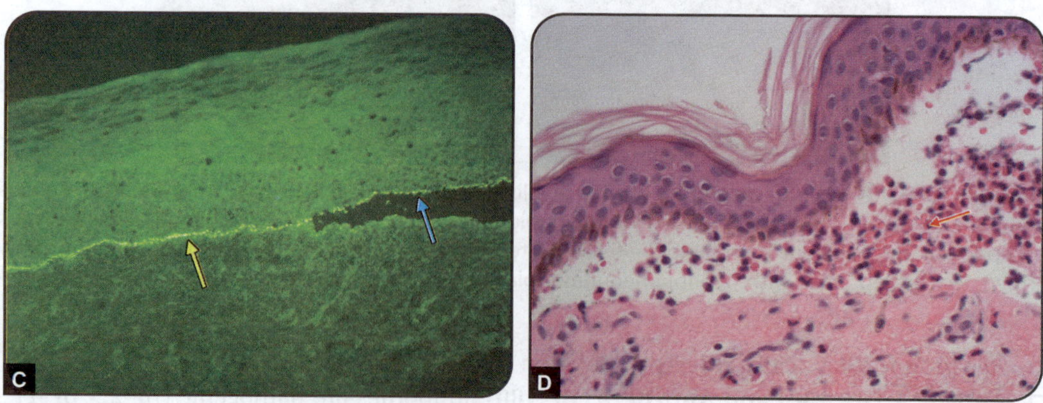

Figs. 8C and D: (C) DIF of BP—Linear DEJ deposits of IgG/C3 (yellow arrow). After keeping the skin biopsy sample in saturated solution of salt (salt-split technique), the DEJ splits at the junction of lamina lucida and lamina densa and the linear fluorescence is then seen on the roof of the split (blue arrow) as the stain fluoresce BP-1 or BP-2 which is at the roof area. If this was a case of EBA—the linear fluorescence would have been seen on the floor of the split (as it would stain the collagen 7 which is below); (D) Histopathology in BP: Subepidermal blister with eosinophils in the blister cavity (red arrow)

- **Treatment:**
  - BP is usually **self-limited** over a 5–6-year period (contrast to PV)
  - **Topical steroids are very effective**, low-dose prednisolone (contrast to PV where high-dose prednisolone is given), tetracycline + niacinamide combination (as an anti-inflammatory), dapsone (as an anti-eosinophilic and anti-neutrophilic agent), azathioprine, mycophenolate mofetil.

Pick-up words in MCQs on BP
- Elderly patients, tense itchy blisters, blisters coming on red skin

Pemphigoid Gestationis (Herpes Gestationis)

- The word can be split into "pemphigoid" + "gestation"—indicating BP in pregnancy. The word "herpes" is incorrect—no relation to herpes
- Typically, the site of involvement is **periumbilical**
- **Resolves after delivery**

Dermatitis Herpetiformis (DH)

- Misnomer—not related to herpes
- Extremely distressing and **severely itchy** disease characterized by grouped, symmetrical papulovesicles on **extensor surfaces (e.g., elbow)** (Figs. 9A and B)
- Due to **severe itch, intact blisters are rarely seen—excoriations (scratch marks) are more common**

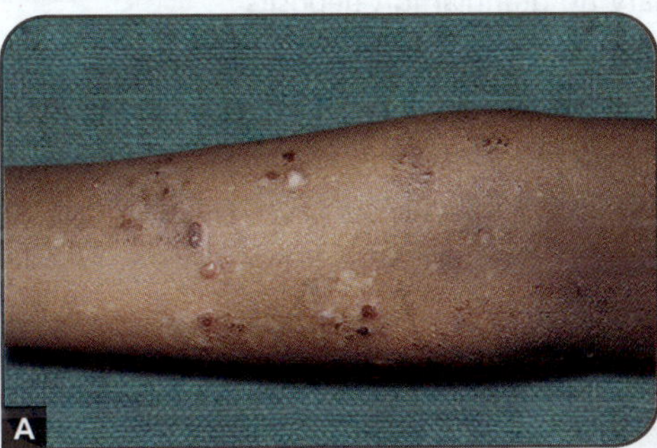

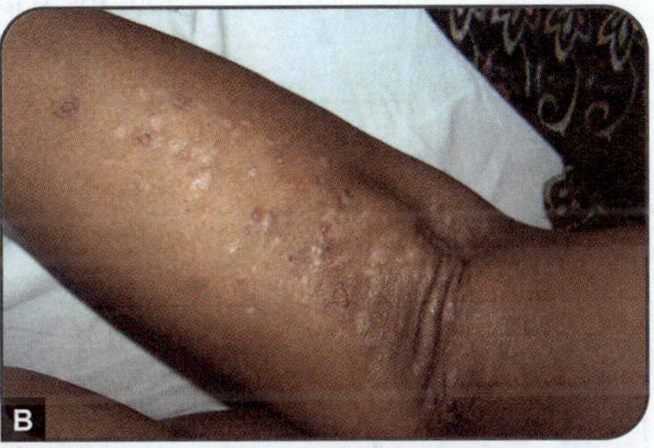

Figs. 9A and B: (A) Small, tense blisters, with excoriation and crusting at elbows; (B) Another patient with small tense blisters at elbow, many have healed with hypopigmentation

- 70–100% patients of DH have underlying **coeliac disease (gluten-sensitive enteropathy)**
- **Potassium iodide and gluten (found in cereals except for rice and corn) flares the disease**
- **IgA antibodies** against **epidermal transglutaminase (TTG)** which are present in the papillary tip are pathogenic (see in Figure 10)
- **Investigation:**
  - Circulating IgA antibodies against the smooth muscle cell endomysium (**anti-endomysial antibodies**) and **IgA antibodies against TTG are present**

- Histopathology—Neutrophils accumulate in the dermal papillae (**papillary tip micro-abscess**), subepidermal blister (Figs. 9C and D)
- Treatment—**Dapsone is the DOC** (acts as a neutrophil remover from papilla) along with a **gluten-free diet** (to avoid wheat, barley, and rye). The improvement with dapsone is so dramatic (in 1-2 days), that the response can be used to confirm the diagnosis.

Pick-up words in MCQs on DH

- Severe itching, elbows, extensor involvement, exacerbation with certain foods

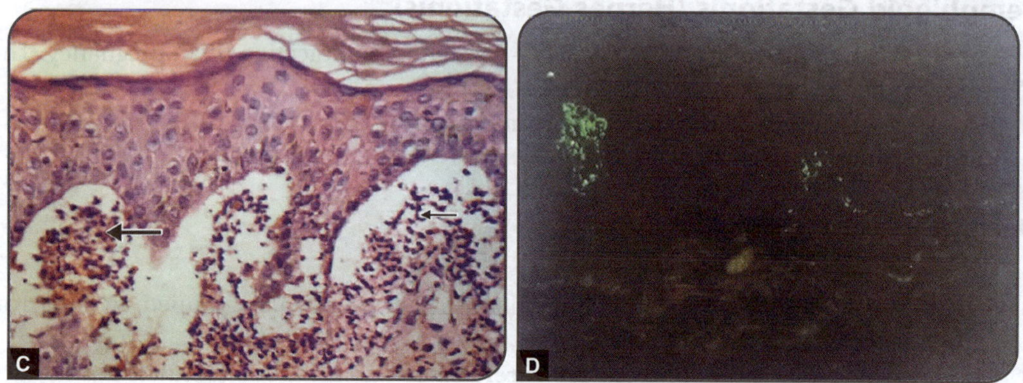

Figs. 9C and D: (C) Histopathology in DH—Note the papillary tip neutrophils and split (black arrows); (D) DIF of DH—Note the papillary tip granular IgA deposits

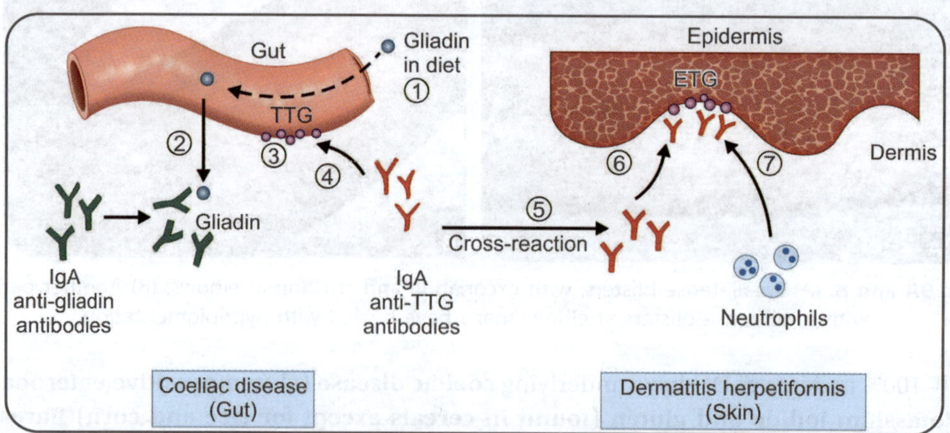

Fig. 10: Pathogenesis of DH—Intake of gliadin containing food (1). Absorption of gliadin into tissue through the gut (2). Formation of IgA anti-gliadin antibodies causing inflammation (3). Tissue transglutaminase (TTG 3) in gut triggers formation of IgA anti-TTG antibodies (4). This anti-TTG cross-reacts with the skin (5) which further targets epidermal transglutaminase-ETG at the tip of dermal papillae (6) since TTG resembles ETG. Neutrophils then aggregate at papillary tip creating papillary tip neutrophil aggregates increasing the dermal inflammation and causing papillary tip blisters (7)

Linear IgA Bullous Dermatosis (LAD)

- Called **chronic bullous disorder of childhood (CBDC)**, if the same disease occurs in children
- Vesicles can resemble DH or BP
- **"String of pearls" or "cluster of jewels" appearance**: Tense blisters form a ring resembling a cluster of jewels/string of pearls (Figs. 11A and B). Common sites of involvement are perineum and perioral areas

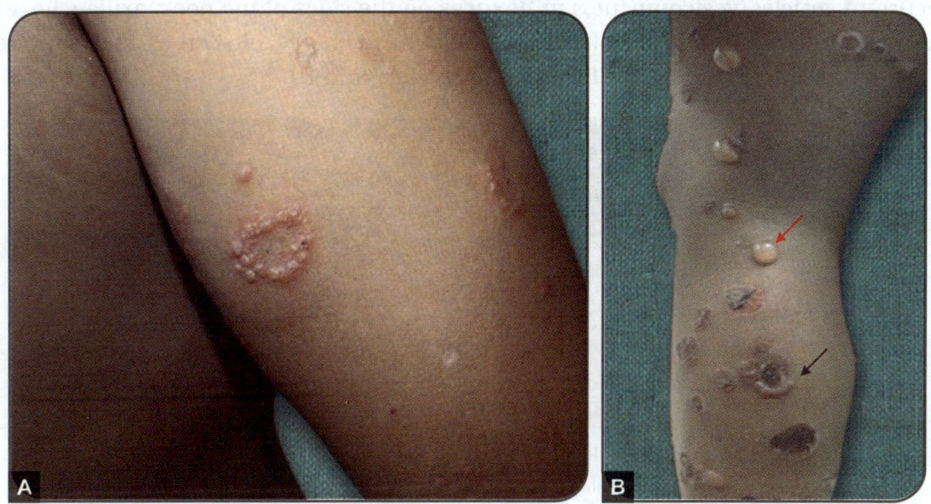

Figs. 11A and B: (A) "String of pearls appearance"; (B) Tense blister (red arrow), blister in a circle at the periphery (string of pearls)

- Mucous membrane involvement in 50% cases
- **Antibody is against LAD antigen (BP-120), BP-1 (BP-230) and BP-2 (BP-180)**
- Histopathology—**Subepidermal blister**
- Treatment—**Dapsone is the drug of choice.**

INHERITED BLISTERING DISORDERS

Hailey-Hailey Disease (Benign Familial Pemphigus)

- Hailey-Hailey disease (HHD) is an autosomal-dominant disorder and is due to a **genetic defect in a calcium pump in golgi apparatus in keratinocyte.** The gene defect is in **calcium ATPase (*ATP2C1*) gene** (ATP2C1 is present in the basal and suprabasal layer and encodes an ATP-powered calcium pump which is essential for desmosome function in suprabasal layer and, hence, keratinocyte adhesion to each other → hence, lack of this pump causes keratinocyte separation **[acantholysis]** and blistering in suprabasal epidermis).

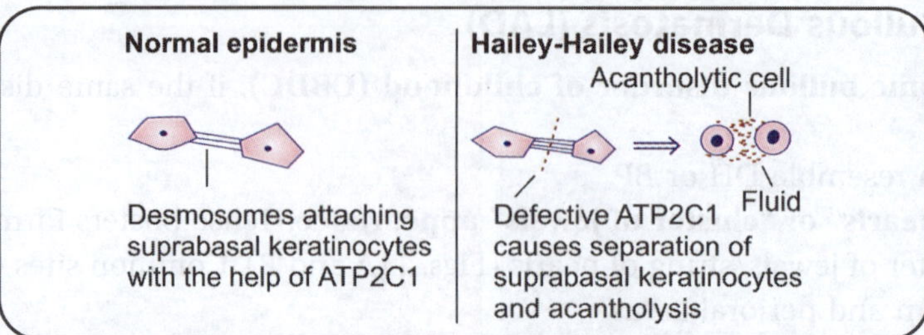

- Recurrent vesicles/vesicopustules in **flexures** on the sides of the neck, axillae, flexures of groin and inframammary area (Usually, intact blisters are not seen as they rupture due to friction in flexures to create **fissures**) (Figs. 12A and B)

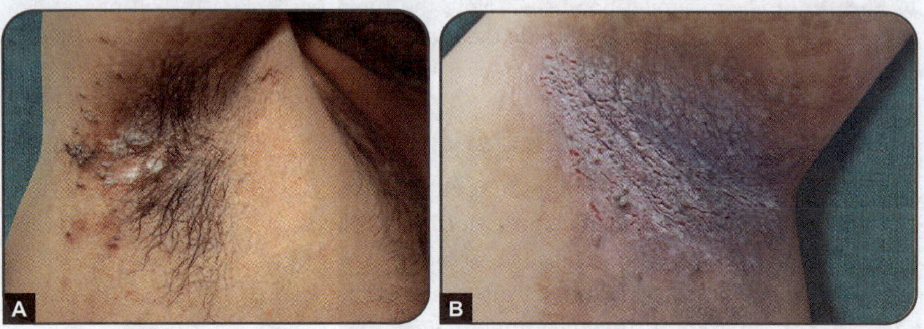

Figs. 12A and B: (A) Hailey-Hailey disease—Vesicopustules in axilla; (B) Hailey-Hailey disease—Fissured plaques in axilla

- Presents between the 2nd–4th decades of life
- Superimposed bacterial/candidal infections. **Koebner's phenomenon may occur**
- Histopathology—**Suprabasal split due to acantholysis**. Typically, however, the acantholysis is incomplete, and separated keratinocytes are still partially connected to each other, giving an **appearance of a broken brick wall (dilapidated brick wall appearance—"dilapidated = broken")** (Figs. 12C and D).
- Treatment—Triggers such as heat, sweating, and friction should be minimized. Systemic/topical antibiotics (for Staphylococcus aureus), Corticosteroids—for inflammation.

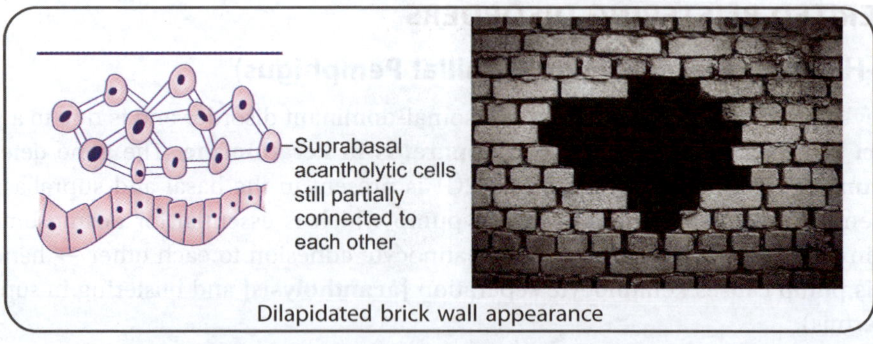

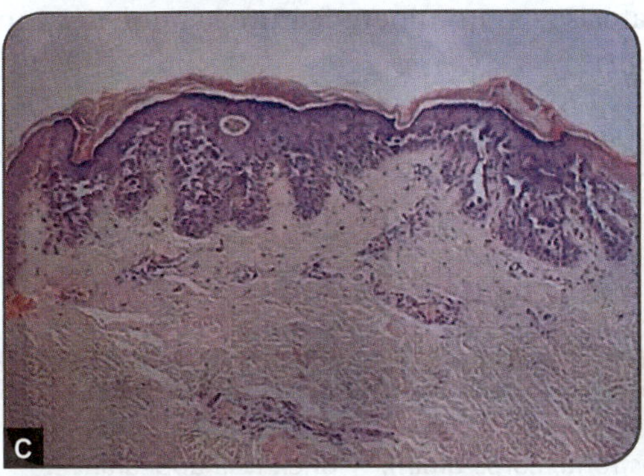

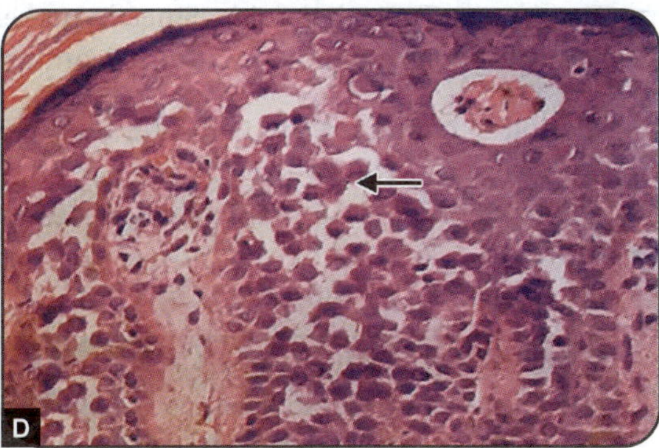

Figs. 12C and D: (C) Low magnification view—Note the suprabasal split; (D) High power view—Note the partially connected acantholytic cells inside the suprabasal split (black arrow)- Dilapidated brick wall appearance

Darier's Disease (Keratosis Follicularis)

- **Autosomal dominant genetic defect in a calcium pump in the keratinocyte endoplasmic reticulum. The gene defect is in calcium ATPase (*ATP2A2*) gene.**
- Like ATP2C1 in HHD, ATP2A2 is also present in the basal and suprabasal layer and encodes an ATP-powered calcium pump essential for desmosome function in suprabasal layer and hence keratinocyte adhesion to each other → hence, lack of this pump causes keratinocyte separation (acantholysis) and blistering in suprabasal epidermis. The difference from HHD is that this **acantholysis classically triggers a process of "dyskeratosis"**—which means abnormal premature keratinization in epidermis (for more on dyskeratosis-see Chapter 2).
- The abnormal keratinization then presents clinically as **keratotic papules in a seborrheic distribution (called "dirty-warty"** papules). It varies from HHD clinically since it **does not present clinically as a blister but as these keratotic papules** (Figs. 13A and B).

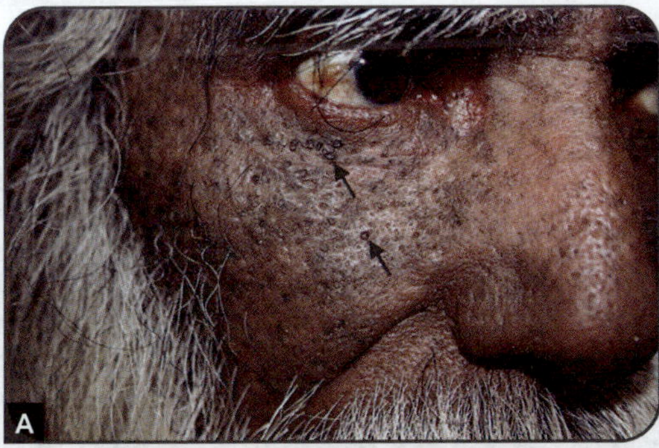

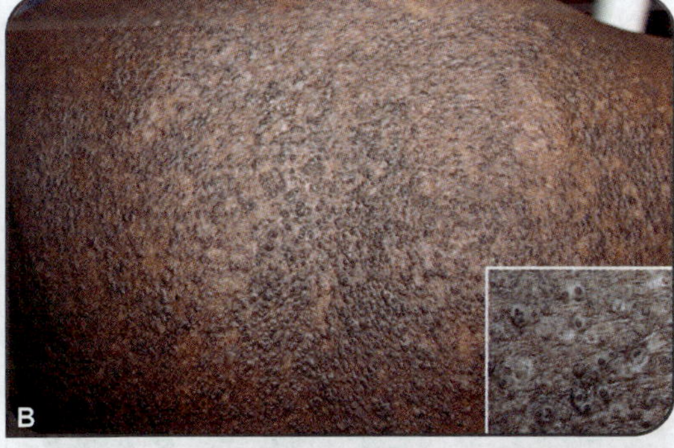

Figs. 13A and B: (A) Darier disease—Hyperkeratotic papules on face (seborrheic area); (B) Darier disease—Hyperkeratotic papules on upper back (seborrheic area) with close-up of dirty-warty papules (inset)

- Treatment—Topical steroids. Since hyperkeratosis is a prominent feature keratolytics can be given (oral retinoids—Acitretin/Isotretinoin)

> Period of contraception with oral retinoids (since it is teratogenic)
> - Acitretin—Till 2 years after the last dose
> - Isotretinoin—Till 1 month after the last dose

Investigations in suprabasal blisters

	Pemphigus vulgaris	Darier's disease	Hailey-Hailey disease
Histopathological features	Acantholysis, row of tombstones	Acantholysis, dyskeratosis (corps rond, corps grain), hyperkeratosis	Acantholysis, dilapidated brick-wall appearance
DIF	Positive	Negative	Negative

Congenital Epidermolysis Bullosa (EB)

- EB is a group **of genetic disorders sharing common symptoms of blisters coming after physical injury ("trauma-induced blisters")**. Hence, blisters are seen in **trauma-prone areas** like **hands, feet, elbows, knees at birth and throughout life**
- **3 types—Epidermolysis bullosa simplex (EBS), epidermolysis bullosa junctional (EBJ) and epidermolysis bullosa dystrophica (EBD)**
- Diagnosis—Electron microscopy is required. **DIF is negative**
- **EBS—Keratin 5 (K5) and Keratin 14 (K14)** which are present normally in basal layer are defective (these keratins provide strength to basal layer). Hence, with the defect of these keratins, the basal layer is fragile and breaks easily, creating a split in basal layer (intra-basal blisters). Since it is an **epidermal blister—blisters do not leave scars** (Fig. 14A)
- **EBJ—Laminin** which is normally present in the dermoepidermal junction (lamina lucida) **is defective** causing damage **and split in the lamina lucida with DEJ blister (hence called EB junctional)**. Extensive blisters form with erosions on rupture. Perioral involvement is frequent (Figs. 14B and C)

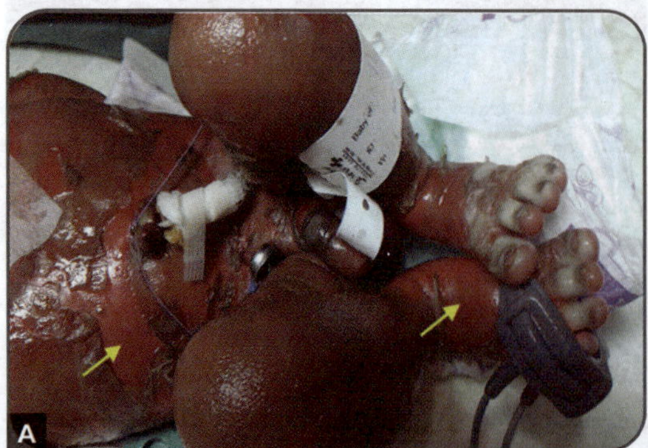

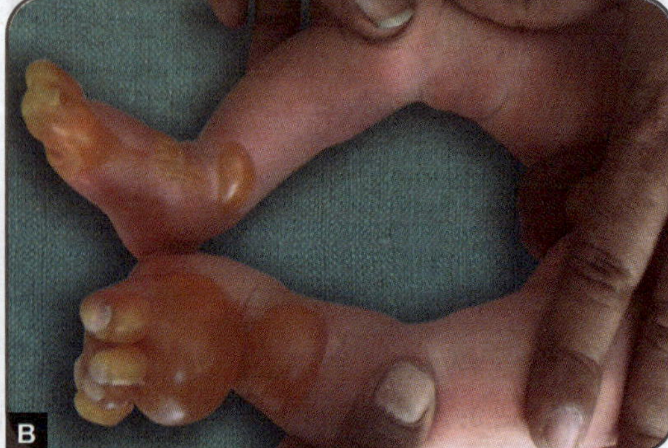

Figs. 14A and B

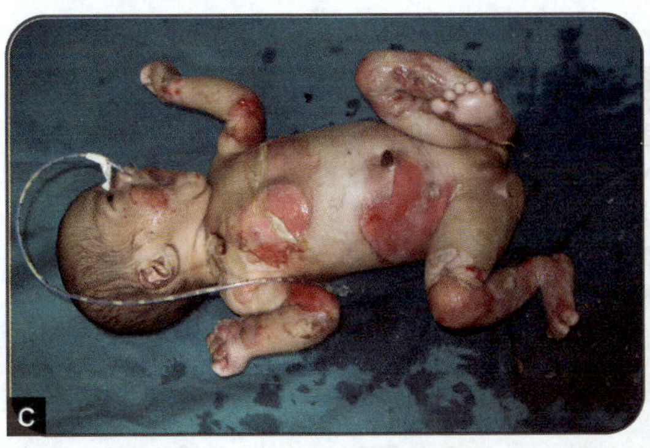

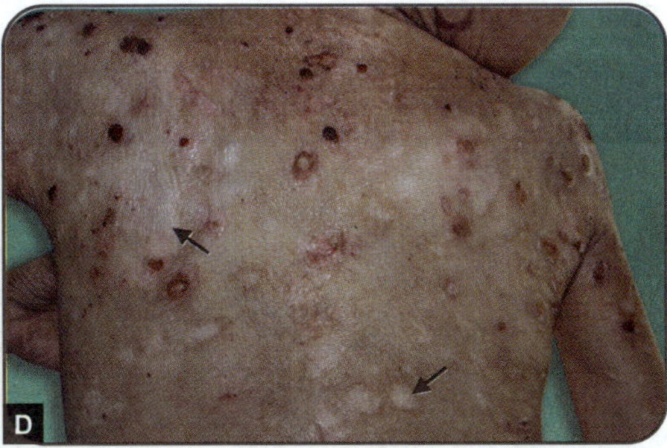

Figs. 14A to D: (A) EBS—superficial erosions (due to burst flaccid blisters) at birth, will heal without scars; (B) Trauma-induced blisters in EB; (C) EBJ—Extensive blistering and erosions with perioral lesion, nail lossh; (D) EBD—Cutaneous scarring (black arrows) after healing of blisters

- **EBD—Collagen 7** in the anchoring fibril is defective since birth. Tense blisters at trauma-prone sites heal with scarring and milia (since it is a dermal blister). The mucous membranes are frequently involved (Fig. 14D).

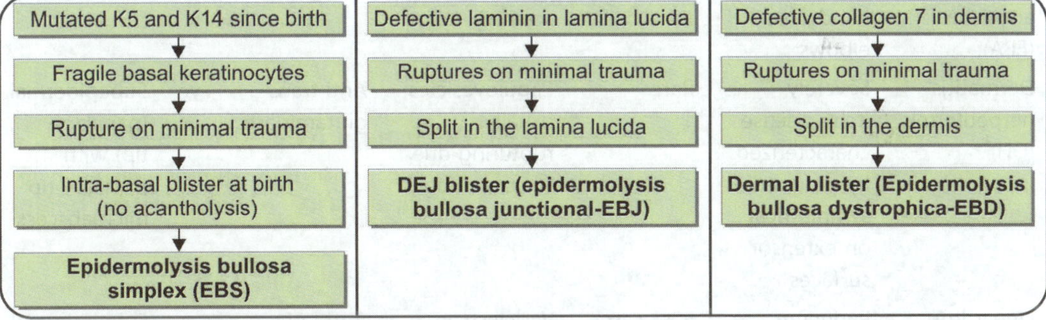

Summary

Disease	Skin involvement	Mucosal involvement	Lesions	Pathology	DIF	Histopathology
Pemphigus vulgaris (PV)	Generalized	Yes	Flaccid blisters, erosions	Anti-Dsg 3 ± Anti-Dsg 1	+ve	Suprabasal split with acantholysis
Pemphigus vegetans	Flexural	Yes	Flaccid blisters, erosions and Cauliflower-like plaques	Anti-Dsg 3 ± Anti-Dsg 1	+ve	Suprabasal split with acantholysis
Pemphigus foliaceus (PF)	Seborrheic areas	No	Scales, crusts	Anti-Dsg 1	+ve	Subcorneal split with acantholysis

Contd...

Contd…

Disease	Skin involvement	Mucosal involvement	Lesions	Pathology	DIF	Histopathology
Paraneoplastic pemphigus	Upper body, palmoplantar	Yes (very severe)	Polymorphous bullae, erosions, "target lesions", lichen planus-like	Anti-Dsg 1, Anti-Dsg 3, Anti-BP-1, Anti-desmoplakin	+ve	Suprabasal blister, basal cell degeneration, band of lymphocytes under DEJ
Bullous pemphigoid (BP)	Groin, axilla, trunk, thighs, limbs	Usually no	Tense, itchy, sometimes hemorrhagic blisters often on red/urticarial background	Anti-BP2 > Anti-BP1	+ve	Subepidermal with eosinophils and neutrophils
Epidermolysis bullosa acquisita (EBA)	Trauma-prone areas like hands, feet, elbows	Rare	Tense blisters, skin fragility, scarring, milia	Anti-collagen 7	+ve	Subepidermal
Dermatitis herpetiformis (DH)	Severely itchy disease characterized by grouped, symmetrical on extensor surfaces	Rare	Papulovesicles usually rupturing due to scratching	Anti-trans-glutaminase	+ve	Subepidermal (papillary tip) with papillary tip microabscess
Linear IgA bullous dermatosis (LAD)	Perineum, perioral areas	50% cases	Vesicles can resemble DH or BP. "String of pearls" or "cluster of jewels" appearance	Anti-LAD (BP-120), Anti-BP 2 (BP-180), Anti-BP-1 (BP-230)	+ve	Subepidermal
Hailey-Hailey disease (HHD)	Friction areas (groin/ axilla/neck/ inframammary)	No	Vesicles, vesicopustules, fissures	No antibody. Genetic defect in the calcium ATPase (*ATP2C1*) gene	–ve	Suprabasal split. Dilapidated brick wall appearance

How to diagnose in an MCQ on blisters?

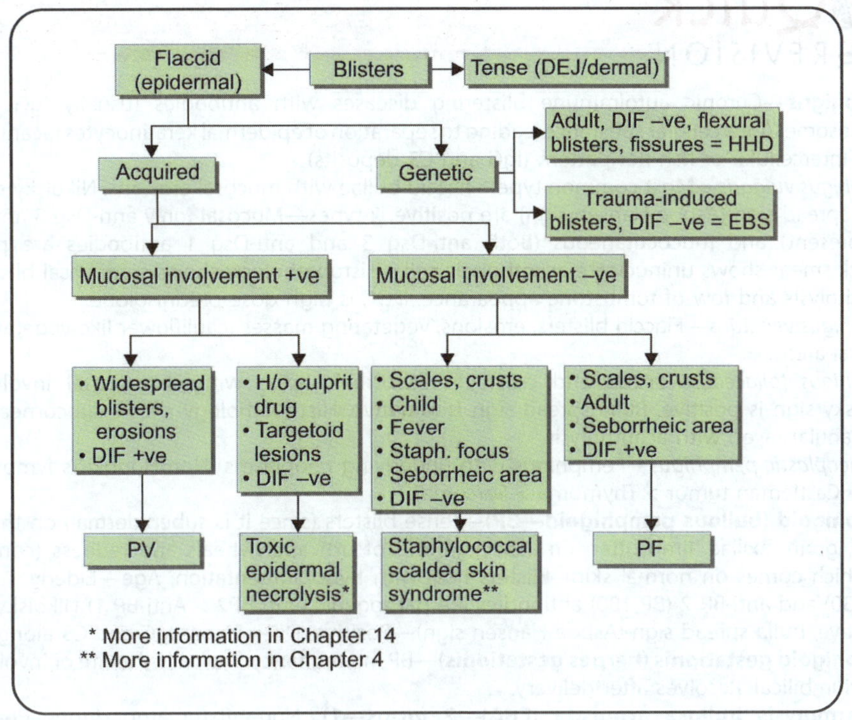

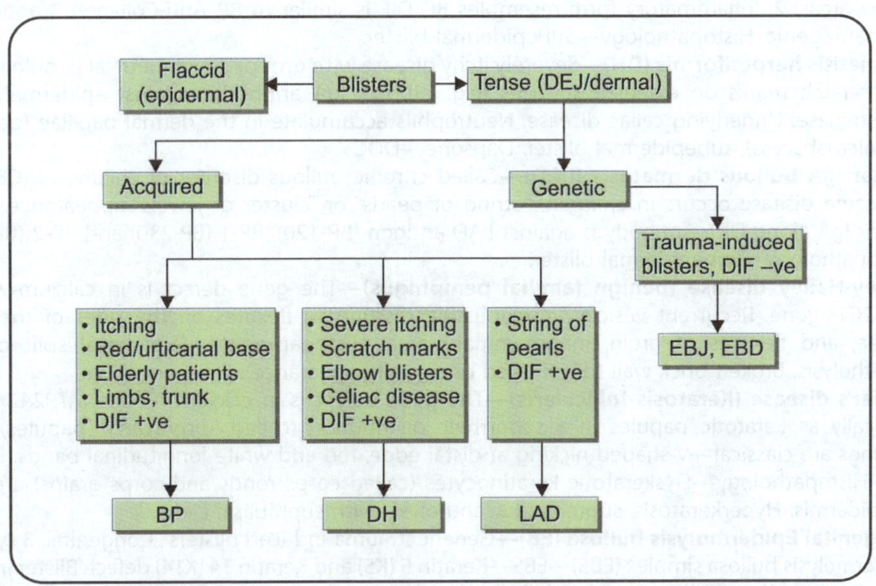

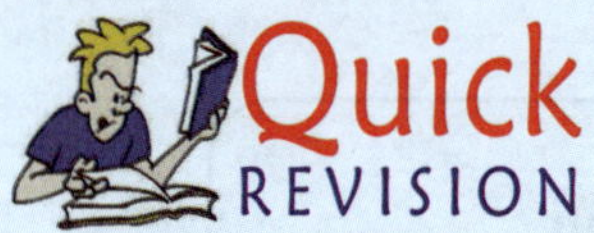

- **Pemphigus**—Chronic autoimmune blistering diseases with antibodies (usually IgG) against desmosomes/Intercellular substance leading to separation of epidermal keratinocytes (acantholysis). DIF—Intercellular or fish-net pattern (IgG and C3 deposits)

  Pemphigus vulgaris—Most common type—flaccid bullae with mucosal erosions. Nikolsky sign and bulla-spread sign (Asboe-Hansen sign) are positive. 2 types—Mucosal (only anti-Dsg 3 antibodies are present) and mucocutaneous (Both anti-Dsg 3 and anti-Dsg 1 antibodies are present). Tzanck smear shows uninucleate acantholytic cells. Histopathology shows suprabasal blister with acantholysis and row of tombstone appearance. DOC is high-dose prednisolone.

  Pemphigus vegetans—Flaccid blisters, erosions, vegetating masses (cauliflower like vegetations) in flexural areas.

  Pemphigus foliaceous—Scales and crusts in seborrheic areas without mucosal involvement. Nikolsky sign is positive. Bulla spread sign is negative. Histopathology shows subcorneal blister (in granular layer) with acantholysis.

  Paraneoplastic pemphigus—Pemphigus with underlying neoplasms (Non Hodgkin's lymphoma > CLL > Castleman tumor > Thymoma > Sarcoma).
- **Pemphigoid (bullous pemphigoid—BP)**—Tense blisters (since it is subepidermal) on the trunk, thigh, groin, axillae, limb often on a background of urticarial wheals and redness (contrast to PV which comes on normal skin). Blisters heal with hypopigmentation. Age—Elderly. Anti-BP-1 (BP-230) and anti-BP 2 (BP-180) antibodies are pathogenic (anti BP2 > Anti-BP 1) Nikolsky sign—Negative, bulla spread sign-(Asboe-Hansen sign)—Positive. DIF—Linear IgG and C3 along DEJ.
- **Pemphigoid gestationis (herpes gestationis)**—BP in pregnancy. Typically the site of involvement is periumbilical. Resolves after delivery.
- **Epidermolysis bullosa acquisita (EBA)—2 forms—1)**. Non-inflammatory form—Resembles epidermolysis bullosa dystrophica (EBD) with skin fragility, scarring, and milia formation in trauma-prone areas; 2. Inflammatory form resembles BP. DIF is similar to BP. Anti-Collagen 7 antibodies are pathogenic. Histopathology—Subepidermal blister.
- **Dermatitis herpetiformis (DH)**—Severely itchy disease with grouped, symmetrical papulovesicles and scratch marks on extensor surfaces (e.g., elbow). IgA antibodies against epidermal trans-glutaminase. Underlying celiac disease. Neutrophils accumulate in the dermal papillae (papillary tip microabscess), subepidermal blister. Dapsone—DOC
- **Linear IgA bullous dermatosis (LAD)**—Called chronic bullous disorder of childhood (CBDC) if the same disease occurs in children. "String of pearls" or "cluster of jewels" appearance. DIF—Linear IgA along DEJ. Antibody is against LAD antigen (BP-120), BP-1 (BP-230) and BP-2 (BP-180). Histopathology—Subepidermal blister.
- **Hailey-Hailey disease (benign familial pemphigus)**—The gene defect is in calcium ATPase (ATP2C1) gene. Recurrent vesicles/vesicopustules/fissures in flexures on the sides of the neck, axillae, and flexures of groin, inframammary area. Histopathology—Suprabasal split due to acantholysis. Broken brick wall (dilapidated brick wall appearance). DIF—negative.
- **Darier's disease (Keratosis follicularis)**—The gene defect is in calcium ATPase (*ATP2A2*) gene. Clinically as keratotic papules in a seborrheic distribution (called "dirty-warty" papules). Nail-findings are classical—V-shaped nicking at distal edge, red and white longitudinal bands. Palmar pits. Histopathology—Dyskeratotic keratinocytes (called corps ronds and corps grains) are seen in epidermis. Hyperkeratosis, suprabasal acantholysis with suprabasal clefts.
- **Congenital Epidermolysis bullosa (EB)**—Genetic "trauma-induced blisters". Congenital. 3 types—Epidermolysis bullosa simplex (EBS)—EBS—Keratin 5 (K5) and Keratin 14 (K14) defect. Blister in basal layer, Epidermolysis bullosa junctional (EBJ)—Absent Laminin causing DEJ blister and epidermolysis bullosa dystrophica (EBD)—Defective collagen 7 causing dermal blister. DIF—negative.

QUESTIONS

1. **A patient has multiple grouped papulovesicular lesions on elbows, knees, buttocks and upper back associated with severe itching. The most likely diagnosis is:**

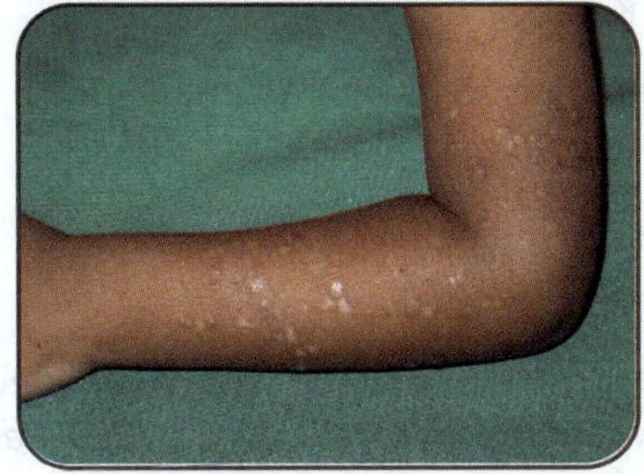

   a. Pemphigus vulgaris
   b. Bullous pemphigoid
   c. Dermatitis herpetiformis
   d. Herpes zoster

2. **A 30-year-old male had severely itchy papulovesicular lesions on extremities, knees, elbows and buttocks for 1 year. Direct immunofluorescence staining of the lesions showed IgA deposition at dermoepidermal junction. The most probable diagnosis is:**
   a. Pemphigus vulgaris
   b. Bullous pemphigoid
   c. Dermatitis herpetiformis
   d. Nummular eczema

3. **A 40-year-old male presents with painful flaccid vesicles on face and oral mucosa with asymmetric distribution. Immunofluorescence shows intercellular IgG deposition in epidermis. Diagnosis is:**
   a. Erythema multiforme
   b. Bullous pemphigoid
   c. Pemphigus vulgaris
   d. Herpes zoster

4. **A middle-aged female has flaccid bullae in the skin and oral erosions. Histopathology shows intraepidermal acantholytic blister. The most likely diagnosis is:**

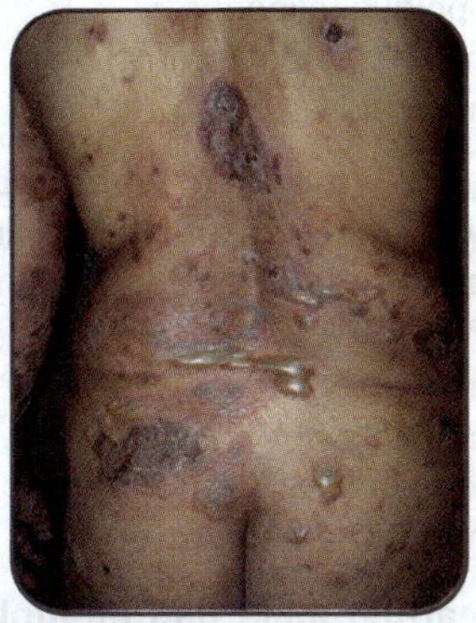

   a. Pemphigus vulgaris
   b. Paraneoplastic pemphigus
   c. Bullous pemphigoid
   d. Dermatitis herpetiformis

5. **A female presents with persistent painful oral lesions and acantholytic cells. Most likely diagnosis is:**
   a. Pemphigus vulgaris
   b. Dermatitis herpetiformis
   c. Epidermolysis bullosa
   d. Bullous pemphigoid

6. **A 50-year-old male presents with erythematous shallow erosions with scales. Oral mucosa is not involved. Immunopathology demonstrates IgG deposition on keratinocytes and auto antibodies against Dsg-1. The diagnosis is:**

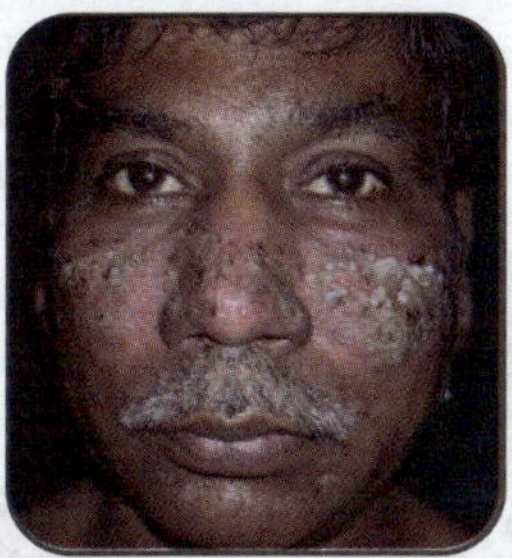

   a. Pemphigus vulgaris
   b. Bullous pemphigoid
   c. Pemphigus foliaceus
   d. Dermatitis herpetiformis

7. A 25-year-old female has palatal ulcers and skin blisters. Most likely diagnosis is:

a. Pemphigus vulgaris
b. Pemphigus foliaceus
c. Dermatitis herpetiformis
d. Pemphigoid

8. An 85-year-old woman with Nikolsky sign negative, blisters on thigh and trunk, lesions come on and off. What is the cause?

a. Pemphigus vulgaris
b. Pemphigoid
c. Lichen planus
d. Dermatitis herpetiformis

9. A 60-year-old male had multiple blisters over the trunk and extremities. Direct immunofluorescence studies showed linear IgG deposits along the basement membrane. Which of the following is the most likely diagnosis?

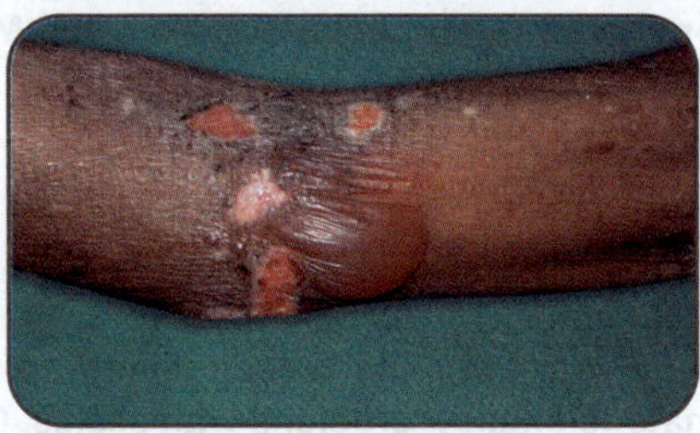

a. Pemphigus vulgaris
b. Bullous pemphigoid
c. Pemphigus foliaceus
d. Dermatitis herpetiformis

10. A patient presented with blisters. His histology is as shown. The diagnosis is: *(AIMS Nov 18)*

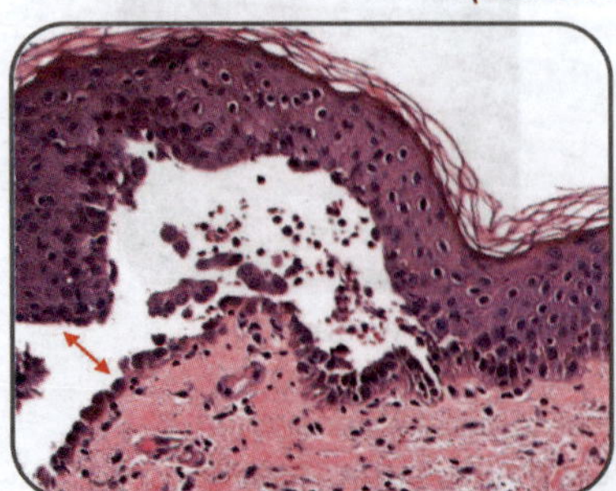

a. Pemphigus vulgaris
b. Leprosy
c. Mycosis fungoides
d. Psoriasis

11. In pemphigus vulgaris, antibodies are present against:

a. Basement membrane
b. Intercellular substance
c. Cell nucleus
d. Keratin

12. Acantholysis is characteristic of:

a. Pemphigus vulgaris
b. Pemphigoid
c. Erythema multiforme
d. Dermatitis herpetiformis

13. Loss of intercellular cohesion between keratinocytes is called as: *(NEET Pattern)*

a. Acanthosis
b. Acantholysis
c. Keratolysis
d. Spongiosis

14. In which of the following diseases, administration of dapsone is used as a therapeutic test?

a. Lepromatous leprosy
b. Pemphigus vulgaris
c. Bullous pemphigoid
d. Dermatitis Herpetiformis

15. Tzanck cell is a: *(NEET Pattern)*

a. Keratinocyte b. Fibroblast
c. Neutrophil d. Lymphocyte

16. Flaccid bullous lesions with oral mucosal lesions. The finding in immunofluorescence is:

a. Fishnet IgG in epidermis
b. Linear IgG in DEJ
c. Granular IgA in dermal papillae
d. Linear IgA in reticular dermis

17. Tense bullous lesions are seen in:

a. Pemphigus vulgaris
b. Pemphigus foliaceous
c. Bullous pemphigoid
d. Pemphigus vegetans

18. Subepidermal bullae on trunk and flexural surface with linear C3/IgG basement membrane deposits are features of:
a. Bullous pemphigoid
b. Pemphigus vulgaris
c. Linear IgA disease
d. Dermatitis herpetiformis

19. Mucosa is never involved in which of the following disorder?
a. Dermatitis herpetiformis
b. Pemphigus foliaceus
c. Epidermolysis bullosa acquisita
d. Toxic epidermal necrolysis

20. One of the following is the treatment of choice for dermatitis herpetiformis:
a. Corticosteroids b. Dapsone
c. Methotrexate d. Retinoids

21. True about dermatitis herpetiformis.
a. Best treated with dapsone.
b. Associated with HPV 6 and 7
c. On flexors predominantly
d. Associated with gluten sensitivity
e. Presents with vesicles

22. In an 8-day-old child with history of consanguinity in the parents, the mother reports blisters and bleeding of the skin at the site of handling and pressure. There was a similar history in the previous child, which proved to be fatal. The diagnosis is:
a. Bullous pemphigoid
b. Congenital syphilis
c. Congenital epidermolysis bullosa
d. Letterer-Siwe disease

23. In congenital dystrophic variety of epidermolysis bullosa, mutation is seen in the gene coding for:
a. Laminin 4 b. Collagen type 7
c. Alpha 6 integrin d. Keratin 14

24. Which of the following shows granular deposition of IgA in dermal papilla?
a. Dermatitis herpetiformis
b. Linear IgA dermatosis
c. Bullous pemphigoid
d. Gestational herpes

25. Skin disease not showing direct immunofluorescence positivity:
a. Darier's disease
b. Hailey-Hailey disease
c. Cicatricial pemphigoid
d. Dermatitis herpetiformis
e. Pemphigus

26. A patient presented with oral mucosal lesions and flaccid blisters over skin. What will be the pattern detected under microscopic examination?
a. Fishnet pattern IgG in epidermis
b. IgG at dermoepidermal junction
c. IgA at dermoepidermal junction
d. IgG in dermis

27. An infant has papulovesicular lesions on palms, soles, face and trunk. The diagnosis would be:
a. Scabies
b. Atopic dermatitis
c. Urticaria
d. Seborrheic dermatitis

28. Disease of dermoepidermal junction is:
a. Pemphigus vulgaris
b. Atopic dermatitis
c. Bullous pemphigoid
d. Staphylococcal scalded skin syndrome

29. Subepidermal splitting is not found in:
a. Bullous pemphigoid
b. Pemphigus foliaceous
c. Dermatitis herpetiformis
d. Burns

30. Bullous skin lesions with "intraepidermal split' are a feature of:
a. Pemphigus vulgaris
b. Pemphigoid
c. Epidermolysis bullosa dystrophica
d. All

31. Intraepidermal blisters are seen in all the following conditions, *except*: *(NEET Pattern)*
a. Pemphigus foliaceus
b. Pemphigus vulgaris
c. Paraneoplastic pemphigus
d. Pemphigoid

32. Blister formation in burn case is:

a. Intraepidermal b. Subepidermal
c. Subdermal d. Subfascial

33. A patient comes with skin and oral lesions. DIF showing fishnet pattern was shown. All are true *except*: *(AIIMS May 17)*

a. Dsg 3 antibodies
b. Dsg 1 antibodies
c. Antibody against hemidesmosome
d. IgG type is the most common

34. Tombstone appearance is seen in:

a. Bullous pemphigoid
b. Pemphigus vulgaris
c. Dermatitis herpetiformis
d. Linear IgA disease

35. Linear deposition of IgG and C3 in lamina lucida is seen in:

a. Dermatitis herpetiformis
b. Pemphigus vulgaris
c. Pemphigus foliaceus
d. Bullous pemphigoid

36. Antibody against BP-120 and BP-180 are seen in:

a. Pemphigus vulgaris
b. Bullous pemphigoid
c. Dermatitis herpetiformis
d. Linear IgA disease

37. Fishnet appearance in immunofluorescence is seen in:

a. Pemphigus vulgaris
b. Bullous pemphigoid
c. Dermatitis herpetiformis
d. Darier disease

38. Which of the following is involved in the pathogenesis of dermatitis herpetiformis?

a. TTG 1 b. TTG 3
c. TTG 6 d. TTG 9

39. Intraepidermal intercellular deposition of IgA on immunofluorescence is seen in:

a. Pemphigus
b. Bullous pemphigoid
c. Epidermolysis bullosa acquisita
d. Subcorneal pustular dermatosis

40. Granular deposition of IgA at dermal papillae on immunofluorescence is seen in:

a. Herpes gestationis
b. Dermatitis herpetiformis
c. Bullous pemphigoid
d. IgA dermatosis of childhood

41. A 60-year-old man presented with itchy tense blisters on urticarial skin. Investigation done for the diagnosis:

a. Direct immunofluorescence
b. Tzanck smear
c. Histopathology
d. Cytopathology

42. Autoantibodies against desmogleins 1 and 3 are seen in:

a. Bullous pemphigoid
b. Bullous systemic lupus erythematosus
c. Pemphigus vulgaris
d. Pemphigus foliaceus

43. A patient came with tense blisters on normal skin as well as over urticarial plaques. What is the diagnosis?

a. Bullous pemphigoid
b. Pemphigus vulgaris
c. Linear IgA disease
d. Dermatitis herpetiformis

44. The characteristic microscopic feature of bullous pemphigoid is:

a. Subepidermal nonacantholytic blister
b. Subcorneal nonacantholytic blister
c. Subcorneal acantholytic blister
d. Subepidermal acantholytic blister

45. Subepidermal blisters with granular deposits of IgA selectively localized to the tips of dermal papillae are a feature of:

a. Dermatitis herpetiformis
b. Pemphigus vulgaris
c. Lichen planus
d. Psoriasis vulgaris

46. Drug of choice in dermatitis herpetiformis:

a. Steroid
b. Phototherapy
c. Dapsone
d. Methotrexate

47. Intraepidermal intercellular deposition of IgG on immunofluorescence is seen in:
a. Pemphigus
b. Bullous pemphigoid
c. Epidermolysis bullosa acquisita
d. Subcorneal pustular dermatosis

48. Bulla in staphylococcal scalded skin syndrome is located:
a. Subepidermal
b. Intraepidermal
c. Mucosa
d. None of the above

49. All are vesiculobullous lesions *except*:
a. Dermatitis herpetiformis
b. Scabies
c. Pemphigus
d. Pemphigoid

50. Subepidermal blisters are:
a. Bullous pemphigoid
b. Pemphigus vulgaris
c. Hailey-Hailey disease
d. Darier's disease
e. Acanthosis nigricans

51. Intraepidermal blisters are seen in:
a. Bullous pemphigoid
b. Pemphigus foliaceus
c. Dermatitis herpetiformis
d. Bullous SLE
e. Bullous impetigo

52. Intraepidermal acantholytic vesicles are seen in:
a. Pemphigus vulgaris
b. Paraneoplastic pemphigus
c. Dermatitis herpetiformis
d. Congenital epidermolysis bullosa
e. Bullous pemphigoid

53. In pemphigus vulgaris, antibodies are present against:
a. Basement membrane
b. Intercellular substance
c. Keratin
d. Cell nucleus

54. A 40-year-old female reported with recurrent episodes of oral ulcers, large areas of denuded skin and flaccid vesiculobullous eruptions. Which is the most important bedside investigation helpful in establishing the diagnosis?

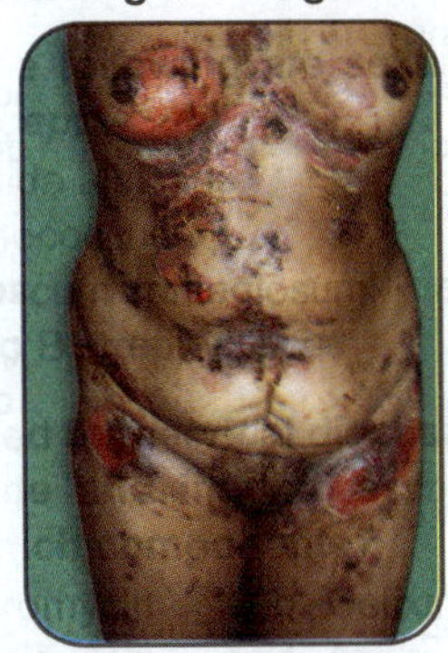

a. Gram staining of the blister fluid
b. Culture and sensitivity
c. Skin biopsy and immunofluorescence
d. Tzanck smear from the floor of bulla

55. Nikolsky sign is positive in all of the following *except*:
a. Staphylococcal scalded skin syndrome
b. Toxic epidermal necrolysis
c. Bullous pemphigoid
d. Pemphigus

56. Dyskeratosis is a feature of:
a. Darier disease
b. Pemphigus vulgaris
c. Psoriasis
d. Bowen's disease
e. Hailey-Hailey disease

57. A patient developed bullae without erythema on elbows, knee and sacral area followed by crust formation, scarring and milia. He had no photosensitivity and negative family history for bullous disease. On DIF, IgG deposition at DEJ with no blood vessel involvement is seen. Probable diagnosis is:
a. Epidermolysis bullosa dystrophica
b. Epidermolysis bullosa acquisita
c. Porphyria cutanea tarda
d. Pemphigoid

58. Commonest/rarest variety of pemphigus:
a. Pemphigus vulgaris/vegetans
b. Pemphigus vegetans/vulgaris
c. Pemphigus foliaceus/erythematosus
d. Pemphigus erythematosus/foliaceus

59. True about pemphigus vulgaris A/E:
a. Subepidermal
b. Autoimmune disease
c. Tzanck smear shows acantholytic cells
d. Antibodies are formed against desmogleins
e. Blister on skin and mucosa

60. A 24-year-old female has flaccid bullae in the skin and persistent painful oral erosions. Histopathology shows intraepidermal acantholytic blister. The most likely diagnosis is:
a. Bullous pemphigoid
b. Erythema multiforme
c. Pemphigus vulgaris
d. Dermatitis herpetiformis

61. Chronic bullous disease of childhood is characterized by all *except*:
a. Mean age of onset <5 years
b. Face and perineum are predominantly involved
c. Cluster of jewel is seen clinically
d. Immunofluorescence shows IgG and C3 complement deposition

62. Mucosal lesions are commonly seen in:
a. Secondary syphilis
b. Dermatitis herpetiformis
c. Psoriasis
d. Pemphigus
e. Porphyria

63. A patient has oral ulcer and skin bullae and large erosions which are slow to heal. The lesion is:
a. Intradermal
b. Suprabasal
c. Subcutaneous
d. Subcorneal

64. A 3-year-old child has high fever along with perioral erosions and scaling. There are a few flaccid blisters on the neck folds and upper back. He has had a furuncle with pus a few days back. There are no mucosal lesions. His Nikolsky is positive. The diagnosis is:
a. Pemphigus foliaceous
b. Pemphigus vulgaris
c. Staphylococcal scalded skin syndrome
d. Toxic epidermal necrolysis

65. Most common site of herpes gestationis is:
a. Periumbilical region
b. Flanks of abdomen
c. Vulva
d. Infraorbital

66. A 65-year-old male with itchy bullae over erythematous areas and normal skin. The diagnosis is:
a. Bullous pemphigoid
b. Dermatitis herpetiformis
c. IgA pemphigus
d. Pemphigus vulgaris

67. A 30-year-old male presents with flaccid bullae and erosions over the oral mucous membrane. The blisters developed painful erosions rupture. What would be the most likely finding on an immunofluorescent examination of the skin biopsy of this patient?
a. Linear IgA deposition in dermoepidermal junction
b. Linear IgG deposition in dermoepidermal junction
c. Fishnet IgG deposition in epidermis
d. Granular deposits of IgA in dermal papillae

68. A 35-year-old female presents with painful blisters over oral mucosa and genital areas. She gives a history of similar lesions in the past. A biopsy from the lesion shows a suprabasal split on histopathology. Immunofluorecence microscopy reveals intercellular IgG deposits. (Image of immunofluorescence was given showing fish-net pattern). What is the most likely diagnosis?
a. Dermatitis herpetiformis
b. Pemphigus vulgaris
c. Behçet's diseases
d. Allergic dermatitis

69. The following diseases can cause bullous lesions in the skin, *except*:
a. Pemphigus
b. Impetigo
c. Toxic epidermal necrolysis
d. Pityriasis rosea

70. Which layer is involved in blister formation in a superficial partial thickness burn? *(AIIMS Nov 2017)*

a. Epidermis
b. Dermis
c. Papillary dermis
d. Reticular dermis

71. A patient comes with lesions the histopathology of which is as shown. The diagnosis is: *(AIIMS May 2017)*

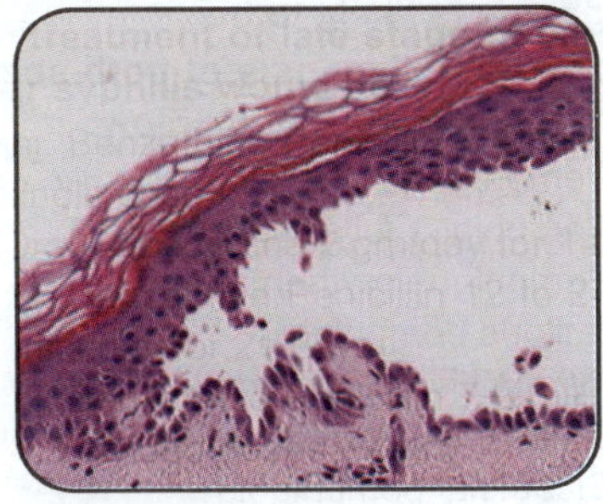

a. Mycosis fungoides
b. Pemphigus vulgaris
c. Lepromatous leprosy
d. Eczema

72. Amongst the following, sub-epidermal disorders is/are:

a. Pemphigus vulgaris
b. Bullous pemphigoid
c. Bullous SLE
d. Pemphigus vegetans
e. Dermatitis herpetiformis

73. Desmosomes is/are associated with:

a. Lichen planus pemphigoides
b. Cardiac arrhythmia
c. Pemphigus
d. Psoriasis
e. Lichen planus

New Questions

74. The following statements are true/false regarding diseases showing a positive Nikolsky sign:

a. Pemphigus
b. Ritter's disease
c. Bullous pemphigoid
d. Epidermolysis bullosa dystrophica
e. Hailey-Hailey disease

75. Arrange the following blistering diseases in skin in the order of their fluid collection levels in skin from top to bottom:

1. Hailey-Hailey disease
2. Cicatricial pemphigoid
3. Epidermolysis bullosa dystrophica
4. Bullous impetigo

a. 1, 2, 3, 4
b. 4, 1, 2, 3
c. 2, 1, 3, 4
d. 1, 2, 4, 3

76. Assertion: Row of tombstones is seen on histology in pemphigus vulgaris
Reason: Hemidesmosomes are not affected in pemphigus vulgaris

a. Both Assertion and Reason are true and Reason is correct explanation of Assertion
b. Both Assertion and Reason are true but Reason is not correct explanation of Assertion
c. Assertion is true and Reason is false
d. Assertion is false and Reason is true
e. Both Assertion and Reason are false

77. Assertion: Bulla spread sign in negative in pemphigus foliaceous
Reason: Scaly presentation is seen in pemphigus foliaceous

a. Both Assertion and Reason are true and Reason is correct explanation of Assertion
b. Both Assertion and Reason are true but Reason is not correct explanation of Assertion
c. Assertion is true and Reason is false
d. Assertion is false and Reason is true
e. Both Assertion and Reason are false

78. Dermal blisters are seen with:

a. Hailey-Hailey disease
b. Staphylococcal toxin disease
c. Burns
d. Bullous SLE

1. If a, b, c are correct
2. If a and c are correct
3. If c and d are correct
4. If all four (a, b, c, & d) are correct

79. Match the direct immunofluorescence findings of column A with best alternative in column B:

Column A	Column B
1. Linear IgG at the DEJ 2. Granular IgA at the tip of dermal papilla 3. Intercellular IgG 4. Negative fluorescence	a. Staphylococcal scalded skin syndrome b. IgA pemphigus c. Cicatricial pemphigoid d. Pemphigus foliaceous e. Linear IgA disease f. Dermatitis herpetiformis

80. Theme and Focus:

Blistering Disease

Clinical vignette:

Case 1

A 30-year-old patient presents mucocutaneous lesions since 5 years. The lesions started in oral mucosa followed by skin lesions. On examination, his skin lesions are raw and painful. There are irregular ulcers noted in oral cavity. Nikolsky sign is positive. His biopsy is likely to be classical of:

Case 2

A 40-year-old male presents with itchy blisters on his body. He often excoriates it. On examination, his blisters are grouped and many scratch marks are seen. He refuses biopsy but rapidly responds to diet modification and a medication given for his condition. The diagnosis is likely to be:

Choose the diagnosis of both scenarios from the options listed below:

a. Pemphigus vulgaris
b. Pemphigus foliaceous
c. Pemphigus erythematosus
d. Bullous pemphigoid
e. Dermatitis herpetiformis
f. Linear IgA disease
g. Cicatricial pemphigoid
h. Hailey-Hailey disease

81. A 65-year-old man comes with itching, urticaria like lesions and bullae on red as well as normal skin. The diagnosis is: ***(INICET Nov 21)***

a. Dermatitis herpetiformis
b. Bullous pemphigoid
c. Linear IgA disease
d. Pemphigus

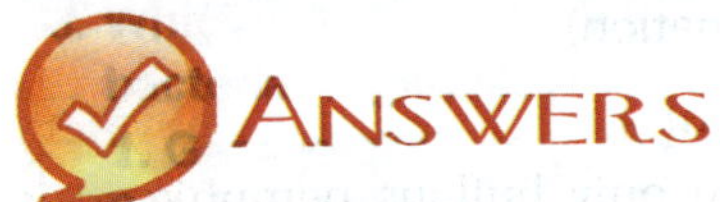

ANSWERS

1. **Ans. (c) Dermatitis herpetiformis** *(Ref: Andrew's Textbook, 11th edn, Page 463)*

   Grouped papulovesicular lesions on elbows and severe itching suggest dermatitis herpetiformis. Pemphigus vulgaris will have painful erosions with mucosal involvement. Bullous pemphigoid will have itchy tense blisters (not "severe" itching) commonly on a red background. Herpes zoster will have dermatomal distribution of painful blisters.

2. **Ans. (c) Dermatitis herpetiformis** *(Ref: Andrew's Textbook, 11th edn, Page 464)*

   Severely itchy papulovesicular lesions on extremities, knees, elbows and buttocks suggest DH. IgA deposits at the dermal papilla are classical.

3. **Ans. (c) Pemphigus vulgaris** *(Ref: Fitzpatrick's Textbook, 8th edn, Page 589)*

   Painful blisters with mucosal involvement are typical of pemphigus vulgaris. IgG in intercellular pattern (fish-net) is seen on DIF. Bullous pemphigoid does not have mucosal lesions and shows IgG in a linear pattern along DEJ.

4. **Ans. (a) Pemphigus vulgaris** *(Ref: Fitzpatrick's Textbook, 8th edn, Page 589)*

   Flaccid bullae in the skin and oral erosions suggest mucocutaneous pemphigus vulgaris. Suprabasal acantholysis is typical.

5. **Ans. (a) Pemphigus vulgaris** *(Ref: Fitzpatrick's Textbook, 8th edn, Page 591)*

   Painful oral lesions with acantholysis points to mucosal pemphigus vulgaris.

6. **Ans. (c) Pemphigus foliaceus** *(Ref: Andrew's Textbook, 11th edn, Page 452)*

   Shallow erosions point to a superficial blister (e.g., PF). Absent oral involvement, scales, IgG deposition on keratinocytes and auto antibodies against Dsg-1 also point to PF.

7. **Ans. (a) Pemphigus vulgaris**

   The question suggests mucocutaneous PV.

8. **Ans. (b) Pemphigoid**

   Nikolsky's sign negative suggests subepidermal blisters. Blisters on thigh and trunk are common in pemphigoid.

9. **Ans. (b) Bullous pemphigoid** *(Ref: Andrew's Textbook, 11th edn, Page 455)*

   Old age (60 years), blisters over the trunk and extremities and DIF showing linear IgG deposit suggests bullous pemphigoid.

10. **Ans. (a) Pemphigus vulgaris** (See page 208 for explanation)

11. **Ans. (b) Intercellular substance**

    Intercellular substance (desmosome) is the target in pemphigus.

12. **Ans. (a) Pemphigus vulgaris** (See page 208 for explanation)

13. **Ans. (b) Acantholysis** *(Ref: Andrew's Textbook, 11th edn, Page 450)*

14. **Ans. (d) Dermatitis Herpetiformis** (See page 214 for explanation)

15. **Ans. (a) Keratinocyte**

16. **Ans. (a) Fishnet IgG in epidermis** (See page 206 for explanation)

17. **Ans. (c) Bullous pemphigoid** (See page 211 for explanation)

    Tense blisters point to junctional/dermal blisters. Here only bullous pemphigoid is junctional.

18. **Ans. (a) Bullous pemphigoid** (See page 211 for explanation)

19. **Ans. (b) Pemphigus foliaceus** *(Ref: Andrew's Textbook, 11th edn, Page 452)*

20. **Ans. (b) Dapsone** *(Ref: Fitzpatrick's Textbook, 8th edn, Page 648)*

21. **Ans. (a, d, e) Best treated with dapsone; Associated with gluten sensitivity; Presents with vesicles**

22. **Ans. (c) Congenital epidermolysis bullosa** (See page 219 for explanation)

    Blisters and bleeding of the skin at the site of handling and pressure suggest EB.

23. **Ans. (b) Collagen type 7** *(Ref: Fitzpatrick's Textbook, 8th edn, Page 659)*

24. **Ans. (a) Dermatitis herpetiformis** *(Ref: Andrew's Textbook, 11th edn, Page 464)*

25. **Ans. (a, b) Darier's disease; Hailey-Hailey disease** (See page 217–218 for explanation)

26. **Ans. (a) Fishnet pattern IgG in epidermis** (See page 206 for explanation)

27. **Ans. (a) Scabies**

    Infantile scabies classical has papulovesicular lesions on palms and soles along with facial involvement. For more information on this topic, see Chapter 7

28. **Ans. (c) Bullous pemphigoid**

29. **Ans. (b) Pemphigus foliaceus**

30. **Ans. (a) Pemphigus vulgaris**

31. **Ans. (d) Pemphigoid**

32. **Ans. (b) Subepidermal** *(Ref: Rook's Textbook of Dermatology, 9th edn, Page 126.2)*

33. **Ans. (c) Antibody against hemidesmosome**

    The questions is of pemphigus vulgaris (mucocutaneous variety). Hemidesmosomes are structures which attach the basal keratinocytes to the DEJ. Typically BP-1 is present in hemidesmosome. Bullous pemphigoid has antibody against hemidesmosome. In pemphigus the antibodies are against desmosomes and not hemidesmosomes. The question is of mucocutaneous pemphigus vulgaris. Hence, both Dsg 3 and Dsg 1 antibodies both would be seen (IgG type). IgG along the basement membrane is not seen in pemphigus vulgaris.

34. **Ans. (b) Pemphigus vulgaris** *(Ref: Andrew's Textbook, 11th edn, Page 450)*

35. **Ans. (d) Bullous pemphigoid** *(Ref: Andrew's Textbook, 11th edn, Page 455)*

36. **Ans. (d) Linear IgA disease** *(Ref: Fitzpatrick's Textbook, 8th edn, Page 625)*

37. **Ans. (a) Pemphigus vulgaris**

38. **Ans. (b) TTG 3**

39. Ans. (a) Pemphigus

This is a rare type of pemphigus where there is IgA deposition in a fishnet/intercellular pattern in epidermis (called IgA pemphigus). Usually IgG is deposited in epidermis in pemphigus.

40. Ans. (b) Dermatitis herpetiformis

41. Ans. (a) Direct immunofluorescence *(Ref: Fitzpatrick's Textbook, 8th edn, Page 613)*

The question refers to BP. DIF would show IgG and C3 in a linear pattern along DEJ.

42. Ans. (c) Pemphigus vulgaris

The question points to mucocutaneous PV.

43. Ans. (a) Bullous pemphigoid *(Ref: Fitzpatrick's Textbook, 8th edn, Page 612)*

44. Ans. (a) Subepidermal nonacantholytic blister

(Ref: Fitzpatrick's Textbook, 8th edn, Page 613)

Option c points to pemphigus foliaceus.

45. Ans. (a) Dermatitis herpetiformis (See page 214 for explanation)

46. Ans. (c) Dapsone *(Ref: Andrew's Textbook, 11th edn, Page 464)*

47. Ans. (a) Pemphigus

48. Ans. (b) Intraepidermal

49. Ans. (b) Scabies

Adult scabies does not have vesicles (only infantile scabies has vesiculobullous lesions)

50. Ans. (a) Bullous pemphigoid

51. Ans. (b, e) Pemphigus foliaceus; Bullous impetigo

52. Ans. (a, b) Pemphigus vulgaris; Paraneoplastic pemphigus

53. Ans. (b) Intercellular substance

Intercellular substance refers to desmosomes.

54. Ans. (d) Tzanck smear from the floor of bulla

Oral ulcers, large areas of denuded skin and flaccid vesiculobullous eruptions suggest mucocutaneous PV. Tzanck smear is a useful bedside test. Biopsy and immunofluorescence are also done but are not bedside tests.

55. Ans. (c) Bullous pemphigoid

56. Ans. (a, d) Darier disease; Bowen's disease

Dyskeratosis refers to an abnormality in the process of epidermal cell keratinization. Seen in malignant diseases (like squamous cell carcinoma), premalignant diseases (like Bowen's disease, actinic keratosis), Darier disease (here the dyskeratotic keratinocytes are called corps ronds and corps grains).

57. Ans. (b) Epidermolysis bullosa acquisita

Blisters on elbows, knee and sacral area (trauma areas) suggests epidermolysis bullosa. Scarring and milia suggests dermal/junctional disease. DIF being positive suggests EB acquisita. Porphyria cutanea tarda has dermal blisters but has photosensitivity and blood vessel involvement. EB dystrophica will have a positive family history and negative DIF.

58. Ans. (a) Pemphigus vulgaris/vegetans

59. Ans. (a) Subepidermal

60. Ans. (c) Pemphigus vulgaris

61. Ans. (d) Immunofluorescence shows IgG and C3 complement deposition (See page 215 for explanation)

62. Ans. (a, d) Secondary syphilis; Pemphigus

63. Ans. (b) Suprabasal

The diagnosis is mucocutaneous PV.

64. Ans. (c) Staphylococcal scalded skin syndrome (See page 84-Chapter 4 for explanation)

65. Ans. (a) Periumbilical region (See page 213 for explanation)

66. Ans. (a) Bullous pemphigoid (See page 211 for explanation)

Old age with itchy bullae over erythematous areas, all suggest BP.

67. Ans. (c) Fishnet IgG deposition in epidermis

Flaccid bullae and erosions over the oral mucous membrane suggest PV.

68. Ans. (b) Pemphigus vulgaris

69. Ans. (d) Pityriasis rosea

70. Ans. (c) Papillary dermis

1st degree burns have only epidermal involvement (no blistering). 2nd degree burn (also known as partial thickness burns) have both epidermal and dermal involvement and in turn are of 2 types- a) Superficial 2nd degree—also called superficial partial thickness extending till the papillary dermis and b) Deep 2nd degree—also called deep partial thickness extending till reticular dermis. Third degree (full thickness) extend till deep dermis and even involves deeper structures.

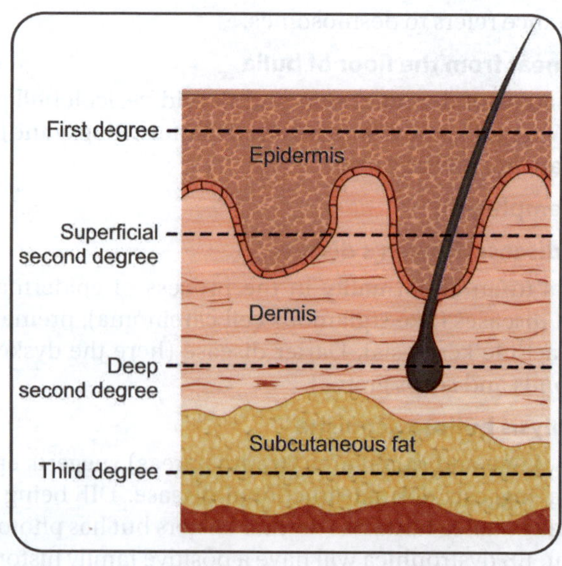

71. Ans. (b) Pemphigus vulgaris. Can clearly see a suprabasal split with row of tombstones

72. Ans. (b, c, e) Bullous pemphigoid; Bullous SLE; Dermatitis herpetiformis

Pemphigus vulgaris causes suprabasal blisters with acantholysis. Pemphigus vegetans is a variant of pemphigus vulgaris. BP/Bullous SLE/DH all are subepidermal.

73. Ans. (b, c) Cardiac arrhythmia; Pemphigus

Pemphigus is classically associated with autoimmune desmosomal dysfunction. Desmosomes are also necessary for mechanically coupling and reinforcing cardiomyocytes. Intercellular communication via cardiac desomomes is essential for proper cardiac function. Cardiac arrhythmias result from cardiac desmosomal dysfunction.

New Answers

74. Ans. a-True; b-True; c-False; d-False; e-True

75. Ans. (b) 4, 1, 2, 3

76. Ans. (a) Both Assertion and Reason are true and Reason is correct explanation of Assertion

Since hemidesmosomes are not destroyed in pemphigus vulgaris, the basal cell is still connected to the DEJ. Since, suprabasal desmosomes are destroyed, the basal layer is separated from the upper epidermis giving the row of tombstone appearance on histology.

77. Ans. (a) Both Assertion and Reason are true and Reason is correct explanation of Assertion

Since scaly-crusty presentation is seen in pemphigus foliaceous, bulla spread sign can't be done which needs an intact blister. Hence, this sign is negative in pemphigus foliaceous.

78. Ans. (3) If c and d are correct

79. Ans. 1-c, 2-f, 3-d, 4-a

80. Ans. Case 1: (a) Pemphigus vulgaris

Nikolsky sign positive is s/o epidermal blisters. P. vulgaris has mucocutaneous lesions.

Case 2: (e) Dermatitis herpetiformis

Dermatitis herpetiformis is classically associated with gluten mediated skin inflammation and rapidly responds to dapsone and a gluten free diet. Blisters are typically very itchy.

81. Ans. (b) Bullous pemphigoid

CHAPTER 10

Papulosquamous Disorders

PAPULOSQUAMOUS LESIONS

Papulo = papules, **Squamous** = scale. Includes diseases having papules/plaques with scales.

Causes:

- Psoriasis
- Lichen planus
- Seborrheic dermatitis
- Reiter's disease
- Neoplastic: Mycosis fungoides, Bowen's disease (Squamous cell carcinoma in situ)
- Tinea (refer to chapter 5)
- Eczema (refer to chapter 12)
- Pityriasis Rosea (refer to chapter 6)
- Secondary syphilis (refer to chapter 8)

High Yield Points

Papulosquamous diseases: **TEN SLiPS**

T: **T**inea
E: **E**czema
N: **N**eoplastic (Mycosis fungoides, Squamous cell carcinoma, Bowen's disease)
S: **S**econdary syphilis
Li: **Li**chen planus
P: **P**soriasis, **P**ityriasis rosea
S: **S**eborrheic dermatitis

PSORIASIS

Introduction

- An **itchy,**(MCQ) chronic, recurrent, **immune-mediated,**(MCQ) inflammatory inherited disease
- **Koebner's phenomenon**(MCQ) (linear trauma causes the lesions to increase in the line of trauma) can be seen in 25% patients (see Figure 3)

Pathology

- Genetic predisposition—particularly **HLA Cw6,**(MCQ) B13, B17 (**HLA-B27** is a marker for sacroiliitis—associated psoriasis arthritis and pustular psoriasis)(MCQ)

- Pathogenesis:

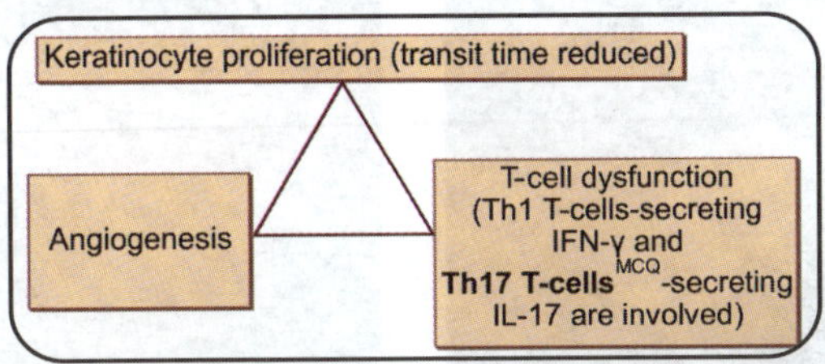

Triggering Factors

1. Infections: Streptococcus in pharynx-**Beta-hemolytic streptococci**(MCQ) of Lancefield groups A, C, and G (typically triggers guttate psoriasis)
2. **Sudden withdrawal of systemic steroids can trigger severe pustular psoriasis** (Hence, systemic steroids are generally not given in psoriasis)
3. Trauma—Seen clinically as Koebner's phenomenon (Fig. 3)
4. **Drugs**(MCQ)**: Beta blockers, NSAIDs, Chloroquine and Lithium**
5. Alcohol, Smoking
6. **Pregnancy**
7. **Winter**
8. Emotional stress
9. Sunlight—Some patients worsen, some improve

Types of Psoriasis

1. **Psoriasis vulgaris (Chronic Plaque Psoriasis):**
   - **Most common type ("Vulgaris" literally means common)**
   - Typically presents as sharply demarcated, erythematous **scaly plaques on extensor aspects** like elbows, knees, knuckles, lower back (Figs. 1A and B).
   - Lesions have a **triad of erythema** (due to new blood vessel synthesis), **thickening** (due to thickened epidermis) and **scale** (due to faulty epidermal keratinization and faulty exfoliation). **Scale is silvery or micaceous** (Fig. 2)(MCQ)

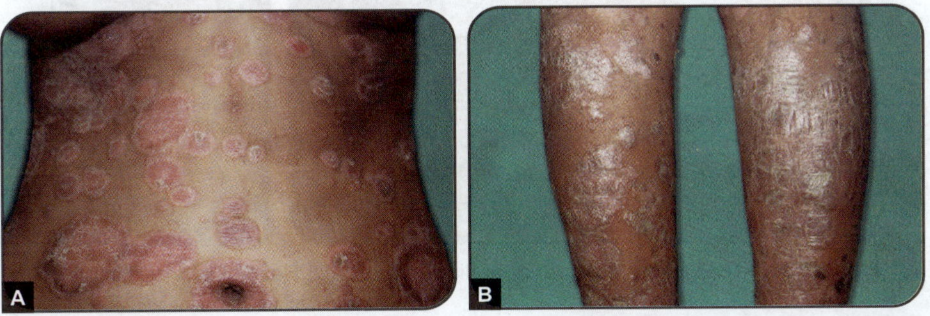

Figs. 1A and B: (A) Erythematous plaques with silvery scales; (B) Erythematous plaques with silvery scales on extensors lower limbs

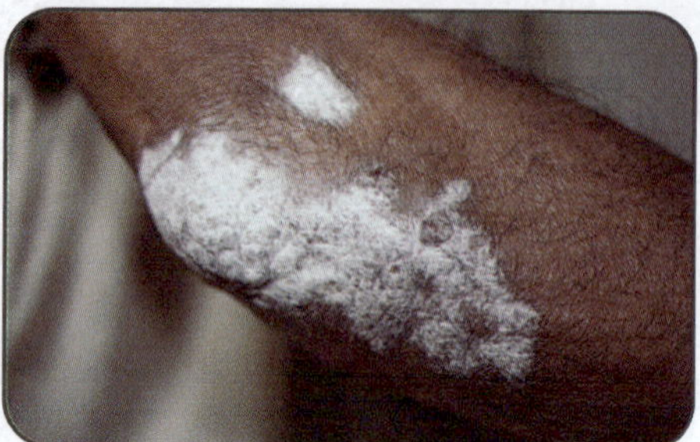

Fig. 2: Classical plaque on elbow extensor with silvery scale

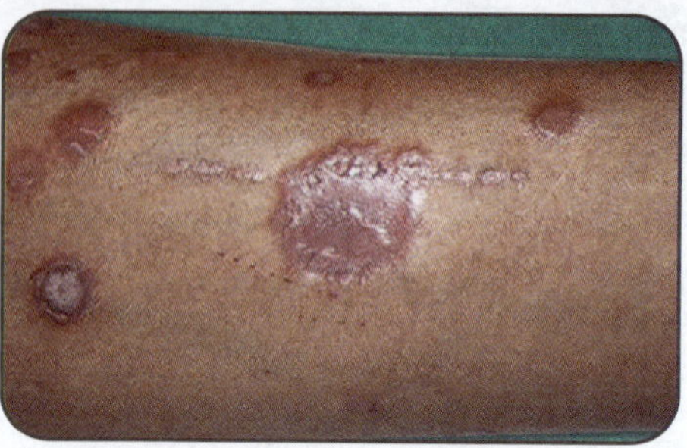

Fig. 3: Koebner's phenomenon. Note lesions increasing in scratched area

2. **Inverse (flexural)**: Lesions on **flexures**, like inframammary area, groins, axillae, etc. (not on extensors). Typically **nonscaly** (Figs. 4A to D)

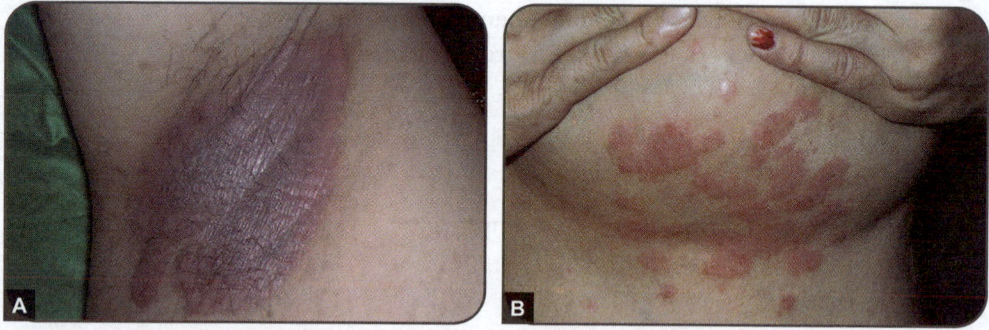

Figs. 4A and B: (A) Erythematous, nonscaly, shiny plaque-axilla; (B) Erythematous shiny nonscaly plaque-inframammary

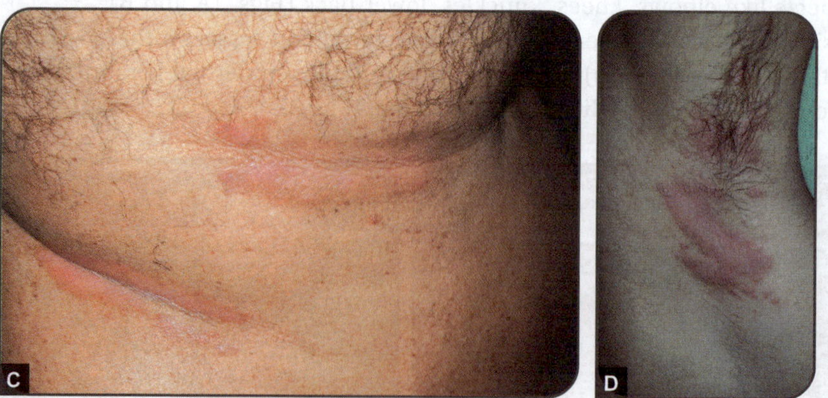

Figs. 4C and D: (C) Note absence of scaling in folds; (D) Flexural psoriasis in axilla

3. **Nail psoriasis**: 10–80% of psoriatic patients. Patients with nail involvement have an increased incidence of psoriatic arthritis.

Features of nail psoriasis:

Oil drop or Salmon patch • A translucent, yellow-red discoloration in the nail bed resembling a drop of oil beneath the nail plate. **Pathognomonic** of nail psoriasis (Fig. 5B)(MCQ)	**Subungual hyperkeratosis** • Excessive deposits of keratin on the nail bed. But there is no "tunneling" ("tunnel formations" in the subungual tissue indicates onychomycosis) (Fig. 5B)(MCQ)
Nail plate pitting • **Most common feature**(MCQ) • Pattern is **random**, deep and **irregular** (Fig. 5A) • Also called "**thimble pits**" • Pit is due to involvement of the **proximal nail matrix**(MCQ)	**Onycholysis** • Separation of the nail plate from its underlying attachment to the nail bed (secondary to subungual hyperkeratosis) (Fig. 5B)
Leuconychia (white streaks on nail)	Splinter hemorrhages (Fig. 5B)

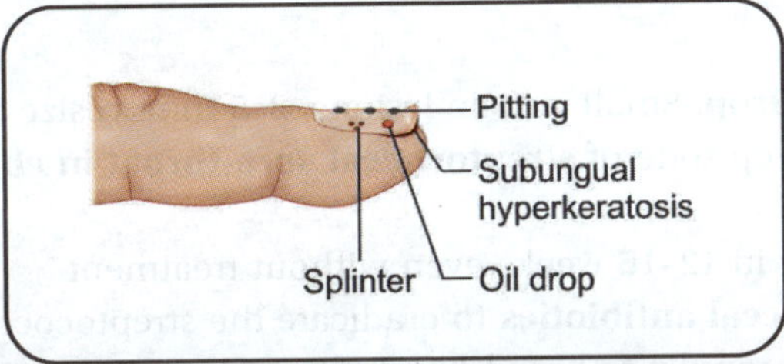

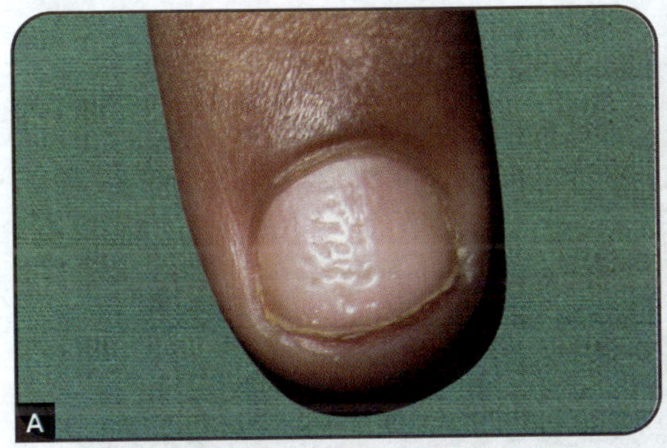

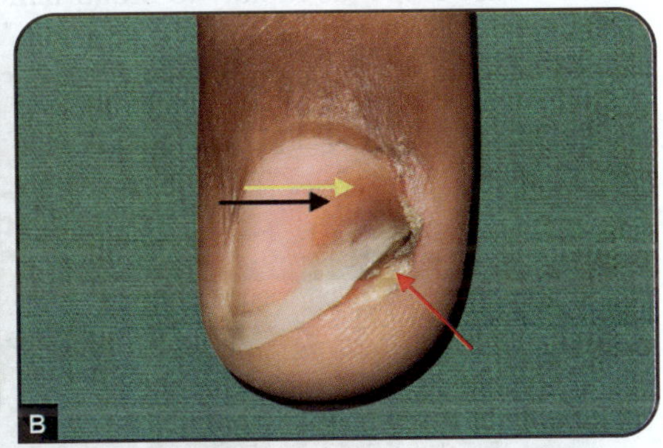

Figs. 5A and B: (A) Irregular, random, deep nail pits; (B) Salmon patch (black arrow), splinter hemorrhage (yellow arrow), subungual hyperkeratosis (red arrow)

High Yield Points

Nail-**POLISH**
P = **P**itting
O = **O**il drop, **O**nycholysis
L = **L**euconychia
I = **I**rregular (pits)
S = **S**plinter hemorrhage
H = **H**yperkeratosis (subungual)

4. **Sebo-psoriasis** (Psoriasis in seborrheic area)
   - In seborrheic areas like scalp, face, retroauricular area, central chest and upper back (Figs. 6A and B).

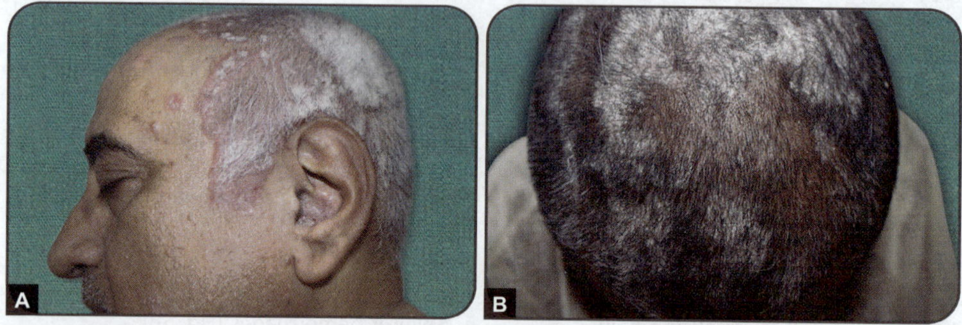

Figs. 6A and B: (A) Erythematous plaques with silvery scales on scalp, ear lobes; (B) Silvery scales on scalp

5. **Guttate psoriasis**
   - **"Guttate"= rain drop**. Small guttate lesions, 2–5 mm in size (Figs. 7A and B)
   - Typically after an episode of **streptococcal sore-throat in children**.
   - Treatment
     - **Self-resolving** in 12–16 weeks even without treatment
     - **Antistreptococcal antibiotics** to eradicate the streptococcal carriage
     - Also responds rapidly to broad-band ultraviolet B.

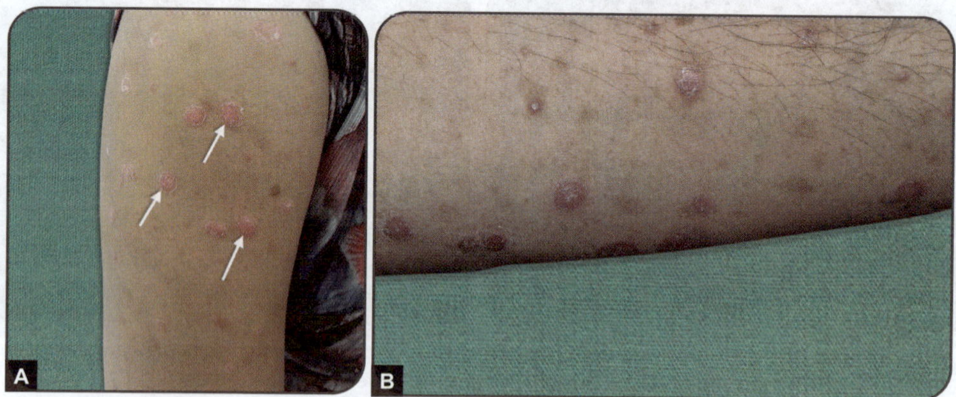

Figs. 7A and B: (A) Small, guttate lesions; (B) Close-up of the guttate lesions

6. **Pustular psoriasis**
   - Often gets **triggered by stoppage of systemic steroids**(MCQ) **(hence, steroids are usually avoided in any psoriasis patient)**
   - **Von Zumbusch type**(MCQ): Severe, acute form. Starts as fever followed by sudden eruption of **sterile pustules** (i.e. pus will not grow organisms). Repeated such waves of pus which fuse to form "**lakes of pus**" or "**sheets of pus**" on skin occurs(MCQ) (Figs. 8A to D)

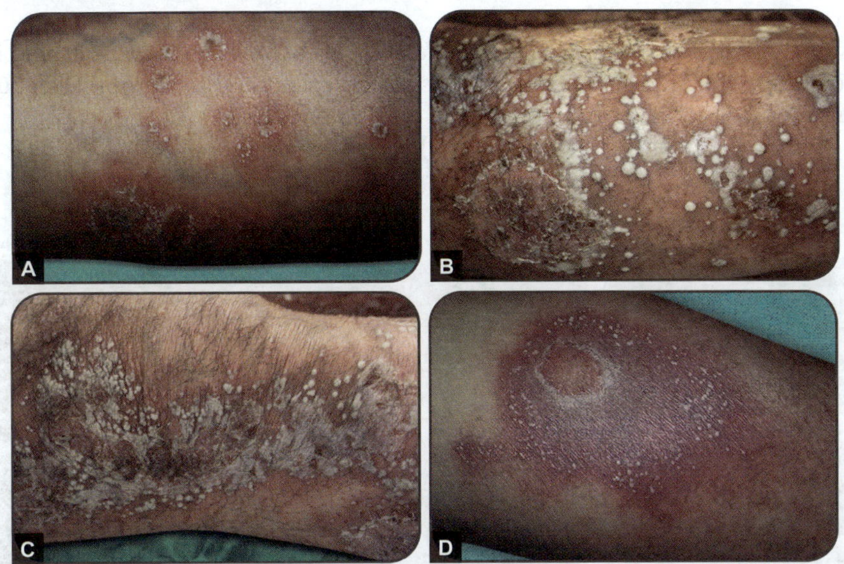

Figs. 8A to D: (A) Von-Zumbusch type-generalized sterile pustules on an erythematous base; (B) Close-up; (C) Note the fusion of pustules to form "lakes of pus"; (D) Pustules over an erythematous plaque of psoriasis

- **Von Zumbusch in pregnancy is called Impetigo herpetiformis**: Usually occurs in the last trimester and usually resolves after delivery, only to recur in subsequent pregnancies (Figs. 9A and B).

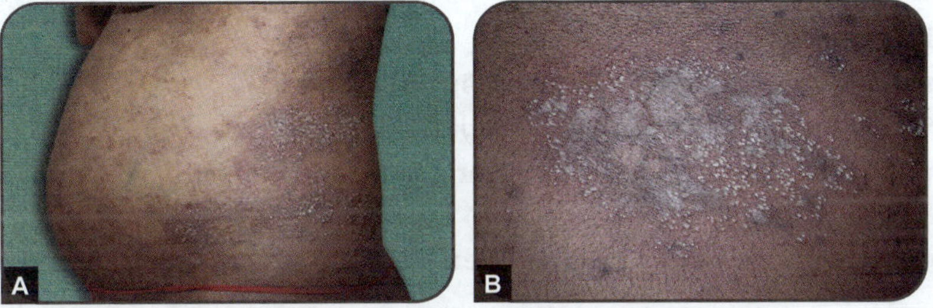

Figs. 9A and B: (A) Impetigo herpetiformis (pregnant women with pustular psoriasis); (B) Close-up showing fusion of pus in the center (lake of pus)

- **Treatment**

1st line	2nd line
• **Acitretin** (DOC)(MCQ) • Methotrexate(MCQ) • **Cyclosporine**(MCQ) ***In impetigo herpetiformis-DOC is systemic steroids but DOC will be cyclosporine if MCQ mentions any contraindication for steroids (e.g. diabetes)**	Biologicals (TNF-alpha inhibitors)

High Yield Points

Pick-up words in an MCQ: "Lake of pus" or "sheet of pus" always indicates Von Zumbusch/Impetigo herpetiformis

7. **Erythrodermic psoriasis**
   - Lesions increase, **lose their margins**, fuse with each other and **>90% gets involved**. (More than 90% involvement in any disease is called erythroderma) (Fig. 10A)
   - **Treatment**
     - **Methotrexate is the DOC** (Fig. 10B)
     - **Cyclosporine** (in life threatening erythroderma for rapid control)
     - Acitretin.

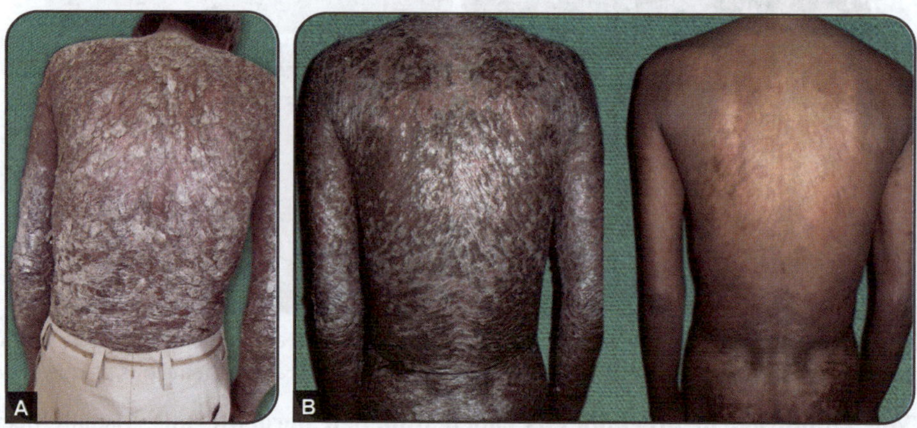

Figs. 10A and B: (A) Erythematous scaly plaques involving more than 90% body surface; (B) Before and after treatment with methotrexate

8. **Psoriatic arthritis**
   - **Seronegative spondyloarthropathy** (Figs. 11A and B)
   - **5–30%** of patients with cutaneous psoriasis[MCQ]
   - Nail psoriasis increases the risk of psoriatic arthritis. Most have cutaneous psoriasis preceding joint involvement
   - Associated with **HLA-B27**. Patients often have associated enthesitis and dactylitis

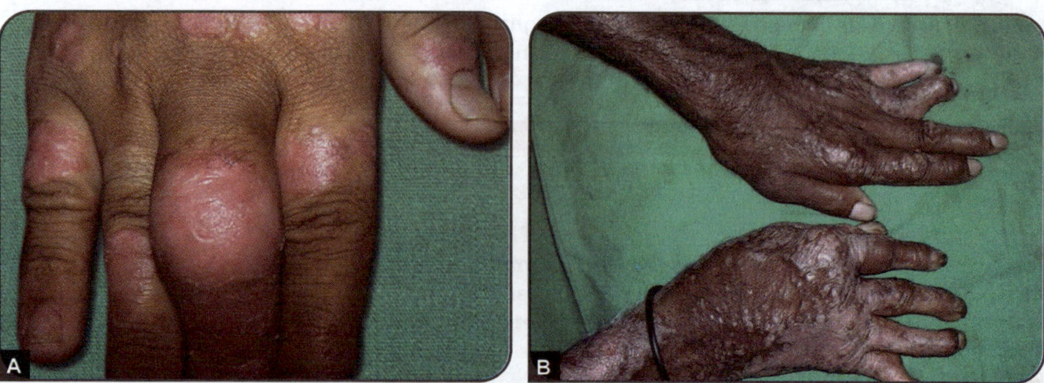

Figs. 11A and B: (A) PIP involvement with overlying psoriatic plaques; (B) Arthritis mutilans

- **Treatment**

1st line	2nd line
NSAIDs **Methotrexate-DOC** Sulfasalazine Leflunomide	Biologicals (TNF-alpha inhibitors)—If 1st line fails—Most efficacious but not the DOC in India due to cost and side-effect profile

9. **Palmoplantar psoriasis**
   - Scaly plaques are seen on palm and soles (Fig. 12)

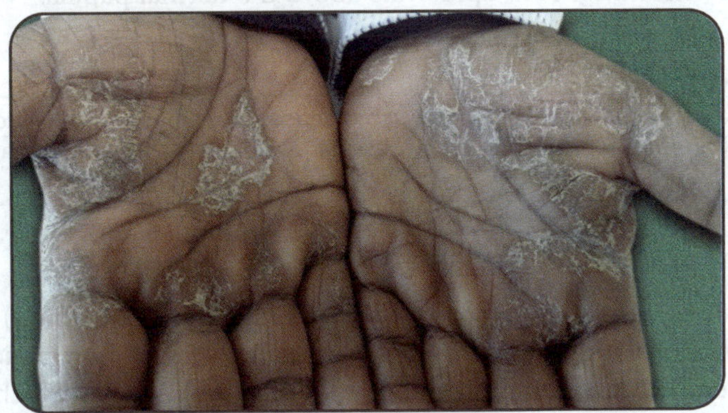

Fig. 12: Scaly plaques on palm and soles

High Yield Points

Types of psoriasis: **Got-A-PEPSI**
Got = **Got**tate (Guttate)
A = **A**rthritis
P = **P**laque (chronic plaque type)
E = **E**rythrodermic
P = **P**ustular
S = **S**ebopsoriasis
I = **I**nverse

Histopathology

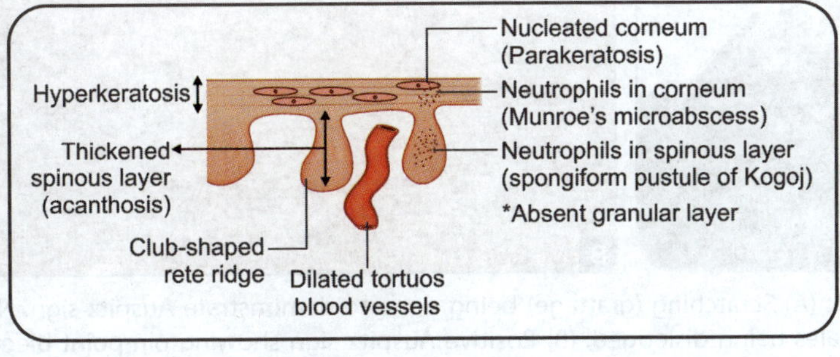

1. Regular elongation of rete ridges (rete ridges are narrow towards the surface and broad at the base)
2. **Acanthosis**: Thickening of stratum spinosum
3. **Parakeratosis (Nuclei in stratum corneum)**, **Hyperkeratosis**
4. **Absent granular cell layer**
5. Formation of **spongiform pustules of Kogoj** (Neutrophils accumulating in stratum spinosum)
6. **Munro microabscess** (Neutrophils accumulating in stratum corneum)
7. Capillary vessels within the superficial dermis are dilated and tortuous
8. **Suprapapillary thinning**: Thin epidermis above the dermal papilla.

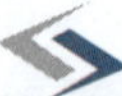

Extra-Edge Point

Psoriasis can be associated with **cardiovascular diseases**, e.g. myocardial infarctions, pulmonary emboli, peripheral arterial disease and cerebrovascular accidents—all due to high-risk of metabolic syndrome.

Auspitz Sign

If the superficial silvery scales are removed via scratching (**grattage method**) (Fig. 13A), scales while coming off attach together, as if one has scratched on a **wax candle (wax-candle scales**). Subsequently, a membrane (**Bulkeley membrane**) is seen, which when removed classical **pinpoint bleeding (Auspitz sign)** is seen (Fig. 13B). Auspitz sign is the clinical reflection of elongated vessels in the dermal papillae together with thinning of the suprapapillary epidermis.

**Note:* Auspitz sign is not seen in all types of psoriasis (Absent in pustular psoriasis)

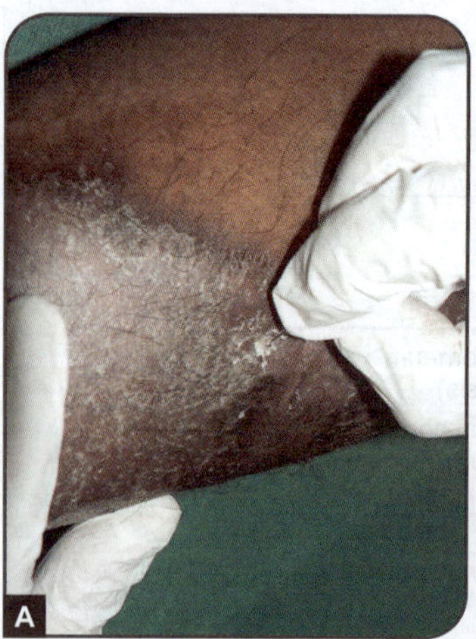

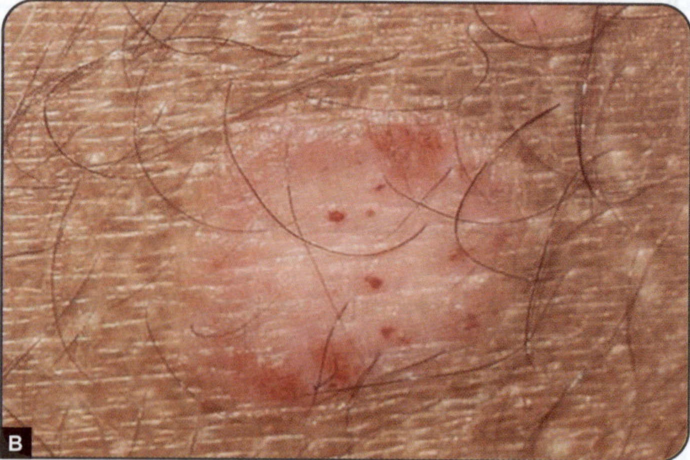

Figs. 13A and B: (A) Scratching (grattage) being done to demonstrate Auspitz sign. Note the candle-wax like scales being dislodged; (B) Positive Auspitz sign showing pin-point bleeding point

Treatment Protocol for Psoriasis

Topical If <10% body surface involved	Phototherapy 10–30% involvement	Systemic If >30% body surface involved
• **Steroids** • **Calcipotriol- Vitamin D derivative** (Vitamin D derivate reduces keratinocytes proliferation)- Preferred over steroids due to less side effects	• PUVA (Psoralens + UVA) • UVB (both narrow band and broad band UVB) PUVA is more effective than UVB, but has more side effects	• **Methotrexate** a. **DOC for psoriatic arthritis** b. **DOC for erythrodermic psoriasis** c. **DOC in chronic plaque psoriasis** Side effects: Hepatotoxic, bone marrow suppression, nausea • **Acitretin** a. **DOC for Pustular psoriasis**
Tacrolimus(PGI Nov 15) useful on facial psoriasis as it has less risk of atrophy than steroids on face		b. Less effective in chronic plaque psoriasis (Though when Retinoids are combined with PUVA, called Re-PUVA = Retinoid + PUVA—it is more effective) c. **DOC in psoriasis in HIV**-as it has no immunosuppressive property Side effects: Dyslipidemia, Liver abnormalities • **Cyclosporine (calcineurin inhibitor)** 2.5–5 mg/kg/day – Used in severe life-threatening erythrodermic psoriasis (as it is the fastest drug to act in psoriasis) – **Useful for Impetigo herpetiformis** – DOC in severe psoriasis Side effects: Nephrotoxic, hypertensive • **Systemic Steroids** – **DOC for Impetigo herpetiformis** (other drugs for impetigo herpetiformis are cyclosporine and biologics) – **DOC for psoriatic erythroderma in pregnancy** • Biologics (Etanercept, Infliximab, Adalimumab, Ustekinumab) – Useful for severe psoriasis not responding to conventional medications – TNF-α inhibitors—DOC for arthritis mutilans Fumaric acid

High Yield Points

Psoriasis

P = **P**laques/**P**inpoint bleed (Auspitz sign)/**P**hysical injury (Koebner phenomenon)/**P**ruritus
S = **S**ilver Scale/**S**calp involvement
O = **O**nycholysis/**O**il spots
R = **R**ed spot on nail (salmon patch)
I = **I**tching
A = **A**rthritis/**A**bscess (Munro)
S = **S**tratum corneum with nuclei, neutrophils
I = **I**mmunological abnormality
S = **S**tratum granulosum absent/**S**tratum Spinosum thickening/**S**uprapapillary thinning

LICHEN PLANUS (LP)

Introduction

- Lichen planus word is derived from ***leichen*, "tree moss" and *planus*—"flat"**. Tree moss is purple; hence **purple** lesions. Also flat lesions occur
- **Autoimmune**, inflammatory disease of skin, mucosa and hair follicles
- **5P's—Purple (violaceous), Polygonal, Pruritic, Plane topped (flat), Papules** (Figs. 14A and B)
- On the surface, **white criss-cross streaks (Wickham striae)** are seen especially, if a thin layer of oil is applied to the surface—**classical feature**
- **Flexural predisposition**(MCQ) (Contrast to psoriasis which has extensor distribution) (Fig. 15A)
- Even though itching is prominent, patients will rub (not scratch) the lesions. Hence, excoriation (scratch marks) not seen
- Association with liver disorders—**HCV**, **HBV**, primary biliary cirrhosis
- **Koebner's phenomenon** (Fig. 15B)
- **Usually self-limiting within 1 or 2 years** and **heals leaving hyperpigmentation** (Fig. 15C)(MCQ).

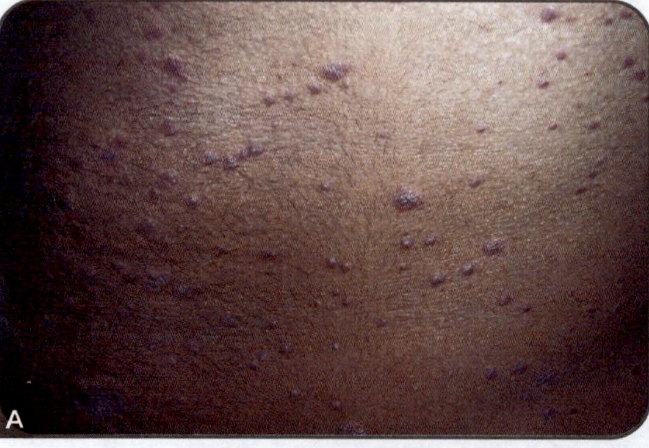

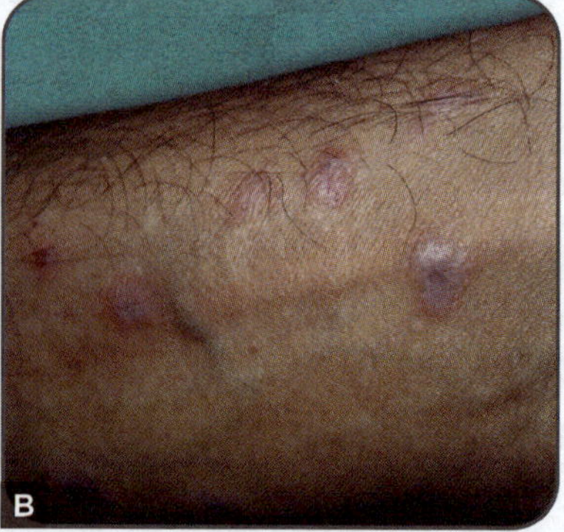

Figs. 14A and B: (A) Widespread acute violaceous lesions; (B) Close-up showing purple, polygonal, flat-topped papule

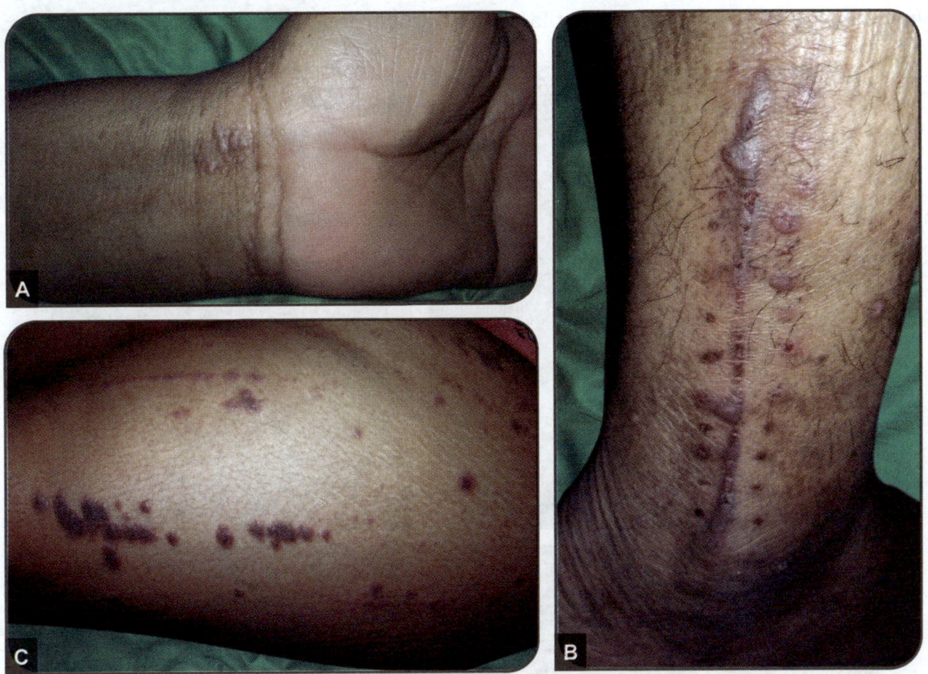

Figs. 15A to C: (A) Flexural distribution on wrist; (B) Koebner's phenomenon in lichen planus on surgical incision site; (C) Lesions healing with hyperpigmentation

Triggering Factors

- Drugs—Antimicrobials, antihypertensives, antimalarials, antidepressants, anticonvulsants
- **Dental amalgam**—Mercury in dental filling (amalgam) can trigger oral LP.

Types of LP

1. **Acute widespread lichen planus**
   - Sudden widespread violaceous papules and plaques (Figs. 14A and B)
2. **Nail LP**
   - 10% of patients. **Pterygium (dorsal pterygium)-Most classical feature.** The proximal nail-**fold fuses with the proximal portion of the nail-bed** (Fig. 16A)
   - **Thinning of nail plate—most common finding** (Fig. 16B)
   - Longitudinal ridging (Fig. 16D)
   - Subungual hyperkeratosis
   - **Tenting or pup-tent sign** is a result of nail bed involvement that elevates the nail plate in a tent shape (Fig. 16C)
   - **Twenty nail dystrophy (Trachyonychia).**

*Other causes of trachyonychia—Alopecia areata and psoriasis

3. **Hypertrophic LP**—Hypertrophic plaques on lower legs (Figs. 17A and B)

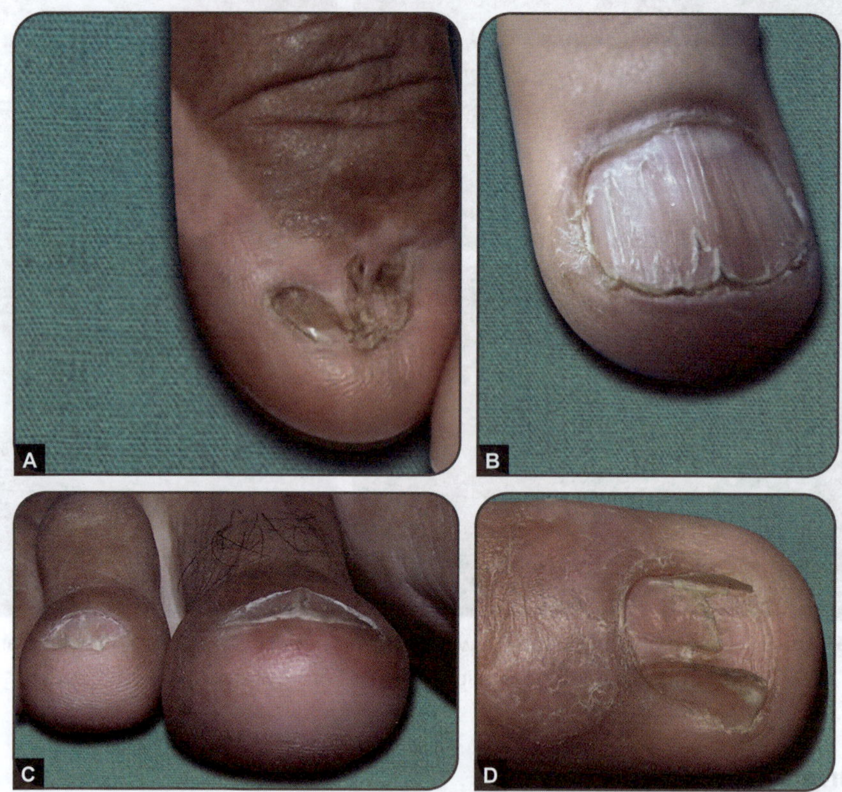

Figs. 16A to D: (A) Pterygium—Note the fusion of proximal nail-fold onto nail bed; (B) Thinning of nail plate; (C) Tenting of great toe nail. Note thinning of the 2nd toe nail plate; (D) Longitudinal ridging

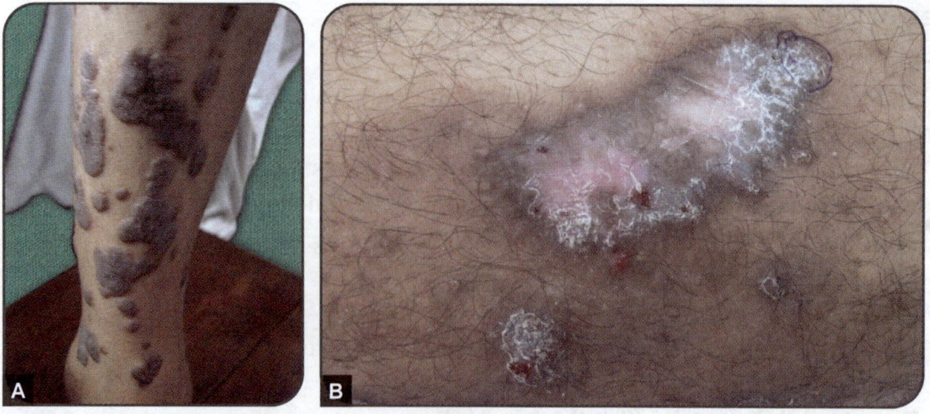

Figs. 17A and B: (A) Hypertrophic lesions on lower legs; (B) Close-up of a hypertrophic lesion. Note the criss-cross white Wickham striae

4. **Oral LP**
   - In up to 30–70% patients with cutaneous LP
   - **Dental filling (Dental amalgam) can be causative. Mercury** in this amalgam can cause oral LP at area of contact onto the buccal mucosa (Fig. 18B)
   - **Commonest form is the reticulate/lacy pattern** (buccal mucosa is the m/c site) (Figs. 18A, B and D)
   - **Ulcerative/Erosive form- rare but has premalignant potential** (Fig. 18C).

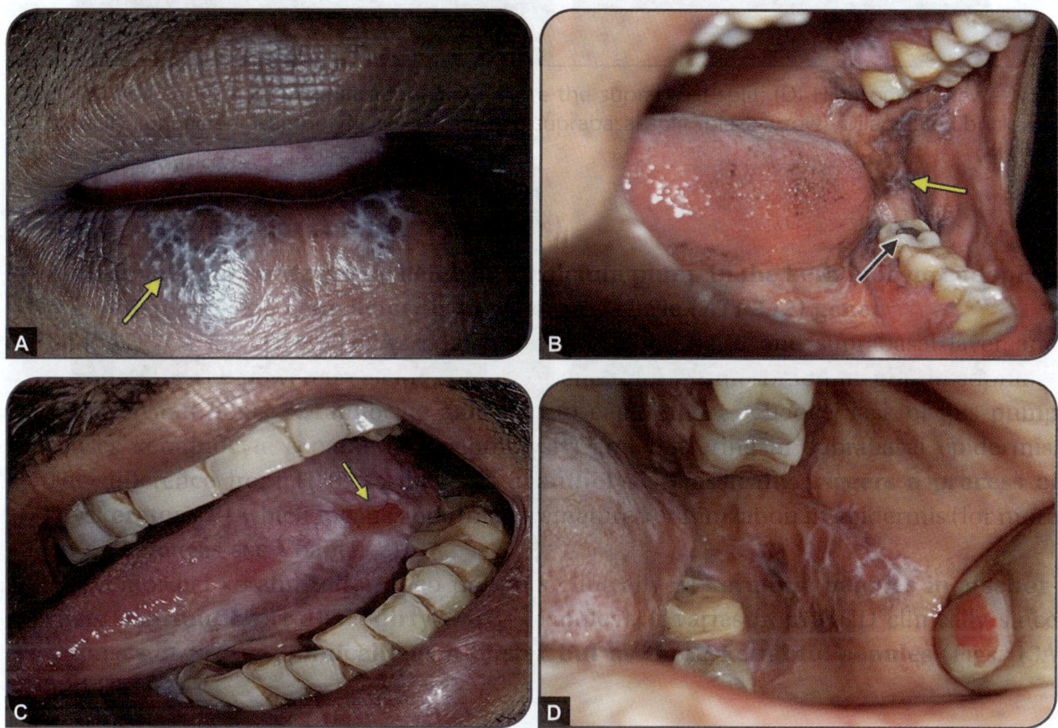

Figs. 18A to D: (A) White lacy lichen planus on lower lip; (B) White lacy lichen planus (yellow arrow). Note the dental filling nearby (black arrow); (C) Oral ulcerative lichen planus (yellow arrow); (D) Oral lacy LP- note the reticulate, criss-cross white pattern

*Leukoplakia is the most common premalignant lesion in the oral cavity(MCQ)

5. **Follicular LP (Lichen planopilaris, Pseudopelade)**—LP of hair follicles causing inflammation and scarring. Multiple areas of **scarring alopecia** are seen on scalp with **perifollicular blue-grey macules** (Figs. 19A to D). The scarring is patchy and irregular giving a "footprint in snow appearance"
6. **Actinic LP**—Actinic = Sun. This is a type of LP triggered by sun exposure (Figs. 20A and B)

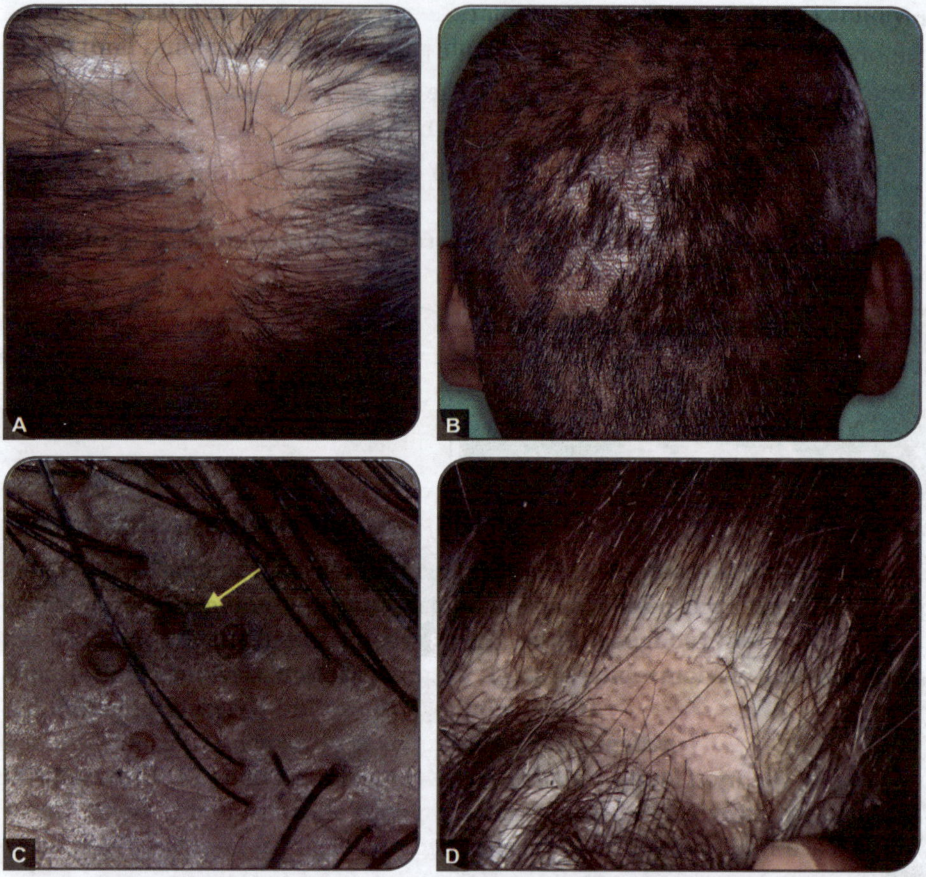

Figs. 19A to D: (A) Scarring on scalp, hair loss, follicular prominence; (B) Scarring in a patchy distribution on scalp ("footprint in snow" appearance); (C) Perifollicular blue gray macules on higher magnification (yellow arrow); (D) Alopecia in lichen planopilaris. Note the perifollicular pigmented macules

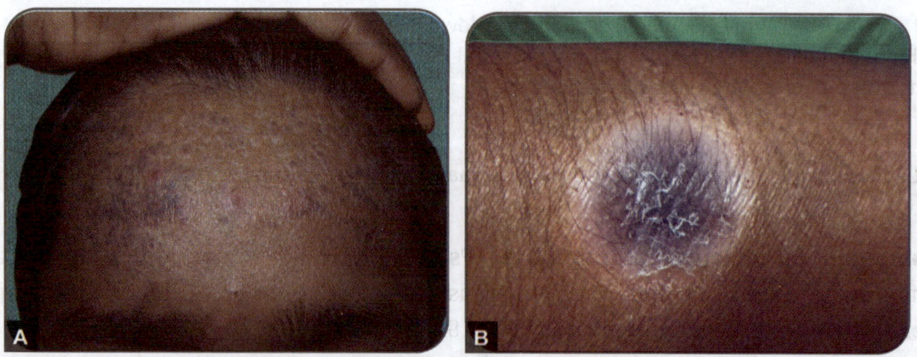

Figs. 20A and B: (A) Violaceous macules on forehead with surrounding hypopigmentation; (B) Close-up purple patch with surrounding hypopigmentation, Wickham striae in the center

7. **Lichen planus pigmentosus (LPP)**: Pigmented dark-brown macules predominantly affecting exposed skin like the face and neck (Figs. 21A to C)

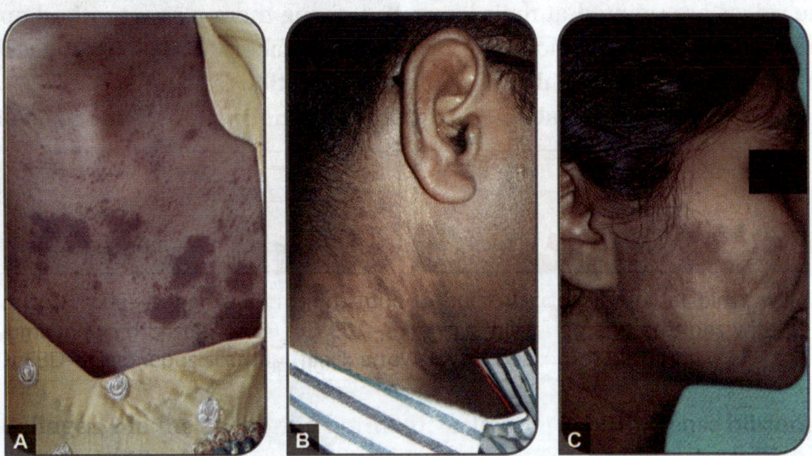

Figs. 21A to C: Hyperpigmented patches on exposed areas

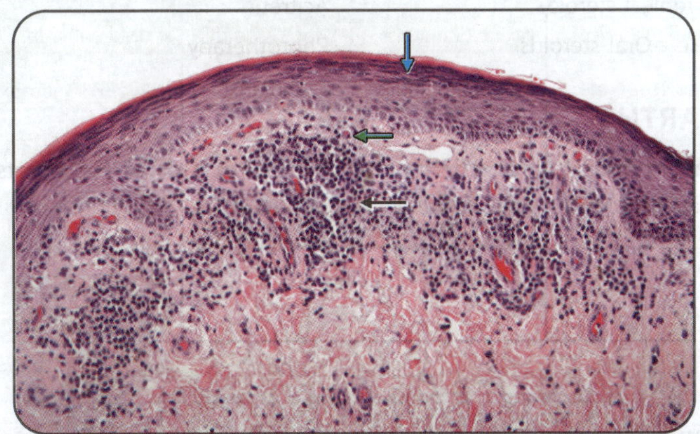

Fig. 21D: Histopathology of LP: Note the dense band of lymphocytes under DEJ (black arrow), hypergranulosis (blue arrow), Civatte bodies (green arrow)

Histopathology (Fig. 21D)

- The earliest pathological change is **basal epidermal cell destruction** (also called as **vacuolization of the basal layer, liquefaction of the basal layer** due to basal keratinocytes being destroyed by dermal CD-8+ lymphocytes—**Classical of lichen planus**). These necrotic/apoptotic keratinocytes are called as **colloid bodies, cytoid bodies or civatte bodies.** Due to autoimmune basal layer destruction and liquefaction, the basal degenerated keratinocytes may fall down and be seen in the dermis.
- Due to autoimmune basal layer destruction and liquefaction, the **basal melanocytes may also fall down into the dermis (pigment will be seen in the upper dermis—called pigment incontinence**[MCQ]**)**

- Hyperkeratosis
- Wedge-shaped **hypergranulosis** (responsible for the clinical appearance of Wickham striae)
- The rete ridges are pointed at their lower end-giving them a **saw-toothed appearance**
- Clefts at dermoepidermal junction, probably an artifact (**Max-Joseph spaces**)
- **Band of lymphocytes at the dermoepidermal junction**(MCQ)
- **Band of lymphocytes + Basal cell destruction/vacuolization = Interface dermatitis.**

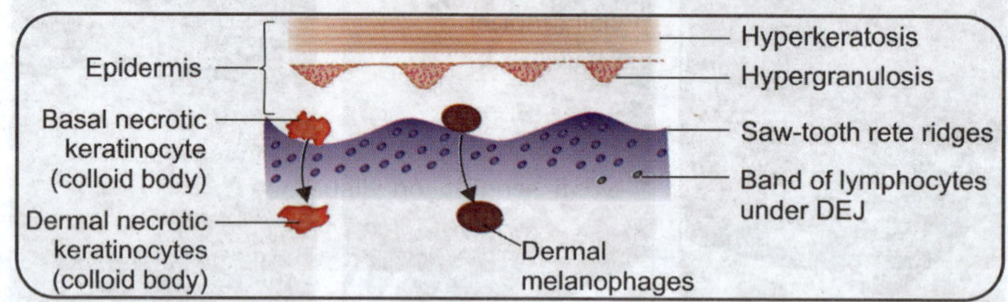

Treatment

1st line	2nd line
Limited disease—Topical steroids	Acitretin
Widespread disease—Oral steroids	Phototherapy

REACTIVE ARTHRITIS/REITER'S DISEASE

- **Classical triad of arthritis, urethritis and conjunctivitis**. Skin also gets involved

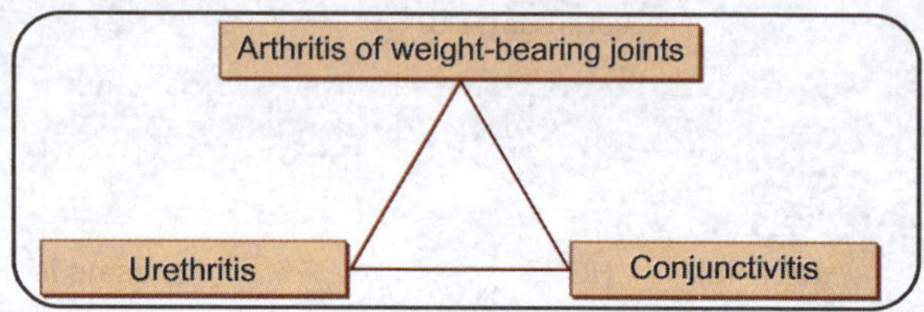

- **HLA-B27** is an association
- **Two forms:**
  1. **Sexually transmitted**: Symptoms emerge after exposure to **chlamydia trachomatis (m/c cause)**(MCQ), ureaplasma through sexual route
  2. **Post-enteric infection**—Symptoms emerge after exposure to shigella, salmonella, yersinia, campylobacter
- Asymmetric arthritis of **large weight bearing joints** or axial sacroiliac arthritis follows after 1–4 weeks of pathogen entry, hence called **reactive arthritis. Enthesitis of Achilles tendon and plantar fascia is the hallmark of the disease**
- Eye involvement—Conjunctivitis, iritis/anterior uveitis.
- **Cutaneous features:**
  - Hyperkeratotic lesions on skin, palms or soles (**keratoderma blenorrhagica**(MCQ)— "kerato" = keratin, "derma" = skin, "bleno" = pus, "rrhagica" = oozing-Keratotic lesions on palms, soles which ooze pus) (Figs. 22A to C)

- **Circinate balanitis**—Inflammation of glans penis with circinate (ring-like) lesions (Fig. 22D)

- Treatment—Mucocutaneous lesions clear with topical steroids. Joint disease—NSAIDs, methotrexate, sulfasalazine, TNF-α antagonists. Doxycycline may help to eradicate chlamydia.

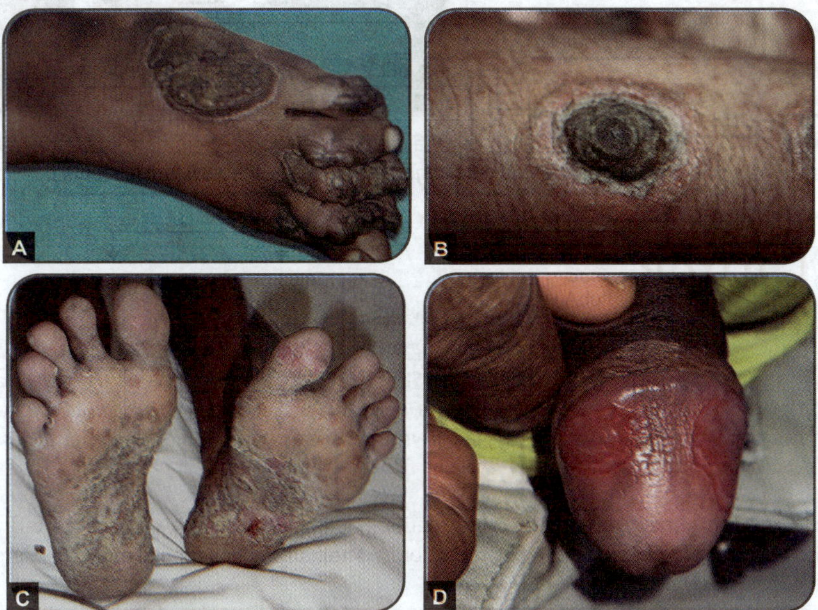

Figs. 22A to D: (A) Hyperkeratotic plaques; (B) Close-up of the thick hyperkeratotic plaques; (C) Keratotic plaques on soles oozing pus (Keratoderma blenorrhagica); (D) Circinate balanitis. Note the ring shaped lesions with glans inflammation

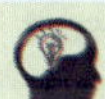

Aid to Remember

- "**CUBIKA**"—**C**onjunctivitis, **U**rethritis, **B**alanitis circinata, **I**ritis, **K**eratoderma blenorrhagica, **A**rthritis
- "**Can't see, Can't pee, Can't bend my knee**"—clinical manifestations

SEBORRHEIC DERMATITIS (SD)

- Recurring dermatitis of seborrheic areas-scalp, face, chest, etc. (seborrheic areas) (Figs. 23A to C)
- Erythematous scaly patches of sebaceous glands
- If there is no inflammation, it is called **dandruff or pityriasis capitis** and if there is inflammation and itching, it is referred to as **seborrheic dermatitis**
- **Lipophilic yeasts** (**Malassezia**—previously known as Pityrosporum) are associated
- The scale has a **yellow, greasy appearance** (Figs. 23B and C)
- **Severe SD is seen in HIV and Parkinson's disease.** SD in infants is called **cradle cap**
- Treatment is with antifungal shampoos containing ketoconazole, ciclopirox, selenium sulfide, coal tar.

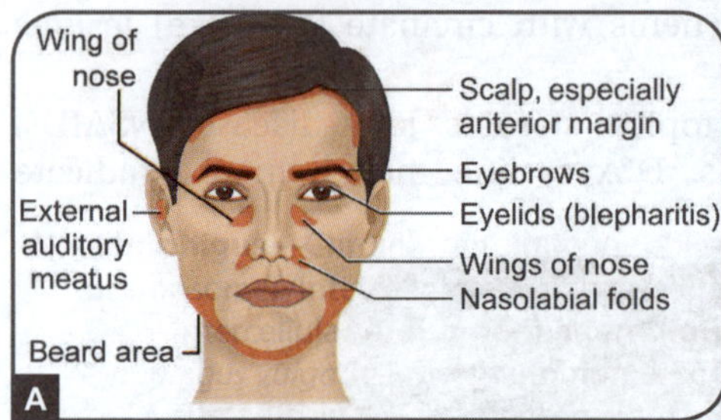

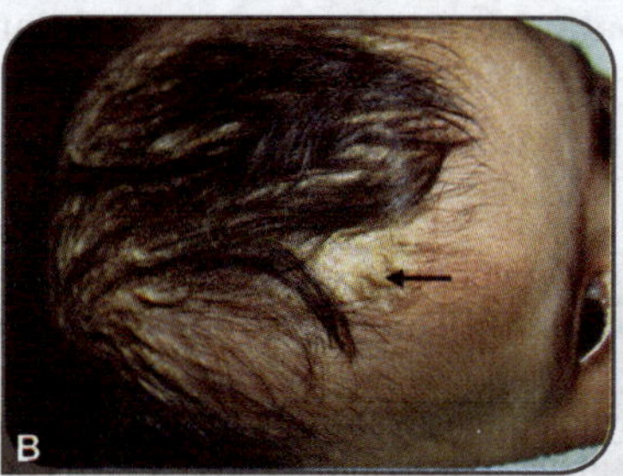

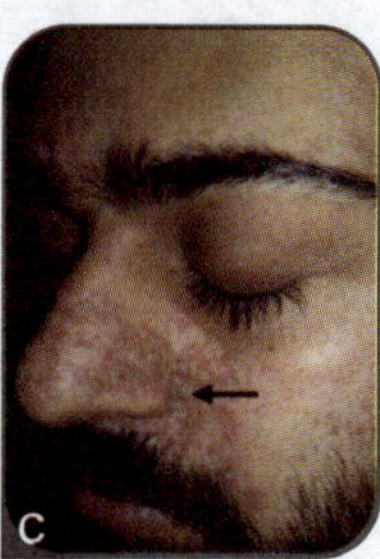

Figs. 23A to C: (A) Schematic representation of areas affected in seborrheic dermatitis; (B) Yellow, greasy scales on scalp in an infant (cradle cap); (C) Yellow greasy scales— nasolabial folds, nose, inner eyebrows

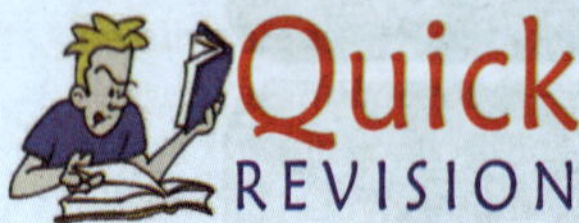

- **Papulosquamous lesions**—Mnemonic: **TEN SLIPS (T**: **T**inea, **E**: **E**czema, **N**: **N**eoplastic [Mycosis fungoides, Squamous cell carcinoma, Bowen's disease], **S**: **S**econdary syphilis, **Li**: **Li**chen planus, **P**: **P**soriasis, **P**arapsoriasis, **P**ityriasis rosea, **P**ityriasis rubra pilaris, **P**ityriasis lichenoides chronica, **S**: **S**eborrheic dermatitis)
- **Psoriasis**
  - Itchy, autoimmune disorder. T-cell dysfunction (Th1 and Th17). HLA-Cw6 associated. Koebner's phenomenon + Triggers—Systemic steroids, streptococcus, drugs (beta blockers, lithium, Chloroquine, NSAIDs)
  - **Psoriasis vulgaris**—M/c type, silvery scales on extensors. **Guttate**—Small rain drop like lesions (treatment is antibiotics). **Sebopsoriasis**- on seborrheic areas. **Flexural**—No scales. **Pustular psoriasis (Von Zumbusch)** has "lakes" or "sheets of pus" on skin. Von Zumbusch in pregnancy is called Impetigo herpetiformis. **Nail**—pitting (m/c), salmon patch/oil drop (pathognomic). **Arthritis**—DIP involvement (most classical), asymmetrical oligoarticular (m/c). **Auspitz sign, Grattage test** useful for diagnosis. **Histopathology**—Parakeratosis, Hyperkeratosis, absent granular layer, spongiform pustules (classical), Munro microabscess (classical).
  - **Treatment**—Topically calcipotriol is the DOC. Erythrodermic and Psoriatic arthritis—Methotrexate is DOC. Von-Zumbusch-Acitretin is the DOC. Impetigo herpetiformis—Steroid is the DOC (if mentioned diabetes—cyclosporine is the DOC).
- **Lichen planus**
  - Autoimmune disease. 5 Ps-Purple, Polygonal, Pruritic, Plane topped (flat), Papules
  - Wickham striae on putting oil on lesions. Association with HBV, HCV, dental amalgam. Flexural predisposition. Heals with hyperpigmentation. Koebner's phenomenon
  - **Nail**—Pterygium, thinning of nail, longitudinal ridging, trachyonychia. **Oral**—Lacy, reticular plaques (ulcerative form-premalignant). **Lichen planopilaris**—scarring alopecia. **Histopathology**—Basal cell degeneration (most diagnostic), hypergranulosis, band of lymphocytes, interface dermatitis, Civatte/Colloid/Cytoid bodies (necrotic keratinocytes).
- Reactive arthritis/Reiter's disease
  - Classical triad of arthritis, urethritis and conjunctivitis. Postsexual (m/c cause chlamydia) or postenteric. Cutaneous features- keratoderma blenorrhagica, Circinate balanitis, Hyperkeratotic skin plaques
- **Seborrheic dermatitis**—Yellow, greasy scales on seborrheic areas, severe in HIV and Parkinson's disease. Treatment by azoles, selenium sulphide, ciclopirox olamine.

QUESTIONS

1. All are causes of papulosquamous lesions *except*:

a. Psoriasis
b. Parapsoriasis
c. Basal cell carcinoma
d. Mycosis fungoides
e. Syphilis

2. All of the following may lead to plaque formation *except*:

a. Psoriasis
b. Lichen planus
c. Pityriasis rosea
d. Pemphigus

3. An important feature of psoriasis is:

a. Crusting
b. Scaling
c. Oozing
d. Erythema

4. A 30-year-old male presented with silvery scales on elbow and knee that bleed on removal. The probable diagnosis is:

a. Pityriasis rosea
b. Seborrheic dermatitis
c. Psoriasis
d. Secondary syphilis

5. A male presents with a violaceous papule which is pruritic. There is pterygium of nail with cicatricial alopecia. Diagnosis is:

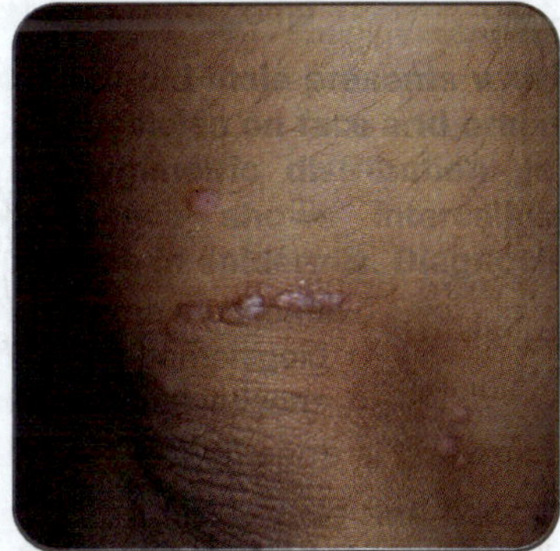

a. Psoriasis
b. Pityriasis rosea
c. Lichen planus
d. Seborrheic dermatitis

6. An adult presents with severe dandruff and greasy yellow scales on scalp. Diagnosis is:

a. Seborrheic dermatitis
b. Pityriasis rubra pilaris
c. Pityriasis rosea
d. Lichen planus

7. A child is presenting with erythematous follicular papules on trunk. There are areas of normal skin within the lesions. There is thickening of palms and soles. This child is suffering from:

a. Pityriasis rosea
b. Pityriasis rubra pilaris
c. Psoriasis
d. Seborrheic dermatitis

8. A patient presented with scarring alopecia, thinned nails, hyperpigmented macular lesions over the trunk and oral mucosa. The diagnosis is:

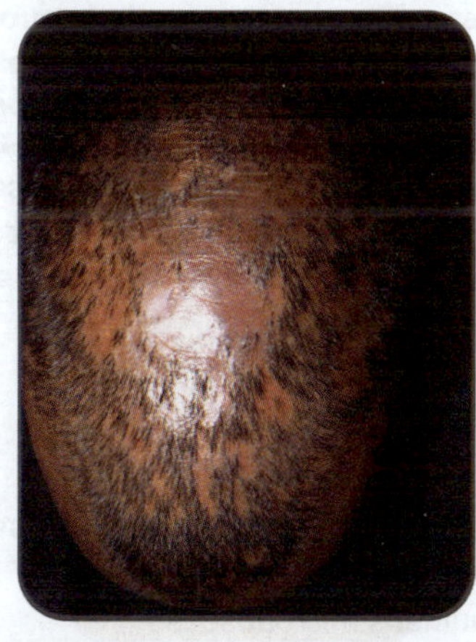

a. Psoriasis
b. Leprosy
c. Lichen planus
d. Pemphigus

9. A young male presented with lacy lesions on tongue since a month with elongation of nail-fold onto the nail-bed. What is the diagnosis?

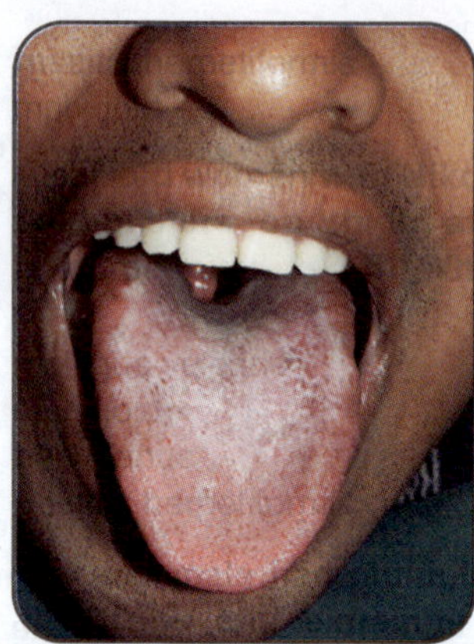

a. Psoriasis
b. Geographic tongue
c. Lichen planus
d. Candidiasis

10. Multiple erythematous annular lesions with peripheral collarette of scales arranged predominantly on trunk are seen in:

a. Pityriasis versicolor
b. Pityriasis rubra pilaris
c. Pityriasis rosea
d. Pityriasis lichenoides chronica

11. A 16-year-old boy presented with asymptomatic, multiple erythematous annular lesions with a collarette of scales at periphery of the lesions present on the trunk. The most likely diagnosis is:

a. Pityriasis versicolor *(AI 05)*
b. Pityriasis alba
c. Pityriasis rosea
d. Pityriasis rubra pilaris

12. Which of the following is seen in psoriasis?

a. Pautrier's microabscess
b. Micro-Munroe abscess
c. Grenz zone
d. Hyperkeratosis
e. Suprapapillary thinning

13. All are true about psoriasis *except*:

a. Pruritic
b. Pitting of nails
c. Joint involvement in 2–5%
d. Parakeratosis and acanthosis
e. Munro's microabscess

14. Typical silvery scales of psoriasis are absent in:

a. Scalp b. Knee
c. Groin d. Elbow

15. Common site involvement in psoriasis is:

a. Scalp b. Nail
c. CNS d. Joints

16. A patient presents with erythematous scaly lesions on extensor aspect of elbows and knee. The clinical diagnosis is assisted by:

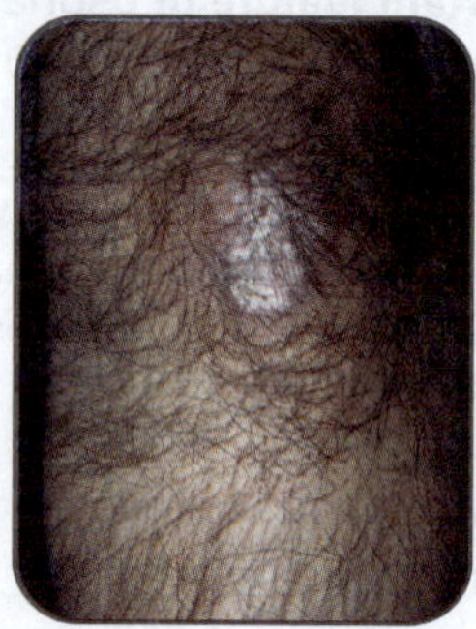

a. Auspitz sign b. KOH smear
c. Tzanck smear d. Skin biopsy

17. Most common type of psoriasis:

a. Pustular psoriasis
b. Psoriasis vulgaris
c. Flexural psoriasis
d. Penile psoriasis

18. This type of psoriasis is commonly seen in children and may follow a streptococcal sore throat: *(AI 2014)*

a. Guttate b. Stable plaque
c. Pustular d. Arthropathic

19. Grattage test is done in:

a. Tinea capitis
b. Lichen planus
c. Pemphigus vulgaris
d. Psoriasis

20. Auspitz sign is characteristically seen in:
- a. Plaque psoriasis
- b. Pustular psoriasis
- c. Lichen planus
- d. Inverse psoriasis

21. A patient with psoriasis was started on systemic steroids. After stopping the treatment, patient developed universally red scaly skin with plaques losing their margins all over his body. The most likely cause is:
- a. Drug-induced reaction
- b. Pustular psoriasis
- c. Bacterial infection
- d. Erythrodermic psoriasis

22. A patient with psoriasis was started on systemic steroids. After stopping treatment, the patient developed generalized pustules all over the body. The cause is most likely to be:

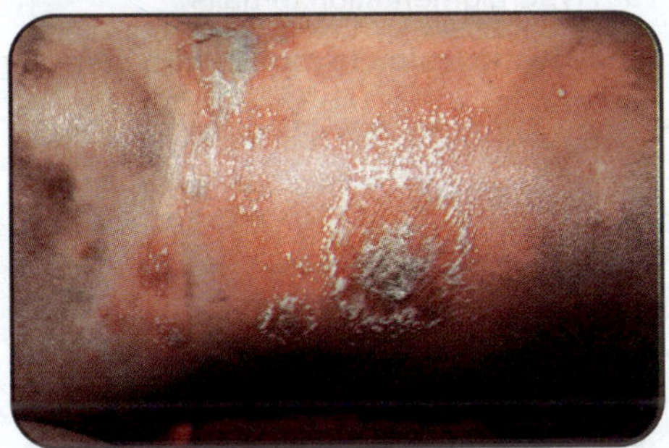

- a. Drug-induced reaction
- b. Pustular psoriasis
- c. Bacterial infections
- d. Septicemia

23. Wickham striae is seen in:
- a. Hairy leukoplakia
- b. Oral lichen planus
- c. Lichen sclerosis
- d. Psoriasis

24. Bleeding spots seen on removal of scales in psoriasis is called as:
- a. Auspitz sign
- b. Punctate hemorrhage
- c. Nikolsky sign
- d. Darier sign

25. Vitamin D analogue calcipotriol is useful in the treatment of:
- a. Cutaneous tuberculosis
- b. Psoriasis
- c. Pemphigus
- d. Leprosy

26. Treatment of choice in pustular psoriasis is:
- a. Thalidomide
- b. Retinoids
- c. Hydroxyurea
- d. Methotrexate

27. Treatment of choice in pustular psoriasis:
- a. Psoralen + UV therapy
- b. Systemic steroid
- c. Methotrexate
- d. Estrogen

28. DOC for a pregnant woman in 2nd trimester with pustular psoriasis is:
- a. Prednisolone
- b. Dapsone
- c. Acitretin
- d. Methotrexate

29. The treatment of choice for erythrodermic psoriasis is:
- a. Corticosteroids
- b. Methotrexate
- c. Coaltar topically
- d. Topical corticosteroids

30. A primigravida female presented with erythematous skin changes and lesion with multiple pus lakes. Which of the following should be the most appropriate?
- a. Corticosteroids
- b. Acitretin
- c. Psoralen + PUVA
- d. PUVA

31. Drug of choice for impetigo herpetiformis is:
- a. Prednisolone
- b. Dapsone
- c. Acitretin
- d. Methotrexate

32. The best indication of giving corticosteroids in pustular psoriasis is:
- a. Psoriatic erythroderma with pregnancy
- b. Psoriasis in a patient with alcoholic cirrhosis
- c. Moderate arthritis
- d. Extensive lesions

33. The only definitive indication of systemic steroids in psoriasis is:
a. Pustular psoriasis
b. Impetigo herpetiformis
c. Psoriatic arthropathy
d. Erythroderma

34. Psoriasis is exacerbated by:
a. Lithium
b. B-blockers
c. Antimalarials
d. All of the above

35. Itchy polygonal violaceous papules are seen in:
a. Psoriasis b. Pemphigus
c. Lichen planus d. Pityriasis rosea

36. Purple papule followed by hyperpigmentation on resolution is seen in:
a. Addison's disease
b. Diabetes mellitus
c. Hypothyroidism
d. Lichen planus

37. Not a histological feature of lichen planus:
a. Acanthosis
b. Hyperkeratosis
c. Neutrophils in stratum corneum
d. Pigment incontinence

38. The most characteristic finding in lichen planus is:
a. Civatte bodies
b. Basal cell degeneration
c. Thinning of nail plate
d. Violaceous lesions

39. A patient presents with flat-topped violaceous papules, thinning of nail and onycholysis. Microscopic finding would be:
a. Basal cell degeneration
b. Epidermal bulla
c. Acantholysis
d. Prominent nuclei in corneum

40. Basal cell degeneration is seen in:
a. Lichen planus b. Psoriasis
c. Pemphigus d. DLE

41. Max Joseph's space is a histopathological feature of:
a. Psoriasis vulgaris
b. Lichen planus
c. Pityriasis rosea
d. Parapsoriasis

42. Wickham striae is classically seen in:
a. Lichen nitidus
b. Lichenoid eruption
c. Lichen striatus
d. Lichen planus

43. Most characteristic feature of lichen planus is:
a. Thinning of nail plate
b. Nonscarring alopecia
c. Violaceous lesion on skin and mucous membrane
d. Wickham striae

44. Characteristic nail-finding in lichen planus:
a. Pitting
b. Pterygium
c. Beau's lines
d. Hyperpigmentation of nails

45. Lacy white lesion in mouth with pterygium is seen in:
a. Psoriasis
b. Pityriasis alba
c. Lichen planus
d. Leprosy

46. Irregular pitting is seen in:
a. Psoriasis
b. Alopecia areata
c. Lichen planus
d. Eczema

47. Regarding lichen planus, all are true *except*:
a. Hypopigmentation in residual disease
b. Lymphocytic infiltration
c. Itchy, polygonal, purple, papule
d. Skin, hair and oral mucosa commonly involved

48. Cicatricing alopecia with perifollicular blue-gray patches are most commonly associated with:
a. Pitting of nails
b. Whitish lesions in the buccal mucosa
c. Arthritis
d. Discoid plaques in the face

49. All of the following drugs can worsen psoriatic lesions *except:*
a. Chloroquine
b. Beta-blockers
c. Acitretin
d. Lithium

50. Treatment of choice for acute widespread lichen planus:
a. Topical corticosteroids
b. Systemic corticosteroids
c. Antihistaminics
d. Acitretin

51. All of the following regarding widespread lichen planus are true *except*:
a. Involves mucous membrane
b. Associated with Hepatitis C
c. Topical calcipotriol is the mainstay of therapy
d. Spontaneous remission in 1 to 2 years

52. Pityriasis rosea—true is:
a. Self-limiting
b. Chronic relapsing
c. Life-threatening infection
d. Caused by dermatophytes

53. Annular herald patch is seen in:
a. Psoriasis
b. Pityriasis alba
c. Pityriasis rosea
d. Nocardiosis

54. Hanging curtain sign is seen in:
a. Pityriasis alba
b. Pityriasis versicolor
c. Pityriasis rubra
d. Pityriasis rosea

55. Which viral association is found in pityriasis rosea?
a. HHV 7
b. CMV
c. Varicella Zoster
d. EBV

56. Which of the following is/are not a type of lichen planus:
a. Hypertrophic
b. Lichen nitidus
c. Lichen scrofulosorum
d. Ulcerative
e. Bullous

57. The most common association with irregular pitting of nails and onycholysis is:
a. Violaceous papules
b. Well-defined scaly plaques
c. Cicatricial alopecia
d. Polygonal papule

58. In a patient of psoriasis, acitretin is used. Pick the incorrect statement *(Recent NEET pattern)*
a. It is not teratogenic
b. Patient can donate blood during treatment
c. It has long elimination time
d. Can cause hyperlipidemia

59. Which of the following nail changes are NOT correctly matched?
a. Lichen planus and dorsal pterygium
b. Systemic sclerosis and ventral pterygium
c. Psoriasis and irregular pitting
d. Alopecia areata and irregular pitting

60. A 22-year-old male patient presents with hyperkeratotic yellow waxy plaques on palms and soles. He also complaints of pain the right knee and ankle. The diagnosis is: *(PGI Nov 18)*
a. Reactive arthritis
b. Metastatic gonorrhoea
c. Psoriasis
d. Secondary syphilis
e. Rheumatoid arthritis

61. Which of the following is not a type of lichen planus?
a. Lichen scrofulosorum
b. Lichen planopilaris
c. Lichen hypertrophica
d. Lichen pigmentosa

62. Drugs used in psoriasis:
a. Methotrexate
b. Vincristine
c. High-dose steroids
d. Infliximab
e. Cisplatin

63. The treatment for a pregnant diabetic patient with lakes of pus on skin is:
a. Cyclosporine
b. Azathioprine
c. Retinoids
d. Methotrexate

64. What is not seen in lichen planus?
a. Excoriation marks
b. Purplish papules
c. Lacy white lines in buccal mucosa
d. Koebenerization

65. Pick the incorrect match: *(UPSC 2016)*
a. Nikolsky sign-pemphigus
b. Erythema multiforme—Stevens Johnson syndrome
c. Erythema nodosum—leprosy
d. Onycholysis—psoriasis

66. Most characteristic sign of psoriasis on histopathology is:
a. Munro's microabscess
b. Parakaratosis
c. Supra papillary thinning of epidermis
d. Elongation of rete ridges

67. Lichen planus associated with all *except*:
a. Pterygium
b. Thickened nail
c. Trachyonychia
d. Tented nail

68. A patient of psoriatic arthritis not tolerating methotrexate. It was changed to a drug which caused a skin rash and was hepatotoxic. The likely drug is:
a. Leflunomide
b. Sulfasalazine
c. Azathioprine
d. Infliximab

69. The treatment of choice for erythrodermic psoriasis is:
a. Topical steroids
b. Oral steroids
c. Methotrexate
d. Coal tar

70. Lady with bilateral buccal reticulate white streaks. Pain increases on spicy food intake. There is no h/o tobacco but show amalgam on 3rd molar tooth. The likely diagnosis is:
a. Lichen planus
b. Leukoplakia
c. Aphthous stomatitis
d. Candida

71. A 3-month-old infant is having thick scales on scalp with dandruff. Erythematous scaly lesions on nasolabial folds are also present. Diagnosis is:
a. Atopic dermatitis
b. Seborrheic dermatitis
c. Xerotic eczema
d. Napkin dermatitis

New Questions

72. A patient presents with recurrent itchy, erythematous plaques over scalp and sacral area. There is history of joint pains. Nail findings are as shown. The likely diagnosis is: *(INICET Nov 22)*

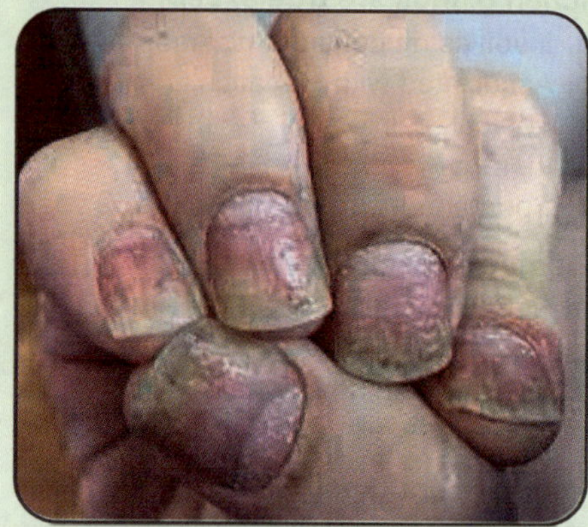

a. Psoriasis
b. Lichen planus
c. Alopecia areata
d. Tinea

73. Pick the papulosquamous lesions:
a. Lichen planus
b. Rosacea
c. Seborrheic dermatitis
d. Eczema
e. Hailey-Hailey disease

74. Arrange the following stages of doing an Auspitz sign in order of their time of occurrence in the test (from earliest to last):
1. Silvery scales
2. Grattage
3. Pin point bleed
4. Bulkeley membrane
a. 1, 2, 4, 3
b. 1, 4, 2, 3
c. 1, 2, 3, 4
d. 1, 4, 3, 2

75. Assertion: Dermal melanin is seen in lichen planus
Reason: Wedge-shaped hypergranulosis is seen in lichen planus

a. Both Assertion and Reason are true and Reason is correct explanation of Assertion
b. Both Assertion and Reason are true but Reason is not correct explanation of Assertion
c. Assertion is true and Reason is false
d. Assertion is false and Reason is true
e. Both Assertion and Reason are false

76. Features of nail psoriasis are:

a. Onycholysis
b. Splinter hemorrhage
c. Thickened nail plate
d. Subungual hyperkeratosis

1. If a, c, d are correct
2. If a and c are correct
3. If c and d are correct
4. If all four (a, b, c, & d) are correct

77. Match column A with best alternative in column B:

Column A	Column B
1. Lichen planus 2. Reactive arthritis 3. Seborrheic dermatitis 4. Pityriasis rubra pilaris	a. Cradle cap b. Silvery scalp scales c. Foot print in snow pattern d. Circinate balanitis e. Follicular keratosis f. Hypopigmented lesions

78. Arrange the following oral lesions in the order of their malignancy potential (from most to least):

1. Oral Erythroplasia
2. Oral ulcerative lichen planus
3. Oral Non homogenous leukoplakia
4. Oral lacy lichen planus

a. 1, 3, 2, 4
b. 4, 1, 2, 3
c. 1, 2, 3, 4
d. 1, 2, 4, 3

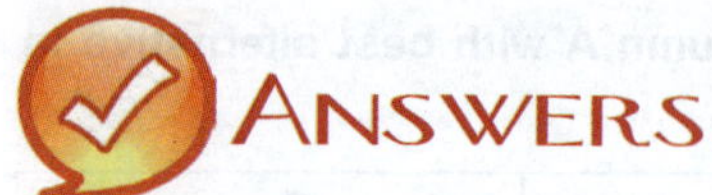

1. **Ans. (c) Basal cell carcinoma** (See page 238 for explanation)
2. **Ans. (d) Pemphigus**
   Pemphigus typically presents as fluid-filled lesions, not as plaques (The word "pemphigus" is derived from the word "pemphix" meaning "blister").
3. **Ans. (b) Scaling**
   Typically the scales are said to be silvery or micaceous. Oozing is typical of eczema.
4. **Ans. (c) Psoriasis** (See page 239 for explanation)
   Typical extensor disease, silvery scales and Auspitz sign.
5. **Ans. (c) Lichen planus** *(Ref: Fitzpatrick's Textbook, 8th edn, Page 296)*
   Violaceous (purple) papules with pruritus suggests LP (Remember the 5 Ps of LP).
6. **Ans. (a) Seborrheic dermatitis** *(Ref: Fitzpatrick's Textbook, 8th edn, Page 259)*
   Greasy, yellow scales point to seborrheic dermatitis.
7. **Ans. (b) Pityriasis rubra pilaris** *(Ref: Andrew's Textbook, 11th edn, Page 206)*
   Erythematous follicular papules, areas of normal skin within the lesion and thickening of palms and soles typically indicate PRP.
8. **Ans. (c) Lichen planus** *(Ref: Fitzpatrick's Textbook, 8th edn, Page 304)*
   Scarring alopecia, thinned nails, hyperpigmented macular lesions indicate LP. Psoriasis causes thickened nails.
9. **Ans. (c) Lichen planus** (See page 252 for explanation)
   The nail-findings are classical of pterygium. Lacy oral lesions indicate oral lichen planus.
10. **Ans. (c) Pityriasis rosea** (See page 134-Chapter 6 for explanation)
    Refer to chapter on viral infections for information.
11. **Ans. (c) Pityriasis rosea** (See page 134-Chapter 6 for explanation)
    Refer to chapter on viral infections for information.
12. **Ans. (b, d, e) Micro's microabscess; Hyperkeratosis; Suprapapillary thinning**
    (Ref: Mckee's Pathology of Skin, 4th edn, Page 207)
    Pautrier's microabscess is seen in cutaneous T-cell lymphoma. Grenz zone is seen in leprosy.
13. **Ans. (c) Joint involvement in 2–5%** (See page 245 for explanation)
    5-30% patients of psoriasis have psoriatic arthritis.
14. **Ans. (c) Groin** (See page 240 for explanation)
    Groin is a flexure. Flexural psoriasis is nonscaly.
15. **Ans. (a) Scalp**
16. **Ans. (a) Auspitz sign**

17. Ans. (b) Psoriasis vulgaris

18. Ans. (a) Guttate

19. Ans. (d) Psoriasis

20. Ans. (a) Plaque psoriasis

Auspitz sign is classically seen in chronic plaque psoriasis. It is not seen in flexural (inverse) psoriasis, pustular psoriasis.

21. Ans. (d) Erythrodermic psoriasis

Erythroderma is classically due to sudden withdrawal of systemic steroids in psoriasis and involves more than 90% skin surface.

22. Ans. (b) Pustular psoriasis

Generalized pustular psoriasis is an unstable form of psoriasis and can be precipitated by withdrawal of systemic steroids.

23. Ans. (b) Oral lichen planus

24. Ans. (a) Auspitz sign

25. Ans. (b) Psoriasis

26. Ans. (b) Retinoids *(Ref: Rook's Textbook of Dermatology, 9th edn, Page 35.37)*

Oral acitretin is the DOC for pustular psoriasis, though even methotrexate is effective.

27. Ans. (c) Methotrexate *(Ref: Rook's Textbook of Dermatology, 9th edn, Pg 35.37)*

Here, methotrexate will be the best answer.

28. Ans. (a) Prednisolone *(Ref: Rook's Textbook of Dermatology, 9th edn, Pg 35.37)*

29. Ans. (b) Methotrexate *(Ref: Fitzpatrick's Textbook, 8th edn, Page 223)*

30. Ans. (a) Corticosteroids (See page 244 for explanation)

31. Ans. (a) Prednisolone

32. Ans. (a) Psoriatic erythroderma with pregnancy

Steroids are indicated in psoriasis of pregnancy (pustular or erythrodermic variant in pregnancy).

33. Ans. (b) Impetigo herpetiformis

34. Ans. (d) All of the above

35. Ans. (c) Lichen planus

36. Ans. (d) Lichen planus

37. Ans. (c) Neutrophils in stratum corneum

Neutrophils in corneum (Munro's microabscesses) are typical of psoriasis. Basal cell damage leads to "incontinence" of melanin into the papillary dermis and is seen in lichen planus.

38. Ans. (b) Basal cell degeneration *(Ref: Mckee's Pathology of Skin, 4th edn, Page 225)*

Basal cell destruction also called liquifactive degeneration is a classical feature of lichen planus.

39. Ans. (a) Basal cell degeneration

40. Ans. (a) Lichen planus

41. Ans. (b) Lichen planus

42. Ans. (d) Lichen planus

43. Ans. (d) Wickham striae *(Ref: Andrew's Textbook, 11th edn, Page 213)*

44. Ans. (b) Pterygium *(Ref: Andrew's Textbook, 11th edn, Page 213)*

45. Ans. (c) Lichen planus

46. Ans. (a) Psoriasis

47. Ans. (a) Hypopigmentation in residual disease

Hyperpigmentation is left behind after resolution of lichen planus lesions.

48. Ans. (b) Whitish lesions in the buccal mucosa

Perifollicular blue-gray macules suggest lichen planopilaris (LP of hair follicles). Whitish lesions in the buccal mucosa suggest coexisting oral lichen planus.

49. Ans. (c) Acitretin

It is the treatment.

50. Ans. (b) Systemic corticosteroids *(Ref: Rook's Textbook of dermatology, 9th edn, Page 37.16)*

51. Ans. (c) Topical calcipotriol are the mainstay of therapy

Systemic steroids are the mainstay for widespread lichen planus.

52. Ans. (a) Self-limiting (See page 134-Chapter 6 for explanation)

53. Ans. (c) Pityriasis rosea (See page 134-Chapter 6 for explanation)

54. Ans. (d) Pityriasis rosea (See page 134-Chapter 6 for explanation)

55. Ans. (a) HHV 7 (See page 134-Chapter 6 for explanation)

56. Ans. (b) Lichen nitidus; (c) Lichen scrofulosorum

57. Ans. (b) Well-defined scaly plaques

Irregular pitting is a feature of psoriasis.

58. Ans. (a) It is not teratogenic

59. Ans. (d) Alopecia areata and irregular pitting

60. Ans. (a) Reactive arthritis

61. Ans. (a) Lichen scrofulosorum

Lichen scrofulosorum is a type of tuberculid (see chapter on tuberculosis).

62. Ans. (a, d) Methotrexate; Infliximab (See page 248 for explanation)

63. Ans. (a) Cyclosporine (See page 243 for explanation)

64. Ans. (a) Excoriation marks (See page 249 for explanation)

65. Ans. (c) Erythema nodosum—leprosy

Nikolsky sign is explained in the chapter on blistering disorders. Erythema multiforme is explained in the chapter on drug eruption. Erythema nodosum leprosum is seen in leprosy and not erythema nodosum.

66. Ans. (a) Munro's microabscess (See page 247 for explanation)

67. Ans. (b) Thickened nail

Lichen planus of nail will cause thinning, not thickening of nail-plate.

68. Ans. (a) Leflunomide

69. Ans. (c) Methotrexate

70. Ans. (a) Lichen planus (See page 252 for explanation)

71. Ans. (b) Seborrheic dermatitis

New Answers

72. Ans. (a) Psoriasis

73. Ans. a-True; b-False; c-True; d-True; e-False

74. Ans. (a) 1, 2, 4, 3

75. Ans. (b) Both Assertion and Reason are true but Reason is not correct explanation of Assertion

Dermal melanin is due to liquefaction of DEJ and not due to hypergranulosis.

76. Ans. (4) If all four (a, b, c, & d) are correct

77. Ans. 1-c; 2-d; 3-a; 4-e

78. Ans. (a) 1, 3, 2, 4

CHAPTER 11

Disorders of Adnexae/Appendages

ACNE VULGARIS

Introduction

- Chronic inflammatory disease of **pilosebaceous follicles**(MCQ)—typically on face, neck, upper trunk and upper arms
- Typical lesions—**comedones**,(MCQ) papules, pustules, nodules, scars
- Triggers—puberty, **PCOD**,(MCQ) oily skin, summer, drugs, menses, cosmetics.

Sebaceous Glands

- Holocrine glands occurring in conjunction with hair follicle known as pilosebaceous unit.
- Present all over the body except palms and soles.
- Scalp and face, interscapular area, sternal area and periumbilical area are main seborrheic areas. Produce secretion sebum, made up of mainly squalene, fatty acids, cholesterol esters, wax and wax esters.

Pathogenesis (Fig. 1)(MCQ)

- Hyperkeratinization of follicle
- **Bacterial proliferation** (*cutibacterium acnes*), **Inflammation**

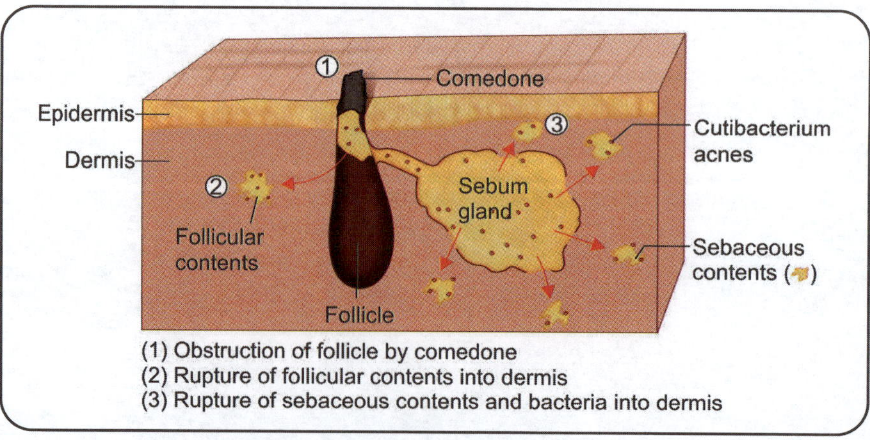

Fig. 1: Pathogenesis of acne vulgaris

- Excess sebum production
- **Hormonal factors**—Androgen stimulation, insulin resistance, Insulin-growth factor-1 (IGF-1)[(MCQ)]

Secretion of **Interleukin-1 (IL-1)** triggers keratinocyte proliferation in follicle
↓
Obstruction of the follicle with this increased keratin (**comedone**)
↓
Dilated lower part of the follicle due to obstruction of upper part with comedone
↓
Rupture of dilated follicle—follicular contents (keratin, free fatty acids and triglycerides in sebum, bacteria) into dermis
↓
Inflammation (papules/pustules/nodules/cysts)

Clinical Features

- **Noninflammatory lesions**—comedone (black head, white head)—Defined as a keratin plug of the pilosebaceous duct (Figs. 2A and B). When the keratin plug is exposed to the environment—it turns black and is called black/open comedone and when the keratin plug is inside the follicle, it is called white/closed comedone
- **Inflammatory lesions**—papules, pustules, nodules, cyst (polymorphic lesions) (Figs. 3A to C).

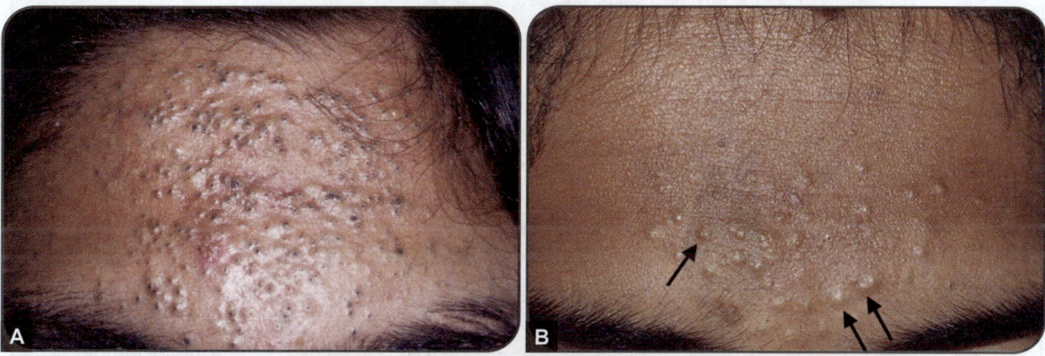

Figs. 2A and B: (A) Black (open) comedones; (B) White (closed) comedones

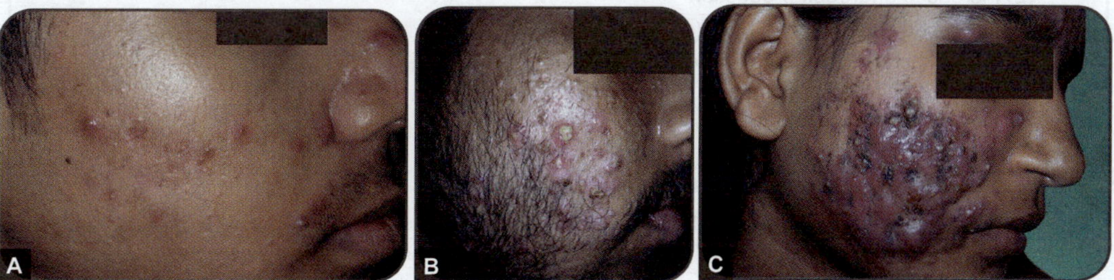

Figs. 3A to C: (A) Mild acne (comedones + papules); (B) Moderate acne (comedones + papules + pustules); (C) Severe nodulocystic acne—comedones + papules + pustules + nodules

Hormonal (endocrine) acne(MCQ)—Acne occurs with an underlying hormonal factor, e.g. PCOD (m/c cause), Late-onset congenital adrenal hyperplasia, Cushing's disease.

- **PCOD acne**—Dihydrotestosterone (DHT) forms from testosterone by action of 5-alpha reductase (5αR). This DHT stimulates the androgen receptor on sebum glands—causing increased sebum production. Follicular androgen receptor stimulation causes growth of hair on chin, beard area (hirsutism) and also keratinization of follicle (comedone)—(Fig. 4).

- **Drug induced acne (acneiform eruptions)**(MCQ)—**Topical/systemic steroids (m/c cause)**, anabolic steroids (danazol, stanozolol), anticonvulsants (carbamazepine, phenytoin, phenobarbitone), AKT (INH, pyrazinamide).

Acneiform eruptions	Acne
Monomorphic lesions (only papules)(MCQ) (Figs. 5A and B)	Polymorphic lesions (comedones, papules, pustules, nodules)
On trunk	On face and trunk
No comedones(MCQ)	Comedones are classical

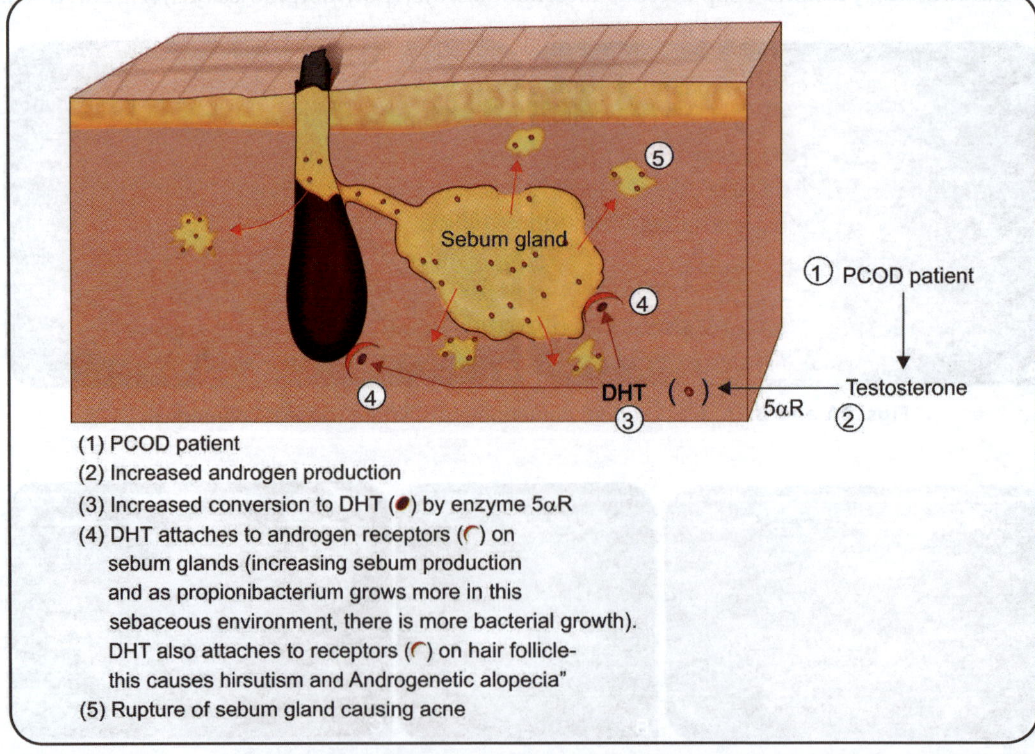

Fig. 4: Pathogenesis of hormonal acne

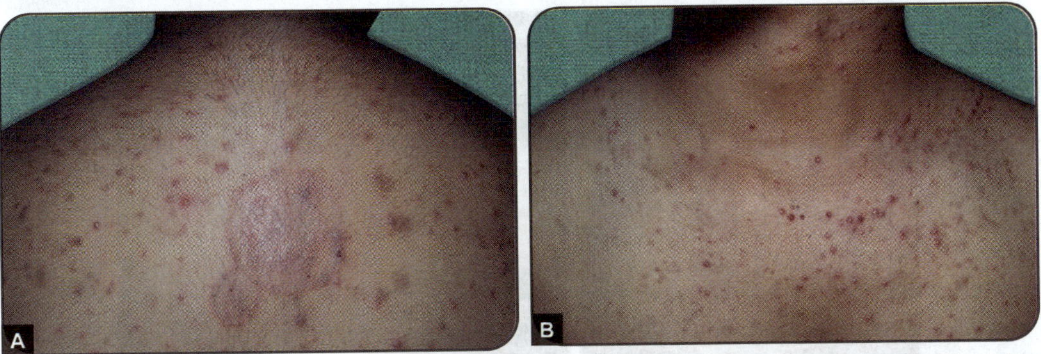

Figs. 5A and B: (A) Multiple monomorphic papules on back. The annular lesion in center is a tinea for which topical steroids were wrongly applied by the patient; (B) Front of the same patient showing monomorphic papules (steroid induced)

- **Food and acne**—Mainly high glycemic index foods and milk causes acne
- **Acne conglobata**(MCQ)—Severe inflammation, extensive inflammatory papules, tender nodules and abscesses. Typically **interconnecting sinuses** form due to fusion of these abscesses, leaving extensive scarring. **Multiple grouped comedones** are also typical. Treatment is **oral isotretinoin + systemic steroids** (to reduce inflammation)

Treatment

1. **Primarily comedonal acne**
   - Topical retinoids (adapalene > tretinoin)
     - Mechanism of action of topical retinoids—Reduce abnormal keratinization within the pilosebaceous duct by its keratolytic action—"unplugs the follicle"
2. **Mainly papular**
   - Topical retinoids + topical antibiotics (clindamycin, clarithromycin, nadifloxacin, dapsone)
3. **Mainly pustular**
   - Topical retinoids + oral antibiotics (doxycycline, minocycline, azithromycin) ± benzoyl peroxide (benzoyl peroxide is a powerful antibiotic with mild comedolytic action and is **DOC in drug resistant acne**).(MCQ)

   *Minocycline is the **most effective oral antibiotic**,(JIPMER 2016) but has more side-effects like drug induced lupus, bluish-skin pigmentation, drug hypersensitivity syndrome (DHS), hepatitis. Hence, doxycycline should be more preferred

4. **Mainly nodular/nodulocystic/acne conglobata**
   - Oral isotretinoin
     - 0.5 mg/kg/day (total dose of 120–150 mg/kg to be finished) (Figs. 5C and D)
     - **DOC also in recalcitrant pustular acne**(MCQ) (recalcitrant = nonresponding, indicates a situation when pustular acne does not respond to antibiotics)
     - Intralesional steroids can be given into the cyst

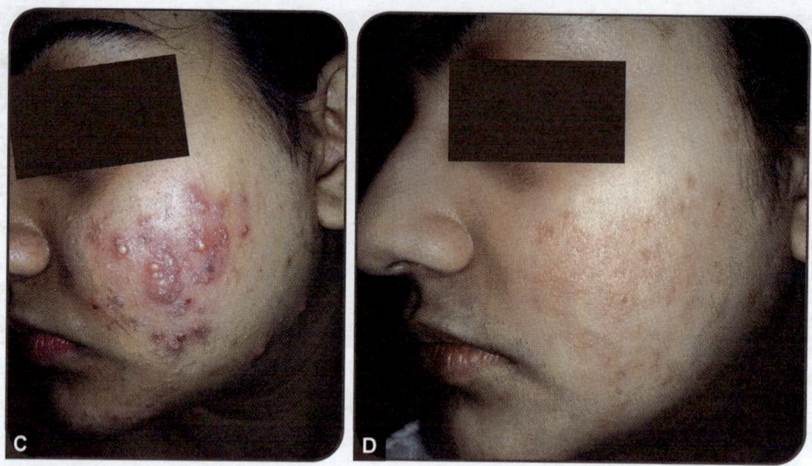

Figs. 5C and D: (C) Grade 4 acne; (D) Same patient after 4 months of oral isotretinoin

- **Side-effects of oral isotretinoin:**
  - Dryness of lips (cheilitis)—m/c(MCQ)
  - Increased lipids
  - Hepatitis
  - Teratogenic(MCQ) **(Period of contraception-till 1 month after stoppage isotretinoin).**

5. **Hormonal acne**
   - Oral contraceptive pills (ethinyl estradiol + cyproterone acetate,(MCQ) Ethinyl estradiol + drospirenone)
   - Spironolactone.

Acne in Pregnancy

- Topical benzoyl peroxide
- Topical erythromycin, topical azelaic acid
- Oral erythromycin.

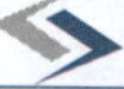

Extra-Edge Point

- **Topical azelaic acid**—Comedolytic and antimicrobial. Since, it is a tyrosinase inhibitor, it also reduces post-acne pigmentation.
- **Lasers (intense pulse light-IPL) and photodynamic therapy**—Light therapy destroys propionibacteria by targeting porphyrins produced by these bacteria.
- **Chemical peels**—Remove the keratin plugs and exfoliates the skin.

ROSACEA

- **Chronic disorder of facial convexities** between 30–50 years of age(MCQ)
- **Triggers**: Sun exposure, hot liquids, spicy food, alcohol, emotional disturbance, exercise.

- **Types:**
  - **Erythemato-telangiectatic rosacea** (ETT)—Facial vascular changes—Redness (flushing) + telangiectasia on central cheeks (Fig. 6A)

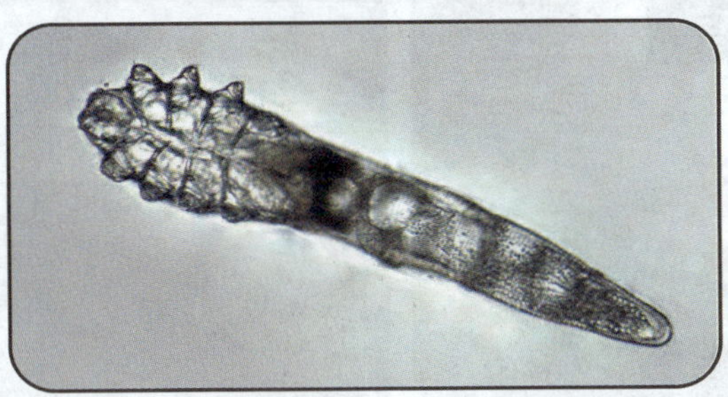

Demodex mite (normal inhabitant of human follicles. Increased number is seen in patients of rosacea)

  - **Papulopustular rosacea** (PPR)—Inflammatory stage- papule + pustule (Fig. 6B)
  - **Phymatous rosacea** (PR)—Hypertrophic stage—"phyma" on skin. Rhinophyma is thickening of the skin of the nose, irregular surface, prominent "pores", appearing like a potato **(potato nose)**. On histology, rhinophyma shows **sebaceous hyperplasia and fibrosis** (Figs. 6D and E).
  - **Ocular rosacea**—Eye involvement due to meibomian gland dysfunction giving a "gritty" feeling in the eyes, blepharitis, recurrent chalazion and conjunctivitis (Fig. 6C).

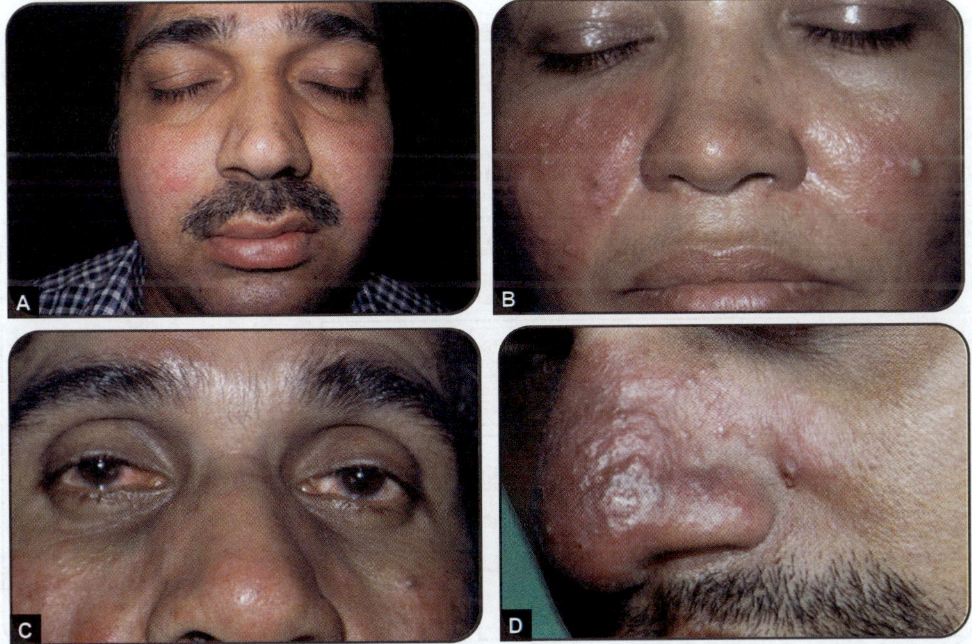

Figs. 6A to D

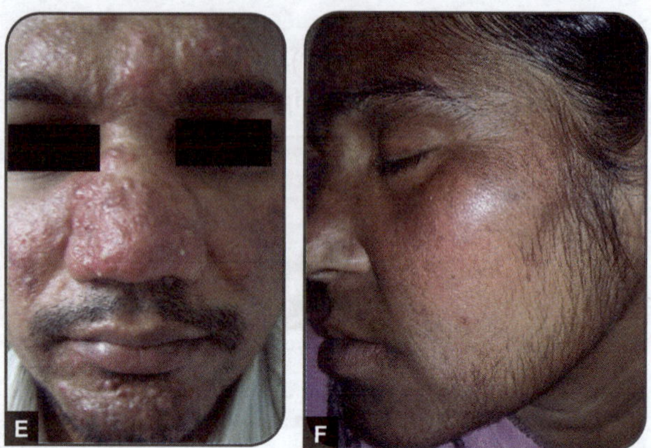

Figs. 6A to F: (A) Flushing on cheeks. Patient was a chronic alcoholic; (B) Papules, pustules on cheek (no comedones); (C) Ocular Rosacea. Note the papulonodules on cheek; (D) Rhinophyma with papules on cheek; (E) Rhinophyma, papulonodules on cheek, chin, forehead; (F) Steroid induced Rosacea. Note the rosacea on cheek for which patient has incorrectly applied steroids. Also note the steroid induced hair growth on beard area

- **Treatment**

  For ETT—Sunscreens—covering both UVA and UVB

  For PPR—Topical metronidazole, topical azelaic acid, low dose oral doxycycline possibly by reducing the microbes reducing microbe driven inflammation

  For PR—Low-dose isotretinoin therapy taken over a period of 2–6 months.

*Topical steroids are contraindicated as they can cause rosacea (Fig. 6F)[MCQ]

Pick-up words in MCQs on rosacea

- Facial flushing, classical triggers, lack of comedones, rarely affecting the trunk differentiates it from acne

Key Chart to help differentiate lesions on face in an MCQ

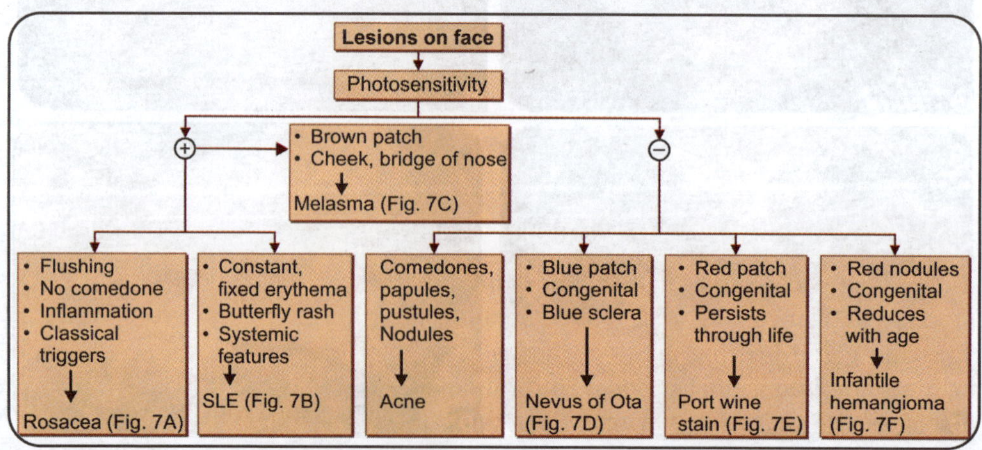

*For more on SLE- see chapter 14, for more on Nevus of Ota-see chapter 13.

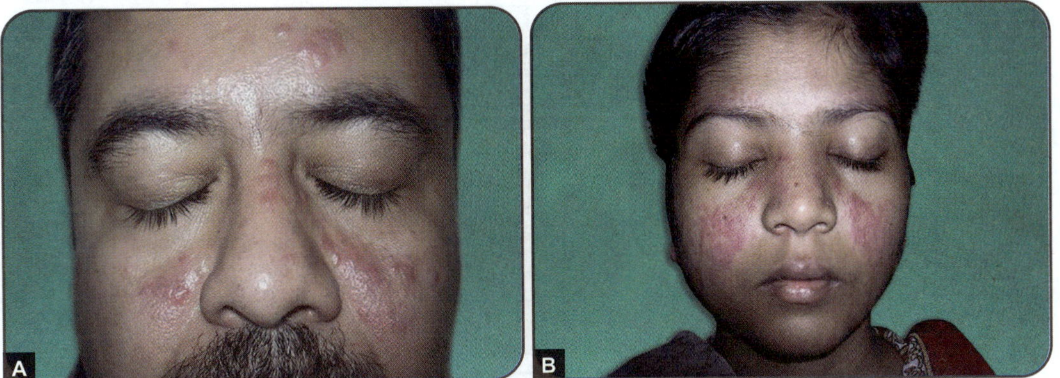

Figs. 7A and B: (A) Papules, mild edema on cheeks, no comedones—rosacea; (B) Butterfly rash—SLE

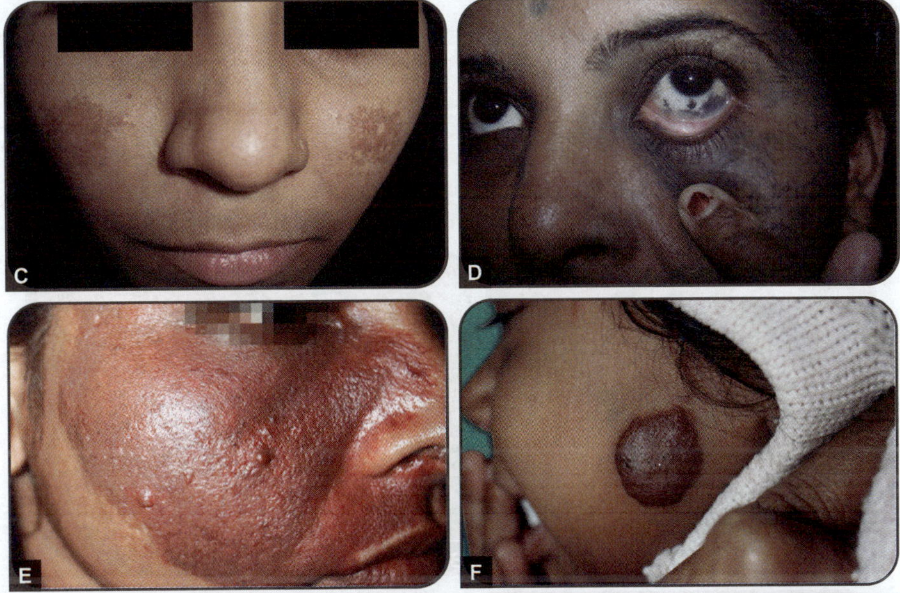

Figs. 7C to F: (C) Brown patches on cheeks—melasma; (D) Blue patch on cheek, congenital, blue sclera—nevus of ota; (E) Red patch, congenital—port wine stain; (F) Red nodule, congenital—Infantile hemangioma

HIDRADENITIS SUPPURATIVA

- A disease of **occlusion of hair follicles and apocrine ducts (Fig. 8)**.
- Presents as comedones, red, tender nodules, abscesses, sinuses and scarring in the **apocrine gland-bearing areas** of the body, most commonly the skin folds—axillary, inguinal and ano-genital regions. Since, lesions resemble acne but are in flexures, the disease is also called **inverse acne** (Figs. 9A to D).
- **Secondary bacterial infection** with *Staphylococcus aureus*, *Streptococcus pyogenes*, and various Gram-negative organisms may occur.

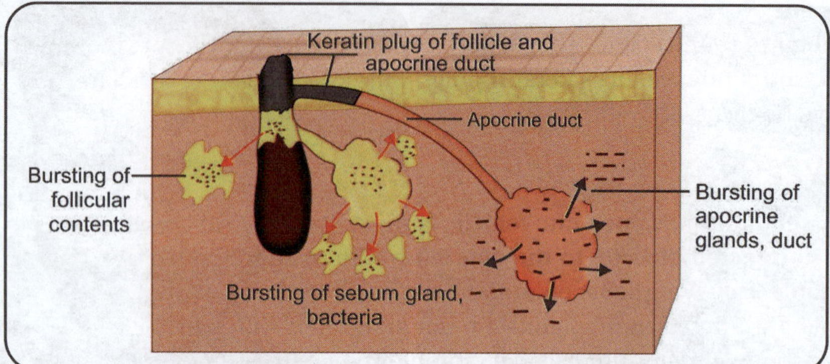

Fig. 8: Pathogenesis of hidradenitis suppurativa—Obstruction of the apocrine apparatus and the follicle causes increased pressure in apocrine glands, apocrine ducts, sebaceous glands and follicle. This causes them to burst into dermis triggering inflammation in areas of skin which have apocrine glands (e.g. axilla, perineum)

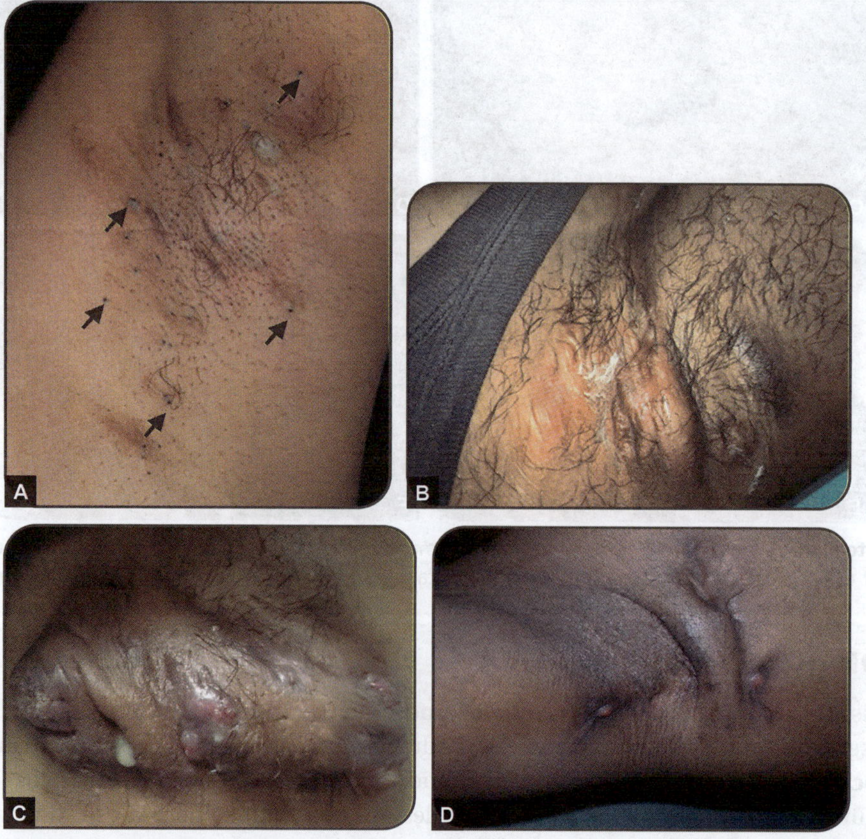

Figs. 9A to D: (A) Early disease—comedones in axilla (black arrows), early scarring; (B) Inflammatory nodules in axilla; (C) Secondary infection with *Staphylococcus*, draining sinuses, scars, inflammation; (D) Scarring due to inflammation

- **Treatment**
  - Antibiotics (tetracycline, amoxicillin, clindamycin, minocycline, rifampicin)
  - Oral isotretinoin reduces keratin plugs. Surgical excision of affected tissue ultimately cures the disease.

FORDYCE SPOTS/FORDYCE DISEASE(MCQ)

- Usually sebum glands open into follicle. Fordyce spots are sebaceous glands in which the duct is **connected directly to the overlying skin or mucosal surface** (Figs. 10A and B).
- Are **ectopic, free lying sebaceous glands**(MCQ)—Commonly on **upper lip, buccal mucosa, penile shaft**. These sebum glands are not associated with hair follicles.
- Fordyce spots on penis are called **Tyson glands.**
- **Asymptomatic—No treatment recquired.**(MCQ)

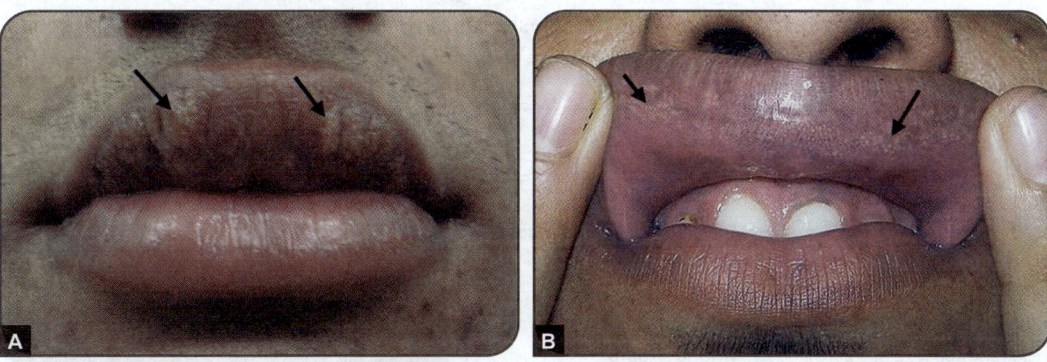

Figs. 10A and B: (A) Yellow papules, yellow colored plaques on upper lip; (B) Yellow papules

FOX–FORDYCE DISEASE (APOCRINE MILIARIA)(MCQ)

- It is due to obstruction of the **follicle by keratin**. Inflammation occurs on the upper part of hair follicles. 90% patients are **females.**
- Characterized by **intensely pruritic, papules in apocrine areas (axillae, areolae)** (Figs. 11A and B).

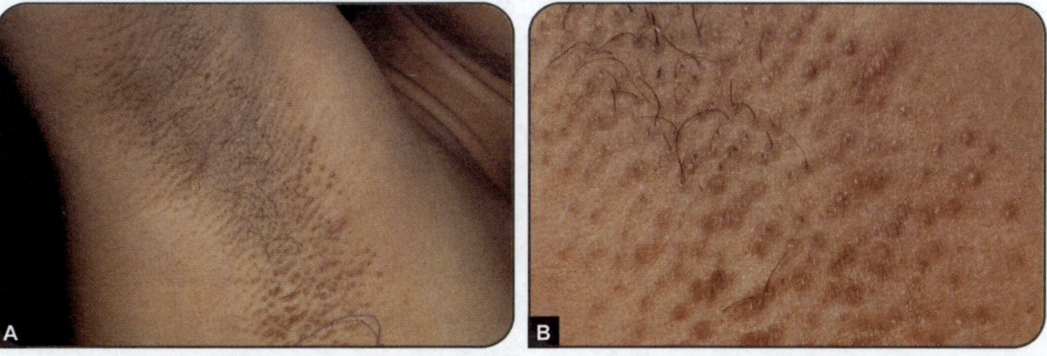

Figs. 11A and B: (A) Multiple inflamed pruritic papules in axillae; (B) Close-up

MILIARIA (PRICKLY HEAT)

- Retention of sweat as a result of **obstruction of eccrine sweat ducts**(MCQ) and consequent rupture of accumulated secretions below the obstruction.
- Common in hot, humid climates.
- ***Staphylococcus epidermidis*** may be an etiological factor. This bacteria produces an extracellular polysaccharide substance which obstructs the delivery of sweat to the skin surface.
- Types depending on the level of obstruction (Fig. 12):
  - **Miliaria crystallina**(MCQ)—"crystal-like" noninflamed, clear vesicles usually after fever. Obstruction of eccrine duct at the level of stratum corneum.
  - **Miliaria rubra**—m/c. Red, inflamed, itchy papules giving a "pricking" sensation. Obstruction at the level of spinous layer of epidermis (Fig. 13).
  - **Miliaria profunda**—Non-pruritic, flesh-colored, deep-seated, whitish papules—Obstruction at DEJ and upper dermis.

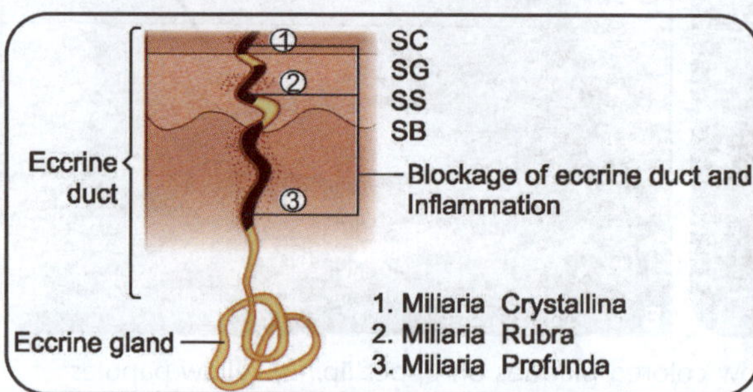

Fig. 12: Miliaria—Diagrammatic representation of various levels of obstruction

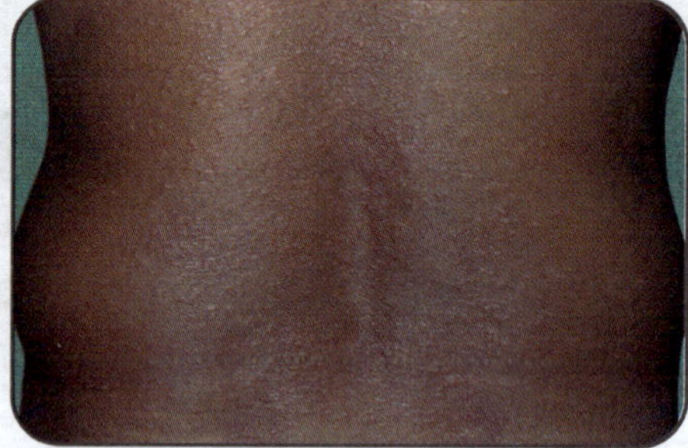

Fig. 13: Multiple, itchy, small papules on trunk

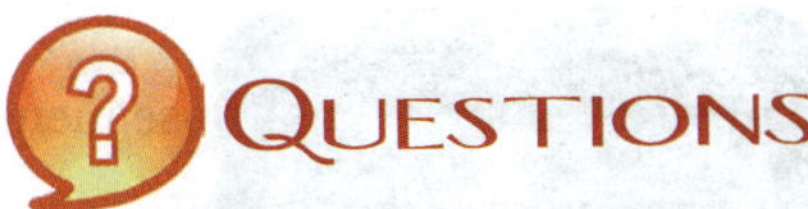

1. **Acne vulgaris involves:**
   a. Pilosebaceous gland
   b. Sebaceous gland
   c. Eccrine gland
   d. Apocrine gland

2. **Not associated with rosacea:**
   a. Photosensitivity
   b. Blepharitis
   c. Flushing
   d. Comedones

3. **A 25-year-old female with nodular acne and hair loss on scalp with increase of central parting. The drug of choice is:**
   a. Oral minocycline
   b. Oral doxycycline
   c. Cyproterone acetate
   d. Oral isotretinoin

4. **What is the ideal period of contraception advisable after treatment with isotretinoin to avoid any teratogenic effects of the drug on the fetus?**
   a. 3 days b. 4 weeks
   c. 3 months d. 3 years

5. **Causative factor for acne are following except:**
   a. Androgen
   b. Oily food
   c. Bacterial proliferation
   d. Hypercornification of duct

6. **Which hormone is responsible for acne?**
   a. Estrogen
   b. Thyroid
   c. Testosterone
   d. Gonadotropins

7. **Causative factor of acne include(s):**
   a. Hypersecretion of sebum
   b. Increased serum IgE
   c. Follicular duct cornification
   d. Increased propionibacterium acnes
   e. Insulin growth factor-1

8. **Treatment of nodulocystic acne on face is:**
   a. Erythromycin b. Tetracycline
   c. Isotretinoin d. Steroids

9. **Recalcitrant acne is treated by:**
   a. Oral erythromycin b. Oral tetracycline
   c. Retinoids d. Steroids

10. **A 24-year-old unmarried woman has multiple nodular, cystic, pustular and comedonal lesions on face, upper back and shoulders for 2 years. The drug of choice is:** *(AI 2006)*
    a. Acitretin b. Isotretinoin
    c. Doxycycline d. Azithromycin

11. **Most common side effect of retinoid is:**
    a. Headache b. Cheilitis
    c. Photosensitivity d. Diarrhea

12. **A teenage girl with moderate acne also has irregular menses. Drug of choice would be:**
    a. Oral isotretinoin
    b. Oral acitretin
    c. Oral minocycline
    d. Cyproterone acetate

13. **A 17-year-old woman with acne has been taking a drug for last two years. She now has blue-black pigmentation of nails. The likely medication causing this would be:**
    a. Tetracycline b. Minocycline
    c. Doxycycline d. Azithromycin

14. **Regarding Fordyce spots, all are true *except:***
    a. Represents internal malignancy
    b. Ectopic sebaceous glands
    c. Presents in axilla
    d. Found in healthy people
    e. Are erythematous

15. **Fordyce disease mainly involves:**
    a. Lips b. Scalp
    c. Neck d. Trunk

16. A face of a lady presents with red macular lesions on central part of face around the cheek and chin with flushing on sun exposure and increasing with emotional disturbance: *(AIIMS May 2015)*

a. Acne vulgaris b. Rosacea
c. SLE d. DLE

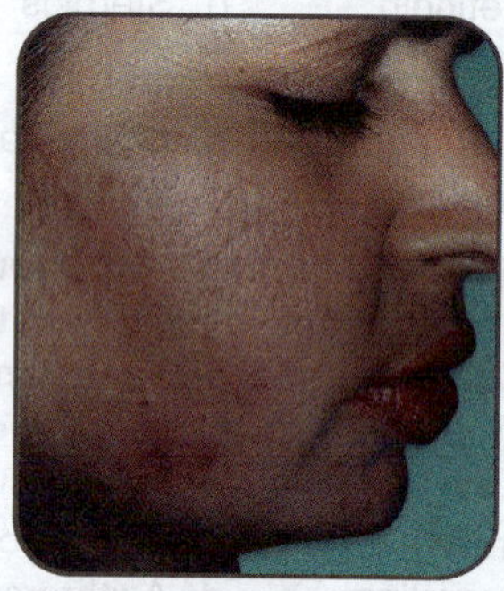

17. A 19-year-old female presents with several comedones, papules and pustules on face and trunk. The appropriate drug of choice for the patient would be:

a. Topical retinoic acid
b. Topical retinoic acid + Oral doxycycline
c. Topical clindamycin
d. Topical azithromycin

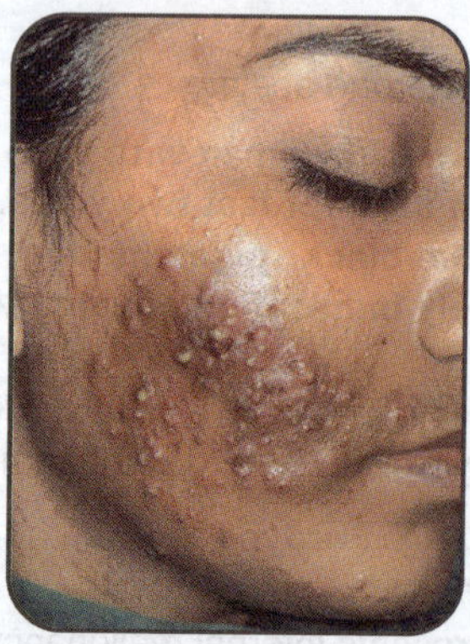

18. A young boy with oily skin presents with acne as shown. What is the appropriate treatment?

a. Oral isotretinoin
b. Oral steroids
c. Topical retinoic acid
d. Topical benzoyl peroxide

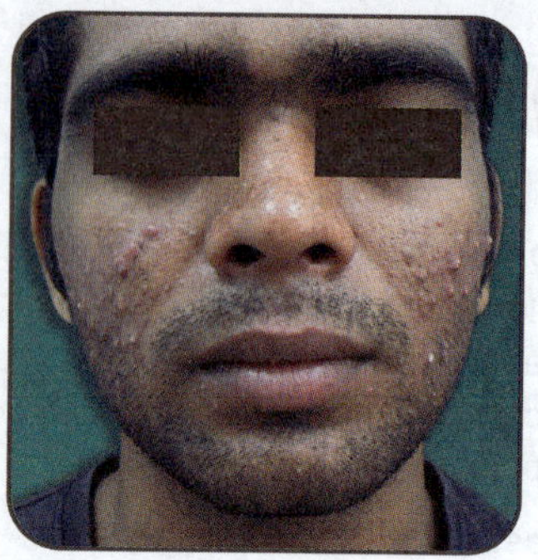

19. Acneiform eruptions are seen with:

a. Tetracycline b. Phenytoin
c. Isoniazid d. Aminoglycoside
e. Quinolone

20. Rhinophyma:

a. A form of rosacea
b. A form of acne vulgaris
c. Affects the scalp
d. A form of dermatofibroma

21. Rhinophyma (potato nose) is:

a. Septal deviation of nose
b. Sweat gland hypertrophy
c. Mucous gland hypertrophy
d. Sebaceous gland hypertrophy

22. A 40-year-old man presents with a 2-year-old h/o erythematous papulopustular lesions on convexities of the face. There in a background of erythema and telangiectasia. The most likely diagnosis is:

a. Acne vulgaris
b. Rosacea
c. SLE
d. Polymorphic light eruption

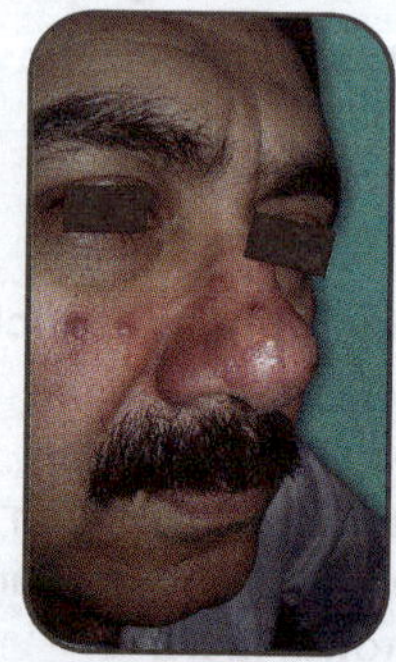

23. Morphological features of rosacea includes:

a. Papules b. Pustules
c. Vesicles d. Telangiectasia
e. Comedones

24. Crystalline miliaria is due to obstruction to:

a. Sebaceous glands
b. Sweat ducts
c. Hair follicles
d. Accessory sweat glands

25. A young male with painful nodulocystic lesions over face and forehead. The best management would be:

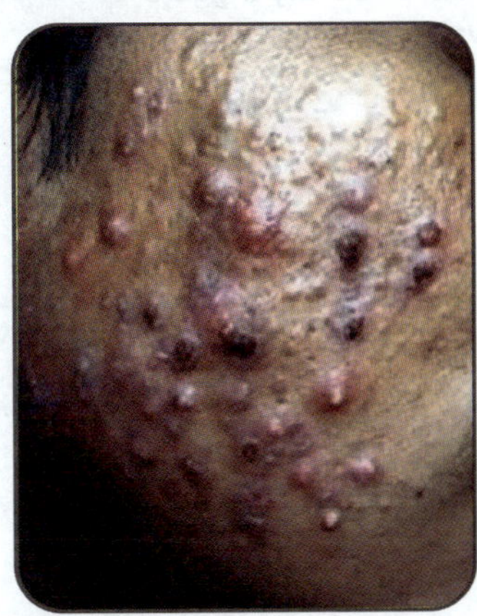

a. Oral Isotretinoin
b. Topical Clindamycin
c. Topical Adapalene
d. Oral Doxycycline

26. In Fox Fordyce disease, true is/are:

a. Common in adult woman
b. Bullous lesions are common
c. Common in areola and axilla
d. Associated with other malignancies
e. Sebaceous disorder

27. Not used in acne:

a. Benzoyl peroxide b. Isotretinoin
c. Adapalene d. Anthralin

28. Causative organism of rosacea is/are:

a. *Propionibacterium acnes*
b. *Malassezia furfur*
c. *Demodex folliculorum*
d. *Staphylococcus aureus*
e. *Candida albicans*

New Questions

29. The following statements are true/false regarding oral isotretinoin use:

a. May be used in rosacea
b. Patients on oral isotretinoin need contraception till they are on the drug
c. Increases staphylococcal aureus colonization
d. Nephrotoxic
e. Drug of choice in hormonal acne

30. Arrange the following areas affected in the descending order of its occurrence in hidradenitis suppurativa:

1. Axilla 2. Inframammary
3. Inguinal 4. Perineal

a. 1, 2, 3, 4
b. 1, 2, 4, 3
c. 1, 3, 4, 2
d. 1, 3, 2, 4

31. Assertion: Oral isotretinoin is very effective in acne
Reason: Patients with acne have sebaceous gland over activity

a. Both Assertion and Reason are true and Reason is correct explanation of Assertion
b. Both Assertion and Reason are true but Reason is not correct explanation of Assertion
c. Assertion is true and Reason is false
d. Assertion is false and Reason is true
e. Both Assertion and Reason are false

32. Match items in column A with best alternative in column B:

Column A	Column B
1. Obstruction of eccrine duct at spinous epidermal level	a. Miliaria crystallina
2. Obstruction of apocrine duct and follicle	b. Fordyce spot
3. Obstruction of pilosebaceous duct	c. Acne vulgaris
4. Obstruction of eccrine duct at DEJ	d. Miliaria rubra
	e. Hidradenitis suppurativa
	f. Miliaria profunda

33. A 20-year-old female, unmarried with history of irregular menses and hirsutism. USG shows increased ovarian volume of 30 mL and 40 mL for ovaries. The initial treatment will be all *except*: *(INICET Nov 21)*

a. Oral contraceptive pills
b. Laparoscopic ovarian drilling
c. Lifestyle modification, weight reduction
d. Spironolactone

34. A 35-year-old obese women presented with acne as given in the image. The lesions are not responding to antibiotics and isotretinoin. What is the next step? *(NEET 2023)*

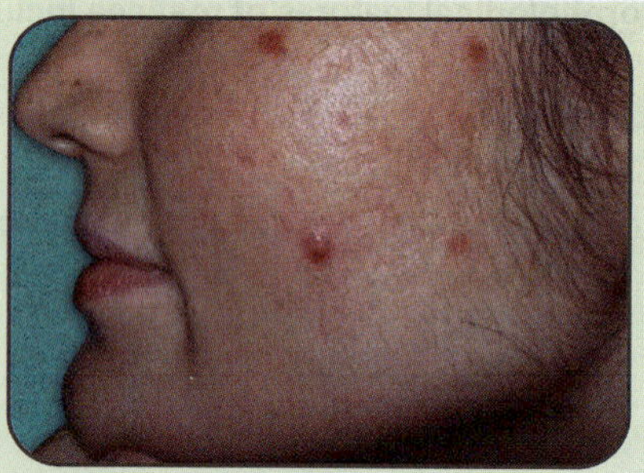

a. Look for resistance to antibiotics
b. Look for triggering drugs
c. Look for dietary triggers
d. Evaluate for hyperandrogenism

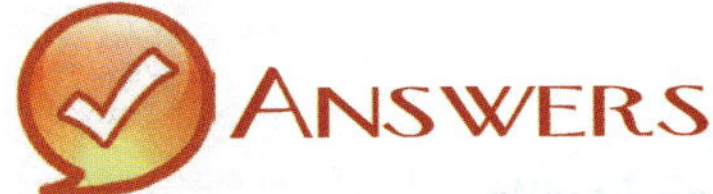

ANSWERS

1. **Ans. (a) Pilosebaceous gland** (See page 269 for explanation)
2. **Ans. (d) Comedones** (See page 274 for explanation)
   Comedones are never seen in rosacea. They help in differentiating rosacea from acne.
3. **Ans. (c) Cyproterone acetate** *(Ref: Fitzpatrick's Textbook, 8th edn, Page 909)*
   Acne with hair loss of central parting (androgenetic alopecia) indicates hormonal acne.
4. **Ans. (b) 4 weeks**
5. **Ans. (b) Oily food** *(Ref: Andrew's Textbook, 11th edn, Page 229)*
6. **Ans. (c) Testosterone** *(Ref: Fitzpatrick's Textbook, 8th edn, Page 899)*
7. **Ans. (a, c, d, e) Hypersecretion of sebum; Follicular duct cornification; Increased propionibacterium acnes; Insulin growth factor-1**
   (Ref: Fitzpatrick's Textbook, 8th edn, Page 898-900)
8. **Ans. (c) Isotretinoin** *(Ref: Rook's Textbook of Dermatology, 9th edn, Pg 90.37)*
9. **Ans. (c) Retinoids** *(Ref: Andrew's Textbook, 11th edn, Page 233)*
   Oral isotretinoin treatment is indicated for severe acne (nodular, acne conglobata) and recalcitrant acne (recalcitrant means poorly responsive acne that improves by less than 50% after 6 months of therapy with combined oral and topical antibiotics).
10. **Ans. (b) Isotretinoin** (See page 273 for explanation)
11. **Ans. (b) Cheilitis** (See page 273 for explanation)
    Almost all patients on oral isotretinoin get dry lips (cheilitis) as it is a powerful sebolytic agent and causes dryness of lips, skin, eyes.
12. **Ans. (d) Cyproterone acetate** *(Ref: Fitzpatrick's Textbook, 8th edn, Page 909)*
13. **Ans. (b) Minocycline** *(Ref: Andrew's Textbook, 11th edn, Page 232)*
14. **Ans. (a, c, e) Represents internal malignancy; Presents in axilla; Are erythematous**
15. **Ans. (a) Lips** (See page 278 for explanation)
16. **Ans. (b) Rosacea** (See page 274 for explanation)
17. **Ans. (b) Topical retinoic acid + Oral doxycycline** (See page 272 for explanation)
    Pustules would indicate the need for oral treatment. This is comedones+papules+pustules.
18. **Ans. (a) Oral isotretinoin** (See page 273 for explanation)
19. **Ans. (b, c) Phenytoin; Isoniazid** *(Ref: Fitzpatrick's Textbook, 8th edn, Page 915)*
20. **Ans. (a) A form of rosacea** (See page 274 for explanation)
21. **Ans. (d) Sebaceous gland hypertrophy** (See page 274 for explanation)
22. **Ans. (b) Rosacea** (See page 274 for explanation)
23. **Ans. (a, b, d) Papules; Pustules; Telangiectasia**

24. Ans. (b) Sweat ducts (See page 279 for explanation)

25. Ans. (a) Oral Isotretinoin

26. Ans. (a, c) Common in adult woman; Common in areola and axilla

27. Ans. (d) Anthralin

28. Ans. (c) *Demodex folliculorum*

New Answers

29. Ans. a-True; b-False; c-True; d-False; e-False

B- Patients need contraception till 1 month after drug discontinuation, D- It is hepatotoxic, E- In hormonal action, androgen blockers are preferred

30. Ans. (c) 1, 3, 4, 2

31. Ans. (a) Both Assertion and Reason are true and Reason is correct explanation of Assertion

32. Ans. 1-d; 2-e; 3-c; 4-f

33. Ans. (c) Lifestyle modification, weight reduction

34. Ans. (d) Evaluate for hyperandrogenism

This is a case of hormonal acne due to PCOD.

CHAPTER 12

Dermatitis

- The word eczema is derived from the Greek work *ekzein*, meaning "to boil". The terms **"Eczema" and "Dermatitis" are synonymous**
- Typically eczema shows spongiosis on histopathology (**spongiotic dermatitis**).
- Two stages:
  1. **Acute stage**: Red, edematous, **oozing plaques** with small, grouped vesicles
  2. **Chronic stage**: **Lichenification.**
- Depending on the etiology
  - **Endogenous eczema:** Where internal constitutional factors predispose the patient, e.g. atopic eczema
  - **Exogenous eczema:** Where external factors are responsible, e.g. contact eczema.

ATOPIC DERMATITIS (AD)

Introduction

- Chronic, inflammatory skin disease
- **Pruritic** with periods of remission and recurrences
- Often associated with **other allergic conditions like asthma and allergic conjunctivitis**
- **Family history** (maternal h/o eczema) is often present
- Strong **genetic predisposition** (**Filaggrin gene mutations** are often present). Filaggrin is responsible for maintaining moisture in skin (**hence all AD patients have dry skin**)
- Immunological factor—**Th-2 disease, Type I hypersensitivity**(MCQ) **(hence serum IgE may be high)**
- **Diagnosis is not by investigations**, but by history and clinical features(MCQ)—**"Hanifin and Rajka criteria"**(MCQ) (see further).

Pathogenesis

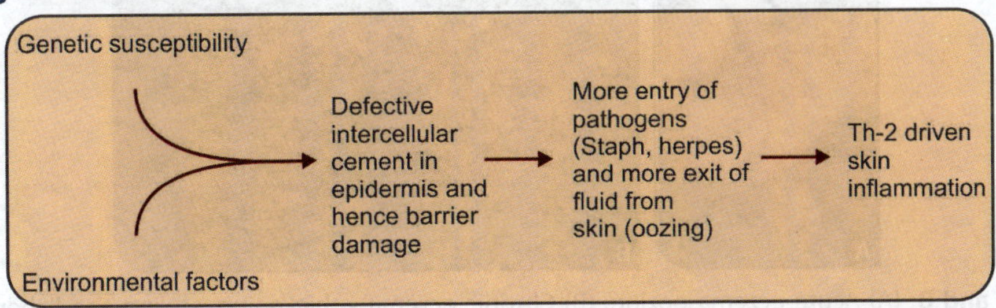

Clinical Manifestations

- Itching is severe and is the **hallmark**(MCQ) of the disease. **Itching often precedes the rash ("the itch that rashes" rather than a "rash which itches". Hence "itch is the disease")**
- A vicious cycle occurs, as pruritus leads to scratching, and scratching causes more itching **(the itch-scratch-itch cycle)**
- **Vascular changes**—perioral, perinasal, and periorbital pallor **("headlight sign")**. Blanching of the skin at the site of stroking with a blunt instrument (**White dermatographism**—For image, see Figure 1D in Chapter 17)
- Triggers: **Winter, woolen clothes, dust mites,**(MCQ) stress, food allergens flare the disease
- As there is reduced intercellular cement, there is epidermal barrier damage, more entry of infections and more water loss from skin (trans-epidermal-water-loss)
- Three stages are seen depending on age groups (Fig. 1)
  1. **Infantile AD**—occurring from 2 months to 2 years of age—**more on extensors**(MCQ)
  2. **Childhood AD**—from 2 to 10 years—**more on flexures**
  3. **Adolescent/adult AD**—more on flexures, hands and feet

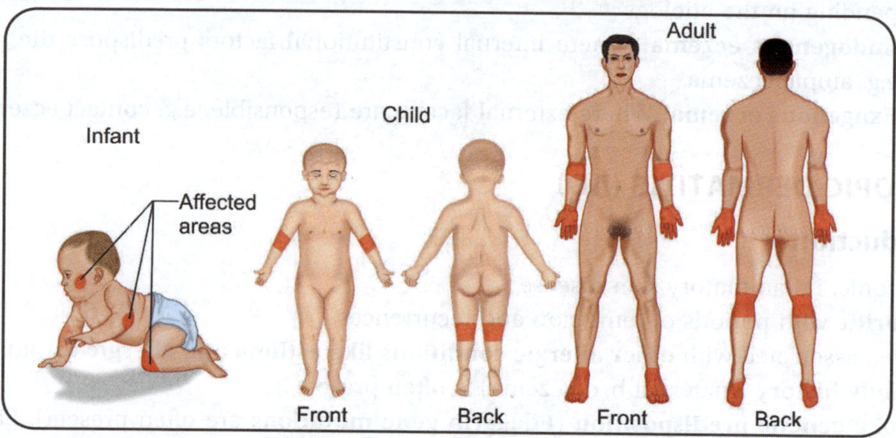

Fig. 1: Distribution of lesions in atopic eczema. Left—infant, Middle—child, Right—adult

Acute stage—Oozing and crusting (Fig. 2A) (**best treated with moist compresses**(MCQ))

Chronic stage—Thickening and scaling (lichenification) (Fig. 2B)—Best treated with ointments

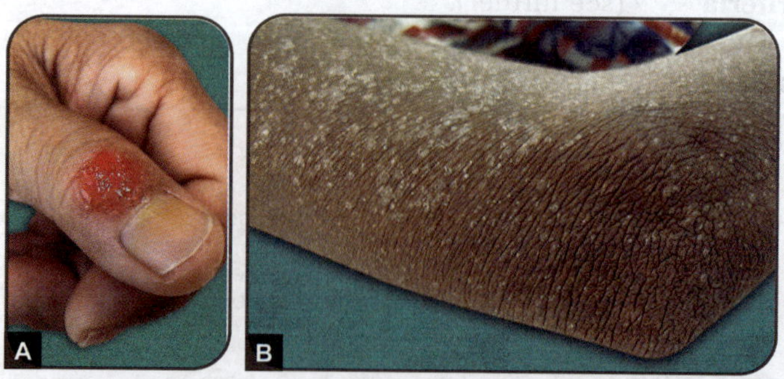

Figs. 2A and B: (A) Acute eczema-oozing; (B) Chronic eczema—thickening, scaling and lichenification

- **Hanifin and Rajka criteria**(AI 13):

Major criteria (Must have 3 of the following)	**Minor criteria** Must have 3: *Only the important ones have been mentioned here
1. Pruritus—HALLMARK of the disease	1. **Dennie-Morgan infraorbital folds**—linear transverse crease under lower eyelid (Fig. 3E)
2. Typical distribution: - Flexural in children and adults —**m/c site is antecubital fossa, knee flexures** (Figs. 3B and C) - Facial and extensor involvement in infancy—**m/c site is face** (Fig. 3A)	2. Ichthyosis (dry skin)/hyperlinear palms (increased skin lines) (Fig. 3F)
3. Chronic relapsing dermatitis	3. Elevated serum IgE
4. Personal or family history of atopic disease (asthma, allergic rhinitis, atopic dermatitis)(MCQ)	4. **Hand/foot eczema** (Fig. 3I)
	5. Dry lips and inflammation (Cheilitis) (Fig. 3J)
	6. **Xerosis (dry skin)** (Fig. 3G)
	7. Eye changes—**Keratoconus,**(MCQ) **anterior subcapsular cataracts**(MCQ)
	8. **White dermatographism**
	9. **Pityriasis alba*** - A form of subclinical dermatitis - Presents as poorly defined, **hypopigmented**, slightly scaly patches on the cheeks, typically in children/young adults (Fig. 3D) - Usually responds to moisturizing (first line) and mild topical steroids (second line) *Note: To differentiate hypopigmented patches on face, see the chart in chapter on fungal infections. 10. Eyelid eczema (Fig. 3H)

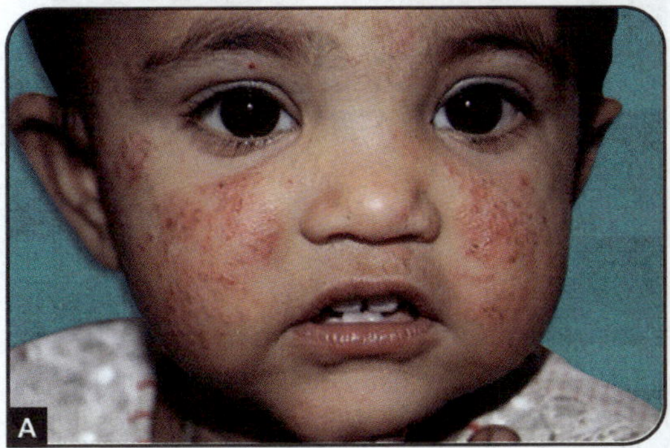

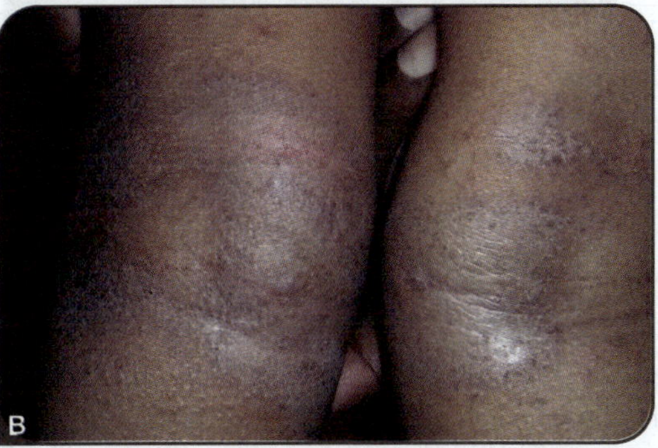

Figs. 3A and B: (A) Eczematous plaques on cheeks—infant; (B) Eczematous plaques on back of knee—child

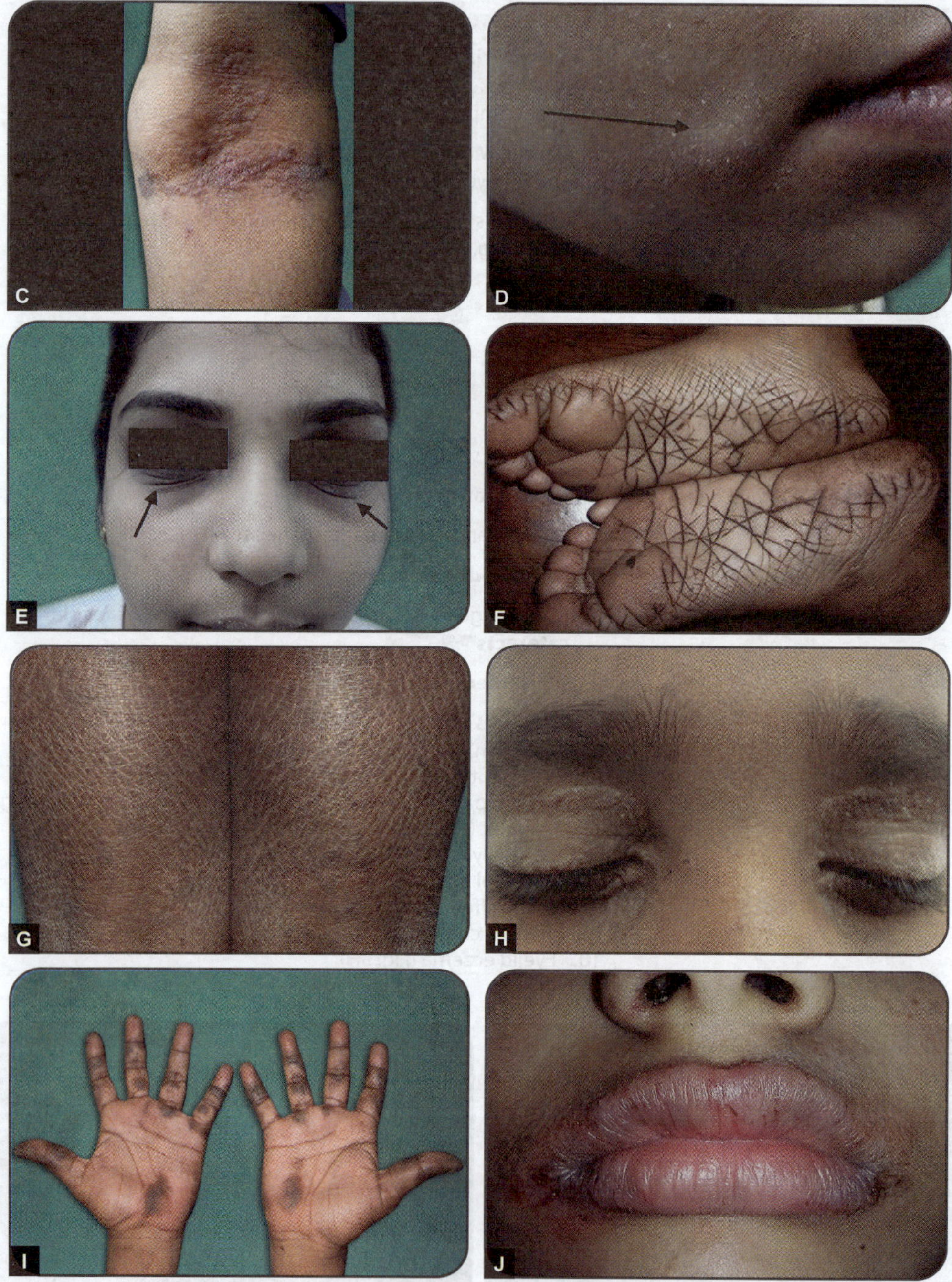

Figs. 3C to J: (C) Eczematous plaque on antecubital fossa—adult; (D) Pityriasis alba—ill-defined hypopigmented patch with scaling (black arrow); (E) Under eyelid skin folds—Dennie-Morgan folds (black arrows); (F) Hyperlinearity on soles; (G) Dry skin, Fish-like scales (ichthyosis vulgaris); (H) Upper eyelid eczema; (I) Hand eczema- hyperpigmented plaques on palm; (J) Lip inflammation (cheilitis)

Treatment

- **General therapy**
  - Barrier repair—Very important to address dryness of skin (xerosis) and an impaired epidermal barrier. This is done by applying moisturizers (Petrolatum and ceramide-based moisturizer)
  - Because of barrier damage, there are microscopic holes in epidermal surface. These allow bacteria (*Staphylococcus aureus*) to colonize the skin (carrier state), hence causing repeated infections. **Prophylactic reduction of nasal staphylococcal carriage is done by "bleach baths" and "topical nasal mupirocin application"**
  - Prevent triggers—Avoid stress, heat, sweating, external irritants and woolen garments
  - Antihistaminics are not effective in controlling itch.
- **Specific therapy**

First line	Second line	Third line (Systemic)
• Moisturizers • **Topical steroids**(MCQ)	• **Topical calcineurin inhibitors** (Tacrolimus/ pimecrolimus)(MCQ)—especially in areas prone for steroid induced atrophy (e.g. face, flexures) • Phototherapy	• Steroids • Azathioprine • Mycophenolate mofetil • Cyclosporine • Methotrexate

CONTACT DERMATITIS

There are two types of contact dermatitis: (1) Irritant contact dermatitis (ICD) and (2) allergic contact dermatitis (ACD).

Irritant Contact Dermatitis

- An inflammatory reaction in the skin due to exposure to a toxic substance (irritant) that causes an eruption in most people who come in contact with it
- **Cumulative irritant dermatitis (Wear and tear dermatitis)**—Due to repeated wet work, soaps and detergents, daily epidermal damage occurs ultimately causing fingertip chapping and inflammation after cumulative exposures
- More common than allergic contact dermatitis.

Allergic Contact Dermatitis

- An inflammatory reaction to a substance (allergen) that causes an eruption in only a few people who come in contact with it (those who have already been sensitized by the molecule previously).

Pathogenesis of allergic contact dermatitis

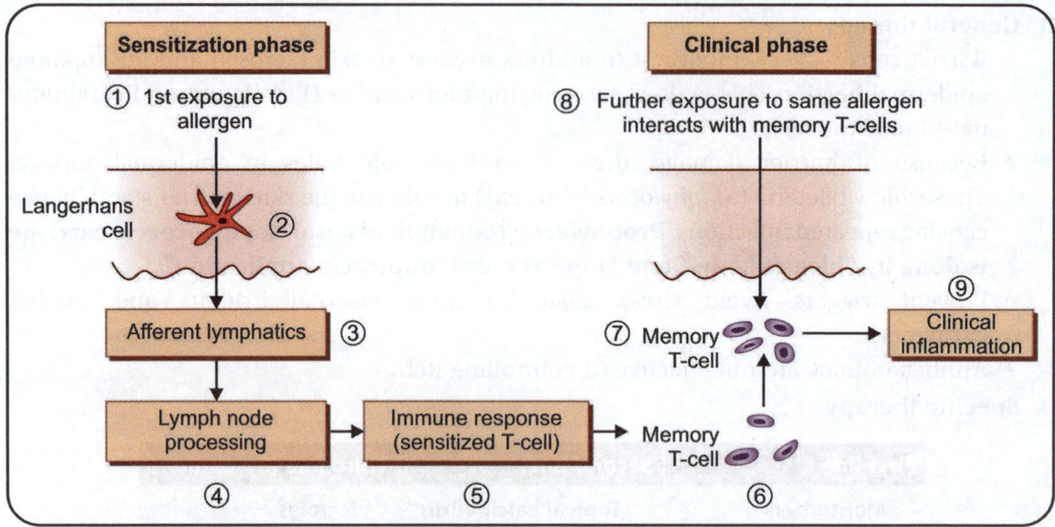

- **Sensitization phase**—The first exposure to the antigen (1) is picked up by Langerhans cells (2), processed by draining lymph nodes (3, 4). Memory T-cells are created from this exposure (5, 6)
- **Clinical phase**—Memory T-cells travel back to the dermis (7) waiting for another exposure to the same antigen (8), upon which clinical disease occurs (9).

ICD	ACD
Not immunological	Immunological Type 4 hypersensitivity
Due to direct toxic effects of strong chemicals	Due to immunological overprocessing of mild chemicals in predisposed persons
No sensitization required, direct clinical phase	Sensitization phase first followed by clinical phase
Inflammation is fast (as immune system processing is not required)	Inflammation takes time to start (as immune system processing is required)
Memory cells not involved(MCQ)	**Memory cells involved**(MCQ)
Most chemicals are irritants, if used in sufficiently high concentrations. Wet work (moist skin) allows more irritants to enter. E.g.: • Alkalis like **soaps and detergents (housewives eczema)-m/c** (Fig. 4A). Acidic corrosives in factory workers (Fig. 4B) • Hairdressors, cooks, caterers, fishing, printing and painting industry, metal workers, construction workers, etc. *Medications called as **"barrier" creams** are available and create a film over the skin protecting the skin from these external irritants	Only some chemicals are allergens (Figs. 4C to F) E.g: • **Nickel**—m/c overall • **Vegetable**—m/c in Indian females(MCQ) • **Paraphenylenediamine (PPD)**—in hair dye Diagnosis—**Patch test**(MCQ)

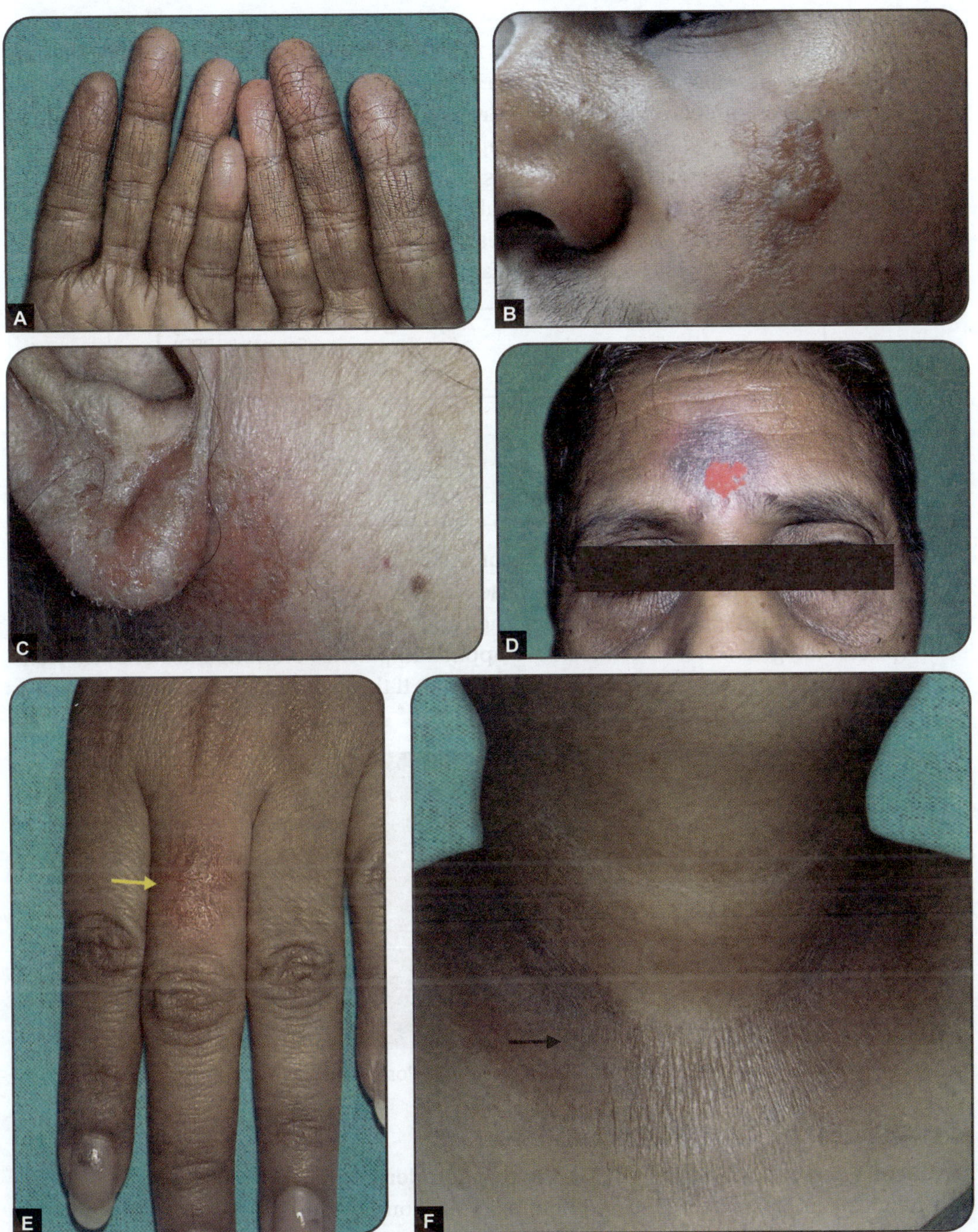

Figs. 4A to F: (A) Fingertip eczema, a form of cumulative ICD presenting as linear fissures and itching on fingertips (housewives' eczema); (B) ICD blister due to accidental corrosive contact; (C) ACD due to metals in earring; (D) ACD due to kumkum; (E) ACD to ring (yellow arrow); (F) ACD to neck jewellery (black arrow)

- **Patch test:**
  - Used to identify exogenous allergens in ACD (**confirmatory test for ACD**),(MCQ) not in endogenous eczema like atopic eczema
  - Patch strips are prepared by putting a drop of the allergen onto aluminium chambers (Finn chambers) and then stuck onto upper back (Fig. 5A).
  - The patches are removed after 48 hours and 3 readings are taken
  - **3 readings**—Immediately after removal of patch (i.e. **2 days**), next at **day 4** (best reading time),(MCQ) and **Day 7** for late reactions (for metals, PPD and neomycin). Red papules, edema and vesicles at a particular area indicates ACD to that chemical (Fig. 5B)

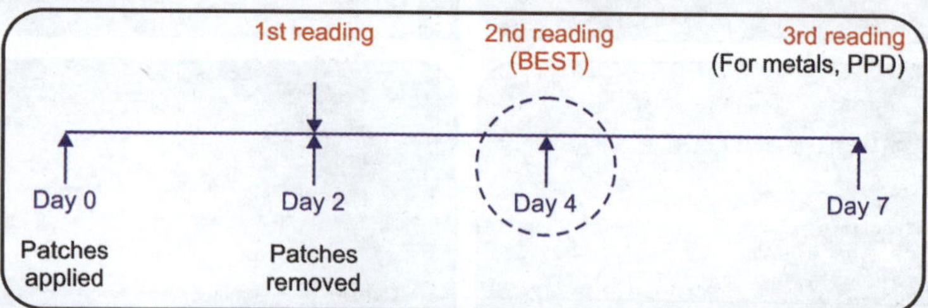

  - Patch test is **not done during periods of active eczema** as the state of hyper-responsiveness during this time can cause false positive reaction at numerous patch sites
  - **Photopatch test**(MCQ): Used to detect chemicals which get activated by sun exposure (photo-allergens). Here chemicals are applied in patches on both sides of back. Half-back is irradiated with UVA, other half covered. If the exposed site becomes positive—indicates photo-allergic eczema.

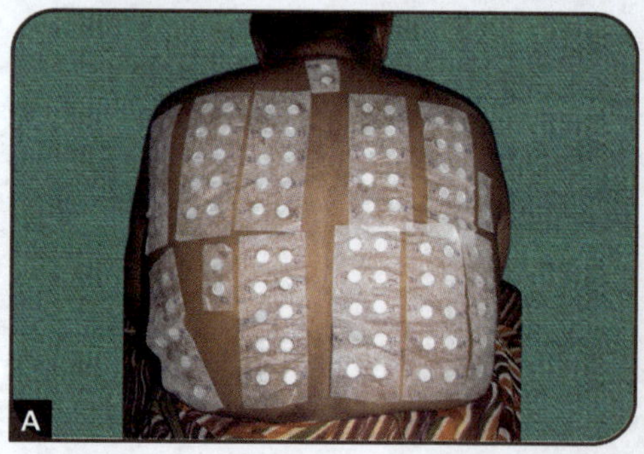

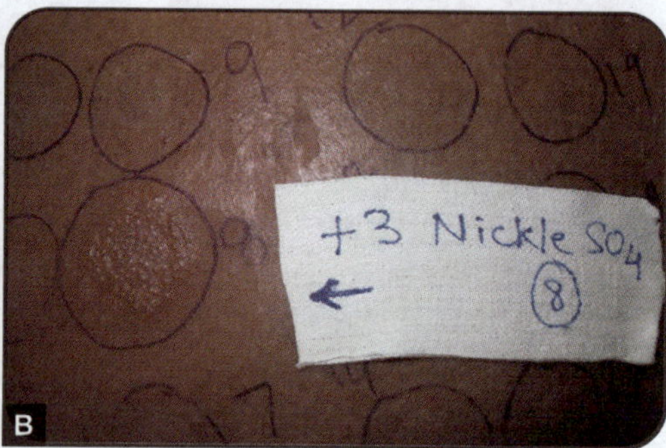

Figs. 5A and B: (A) Patch strips applied on back; (B) Positive nickel reaction at position 8

Special Form of Contact Dermatitis

Air-borne contact dermatitis (ABCD)/Phyto-photodermatitis:

- Chemicals in plants can cause a phototoxic reaction on exposed parts of skin (phyto = plant, photo = light)
- A combination of Type 1 and Type 4 hypersensitivity is postulated
- **Parthenium hysterophorus (congress-grass)**(MCQ)—a plant-weed of family Compositae grows freely in Indian farms (Fig. 6A) (**commonest cause of plant dermatitis in India**).

- Chronic itching, scaling, lichenification (Fig. 6B) is seen on eyelids (air allergens can lodge in eyelids initially), face, nasolabial folds, V-area of the chest. More in summers, less in winters
- Involvement of whole face including eyelids, under the nose, below the chin, neck- **Phyto-photodermatitis.**
- **Diagnosis is by photo-patch test.**
- **Oral steroid is the DOC** for acute management **and Azathioprine**(MCQ) **is the DOC for long-term immunosuppressive management.**

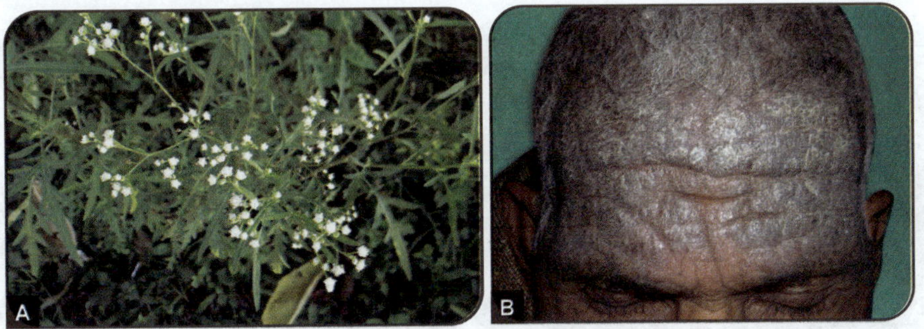

Figs. 6A and B: (A) Parthenium hysterophorus; (B) Lichenification, hyperpigmented papules/plaques on forehead

DISCOID ECZEMA (NUMMULAR ECZEMA)

- Disc = oval or circular, "oid"= like. Hence, circular or oval plaques (like a coin) of eczema with a clearly demarcated edge (Fig. 7A).

ASTEATOTIC ECZEMA (XEROTIC ECZEMA, ECZÉMA CRAQUELÉ)

- An eczema developing in **very dry skin, usually in the elderly** (xerosis = dryness)
- Classically affects the legs, arms and hands of elderly people. Typically a **"crazy-paving" pattern or dry-earth pattern** is observed. Hence, the name **eczéma craquelé** (eczema which appears cracked) (Fig. 7B).
- Management is to restore skin hydration.

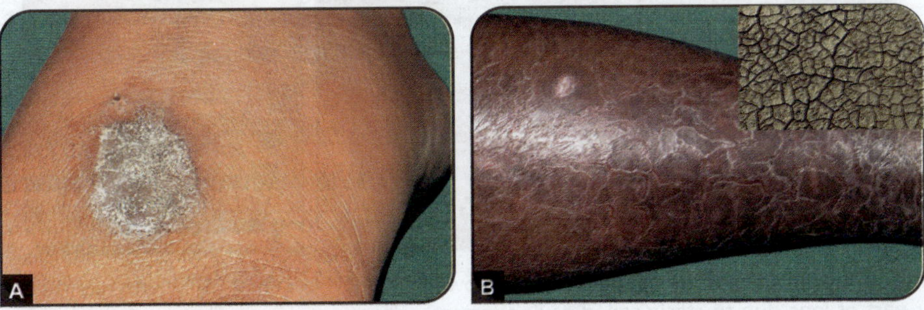

Figs. 7A and B: (A) Discoid eczematous plaque; (B) Asteatotic eczema—Note the cracking like a pavement

POMPHOLYX (DYSHIDROTIC ECZEMA, ACUTE VESICULAR DERMATITIS OF THE HANDS AND FEET)(PGI NOV 15, APPG 15)

- A form of recurrent palmoplantar eczema
- **Intense pruritus**
- **Firm, deep-seated** vesicles (Fig. 8A)
- Begins **on sides on fingers** (Fig. 8B)
- **"Sago-grain-like"** or **"tapioca-like"** lesions
- Association with atopic dermatitis.

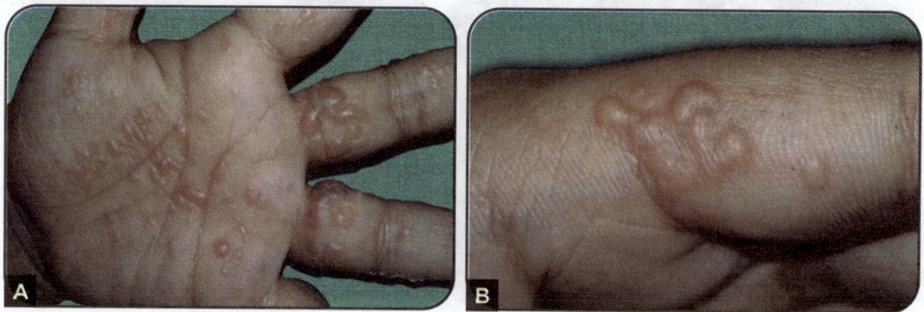

Figs. 8A and B: (A) "Sago-grain-like" deep seated vesicles; (B) Close-up. Typical itchy lesions on sides of finger

STASIS ECZEMA (VENOUS ECZEMA)

- Results from **dysfunctional venous drainage** of the lower legs
- High venous pressure within the calf muscle pump is relayed to cutaneous tissues around ankle. This distends the capillary bed, widens the spaces between endothelial cells and allows fibrinogen, RBCs, WBCs to escape outside the vessels causing inflammation and eczematous changes of overlying skin (Figs. 9A and B).

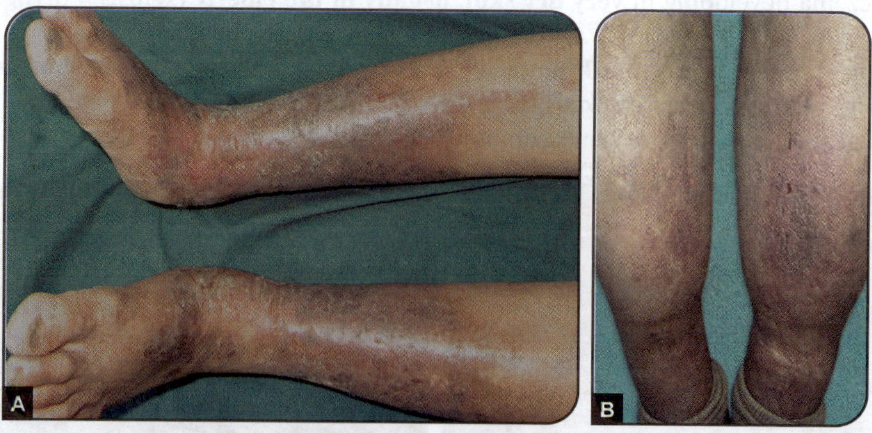

Figs. 9A and B: (A) Eczematous plaques on both lower legs due to stasis; (B) Sclerosis and contraction of lower part of legs due to stasis called as lipodermatosclerosis giving an "Inverted champagne-bottle appearance"

INSECT BITE HYPERSENSITIVITY(MCQ)

- Hypersensitivity reaction to insect bites
- Symmetrically distributed, itchy papules and papulovesicles (Figs. 10A and B)
- **Exposed parts of extremities, increases in monsoon.**(MCQ)

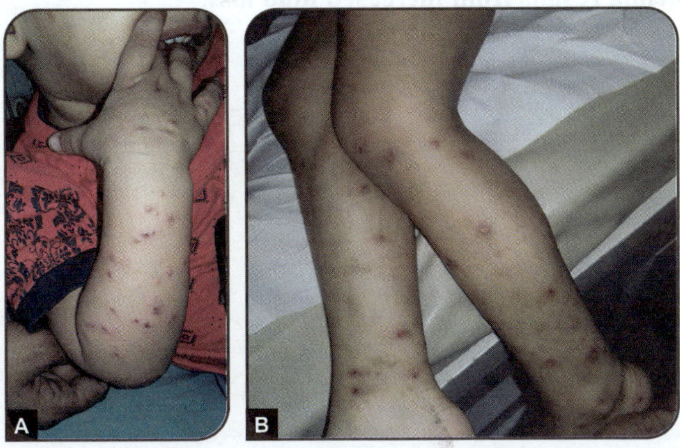

Figs. 10A and B: Papules (few excoriated) on exposed part in a child

ERYTHRODERMA (EXFOLIATIVE DERMATITIS)

- Erythroderma is the term applied to any inflammatory skin disease that affects **more than 90% of the body surface**. Since it causes skin exfoliation and scaling, it is also called as **exfoliative dermatitis.**
- Causes: Psoriasis, eczema (atopic, contact, seborrheic dermatitis), cutaneous T-cell lymphoma/leukemia, Drugs (phenytoin, carbamazepine, gold salts, lithium), pemphigus foliaceous, seborrheic dermatitis, idiopathic.
- First there is **diffuse erythema** (hence the name "**erythro**-derma") then there is **scaling and exfoliation** (hence the name **"exfoliative dermatitis"**) (Fig. 11).

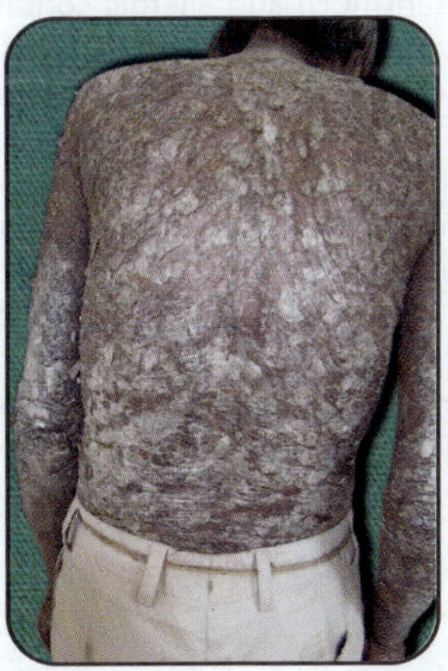

Fig. 11: Diffuse scaling and erythema >90% body surface (erythroderma/exfoliative dermatitis)

- **Complication**: Hemodynamic and metabolic disturbances. Cutaneous vessels are vasodilated (hence the redness of skin)—As blood flow through the skin is increased, there may be **high-output cardiac failure**. The increased skin perfusion may lead to **hypothermia and shivering. Increased loss of scales (which have keratin) causes hypoalbuminemia. Hypovolemia results from increased fluid loss.**

Aid to Remember

Causes of erythroderma—**ID-SCALP**
I: **I**diopathic
D: **D**rugs
S: **S**eborrheic dermatitis
C: **C**ontact eczema
A: **A**topic eczema
L: **L**ymphoma/Leukemia
P: **P**soriasis, **P**emphigus foliaceous

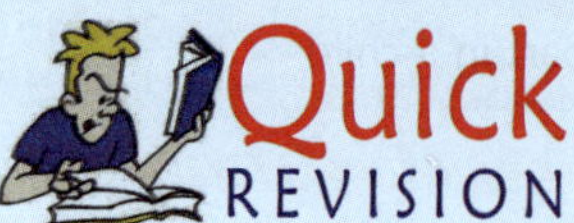

- Eczema typically shows spongiosis on histology. Acute stage presents with oozing while chronic stage presents with lichenification.
- Atopic dermatitis is a chronic inflammatory, recurrent, itchy disease with a positive family history of atopy. Type 1 hypersensitivity: Diagnosis is clinical by the Hanifin and Rajka criteria. Infantile AD is most commonly on extensors (cheeks, elbow and knee extensors) while child and adult disease is flexural (antecubital fossa and knee flexure). Dennie-Morgan undereye folds, Hertoghe's sign, Pityriasis alba, xerosis, white dermatographism, keratoconus, anterior subcapsular cataracts may also occur. Topical steroids and moisturizers are the first line therapies. Topical calcineurin inhibitors (tacrolimus, pimecrolimus), systemic immunosuppressives are also useful.
- Contact dermatitis: 2 types—irritant (ICD) and allergic contact dermatitis (ACD). ICD is universal, immediate and nonimmunological. For example—detergent, soaps. ACD is a type 4 hypersensitivity response involving memory T cell in sensitized individuals. Nickel is the m/c cause of ACD. Parthenium is the m/c cause of ABCD. Patch test is the test of choice for ACD (photopatch test for ABCD). Best reading of patch test is at day 4.
- Discoid eczema is coin shaped (nummular), asteatotic eczema is dry, pavement-like in elderly skin, stasis dermatitis is due to venous leg hypertension.
- Pompholyx has "sago-grain" like deep seated itchy vesicles on palms and soles, begins on sides on fingers and is associated with atopic dermatitis.
- Erythroderma involves >90% skin surface. Causes—Psoriasis, eczema, lymphoma/leukemia, drugs, pityriasis rubra pilaris (mnemonic- ID-SCALP).

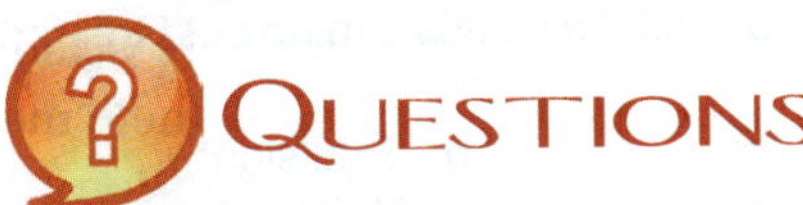

1. **Spongiosis is seen in:**
   a. Acute eczema
   b. Lichen planus
   c. Scabies
   d. Lichen scrofulosorum
2. **Patch tests are used for diagnosis of:**
   a. Contact dermatitis
   b. Seborrheic dermatitis
   c. Atopic dermatitis
   d. Nummular dermatitis
3. **In India, the plant which causes dermatitis most commonly is:**
   a. Parthenium grass
   b. Cotton fibers
   c. Poison ivy
   d. Ragweed
4. **The most common cause for contact dermatitis worldwide is:**
   a. Nickel
   b. Chromium
   c. Gold
   d. Mercury
5. **Most common metal in contact allergic dermatitis is:**
   a. Gold
   b. Silver
   c. Aluminum
   d. Nickel
6. **True about pompholyx is:**
   a. Sagograin lesions
   b. Lesions begin over fingertip
   c. Recurrences are common
   d. Severe episodes are treated with short course steroids
   e. Dyshidrotic eczema
7. **Which of the following is the correct use of barrier creams?**
   a. For contraception
   b. Protection from occupational dermatitis
   c. As mosquito repellents
   d. Protection from contagious diseases
8. **Most common cause of air borne contact dermatitis is:**
   a. Parthenium hysterophorus
   b. Poison ivy
   c. Poison oak
   d. Pollen
9. **Coin shaped eczema is:**
   a. Nummular eczema
   b. Atopic eczema
   c. Infantile eczema
   d. Endogenous eczema
10. **The following are true regarding pompholyx *except*:**
    a. 50% of patients have a history of atopy
    b. Topical corticosteroids are usually helpful
    c. Pruritic "tapioca" vesicles on palms and sides of fingers
    d. They are painful but not pruritic
11. **True about atopic dermatitis are all *except*:**
    a. Pruritus
    b. Scratching
    c. Mica like scales
    d. Xerosis
12. **A 7-year-old Chandu presents with recurrent, scaly, hypopigmented patch on face. Diagnosis is:**
    a. Vitiligo
    b. Indeterminate leprosy
    c. Pityriasis alba
    d. Pityriasis rosea
13. **Hanifin and Rajka is the diagnostic criteria for:**
    a. Atopic dermatitis
    b. Contact dermatitis
    c. Urticaria
    d. Erythroderma
14. **Dennie-Morgan fold is seen in:**
    a. Atopic dermatitis
    b. Seborrheic dermatitis
    c. Contact dermatitis
    d. Dermatomyositis

15. A 45-year-old male presents with itchy papules over face, neck and V area of chest for last three years which are exacerbated in summers and improved in winters. What test will you do to confirm diagnosis? *(AIIMS May 2016)*

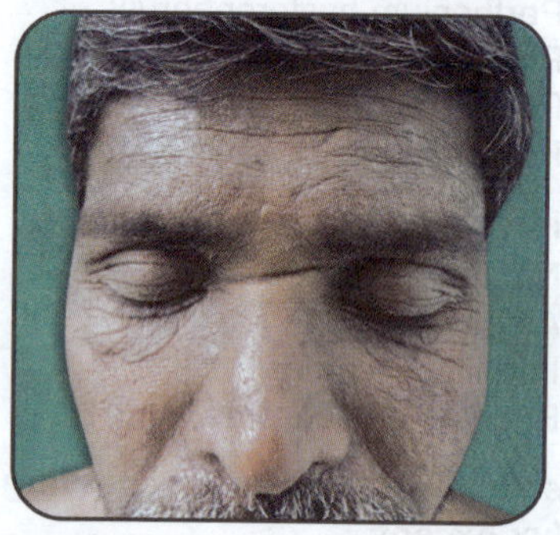

a. Patch test
b. Prick test
c. IgE levels
d. Skin biopsy

16. A 2-year-old child presents with eczematous dermatitis over the extensor surfaces. His mother has the history of bronchial asthma. What should be the most probable diagnosis?

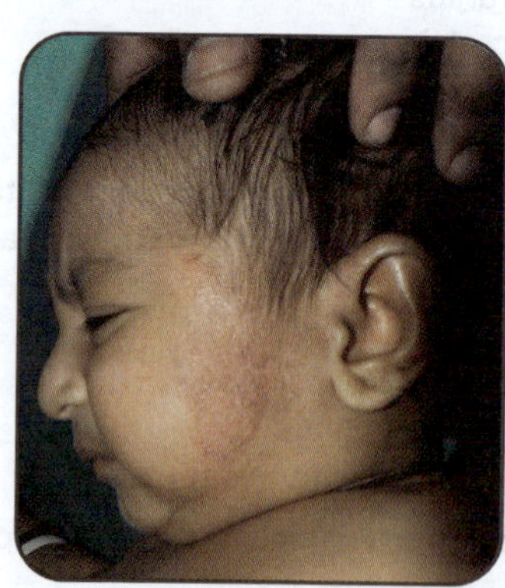

a. Atopic dermatitis
b. Air borne contact dermatitis
c. Seborrheic dermatitis
d. Infantile eczematous dermatitis

17. Treatment of atopic dermatitis includes any of the following *except:*

a. Calcineurin inhibitors
b. Phototherapy
c. Cyclosporine
d. Isotretinoin

18. Acute contact dermatitis can be best treated by:

a. Cream
b. Emulsion
c. Ointment
d. Moist compresses

19. A 25-year-old man presents with recurrent episodes of flexural eczema contact urticaria, recurrent skin infections and severe abdominal cramps and diarrhea upon taking sea foods. He is suffering from:

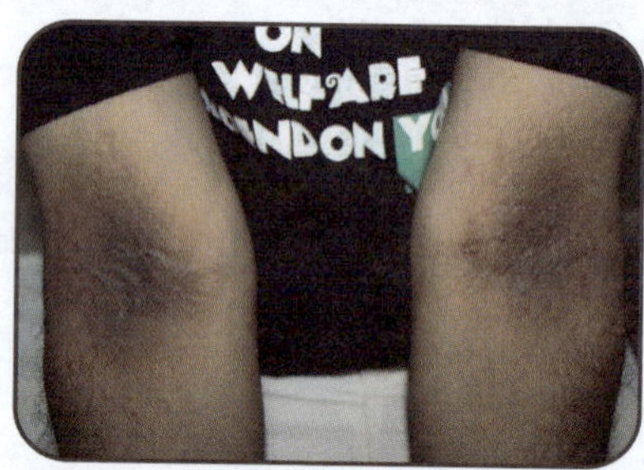

a. Seborrheic dermatitis
b. Atopic dermatitis
c. Airborne contact dermatitis
d. Nummular dermatitis

20. Rakesh, a 3-year-old boy had itchy, excoriated papules on the forehead and the exposed parts of the arms and legs. The disease was most severe in the rainy season and improved completely in winter. Most likely diagnosis is:

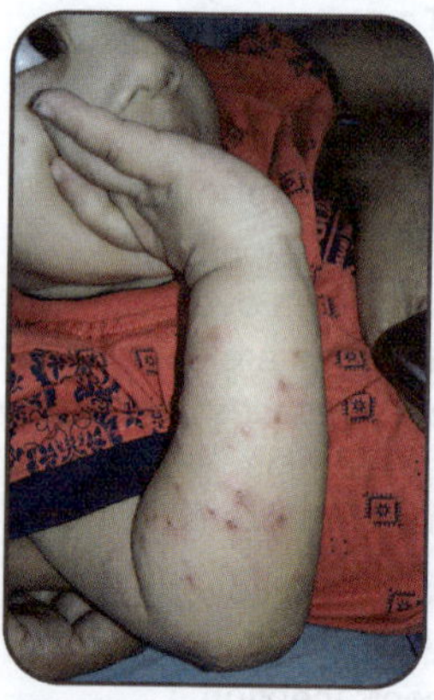

a. Insect bite hypersensitivity
b. Scabies
c. Urticaria
d. Atopic dermatitis

21. **Characteristic of chronic eczema:**
    a. Erythema b. Induration
    c. Lichenification d. Edema

22. **Characteristic feature of Atopic dermatitis is:**
    a. Pruritus
    b. Dennie-Morgan folds
    c. Scaling skin
    d. Rash

23. **"Itch is disease" is true for:**
    a. Atopic dermatitis
    b. Insect bites
    c. Seborrheic dermatitis
    d. Tinea cruris

24. **Dennie-Morgan fold is seen in:**
    a. Dermatomyositis
    b. SLE
    c. Psoriasis vulgaris
    d. Atopic dermatitis

25. **Most common site of atopic dermatitis in an adult is:**
    a. Scalp b. Elbow
    c. Antecubital fossa d. Trunk

26. **Atopic dermatitis is diagnosed by:**
    a. Patch test
    b. Wood lamp
    c. Clinical examination
    d. IgE

27. **Minor clinical feature in diagnosis of atopic dermatitis A/E:**
    a. Dry skin
    b. Pruritus
    c. Dennie-Morgan fold
    d. Pityriasis alba
    e. Dermographism

28. **Most common cause of allergic contact dermatitis in Indian female is:**
    a. Vegetables b. Nail polish
    c. Detergents d. Dyes

29. **Most common precipitant of contact dermatitis is:**
    a. Gold b. Nickel
    c. Silver d. Iron

30. **A patch is applied for allergic contact eczema. The test is best read after:**
    a. 4 hours b. 4 days
    c. 4 weeks d. 4 months

31. **Patch testing is done for:**
    a. Atopic dermatitis
    b. Irritant contact dermatitis
    c. Allergic contact dermatitis
    d. Seborrheic dermatitis

32. **Air-borne contact dermatitis can be diagnosed by:**
    a. Skin biopsy
    b. Patch test
    c. Prick test
    d. Estimation of serum IgE levels

33. **Patch test is done to document:**
    a. Type I hypersensitivity
    b. Delayed type hypersensitivity
    c. Autoimmune disease
    d. Immune-complex deposition

34. **A 55-year-old male with uncontrolled diabetes mellitus and hypertension, developed severe air-borne contact dermatitis. The most appropriate drug for his treatment would be:**
    a. Systemic corticosteroids
    b. Thalidomide
    c. Azathioprine
    d. Cyclosporine

35. **All are the causes of erythroderma *except*:**
    a. Psoriasis
    b. Seborrheic dermatitis
    c. Cutaneous lymphoma
    d. SLE

36. **Which is less seen in atopic dermatitis?**
    a. Anterior subcapsular cataract
    b. Posterior subcapsular cataract
    c. Keratoconus
    d. Hertoghe's sign

37. **Which component of cement causes allergic dermatitis?**
    a. Cobalt b. Nickel
    c. Iron d. Chromate

38. Patch test is a type of:
a. Immediate hypersensitivity
b. Antibody mediated hypersensitivity
c. Immune complex mediated hyper-sensitivity
d. Delayed hypersensitivity

39. Contact dermatitis known as "scourge of India":
a. Detergents
b. Parthenium
c. Nickel
d. Ragweed

40. Contact dermatitis, if suspected can be confirmed by patch testing. Ideally patients should not be on steroids or immunosuppressive, disease should be controlled and test site should not have active lesions. What is the best time schedule to read the results?
a. 1-2 hours after patch application
b. 96 hours after the patch application
c. 72 hours after patch application
d. 48 hours after the patch application

41. A patient comes with exudative lesions in cubital fossa, popliteal fossa and neck. The diagnosis is:
a. Dermatitis herpetiformis
b. Pemphigus
c. Psoriasis
d. Atopic dermatitis

42. Mother has a history of asthma. Her baby developed an erythematous rash on the cheeks as shown. The diagnosis is: *(Recent NEET pattern)*

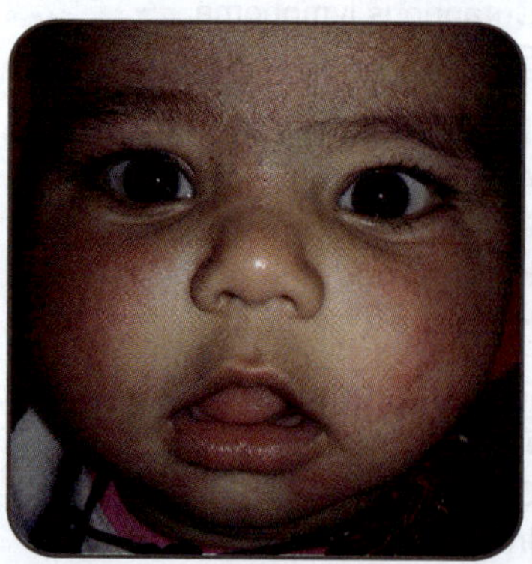

a. Atopic dermatitis
b. Contact dermatitis
c. HHV 6 infection
d. Scrofuloderma

New Questions

43. The following statements are true/false regarding atopic eczema:
a. Serum IgE is measured for diagnosis
b. Barrier defect is seen
c. Filaggrin mutations
d. Acitretin is effective
e. Lichenification occurs in chronic stage

44. Assertion: Patients with atopic eczema have more staphylococcal infections
Reason: Patients with atopic eczema have barrier dysfunction
a. Both Assertion and Reason are true and reason is correct explanation of assertion
b. Both Assertion and Reason are true but reason is not correct explanation of assertion
c. Assertion is true and Reason is false
d. Assertion is false and Reason is true
e. Both Assertion and Reason are false

45. The following agents act as allergens to cause allergic contact dermatitis:
a. Nickel
b. Detergent
c. Potassium dichromate
d. Acids
1. If a, and b are correct
2. If a, c, d are correct
3. If a and c are correct
4. If all four (a, b, c, & d) are correct

46. The following are included in the minor criteria for atopic eczema:
a. Pityriasis alba
b. Ichthyosis vulgaris
c. Family history
d. Serum IgE
1. If a, b, d are correct
2. If a, c, d are correct
3. If a and d are correct
4. If all four (a, b, c, & d) are correct

47. **Match the findings of column A with best alternative in column B:**

Column A	Column B
1. Phytophotodermatitis 2. Housewives eczema 3. Hair dye allergic contact dermatitis 4. Atopic eczema	a. Irritant contact dermatitis b. White dermographism c. Nickel d. Parthenium e. Potassium dichromate f. Paraphenylene Diamine

48. **An adult presents with itchy hyperpigmented plaque with exudation on the flexure of the elbow and back of knee as shown. The diagnosis is:** *(INICET Nov 21)*

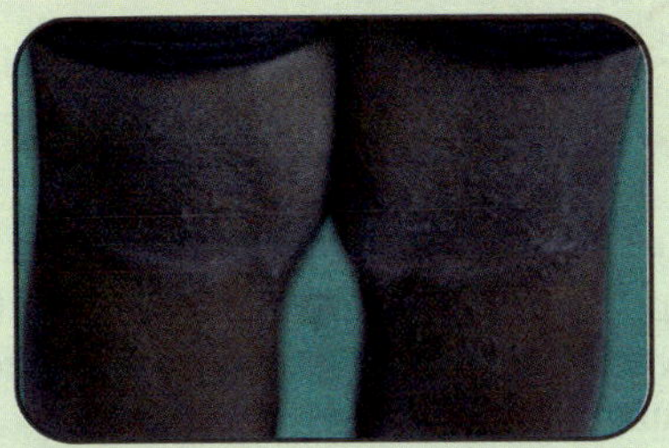

a. Psoriasis
b. Atopic dermatitis
c. Dermatitis herpetiformis
d. Pemphigus

49. **About air born contact dermatitis, the gold standard diagnostic test is:** *(INICET Nov 2020)*

a. Oral provocation test
b. Patch test
c. Radio allergo sorbent test
d. IgE level

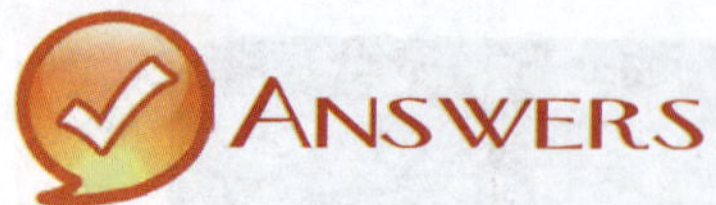

1. **Ans. (a) Acute eczema** *(Ref: Mckee's Pathology of Skin, 4th edn, Page 180)*
   Spongiosis is intercellular edema (edema in between keratinocytes) and is a feature of acute eczema. This fluid may ooze out clinically causing the classical oozing of acute eczemas.
2. **Ans. (a) Contact dermatitis** *(Ref: Andrew's Textbook, 11th edn, Page 91)*
   Patch testing is the confirmatory test for allergic contact eczema.
3. **Ans. (a) Parthenium grass** *(Ref: IADVL Textbook of Dermatology, 3rd edn, Page 564)*
4. **Ans. (a) Nickel** *(Ref: IADVL Textbook of Dermatology, 3rd edn, Page 559, Rook's Textbook of Dermatology, 9th edn, Page 128.19)*
5. **Ans. (d) Nickel** (See page 292 for explanation)
6. **Ans. (a, c, d, e) Sagograin lesions; Recurrences are common; Severe episodes are treated with short course steroids; Dyshidrotic eczema** (See page 295 for explanation)
   Lesions do not begin on finger-tip but on sides of fingers.
7. **Ans. (b) Protection from occupational dermatitis** (See page 290 for explanation)
8. **Ans. (a) Parthenium hysterophorus** (See page 294 for explanation)
9. **Ans. (a) Nummular eczema** *(Ref: Andrew's Textbook, 11th edn, Page 77)*
10. **Ans. (d) They are painful but not pruritic** *(Ref: Andrew's Textbook, 11th edn, Page 73)*
    Pruritus is intense in pompholyx.
11. **Ans. (c) Mica like scales**
    Mica-like scales are seen in psoriasis.
12. **Ans. (c) Pityriasis alba** (See chart on page 101-Chapter 5 for explanation)
    For table on how to differentiate hypopigmented patches on face, see the chapter on fungal infections.
13. **Ans. (a) Atopic dermatitis** (See page 288 for explanation)
14. **Ans. (a) Atopic dermatitis** *(Ref: Andrew's Textbook, 11th edn, Page 63)*
15. **Ans. (a) Patch test**
    The distribution of lesions on exposed area increasing in summers suggests photodermatitis. Photopatch test is done for diagnosis of patch test.
16. **Ans. (a) Atopic dermatitis**
    Eczematous dermatitis over the extensor surfaces with mother's history of bronchial asthma suggests atopic dermatitis.
17. **Ans. (d) Isotretinoin**
    Isotretinoin as a sebolytic agent would dry the skin further in a skin which is already dry due to atopic dermatitis and would be counter-productive.
18. **Ans. (d) Moist compresses**
    Moist compresses help in reducing oozing in acute eczemas.

19. Ans. (b) Atopic dermatitis

Adults with atopic dermatitis have a flexural rash.

20. Ans. (a) Insect bite hypersensitivity (See page 296 for explanation)

Lesions on exposed parts increasing in monsoons point to insect bite hypersensitivity.

21. Ans. (c) Lichenification (See page 288 for explanation)

Due to the chronic scratching and itching in chronic eczema, lichenification occurs.

22. Ans. (a) Pruritus *(Ref: Rook's Textbook of Dermatology, 9th edn, Page 41.14)*

Itching is the hallmark of atopic dermatitis.

23. Ans. (a) Atopic dermatitis *(Ref: Andrew's Textbook, 11th edn, Page 63)*

Itching is central to atopic eczema and rash occurs after itch, rather than the other way around.

24. Ans. (d) Atopic dermatitis *(Ref: Andrew's Textbook, 11th edn, Page 65)*

25. Ans. (c) Antecubital fossa *(Ref: Andrew's Textbook, 11th edn, Page 64, Rook's Textbook of Dermatology, 9th edn, Page 41.19)*

26. Ans. (c) Clinical examination

Clinical criteria (Hanifin and Rajka) and history are used in diagnosis of atopic eczema. Serum IgE is not specific to atopic eczema. Patch test is the test of choice for allergic contact eczema.

27. Ans. (b) Pruritus *(Ref: Andrew's Textbook, 11th edn, Page 63)*

Pruritus is a major criteria, not minor.

28. Ans. (a) Vegetables *(Ref: Goyal S et al. Contact Dermatitis in Housewives—A Clinico-Etiological Study In A Tertiary Care Hospital of Northern India, IJRRMS 2012;2(3))*

The question meant Indian housewives. Vegetables (garlic and onion) were the commonest suspected contact allergens (50%) followed by soap and detergents (40%) and condiments (10%).

Detergents cause irritant contact dermatitis, not allergic contact dermatitis.

29. Ans. (b) Nickel

30. Ans. (b) 4 days *(Ref: Rook's Textbook of Dermatology, 9th edn, Page 128.66)*

31. Ans. (c) Allergic contact dermatitis

32. Ans. (b) Patch test

33. Ans. (b) Delayed type hypersensitivity

34. Ans. (c) Azathioprine

Due to diabetes and hypertension, Azathioprine would be preferred.

35. Ans. (d) SLE (See page 297 for explanation)

36. Ans. (b) Posterior subcapsular cataract (See page 288 for explanation)

37. Ans. (d) Chromate

Occupational contact dermatitis (a) Farmers- Due to plant (Parthenium) (b) Cement/ leather - Due to Potassium dichromate (c) Textile- Due to Azo dyes (d) Hairdressers- Due to ParaPhenylene Diamine (PPD)

38. Ans. (d) Delayed hypersensitivity

39. Ans. (b) Parthenium

Scourge is something which causes great suffering. Parthenium plant causes great suffering in farmers who are exposed to it chronically in fields.

40. Ans. (b) 96 hours after the patch application (See page 293 for explanation)

41. Ans. (d) Atopic dermatitis

Atopic dermatitis is typically in ante-cubital fossa and flexures like popliteal fossa in adults. Also exudation (oozing) is a sign of eczema due to spongiosis. Psoriasis is classically on extensors. Although the variant called as flexural psoriasis has flexural lesions, it will not ooze. Dermatitis herpetiformis will have itchy excoriations and relation to gluten.

42. Ans. (a) Atopic dermatitis

This is the classical image of atopic dermatitis in a child with mother having (a) h/o asthma. Why not: (b) Will have localized lesions on contact area. Mother history would not be present (c) This is Roseola infantum - will have fever with rash (d) Will have lymphadenitis with sinus on neck/axillae

New Answers

43. Ans. a-False; b-True; c-True; d-False; e-True

44. Ans. (a) Both Assertion and Reason are true and Reason is correct explanation of Assertion

45. Ans. (3) If a and c are correct

46. Ans. (1) If a, b, d are correct

47. Ans. 1-d; 2-a; 3-f; 4-b

48. Ans. (b) Atopic dermatitis

49. Ans. (b) Patch test

CHAPTER 13

Disorders of Pigmentation

DISORDERS OF HYPERPIGMENTATION

Depending on the histopatholgical level of melanin in the skin, clinical color varies.

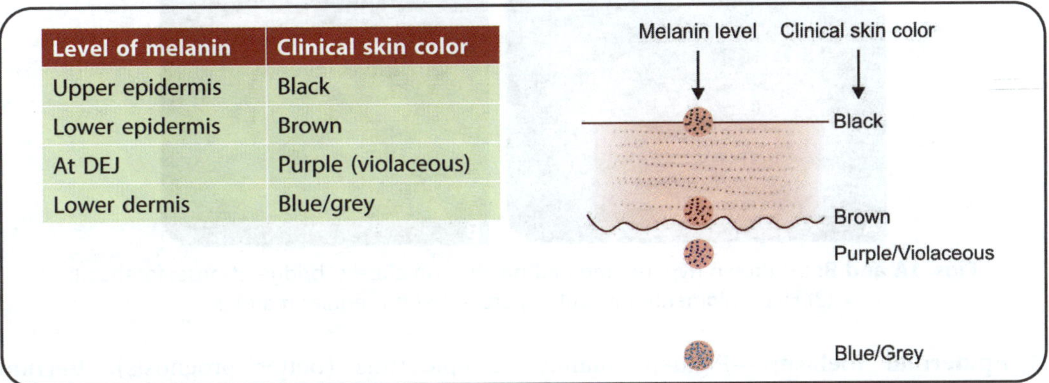

Level of melanin	Clinical skin color
Upper epidermis	Black
Lower epidermis	Brown
At DEJ	Purple (violaceous)
Lower dermis	Blue/grey

There are two types of melanin:

1. Brown-black **eumelanin**
2. Red-brown or yellow **pheomelanin**

Epidermal melanocytic lesions	Dermal/DE junction melanocytic lesions
Melasma	Melasma
Lentigine	Nevus of Ota
Becker's nevus	Nevus of Ito
Café-au-lait macule	Mongolian spot
Endocrine disorders	• Congenital melanocytic nevus • Acquired melanocytic nevus
Freckle	Lichen planus

Melasma(MCQ)

❑ **Sun exposure**(MCQ) is the primary trigger. Hence, lesions are seen on face and **worsens in summer**

- Other triggers—**Female hormones** (hence more common in females), **OCPs,**(MCQ) **pregnancy**(MCQ) in the 3rd trimester (**Melasma in pregnancy is called Chloasma—mask of pregnancy**),(MCQ) hormone replacement therapy (HRT) at menopause
- Presents as **brown patches**(MCQ) of pigmentation, typically on the **malar prominences, bridge of nose and forehead** (Figs. 1A and B)

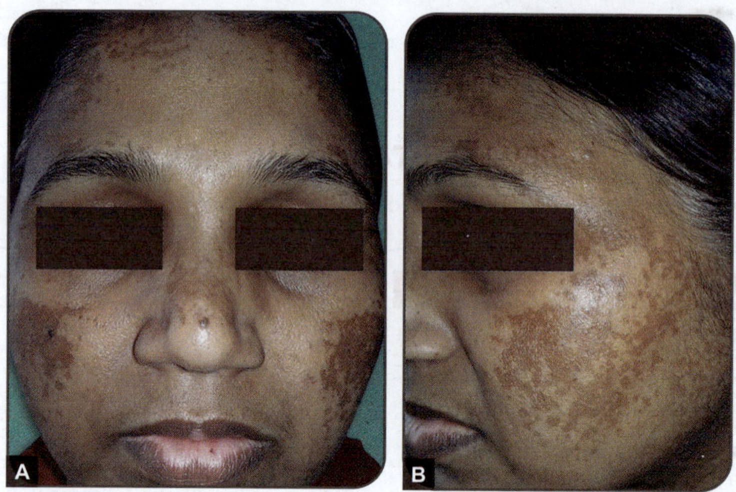

Figs. 1A and B: (A) Brown hyperpigmented patches on cheeks, bridge of nose, forehead; (B) Hyperpigmented macules, patches with irregular margins

- **Epidermal melasma**—Pigment mainly in epidermis (better prognosis), **Dermal melasma**—pigment mainly in dermis (poorer prognosis). **Wood's lamp helps differentiate epidermal (increases on Wood's lamp) from dermal melasma (reduces on Wood's lamp)**
- **Histopathology**: The number of melanocytes is not increased but they are enlarged and more active (**hyperfunctional melanocytes**)
- **Treatment**
  - Melasma is chronic and needs long-term treatment, while **chloasma self-resolves after pregnancy**(MCQ)
  - Sunscreens with a good UVA coverage
  - **Hydroquinone (gold standard)** reduces tyrosinase activity and is often used in 2–4% strength
  - **Kligman regimen**(MCQ) (hydroquinone + tretinoin + topical steroid)—DOC
  - Chemical peels (glycolic acid, trichloroacetic acid, salicylic acid)
  - Kojic acid (tyrosinase inhibitor).

Becker's Nevus

The word "nevus" means "birth-mark". Histopathologically, nevus is an **aggregation of melanocyte clusters**. If the clusters are in epidermis—epidermal melanocytic nevus and if in dermis—dermal melanocytic nevus.

- Becker's nevus is an **epidermal melanocytic nevus**(MCQ)
- Even though called a nevus (birth mark), **onset is in adolescence**
- **Increased sensitivity of androgens**(MCQ) on outer arms, scapular area and chest
- **Hyperpigmentation + increased hair + acne** in these areas (Figs. 2A and B).

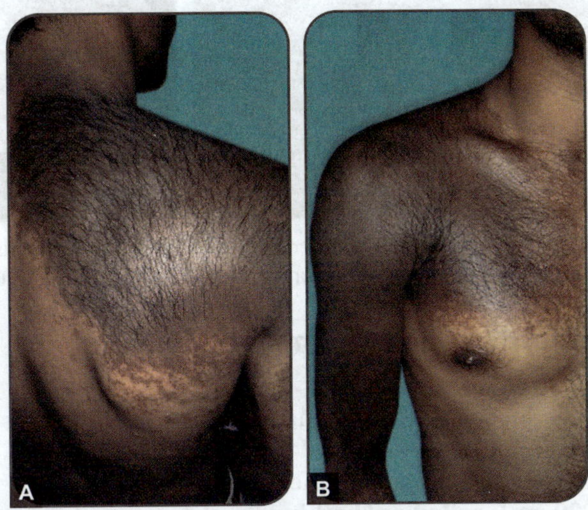

Figs. 2A and B: (A) Brown hyperpigmented macules, patches with hypertrichosis; (B) Anterior chest in the same patient

Acquired Melanocytic Nevi (Common Moles)

Three types, depending on the position of the melanocyte clusters

1. **Junctional**(MCQ)—Nevus cells at the DE junction. Smooth brown macules (Fig. 3A)
2. **Compound**(MCQ)—Nevus cells at DE junction + dermis. Dome shaped, deeply pigmented, sometimes with hair from them (Fig. 3A)
3. **Intradermal**(MCQ)—Nevus cells in the dermis. Dome shaped, but non-pigmented (Fig. 3B)

**Note:* Its not the type, but the number of nevi which determine malignant conversion (more the number, more the chances)

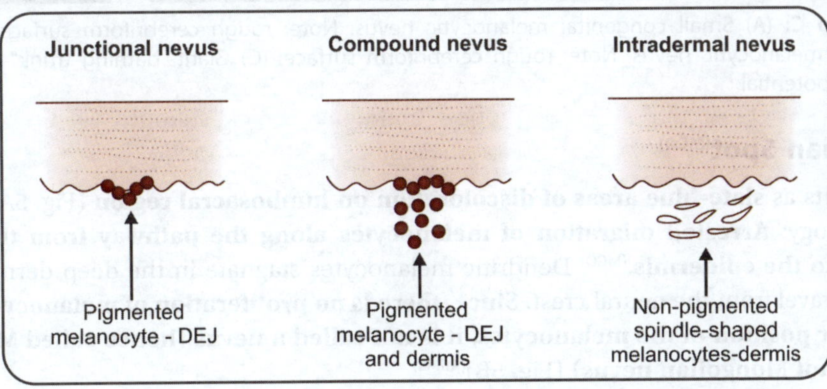

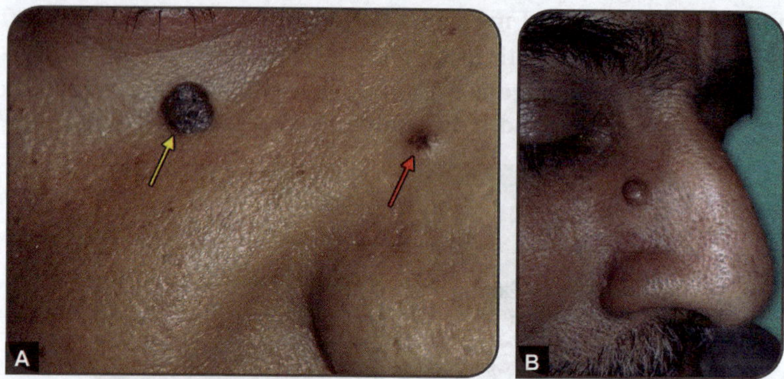

Figs. 3A and B: (A) Dome shaped deeply pigmented lesion (compound nevus)–Yellow arrow, Flat brown macule near nose (junctional nevus)–Red arrow; (B) Non-pigmented nodule (intradermal nevus)

Congenital Melanocytic Lesions (Common Moles)

- Color varies from brown to black
- With age, the lesions can become raised and develop irregularity on surface (**cerebriform appearance**) (Figs. 4A and B).
- Coarse hair often develops on many of the lesions
- **If giant in size (>20 cm), called as "bathing trunk" nevus—has malignant conversion potential** (Fig. 4C).(MCQ)

* Note: It is the size, not the number which determines malignant conversion.

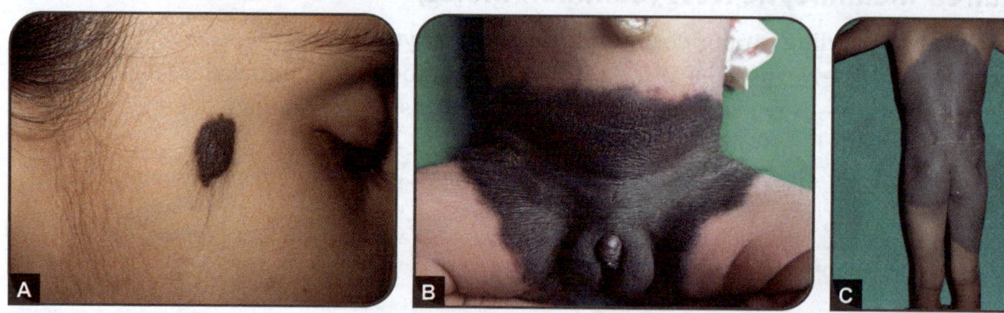

Figs. 4A to C: (A) Small congenital melanocytic nevus. Note: rough cerebriform surface; (B) Large congenital melanocytic nevus. Note: rough cerebriform surface; (C) Giant "bathing trunk" nevus with malignant potential

Mongolian Spot(MCQ)

- Presents as **slate-blue areas of discoloration on lumbosacral region** (Fig. 5A)
- Pathology: **Arrested migration of melanocytes along the pathway from the neural crest to the epidermis.**(MCQ) Dendritic melanocytes stagnate in the deep dermis during their travel from the neural crest. **Since, there is no proliferation of melanocytes, just a deeper position of the melanocytes, it is not called a nevus (hence called Mongolian spot, not Mongolian nevus)** (Fig. 5B)(AIIMS)

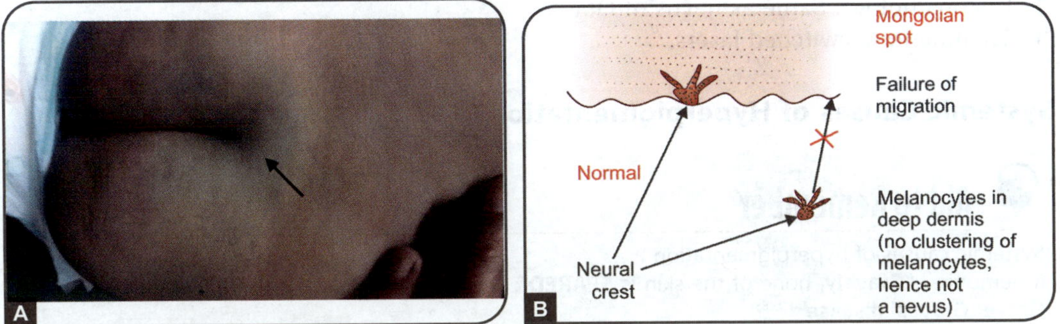

Figs. 5A and B: (A) Blue macules, patches on sacrum (black arrow); (B) Schematic representation of pathology in Mongolian spot

- Histopathology: Melanocytes in **deep reticular dermis (low-dermal)**
- **Treatment:** Spontaneous regression during infancy or childhood, and generally disappear by puberty

Nevus of Ota[(AIIMS May 15)]

- Ill-defined **slate-blue, usually unilateral lesion** situated in the distribution of the **ophthalmic and maxillary divisions of the trigeminal nerve**
- Often with a **blue sclera**, conjunctiva on the same side (Fig. 6A)
- **Histopathology**: Upper and mid dermis have collections of heavily pigmented, spindle-shaped, dendritic melanocytes (Fig. 6B)
- Treatment: Q-switched lasers

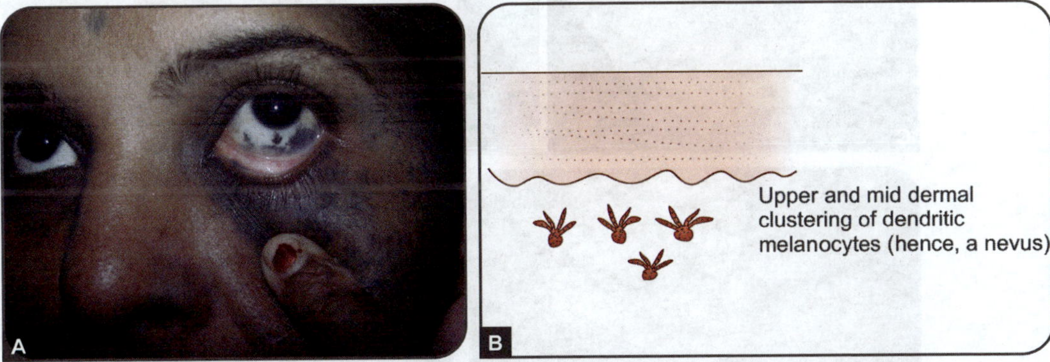

Figs. 6A and B: (A) Bluish macules and patches around eye with scleral pigmentation; (B) Schematic representation of the histopathological feature of nevus of Ota

Nevus of Ito

- Similar to nevus of Ota, an **ill-defined slate-blue, usually unilateral lesion situated in the distribution of the posterior supraclavicular and lateral brachial cutaneous nerve**[(MCQ)]
- Seen on **shoulder and scapular area**

- Histopathology: Same as nevus of Ota
- Treatment: Q-switched lasers.

Systemic Causes of Hyperpigmentation

Aid to Remember

Systemic causes of hyperpigmentation

Mnemonic—"**Gravely**, none of the skin is **SPARED**":

Grave: Graves' disease(AI 93,83)

S: **S**teroid (Cortisol excess—Cushing's syndrome), **S**cleroderma(MCQ) (salt and pepper pigmentation) (Fig. 6D)

P: **P**regnancy, **P**eutz-Jeghers syndrome (Fig. 6C)

A: **A**ddison's disease, **A**rsenic poisoning

R: **R**enal failure

E: **E**xcess iron (hemochromatosis—gray to brown mucocutaneous hyperpigmentation in sun-exposed areas due to **epidermal melanin and to a lesser extent hemosiderin deposits**(MCQ)

D: **D**rugs: Clofazimine [red-brown pigmentation (Fig. 6E)], Minocycline (blue black)

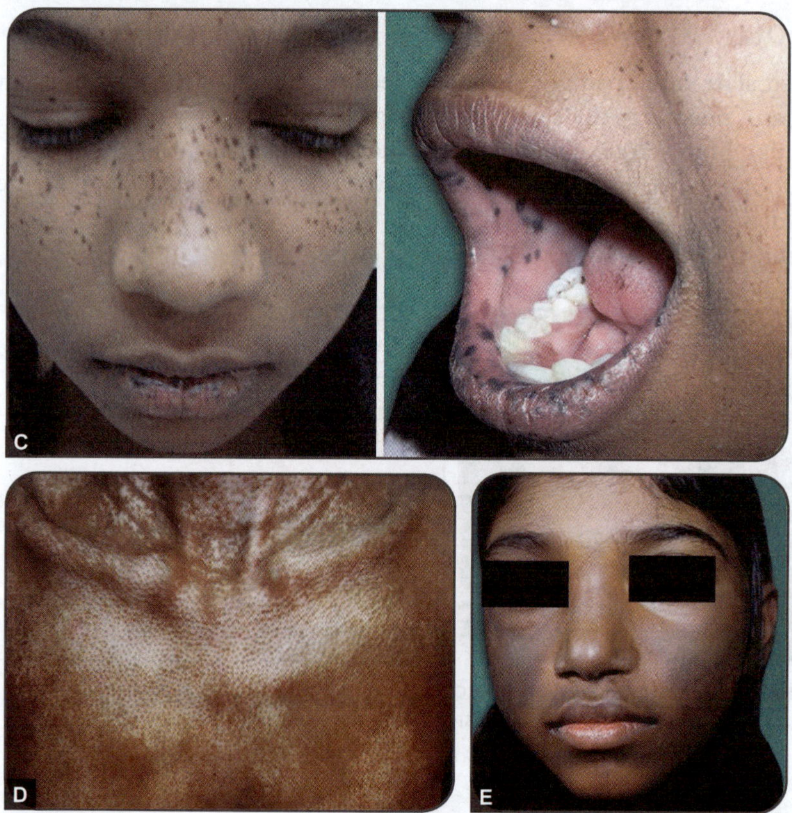

Figs. 6C to E: (C) Peutz-Jeghers syndrome—Pigmented macules (Lentigine) on face and buccal mucosa; (D) Scleroderma—Salt and pepper pigmentation; (E) Clofazimine induced red-brown pigmentation

Key chart to help differentiate lesions on face in an MCQ

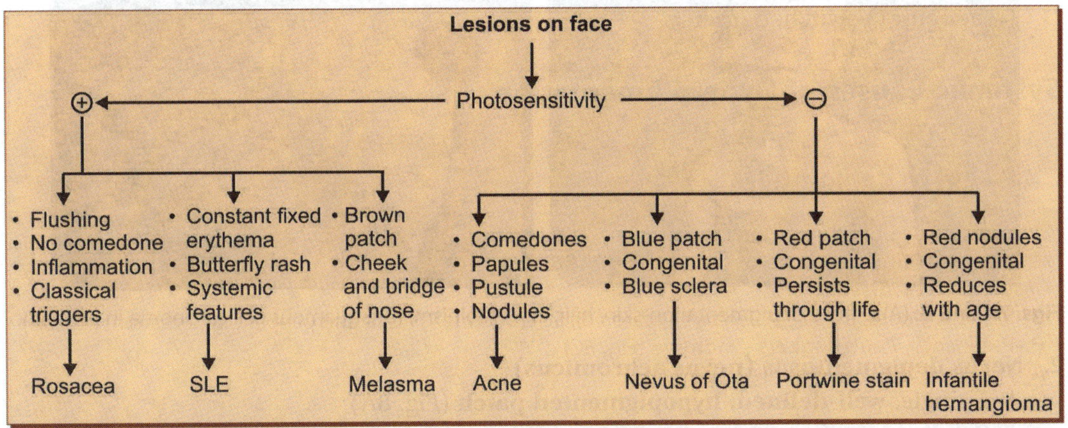

**Note:* For images for these diseases, refer to Chapter 11.

DISORDERS OF HYPOPIGMENTATION/DEPIGMENTATION

Classification

Depending on pathology	Depending on onset
Absent/reduced melanocytes E.g. Vitiligo Piebaldism Contact leucoderma	**Congenital** E.g. Albinism Piebaldism Nevus depigmentosus
Normal melanocytes number but reduced melanin synthesis due to defective tyrosinase activity E.g. Albinism Pityriasis versicolor (see Chapter 5)	**Acquired** E.g. Vitiligo Pityriasis versicolor Contact leucoderma PKDL (see Chapter 7) Hansens disease (see Chapter 3) Pityriasis alba (see Chapter 12)

CONGENITAL

1. **Albinism (Oculocutaneous albinism)**
   - **Autosomal recessive trait. Genetic mutation in tyrosinase** (which helps synthesize melanin) results in congenital loss of melanin.
   - **Depigmented skin, hair and eyes (iris/retina)** (Fig. 7A). Eye involvement: Nystagmus, photophobia. Increased risk of cutaneous malignancies (commonly squamous cell carcinoma) (Fig. 7B)
   - Histopathology: **Normal melanocytes, loss of melanin production.**(MCQ)

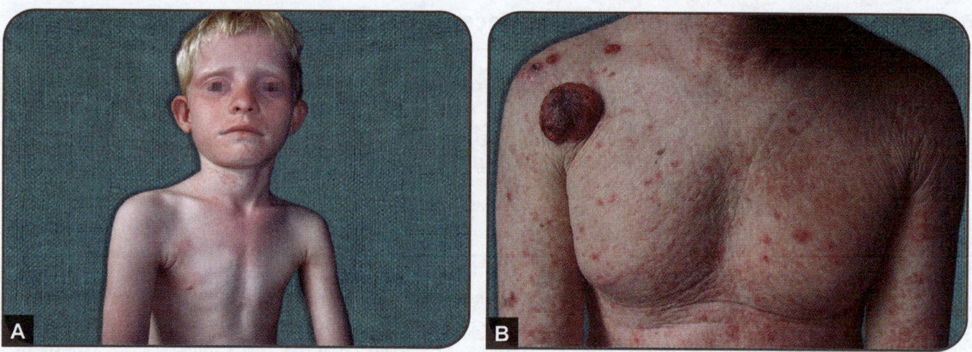

Figs. 7A and B: (A) Diffuse depigmentation-skin, hair, iris—Albinism; (B) Squamous cell carcinoma in an albino

2. **Nevus depigmentosus (nevus achromicus)**
   - A single, **well-defined, hypopigmented patch** (Fig. 8A)
   - **On diascopy (pressing with a glass slide)—the lesion border is not lost and the lesion does not merge into the surrounding skin** (Fig. 8B)
   - **Histopathology:** Normal or reduced number of melanocytes and reduced transfer of melanin from melanocytes into keratinocytes.

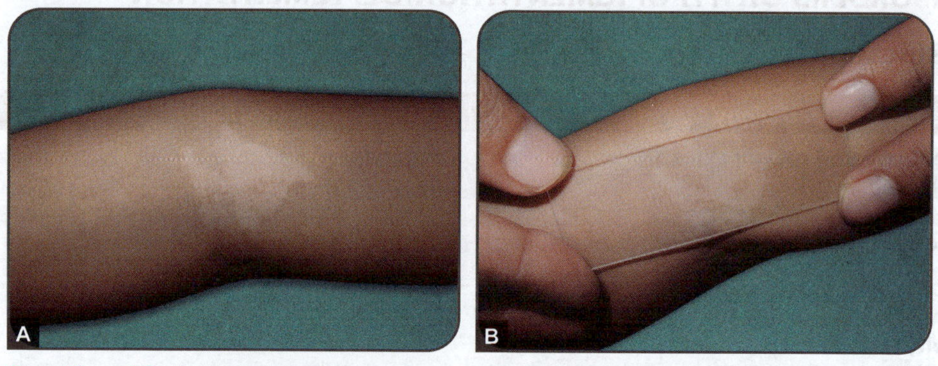

Figs. 8A and B: (A) Well-defined hypopigmented patch; (B) No increase in size on diascopy

Chart on how to differentiate congenital white patches

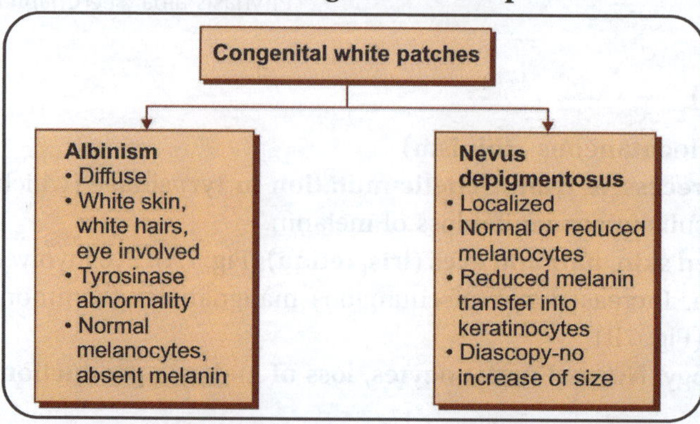

ACQUIRED

Depigmented Lesions

1. **Vitiligo**
   - Pathogenesis:
     - **Neurogenic theory:** Segmental vitiligo is seen along a dermatome (lines along distribution of nerves), suggesting a neural origin—a toxin released at the nerve endings may destroy melanocytes
     - **Autoimmune theory:** Autoimmune destruction of melanocytes (antigen is melanocyte). These self-antigens are picked up by Langerhans cells in epidermis, presented to lymph nodes, melanocyte-specific cytotoxic T cells are formed destroying melanocytes either only in skin or in skin and hair follicles

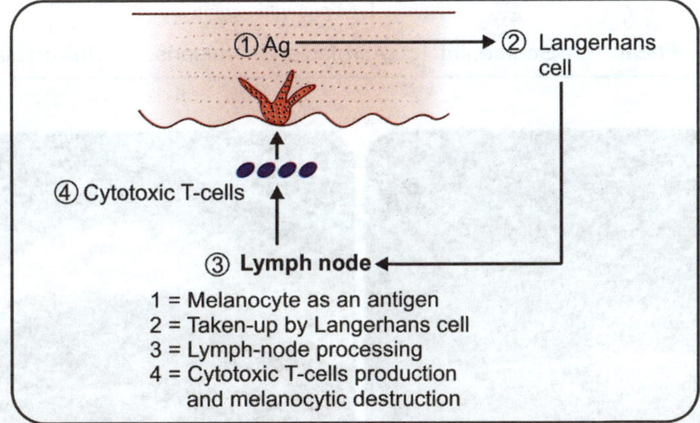

   - Strong genetic predisposition
   - Depigmented **milky-white patches** (initially may be hypopigmented), sometimes with white hairs **(leucotrichia)**—found particularly in areas of repeated friction and pressure points, e.g. dorsa of the hands/fingers, feet, elbows, knees and ankles. **Having white hairs is a poor prognostic sign (since the hair follicle has melanocyte precursors for skin repigmentation)**
   - **Types:**

     Localized:
     - Focal (single or a few macules in one anatomic area) (Fig. 9A)
     - Segmental—Lesions linearly in a segment (Fig. 9B). (Lesions stop growing after initial increase)
     - Mucosal—e.g. lips, genitals (Fig. 9D)
     - Lip-Tip (on lips and finger tips) (Fig. 9C)

     Generalized:
     - Acrofacial—Acro = acral areas (fingers and toes) and face
     - Symmetrical generalized (vitiligo vulgaris)—**most common (remember "vulgaris" means common)** (Fig. 9E)
     - Universal (Figs. 9F and G)

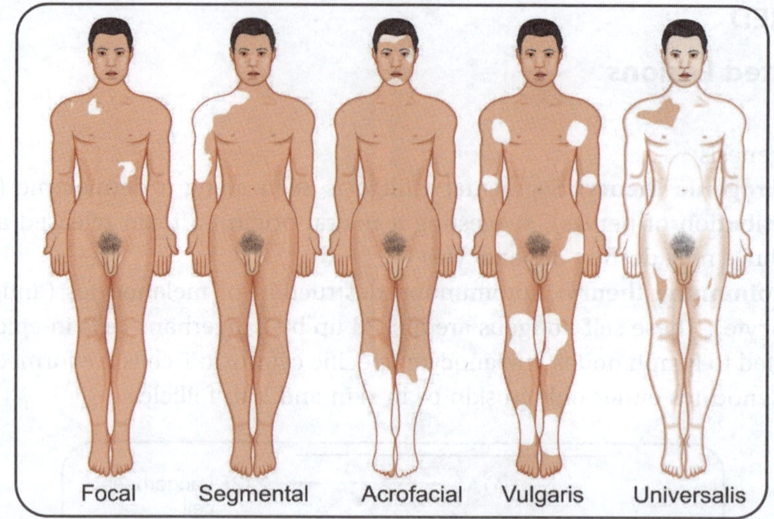

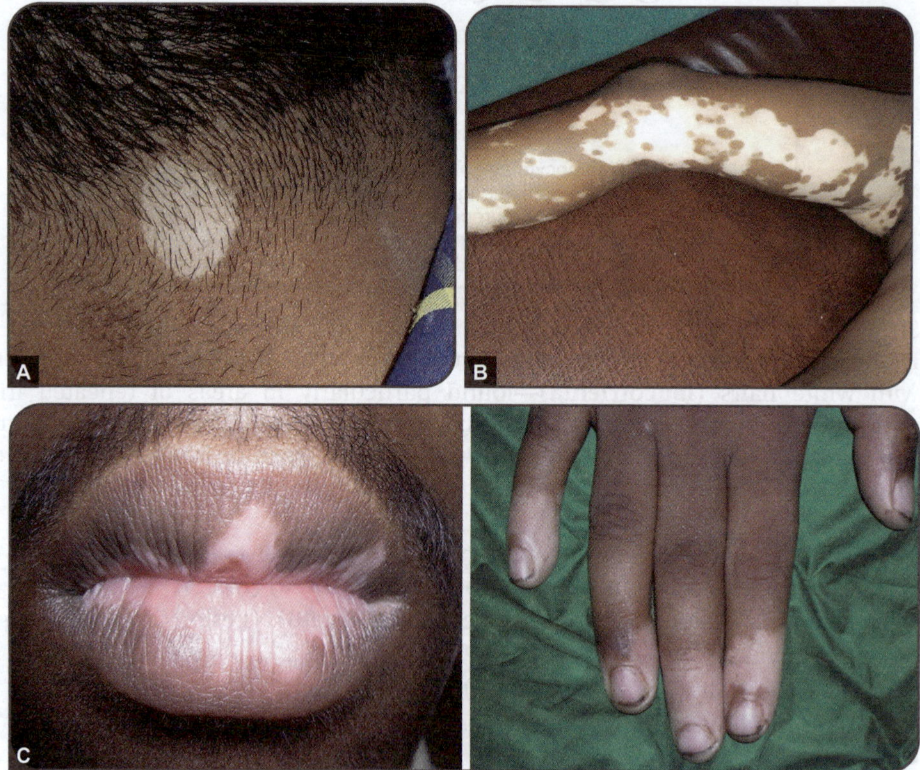

Figs. 9A to C

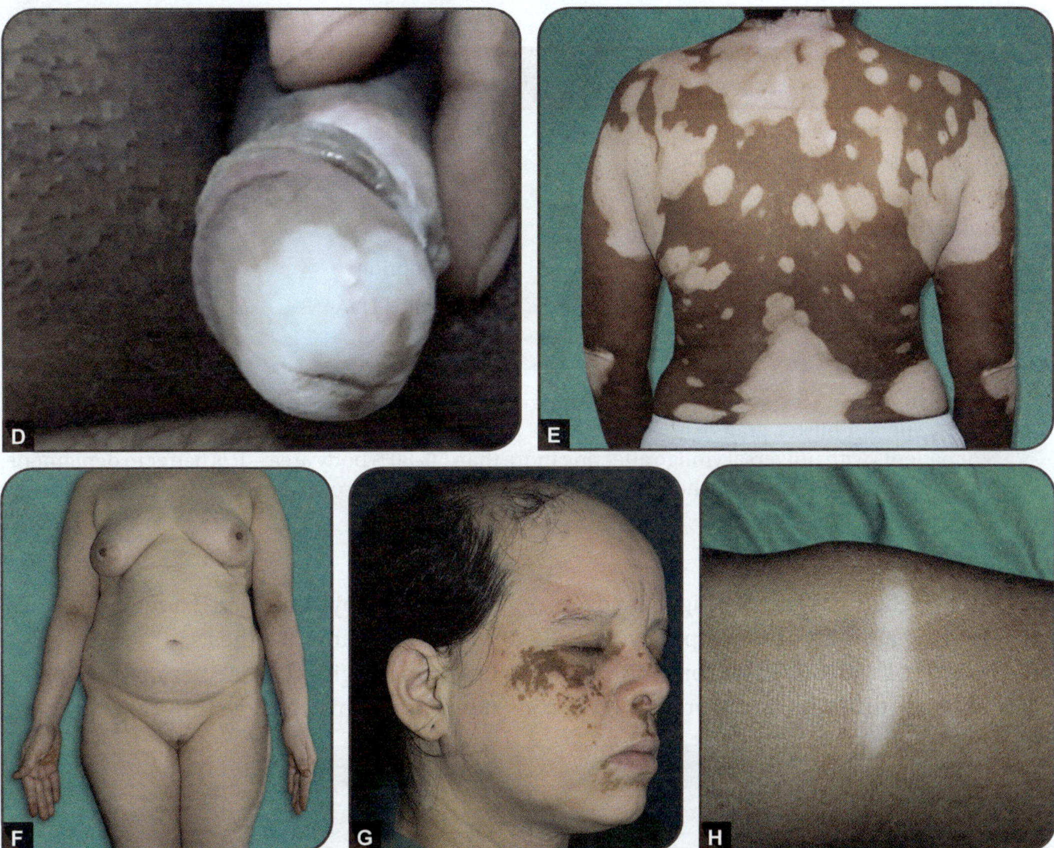

Figs. 9A to H: (A) Focal vitiligo (black hairs); (B) Segmental vitiligo—Depigmented linear/segmental patches; (C) Lip-tip vitiligo; (D) Mucosal vitiligo; (E) Vitiligo vulgaris—symmetrical patches; (F) Universal vitiligo; (G) Few residual areas of normal skin in the same patient as in Figure 10F (treatment would be to depigment the remaining normal skin with melanocyte destroyer creams containing a chemical called as monobenzyl ether of hydroquinone-MBEH); (H) Koebner's phenomenon in vitiligo

- **Associated other autoimmune diseases—Most common associated autoimmune disease is autoimmune thyroid dysfunction**, either hypothyroidism (Hashimoto's thyroiditis) or hyperthyroidism (Grave's disease). Others are type 1 diabetes mellitus, pernicious anemia Addison's disease,(MCQ) SLE,(MCQ) rheumatoid arthritis
- **Koebner's phenomenon positive** (Fig. 9H).
- **Diagnosis**
  - Wood's lamp will give an "ivory-white" color to lesions
  - Histopathology—**Absent melanocytes (autoimmune destruction) and hence absent melanin**

- **Treatment**

<20% involved Topical	>20% involved Systemic
Potent steroids (e.g. betamethasone valerate or clobetasol propionate)—DOC	**Narrow band UVB (best)**(MCQ)
Tacrolimus(MCQ)—for areas prone for steroid induced atrophy—e.g. face	Systemic corticosteroids
Calcipotriol(MCQ)	Azathioprine
Topical PUVA	Systemic PUVA(MCQ)
Excimer laser	

***Surgical option (for stable vitiligo)**—Skin grafting (full-thickness punch grafts, split-thickness grafts, suction blister grafts)

*For patients with universal vitiligo affecting more than 50–80% body area—It is better to depigment remaining normal skin patches by applying melanocyte destroyer creams (**Monobenzylether of hydroquinone-MBEH**)

Phototherapy in Vitiligo

- "Photo"= light. When UV light is given on skin, it acts by removing Langerhans cells, removing autoimmune lymphocytes and stimulating melanin synthesis.
- Either UVA (320-400 nm) or UVB (290-300 nm) can be given. UVA therapy first needs photosensitization with psoralen. UVB does not require this sensitization (Fig. 10).

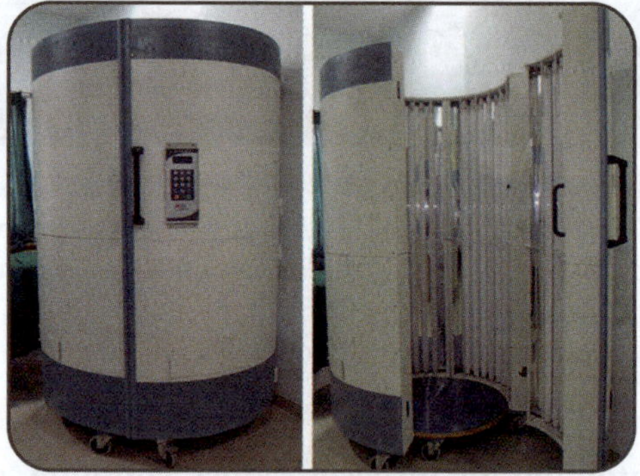

Fig. 10: Phototherapy chamber

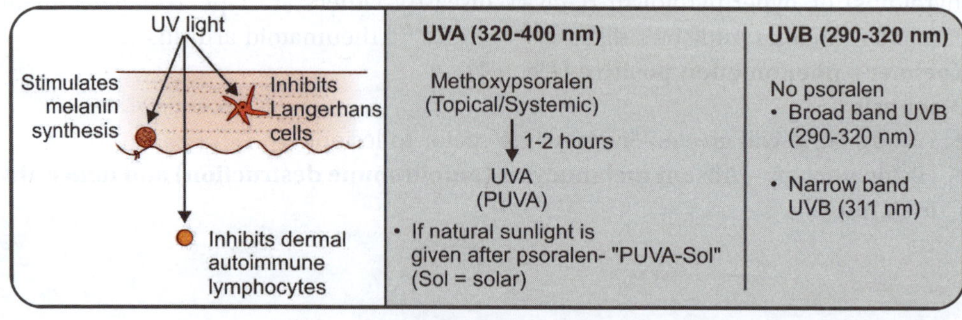

Poor Prognostic Factors

- Extensive
- Long standing
- Vitiligo on bony prominences (Fig. 11B)
- **Leucotrichia** or non-hairy areas (since the hair follicle has melanocyte precursors for skin repigmentation) (Fig. 11A)
- Lip-tip vitiligo (areas devoid of hair)
- Underlying thyroid disease.

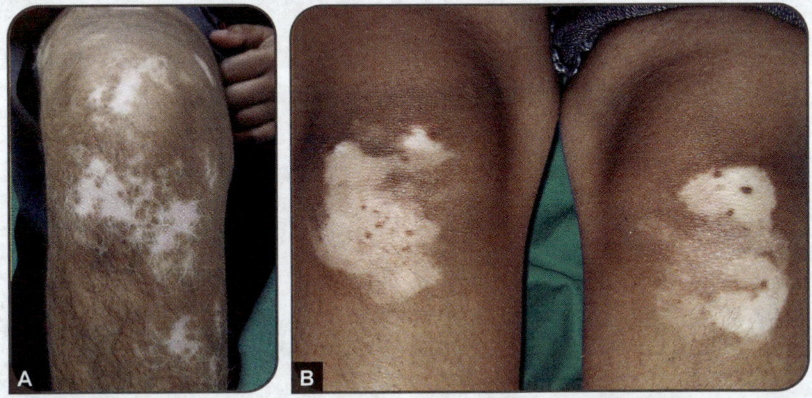

Figs. 11A and B: (A) Leucotrichia—Poor prognosis; (B) Vitiligo on bony prominences—Poor prognosis

2. **Contact leucoderma/chemical leucoderma**
   - With repeated exposure to chemicals which physically destroys melanocytes (not an autoimmune destruction)
   - Caused by derivatives of phenols and catechols, e.g. **paratertiary butyl phenol-PTBP (adhesive in sticker bindi). Mono-benzyl-ether-of hydroquinone-MBEH**, a constituent of rubber in rubber slippers, leather wallets, watch straps, rubber gloves, is a powerful agent causing leucoderma (Figs. 12A to D)
   - Histologically, there is an absence of melanocytes identical to lesions of vitiligo.

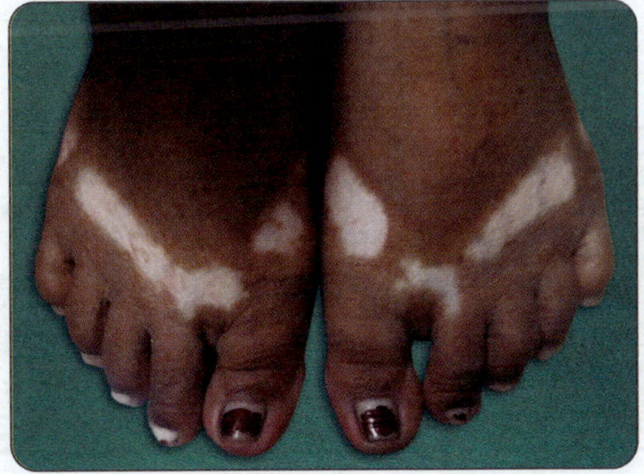

Fig. 12A: Rubber-slipper induced leucoderma

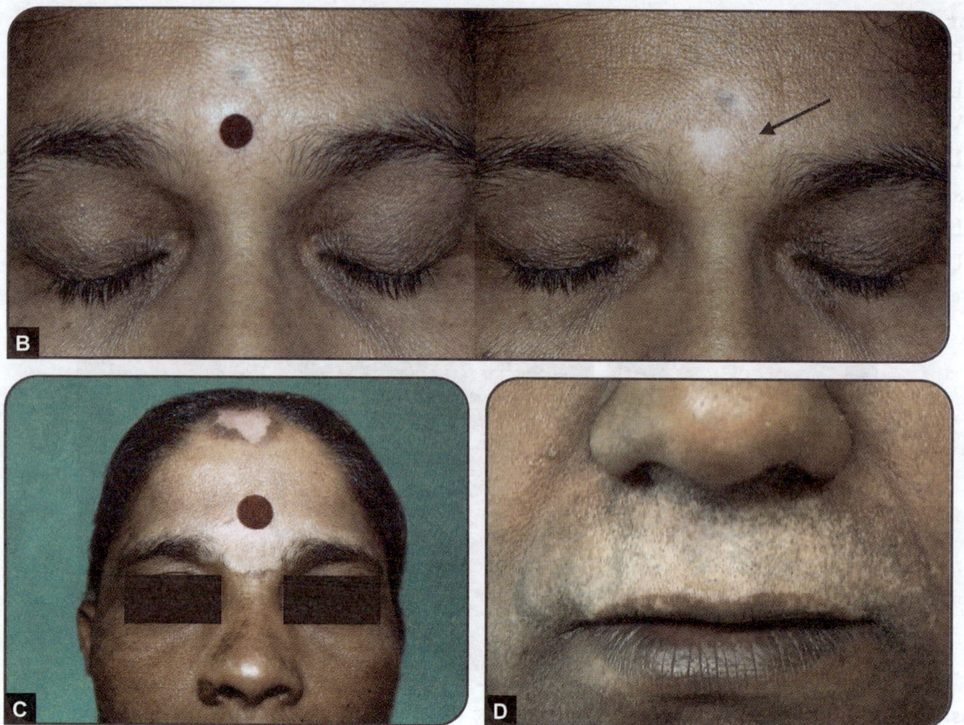

Figs. 12B to D: (B) Bindi-induced leucoderma; (C) Kumkum-induced leucoderma at hair line; (D) Hair dye-induced leucoderma

Hypopigmented Lesion

Chart on how to differentiate various hypopigmented lesions is given below. For details on individual diseases, refer to the respective chapter.

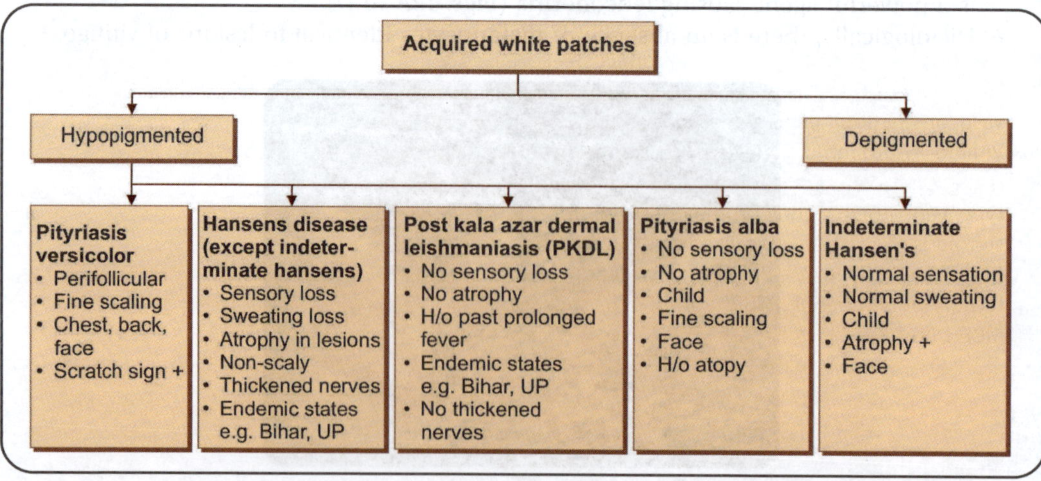

Aid to Remember

Differential diagnosis of white patches (hypopigmented/depigmented) of skin
Mnemonic: "**Vitiligo PATCH**"
Vitiligo
Pityriasis alba/**P**ityriasis versicolor/**P**KDL/**P**iebaldism
Albinism
Tuberous sclerosis (ash-leaf macule)
Congenital birthmarks (nevus depigmentosus/nevus anemicus)
Hansen's disease

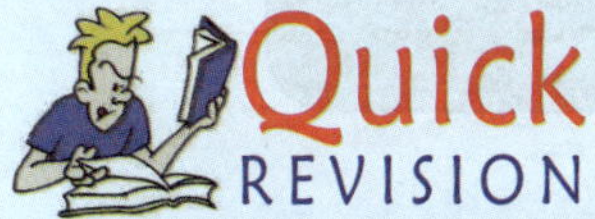

- Epidermal pigmentation—Melasma, Freckles, Café-au-lait macules
- Dermal pigmentation—Melasma, nevus of Ota, Nevus of Ito, Mongolian spot, Congenital and acquired melanocytic nevi
- Melasma—Usually in females. Epidermal or dermal melanin. Brown patches on cheeks, bridge of nose. Melasma in pregnancy = chloasma. Triggered by OCPs, sun, pregnancy. Melasma needs long-term treatment (Kligman regimen-DOC, hydroquinone), chloasma—self-resolving
- Becker's nevus—Hyperpigmentation + acne + hypertrichosis on shoulder, arms. Epidermal melanocytic nevus. Androgen hypersensitivity
- Acquired melanocytic nevus: 3 types—Junctional nevus (nevus cells at DEJ), compound nevus (nevus cells at DEJ and dermis), Intradermal nevus (dermal nevus cells)
- Congenital melanocytic nevus—"bathing trunk nevus" has malignant potential
- Nevus of Ota/Ito—Dermal melanocytic nevi. Ota—Bluish pigmentation on trigeminal area with sclera pigmentation. Ito—Similar bluish pigmentation on shoulder and scapular area
- Mongolian spot—Not a nevus. Deep dermal arrest of melanocytes travelling from neural crest. Bluish pigmentation on lumbosacral region. Self-resolving
- Albinism—Tyrosinase defect. Depigmented skin, hair, eye- normal melanocytes, absent melanin
- Piebaldism—Localized white patches with normal skin areas inside, white fore-lock.
- Nevus depigmentosus (nevus achromicus)—Localized white patches, On diascopy–no change.
- Nevus anemicus—Localized white patches. Not a melanin disorder. Vascular disorder (localized vasoconstriction). Increases on diascopy
- Vitiligo—Autoimmune destruction of melanocytes and hence loss of melanin. Thyroid disorder is the most common underlying association. Koebner's positive. Vitiligo vulgaris—most common type. Leucotrichia, bony prominences, lip-tip, and thyroid disease indicates poor prognosis. Topical steroid is the DOC for localized and NBUVB for extensive disease
- Contact leucoderma—Physical destruction of melanocytes form external chemicals—e.g. Para-tertiary-butyl-phenol, PTBP (adhesive in sticker bindi) and mono-benzyl-ether-of hydroquinone, MBEH (in rubber).

QUESTIONS

1. Hyperpigmentation is not seen in:
a. Addison's disease
b. Cushing's disease
c. Graves's disease
d. Hypothyroidism

2. Hyperpigmented lesions are seen in:
a. Pityriasis alba
b. Melanoma
c. Nevus anemicus
d. Dyskeratosis congenita
e. Lichen planus

3. Which of the following is/are not the cause of hypopigmentation?
a. Leprosy
b. Pinta
c. Syphilis
d. Fixed drug eruption
e. Pityriasis versicolor

4. Hypopigmentation is/are seen in:
a. Vitiligo
b. Pityriasis versicolor
c. Lichen planus
d. Melasma
e. Scleroderma

5. Hypopigmented patches can be seen in:
a. Becker's nevus
b. Freckles
c. Nevus of Ito
d. Nevus of Ota
e. Nevus anemicus

6. Hypo-depigmented lesion seen in:
a. Nevus of Ito
b. Nevus depigmentosus
c. Nevus of Ota
d. Nevus anemicus
e. Freckles

7. A newborn child presents with solitary white well-defined hypopigmented patch on his left thigh. Diagnosis is:

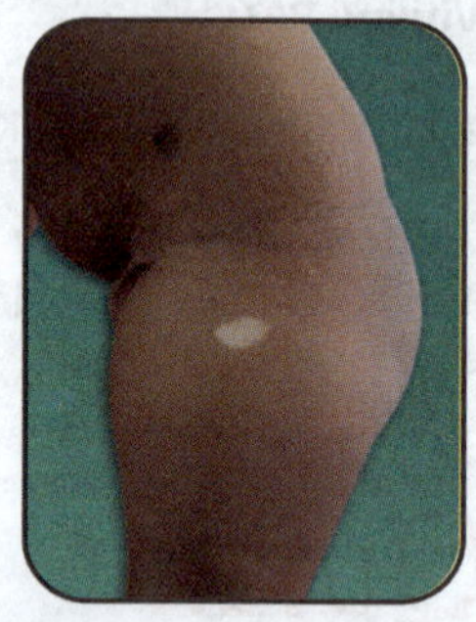

a. Piebaldism
b. Albinism
c. Nevus achromicus
d. Acral vitiligo

8. True about vitiligo are all *except*:
a. Genetic predisposition is known
b. Leucotrichia is associated with good prognosis
c. PUVA is used for treatment
d. Topical steroids give good results

9. An increased incidence of vitiligo is found in:
a. Psoriasis
b. Nutritional deficiency
c. Old age
d. Diabetes mellitus

10. In a patch of vitiligo:
a. Melanin synthesis is inhibited
b. Melanosomes are absent
c. Melanocytes are absent
d. Melanocytes are reduced

11. Psoralen is used in the treatment of:
a. Pemphigus b. Vitiligo
c. Pityriasis alba d. Ichthyosis

12. For vitiligo vulgaris, best treatment is:
a. PUVA b. Steroids
c. Coaltar d. All

13. Skin pigmentation is caused by all *except*:
a. Monobenzyl ether of hydroquinone
b. Dactinomycin
c. Cyclophosphamide
d. Busulphan

14. Rain drop pigmentation is seen in:
a. Chronic lead poisoning
b. Chronic arsenic poisoning
c. Chronic mercury poisoning
d. All of the above

15. State like discoloration of the skin is caused by all these drugs *except*:
a. Chlorpromazine
b. Minocycline
c. Amiodarone
d. Thiacetazone

16. Chronic arsenic poisoning causes all *except*:
a. Rain drop pigmentation
b. Basal cell carcinoma
c. Hirsutism
d. Palmar hyperkeratosis
e. Anemia

17. All of the following are pre-malignant lesions *except*:
a. Giant hairy nevus b. Rhinophyma
c. Actinic keratosis d. Bowen's disease

18. Which of the following is untrue regarding piebaldism?
a. Autosomal dominant condition
b. Amelanotic skin associated with a white forelock
c. Islands of normal or hypermelanotic skin
d. Usually improves with age

19. Hypopigmented lesions are seen in:
a. Melasma
b. Pityriasis alba
c. Lichen planus pigmentosus
d. Urticaria pigmentosa

20. Hypopigmented patches presents in:
a. Nevus of Ota b. Nevus of Ito
c. Nevus anemicus d. Becker's nevus

21. Commonest type of vitiligo:
a. Vulgaris b. Segmental
c. Acrofacial d. Facial

22. Most common endocrine disturbance associated with vitiligo is:
a. Addison's disease
b. Thyroid disease
c. Diabetes insipidus
d. Diabetes mellitus

23. A female has hypopigmented lesion on center of forehead. Agent responsible is:

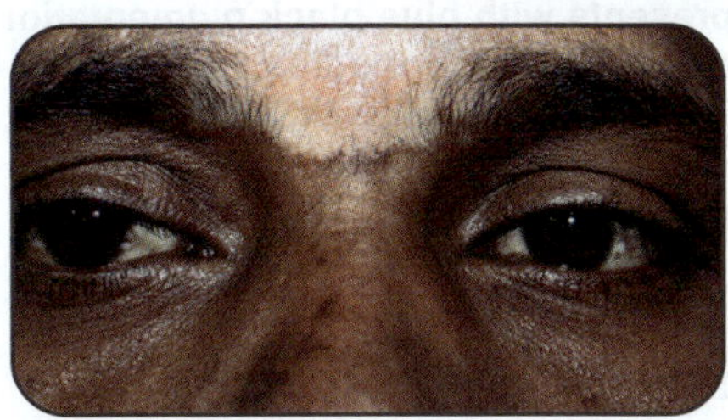

a. Hydroquinone
b. Ether metabolite of hydroquinone
c. Para tertiary butyl catechol
d. Para tertiary butyl phenol

24. A 23-year-old lady develops brown macular lesions over bridge of nose and cheeks following exposure to light. The probable diagnosis is:
a. Chloasma
b. Rosacea
c. Systemic lupus erythematosus
d. Photodermatitis

25. A child had hyperpigmented patch with hair on cheek since birth. The diagnosis is: *(AIIMS May 2017)*

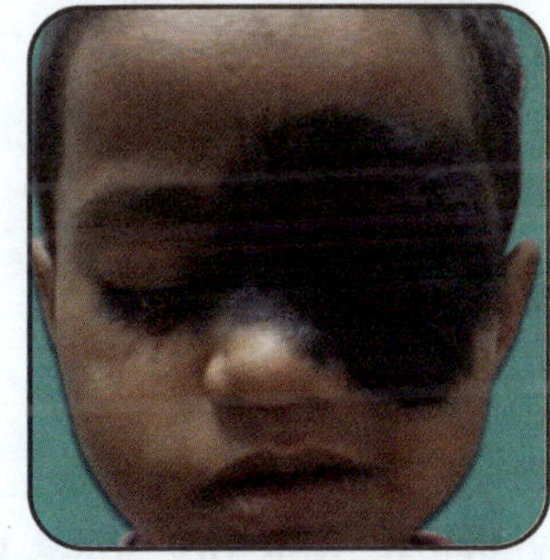

a. Congenital melanocytic nevus
b. Verrucous epidermal nevus
c. Lentigine
d. Melanoacanthoma

26. Diffuse form of hyperpigmentation is seen in:
a. Vitamin B_{12} deficiency
b. Ectopic ACTH secretion
c. Whipple's disease
d. All of the above

27. A 17-year-old girl with acne has been taking a drug for the last 2 years. She now presents with blue black pigmentation of nails. The likely medication causing the above pigmentation is:

a. Tetracycline b. Minocycline
c. Doxycycline d. Azithromycin

28. Topical azelaic acid is used in:

a. Hyperpigmentary disorders
b. Dermatophyte infections
c. Vitiligo
d. Mixed infections

29. Hyperpigmentation in HIV patients is due to:

a. Adrenalin
b. MSH
c. Interferon alpha
d. Interferon beta

30. A young female presents with blue macules on forehead and ocular macules. The diagnosis is: *(AIIMS May 15)*

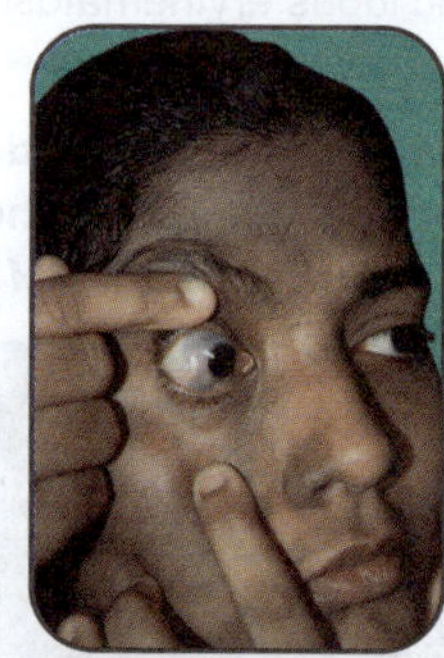

a. Mongolian spot
b. Nevus of Ota
c. Nevus of Ito
d. Becker's nevus

31. A lady comes with two white patches over the neck and chin associated with leucotrichia. The diagnosis is: *(AIIMS May 15)*

a. Segmental vitiligo
b. Acne vulgaris
c. Focal vitiligo
d. Piebaldism

32. A 30-year-old with depigmented patches on the medial aspect foot with feathery margin. The rest of the physical examination is normal. Which of the following drug should not be used in the treatment of this patient? *(AIIMS Nov 15)*

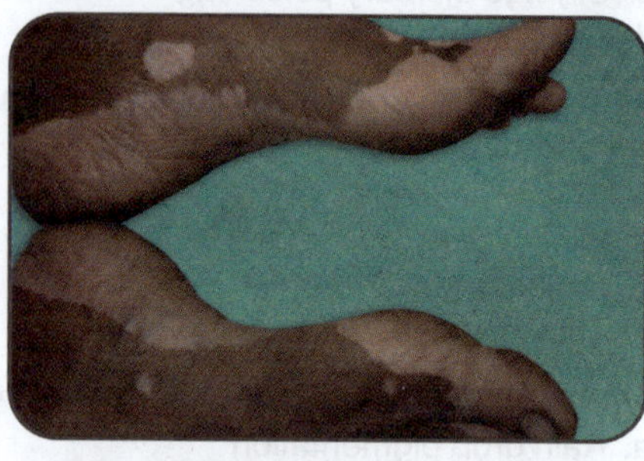

a. Topical clobetasol
b. Topical tretinoin
c. Topical tacrolimus
d. Topical methoxsalen

33. A 40-year-old lady with brown patches on her skin (chin, cheeks, forehead). She's not on any regular medication except birth control pills. She has observed that it has increased after 1st delivery and also after the 2nd delivery. Thyroid function test is normal. Which statement is correct?

a. It's unrelated to OCPs
b. It may fade away with time
c. It might exacerbate with next pregnancy
d. Need other endocrinal evaluation tests

34. Vitiligo is associated with all *except*:

a. Addison's disease
b. Autoimmune polyglandular syndrome
c. Pernicious anemia
d. Crohn's disease

35. Vitiligo is associated with all of the following *except*:

a. Addison's disease
b. Iron deficiency anemia
c. Rheumatoid arthritis
d. Thyrotoxicosis
e. Diabetes mellitus

36. Most common endocrine disturbance associated with vitiligo is:

a. Addison's disease
b. Thyroid disease
c. Diabetes insipidus
d. Diabetes mellitus

37. A 15 cm hyperpigmented macule on an adolescent male undergoes changes such as coarseness, growth of hair, acne. Diagnosis is:

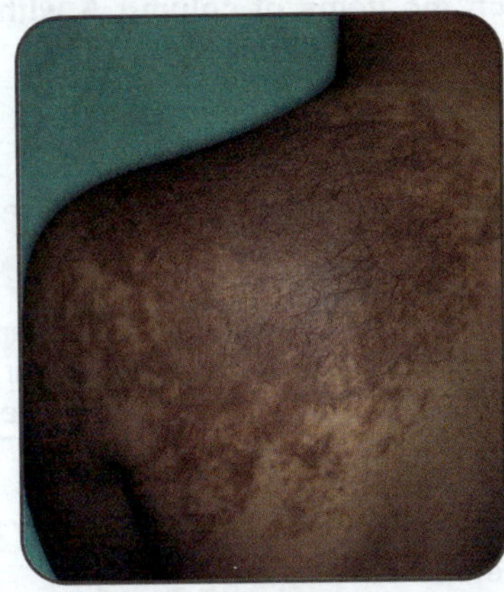

a. Melanocytic nevus
b. Becker's nevus
c. Sebaceous nevus
d. Comedo nevus

38. In nevus of Ota, melanocyte proliferation is found in which part of dermis?

a. Upper to mid dermis
b. Deep dermis
c. Subcutaneous fat
d. Epidermis

39. Which is not a nevus of melanocytes?

a. Becker's nevus b. Nevus of Ota
c. Nevus of Ito d. Mongolian spot

40. Mongolian spots in newborn have their color due to defect in migration of melanocytes from neural crest. This occurs at:

a. Level of neural crest
b. High dermal
c. Low dermal
d. Mid dermal level

41. You diagnose a patient with vitiligo based on history, physical examination and Wood's lamp exam. Which of the following test is also warranted?

a. Full thyroid studies
b. HIV testing
c. HbA1c
d. ANA

42. Malignant transformation to melanoma is common in:

a. Dermal nevus b. Junctional nevus
c. Congenital nevus d. Dysplastic nevus

43. Patient with a unilateral blue brown speckled patch involving her malar face. Biopsy shows increased number of elongated, dendritic melanocyte scattered throughout dermis and normal collagen pattern. Diagnosis is:

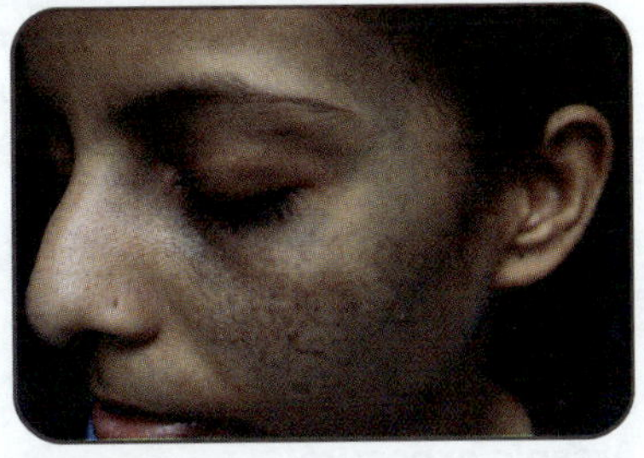

a. Nevus of Ota
b. Blue nevus
c. Hypomelanosis of Ito
d. Sturge-Weber syndrome

44. A female patient presents with the following lesions. The diagnosis is: *(NEET pattern)*

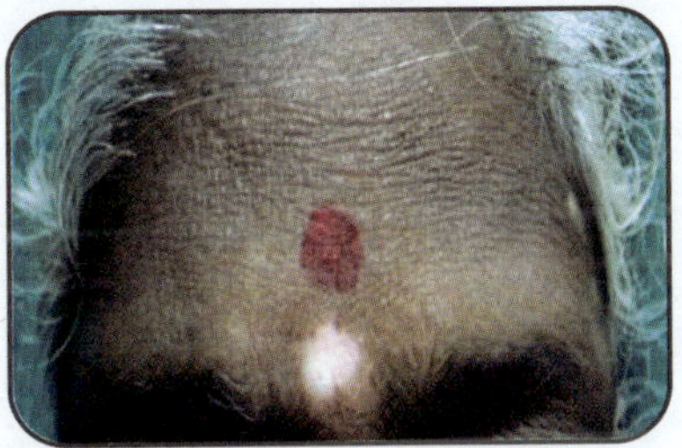

a. Piebaldism
b. Contact leukoderma
c. Vitiligo
d. Pityriasis versicolor

New Questions

45. Which of the following diseases are epidermal melanin diseases? Mention true/false:

a. Lichen planus b. Nevus of Ito
c. Becker's nevus d. Freckle
e. Mongolian spot

46. Assertion: Topical hydroquinone is effective in melasma
Reason: Hydroquinone is a tyrosinase inhibitor
a. Both Assertion and Reason are true and Reason is correct explanation of Assertion
b. Both Assertion and Reason are true but Reason is not correct explanation of Assertion
c. Assertion is true and Reason is false
d. Assertion is false and Reason is true
e. Both Assertion and Reason are false

47. Systemic causes of hyperpigmentation are:
a. Graves' disease
b. Chediak-Higashi syndrome
c. Arsenic exposure
d. Pregnancy
1. If a, b, c are correct
2. If a, c and d are correct
3. If c and d are correct
4. If all four (a, b, c, & d) are correct

48. Match the items of column A with best alternative in column B:

Column A	Column B
1. Mongolian spot	a. Nose area
2. Becker's nevus	b. Buccal mucosa
3. Nevus of ota	c. Cheek area
4. Peutz-Jeghers syndrome	d. Thigh area
	e. Lumbosacral area
	f. Shoulder, upper arms, chest area

49. Which type of vitiligo increases after initially growing? *(INICET May 2024)*
a. Segmental
b. Focal
c. Vitiligo vulgaris
d. Universal

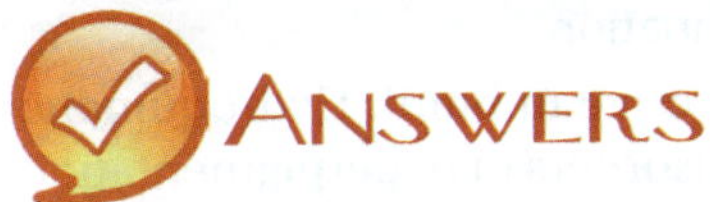

1. **Ans. (d) Hypothyroidism** *(Ref: Andrew's textbook, 11th edn, Page 491)*
2. **Ans. (b, d, e) Melanoma; Dyskeratosis congenita; Lichen planus**

   Dyskeratosis congenita is a rare congenital syndrome characterized by cutaneous poikiloderma (atrophy + hyperpigmentation + hypopigmentation), nail dystrophy, and premalignant leukoplakia.
3. **Ans. (d) Fixed drug eruption**

   The classical manifestation of pinta is depigmented macules resembling vitiligo. Secondary syphilis can cause depigmentation (syphilitic leucoderma).
4. **Ans. (a, b, e) Vitiligo; Pityriasis versicolor; Scleroderma**
5. **Ans. (e) Nevus anemicus** (See page 313 for explanation)
6. **Ans. (b, d) Nevus depigmentosus; Nevus anemicus**
7. **Ans. (c) Nevus achromicus**

   Acral vitiligo is ruled out as the onset in the question is at birth. Piebaldism will be a localized patch. Piebaldism will have a white forelock and areas of normal skin within the white patch. Albinism is not localized, but diffuse.
8. **Ans. (b) Leucotrichia is associated with good prognosis** (See page 315 for explanation)
9. **Ans. (d) Diabetes mellitus** (See page 318 for explanation)
10. **Ans. (c) Melanocytes are absent** (See page 318 for explanation)
11. **Ans. (b) Vitiligo** (See page 319 for explanation)
12. **Ans. (a) PUVA**

    Phototherapy (NB-UVB > PUVA) is the modality of choice for treatment.
13. **Ans. (a) Monobenzyl ether of hydroquinone**

    (Ref: Bolognia Dermatology, 3rd edn, Page 1056-57)
14. **Ans. (b) Chronic arsenic poisoning** (See page 312 for explanation)
15. **Ans. (d) Thiacetazone** *(Ref: Bolognia Dermatology, 3rd edn, Page 1056-57)*
16. **Ans. (c) Hirsutism** *(Ref: Bolognia Dermatology, 3rd edn, Page 1498)*

    Causes alopecia and not hirsutism.
17. **Ans. (b) Rhinophyma**
18. **Ans. (d) Usually improves with age** (See page 313 for explanation)
19. **Ans. (b) Pityriasis alba**
20. **Ans. (c) Nevus anemicus**
21. **Ans. (a) Vulgaris** (See page 316 for explanation)

    The word "vulgaris" means common.
22. **Ans. (b) Thyroid disease** (See page 318 for explanation)

23. Ans. (d) Para tertiary butyl phenol (See page 321 for explanation)

Here they are referring to contact leucoderma due to adhesive in bindi. Hydroquinone causes temporary hypopigmenting effect (hence used in disorders of hyperpigmentation like melasma). Ether metabolite of hydroquinone (mono benzyl ether of hydroquinone-MBEH) in rubber causes permanent depigmentation.

24. Ans. (a) Chloasma

Brown macular pigmentation on cheeks indicates melasma which would have been the best options. In its absence, chloasma would be the best answer (even though by definition, chloasma is melasma in pregnancy). Rosacea, SLE and photodermatitis would not be brown but erythematous.

25. Ans. (a) Congenital melanocytic nevus

Congenital melanocytic nevus is congenital. There is no verrucosity on the lesions neither is it along a blaschko line. Hence not B. Melanoacanthoma is very rare variant of seborrheic keratosis presenting as a deeply Pigmented proliferation of melanocytes and keratinocytes over the head, neck and trunk of elderly people. Hence answer is A.

26. Ans. (d) All of the above

Whipple's disease has malnutrition due to malabsorption. Due to consequent niacin deficiency (pellagra) or vitamin B_{12} deficiency, there is hyperpigmentation. MSH (melanocytes stimulating hormone) is a byproduct of ACTH synthesis, hence ectopic ACTH secretion increased pigmentation.

27. Ans. (b) Minocycline *(Ref: Bolognia Dermatology, 3rd edn, Page 1057)*

28. Ans. (a) Hyperpigmentary disorders

Topical azelaic acid is a tyrosinase inhibitor and is hence used for hyperpigmentary disorders. Since it has comedolytic and anti-inflammatory activity as well, it is also used in acne and rosacea.

29. Ans. (b) MSH *(Ref: Andrew's textbook, 11th edn, Page 846)*

30. Ans. (b) Nevus of Ota (See page 310 for explanation)

31. Ans. (a) Segmental vitiligo

32. Ans. (b) Topical tretinoin

Topical tretinoin is a keratolytic and comedolytic and would have no role in vitiligo. Methoxsalen is a psoralen used for PUVA therapy.

33. Ans. (c) It might exacerbate with next pregnancy

34. Ans. (d) Crohn's disease *(Ref: Andrew's Textbook, 11th edn, Page 855)*

35. Ans. (b) Iron deficiency anemia (See page 318 for explanation)

36. Ans. (b) Thyroid disease *(Ref: Rook's textbook of Dermatology, 9th edn, Page 88.35)*

37. Ans. (b) Becker's nevus (See page 308 for explanation)

38. Ans. (a) Upper to mid dermis (See page 310 for explanation)

39. Ans. (d) Mongolian spot

Nevus is a proliferation of melanocytes. As Mongolian spot does not have a proliferation of melanocytes on histopathology, it is not a nevus.

40. Ans. (c) Low dermal *(Ref: Mckee's Pathology of Skin, 4th edn, Page 1026-7, Rook's Textbook of Dermatology, 9th edn, Page 132.12, Bolognia Dermatology, 3rd edn, Page 1858)*

41. Ans. (a) Full thyroid studies

42. Ans. (d) Dysplastic nevus

43. Ans. (a) Nevus of Ota

44. Ans. (b) Contact leucoderma

This is bindi induced depigmentation. Why not: A: No white forelock, congenital onset, C: Will not be in this circular bindi area pattern, D: Hypopigmented, not depigmented

New Answers

45. Ans. a-False; b-False; c-True; d-True; e-False

46. Ans. (a) Both Assertion and Reason are true and Reason is correct explanation of Assertion

47. Ans. (2) If a, c and d are correct

Chediak-Higashi syndrome is associated with albinism

48. Ans. 1-e; 2-f; 3-c; 4-b

49. Ans. (a) Segmental

CHAPTER 14

Connective Tissue Disorders, Drug Eruptions

CONNECTIVE TISSUE DISORDERS

Lupus Erythematosus

- An autoimmune, connective tissue disease having circulating nonorgan-specific autoantibodies to cell nuclear antigens
- 2 forms—**Discoid lupus erythematosus** (DLE)—purely cutaneous features, **Systemic lupus erythematosus** (SLE)—widespread systemic features

Discoid Lupus Erythematosus (DLE)/Chronic Cutaneous LE (CCLE)

- **Most common type.** Well-defined, **red, discoid** ("Disc" = coin, "oid" = like) **plaques with an adherent scale and peripheral hyperpigmentation**. Later there is **atrophy and scarring** (Figs. 1A and B)
- Favored are the sun exposed sites—**scalp (most common site)**, bridge of the nose, malar areas, lower lip, and ears
- Scalp involvement typically causes **scarring alopecia. Dilated follicular openings**, many with hyperkeratosis may be seen on the scalp (Fig. 1D)
- There is an **adherent scale on the plaque** and when this is pulled-off, its undersurface shows hard pin-like structures attached. These hard plugs are in-fact areas of hyperkeratosis which had earlier occupied underlying dilated hair follicles and have been removed along with the removed scales. These attached plugs look like carpet tacks **(carpet tack or cat's tongue sign)** (Fig. 1C)

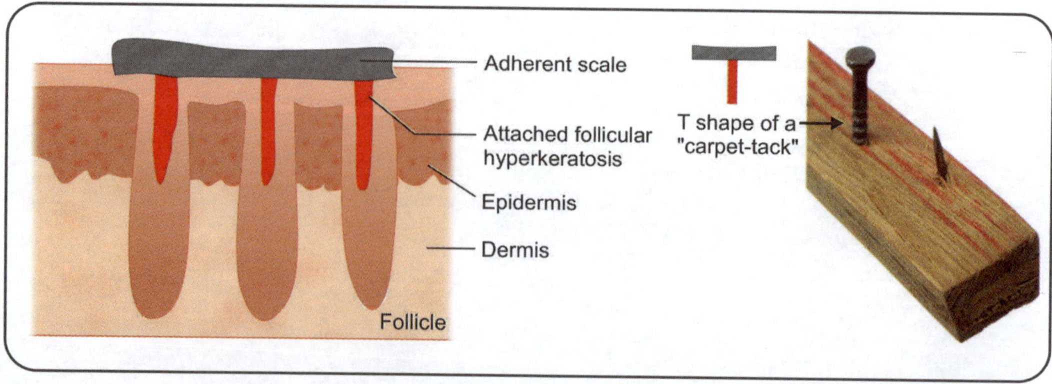

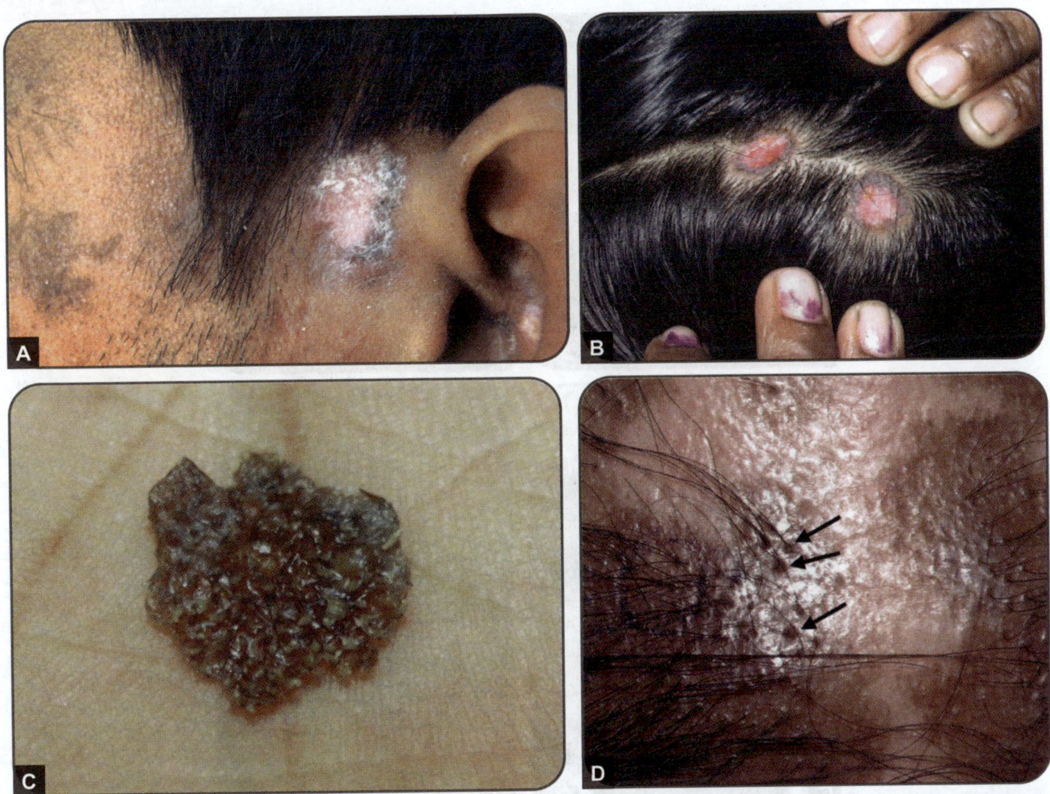

Figs. 1A to D: (A) Atrophic scaly plaque, peripheral hyperpigmentation, also note a smaller lesion in the concha; (B) Atrophic erythematous plaque, peripheral hyperpigmentation, scarring alopecia; (C) Undersurface of a detached carpet-tack scale in DLE showing keratotic plugs attached. These would have been occupying dilated follicles; (D) Dilated follicular orifices on scalp

Systemic Lupus Erythematosus

- Multisystem organ inflammation, e.g. skin, joints and vasculature with immunological abnormalities, more common in females.
- Cutaneous features:
  - **Malar/Butterfly rash—Classical erythematous rash, typically sparing the nasolabial folds. Rash is fixed** (Note the rash of rosacea is intermittent flushing and not constant as in SLE) (Figs. 2A and C).
    (Note: For chart on differentiating lesions on the face by their color, see Chapter 13)
  - Discoid rashes resembling DLE
  - Hair is fragile and thinned-out **(Lupus hairs-** Fig. 2D**). There may be scarring or non-scarring alopecia (Nonscarring > scarring). Note that DLE only causes scarring alopecia**
  - **Painless hard palatal**, buccal, tongue or nasal ulcers (Fig. 2B)
  - **Most common skin manifestation: Photosensitivity > Raynaud phenomenon> malar rash.**
- Most common cause of death in SLE—**Renal**

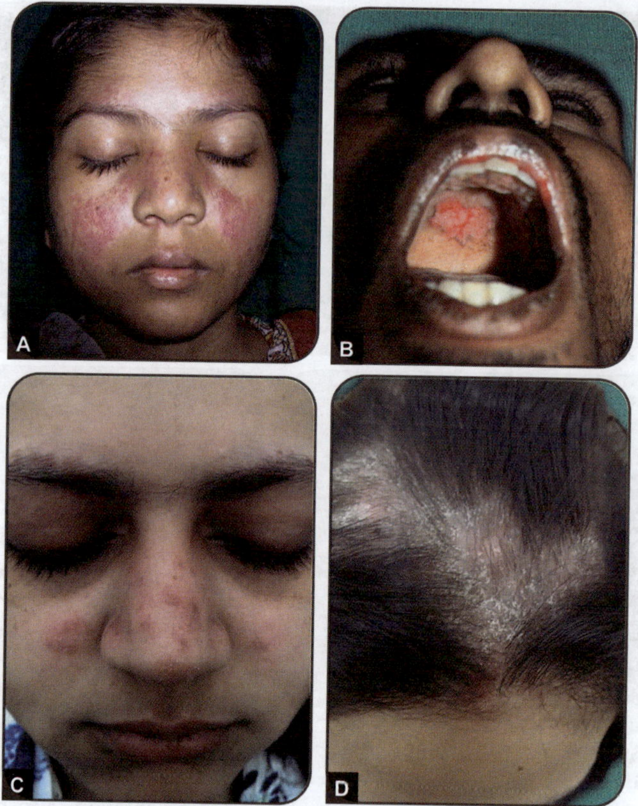

Figs. 2A to D: (A) Malar butterfly rash (note sparing of nasolabial folds); (B) Painless ulcers on hard palate; (C) Malar rash in SLE; (D) Same patient as in 2C- Short broken hairs on frontal scalp (lupus hairs)

- **Investigations:**
  - **Most sensitive antibody**—ANA
  - **Most specific antibody**—anti-Sm (but has low sensitivity—30%)
  - **Best test overall**—anti-dsDNA antibody as it is highly specific (though not as specific as anti-Sm), more sensitive than anti-Sm (60–70%) and also correlates with disease activity and lupus nephritis (anti-Sm does not correlate with disease activity)
  - **Marker of photosensitivity in SLE**—Anti-Ro antibody

Dermatomyositis

- Autoimmune disorder predominantly affecting **skin and proximal skeletal muscle**
- **Classic cutaneous signs**
  - **Heliotrope rash—An erythema with a purple tinge on upper eyelids is pathognomic.** This eyelid rash with eyelid edema often correlates with muscle disease activity (Fig. 3A)
  - **Shawl sign**—Fixed macular erythema on the "V" of the chest, across the shoulders and outer arms (shawl distribution) (Fig. 3B)
  - **Gottron's papule**—Inflammatory, flat-topped, **lichenoid (red-purple) papules** on PIP, DIP and MCP joints are pathognomic (Fig. 3C).

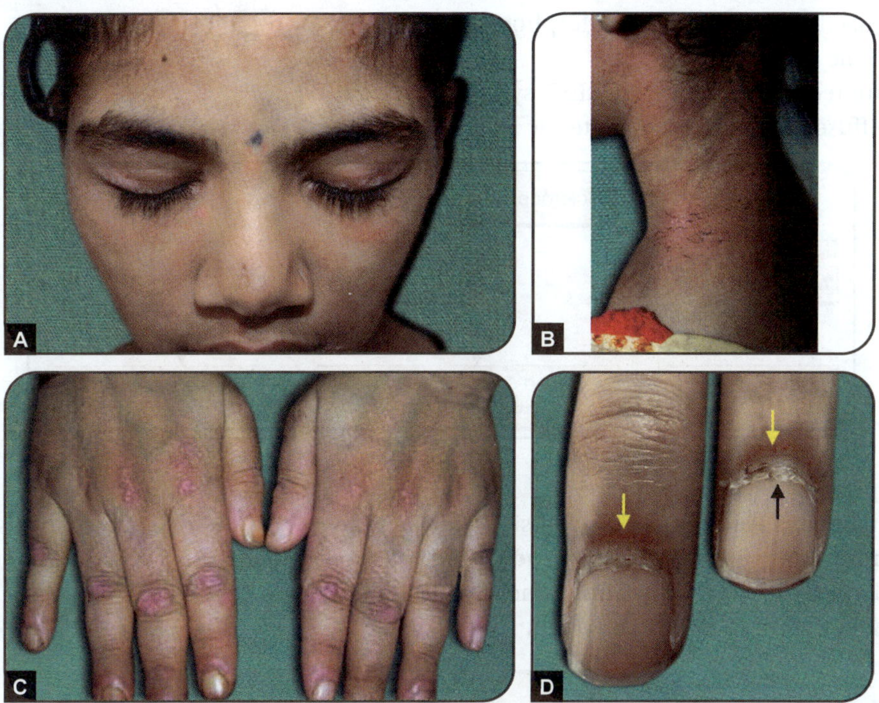

Figs. 3A to D: (A) Violaceous (lilac) erythema on eyelids; (B) Erythema across the shoulder (shawl sign); (C) Violaceous/Lilac-erythema on DIP, PIP and MCP joints; (D) Ragged cuticles (black arrow), nail fold telangiectasia (yellow arrow)

- **Nail fold changes-periungual erythema, dilated capillary loops in the proximal nail fold, damaged ("ragged") cuticle is typical (Fig. 3D)**
- **Gottron's sign**—Lichenoid (red-purple) macules (not papules) on PIP, DIP, MCP joints

  - **Investigations—Gottron's papule, heliotrope rash, shawl sign are associated with anti-Mi 2 antibodies** while **mechanics hand, myositis and interstitial lung disease are associated with anti-Jo-1 antibodies.**

Aid to Remember

- Heliotrope—is a pink-purple tint which is the color of the heliotrope flower. Hence, a purplish rash
- "Helio" also refers to the sun—hence remember it as a photosensitive rash.

Scleroderma

- Characterized by sclerosis or thickening of skin. **HALLMARK is a bound down or hide bound feel of skin which is difficult to pinch**
- Systemic features are common with internal organ fibrosis and associated vascular abnormality. **Raynaud phenomenon is typical** (phases of Raynaud phenomenon—Initial pallor, then cyanosis and finally erythema on digits after cold exposure)

- Localized cutaneous form—Morphoea
- Systemic form:
  - Limited systemic form (CREST syndrome)
  - Diffuse systemic form- Systemic sclerosis

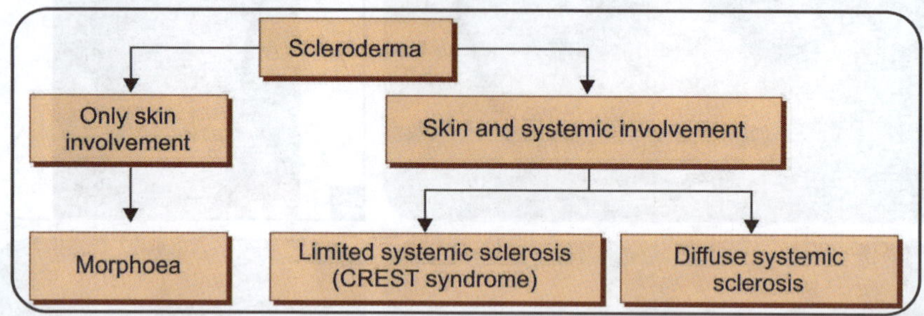

- **Morphoea:**
  - Cutaneous hide-bound sclerosis **(unpinchable)** without systemic involvement. Presents as **violaceous, hard (indurated) plaques**; which soon turn into ivory colored plaques, the surface is shiny, smooth and bound down (Fig. 4)
  - **Most common site is the trunk**

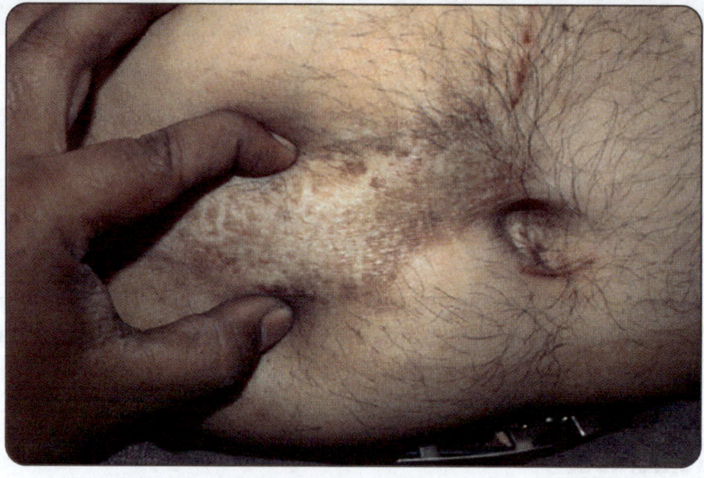

Fig. 4: Unpinchable, bound-down plaque on trunk

- **Diffuse systemic sclerosis (Diffuse SSc)**

  ARA criteria:

  1. **Major criterion**—Skin thickening proximal to the metacarpophalangeal joints (essential criteria).
  2. **At least two minor criteria** consisting of:
     a. Sclerodactyly—Skin thickening of finger with tapered fingers
     b. Digital pitted scarring—Pitted scars on tips of fingers
     c. Bilateral basal pulmonary fibrosis

Features	Diffuse SSc	Limited SSc (CREST syndrome)
Skin involvement	Diffuse involvement—Truncal, face, extremities	Limited acrally (hands, feet) and face
Raynaud phenomenon	**Short history** of Raynaud prior to onset of skin changes	**Long history** of Raynaud before skin disease
Organ involvement	• **Pulmonary fibrosis-most common cause of death** • Renal involvement • Diffuse GI disease • Myocardial involvement • Esophageal dysmotility	• Pulmonary hypertension • Calcinosis • Esophageal dysmotility
Nail-fold capillaries	Nail-fold capillary dilatation and **dropouts**	Only nail fold capillary dilatation without dropouts
Auto-antibodies	**Anti-topoisomerase-1 (anti-Scl-70) antibody +ve**	**Anticentromere (ACA) antibody +ve**

- Important cutaneous features of diffuse SSc

Head and neck	• Expression less face (**Mask-like**) (Fig. 5A) • **Beaked nose/pinched nose**—due to tight skin • Microstomia (purse string mouth/fish-hole mouth) (Fig. 5D) • Perioral radial folds (rhagades) (Fig. 5A) • **Salt and pepper pigmentary abnormality** (both hyper- and hypopigmentation alternatively) (Fig. 5C) • Difficulty in pulling down the lower eyelid (conjunctival sign)
Hands	• Raynaud phenomenon (Fig. 5F) • Sclerodactyly i.e. thin tapering fingers (Fig. 5C) • Loss of pulp of fingertips (Fingerpad sign) • Painful fingertip ulcers healing with pitted scars (Fig. 5B) • Nail fold telangiectasia (Fig. 5E) • Calcinosis is seen around joints

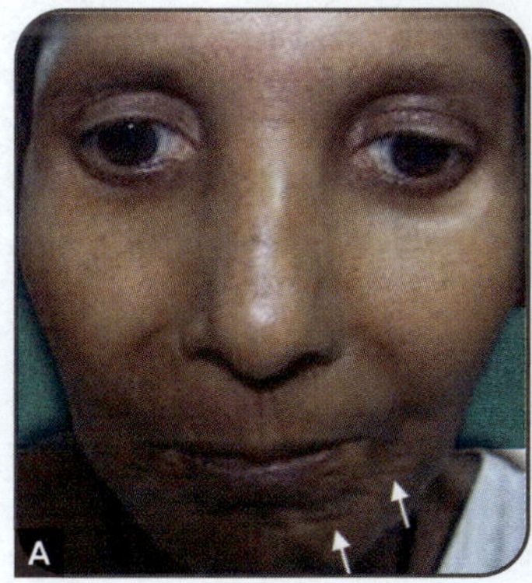

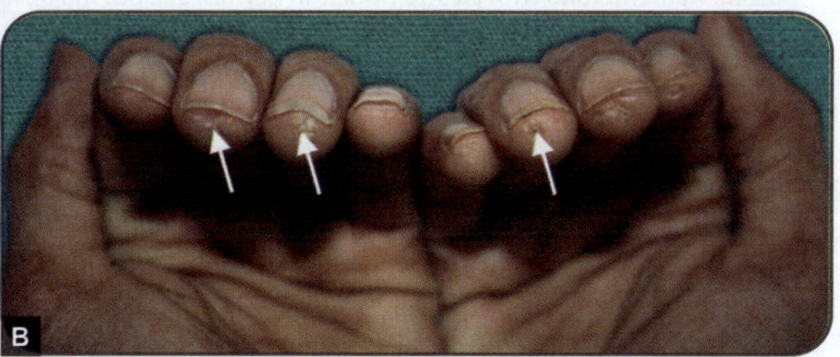

Figs. 5A and B

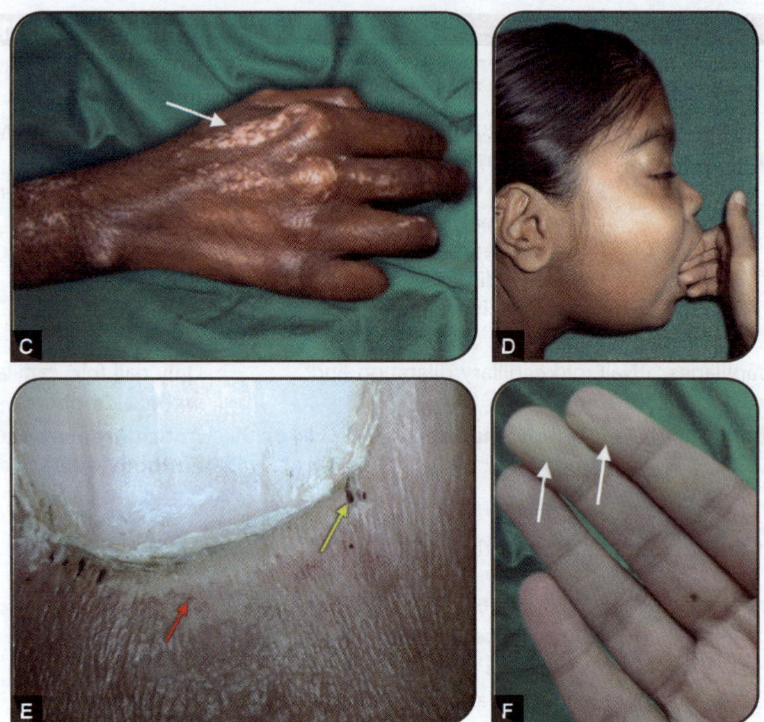

Figs. 5A to F: (A) Mask-like bound down skin on face. Note perioral radial folds—rhagades (white arrows); (B) Pitted finger—tip scars (white arrows); (C) Sclerosed hard-bound extremity, salt and pepper pigmentation on skin (white arrow) and amputated fingers due to digital necrosis (acro-osteolysis); (D) Microstomia; (E) Nail fold in diffuse SSc—Nail fold capillary dilatation (red arrow), hemorrhages (yellow arrow); (F) Pallor (white arrows) after cold exposure at the start of an attack of Raynaud phenomenon

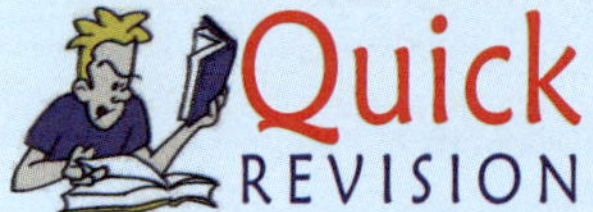

- Lupus erythematosus—DLE has discoid scaly plaques with scarring alopecia on scalp, face, etc. Scales have plugs attached to its surface (carpet-tac sign). Histopathology is interface dermatitis, thickened basement membrane with civatte bodies in dermis. SLE has malar, fixed erythema, photosensitivity (most common skin feature), palatal ulcers. It can cause scarring and non-scarring alopecia. Investigations: Most sensitive—ANA, most specific—Anti-Sm. Anti-dsDNA is used to monitor disease activity.
- Dermatomyositis—Heliotrope periorbital rash, shawl sign, Gottron's papule, nail fold telangiectasia, ragged cuticles, mechanic's hand, photosensitivity.
- Scleroderma—Hallmark is a skin which has a bound-down or hide bound feel which is difficult to pinch. Raynaud phenomenon is typical. Localized cutaneous form—morphoea. Systemic form—limited systemic form (CREST syndrome), diffuse systemic form—systemic sclerosis. Systemic sclerosis has skin thickening proximal to the metacarpophalangeal joints (essential criteria), sclerodactyly, digital pitted scarring and bilateral basal pulmonary fibrosis (minor criteria). Other features—Mask-like face, beaked nose, perioral rhagades, microstomia, salt and pepper pigmentation.

REACTIVE SKIN DISEASES

Erythema Multiforme (EM)

- Classical lesion is **"target lesion"**, also called as **"iris lesion"** and **"bull's eye lesion"**
- **Self-limited**, recurrent disease, each episode lasting 1–4 weeks
- Shows the classic "target" lesion with **three zones**—central dusky purpura; an edematous, pale middle zone; and peripheral erythema. The central area may be bullous (**bullous EM**) (Figs. 6 and 7).

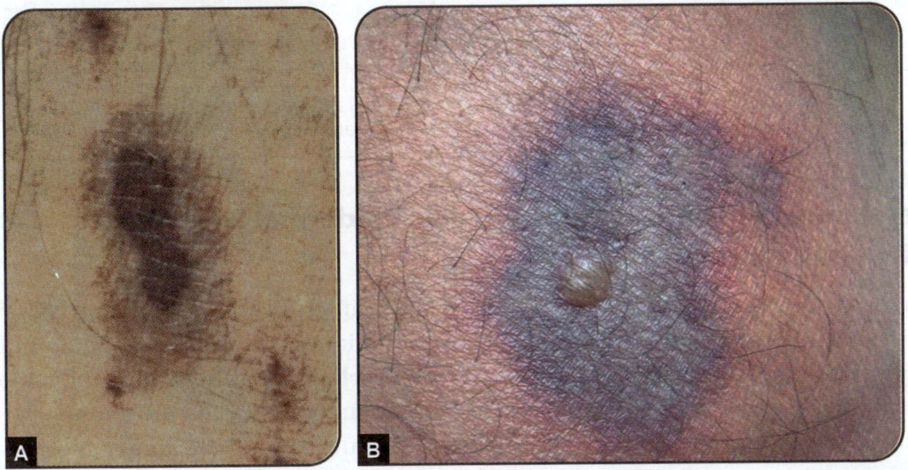

Figs. 6A and B: (A) Typical 3 zone target; (B) Bullous EM—blister in the central zone

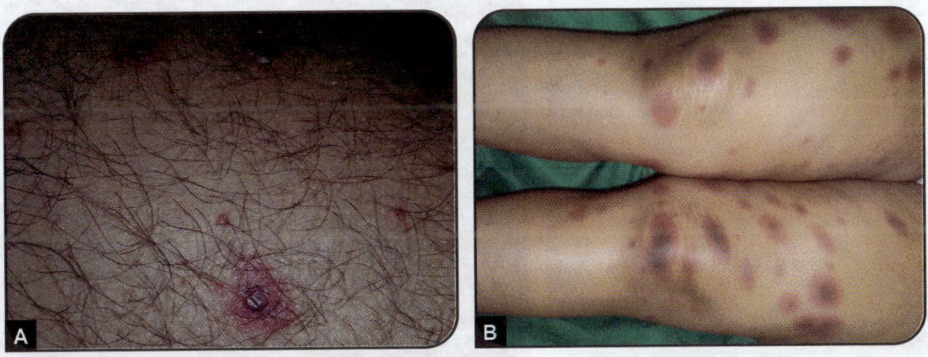

Figs. 7A and B: (A) Bullous EM—Blister in the centre of the EM lesion; (B) Targets on anterior thigh

- Site: **Acral** (palms, hands, elbows, legs, foot), sometimes face (acrofacial)
- Koebner's phenomenon may be seen
- **Etiology: Infections are the most common cause (Herpes simplex virus > mycoplasma)**. The so called "idiopathic" variety often shows HSV-DNA on PCR. **Drugs (antimalarials/sulphonamides) and Leukemia are rare causes**
- **Treatment**—Self resolving. Prevention of future HSV attacks by acyclovir prophylaxis will prevent herpes associated EM

- **Two types: EM Minor and EM major:**
  1. **EM Minor:** m/c type of EM. Few target lesions, no mucosal involvement
  2. **EM Major:** Similar to EM minor, but more extensive target lesions, fever and one mucosa (usually oral) gets involved.

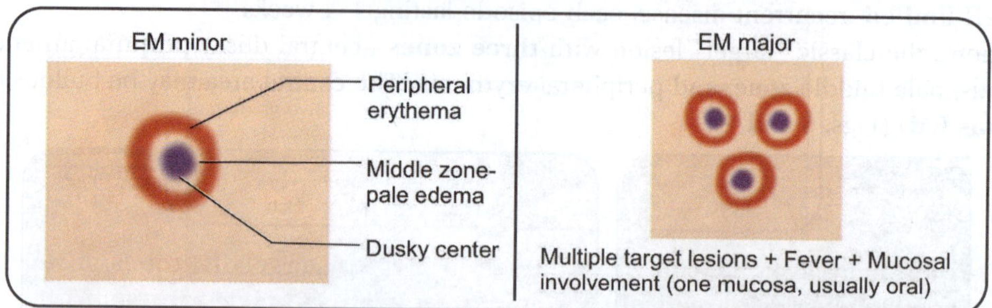

Stevens-Johnson Syndrome (SJS), Toxic Epidermal Necrolysis (Lyell's Syndrome)

- Usually **drug is the cause** (85% cases). Mycoplasma and HSV are less common causes (contrast with EM). Common drugs responsible are antibiotics (**sulpha group, penicillin**), nevirapine, **lamotrigine, NSAIDs (oxicam group), carbamazepine**, phenytoin, allopurinol
- Starts within 8 weeks (average 4 days–30 days) of initiation of the drug
- Instead of target (3 zones), **targetoid lesions** (2 zones-central duskiness and peripheral erythema) are seen (Figs. 8A and B)

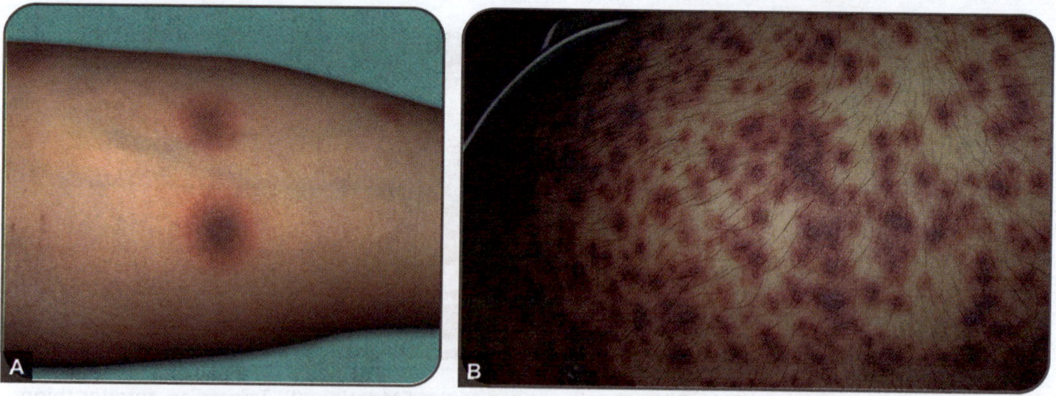

Figs. 8A and B: (A) Targetoid lesions (2 zones); (B) Multiple targetoid lesions (note central duskiness and peripheral erythema)

- **Three types—Stevens-Johnson syndrome, toxic epidermal necrolysis (TEN) and SJS-TEN overlap cases**
  - **SJS**—<10% body surface area (BSA) involved, **SJS-TEN overlap cases**-10-30% BSA involvement , and **TEN** >30% BSA involvement
- Skin lesions + mucosal involvement + systemic features (fever, hepatitis, eosinophilia)

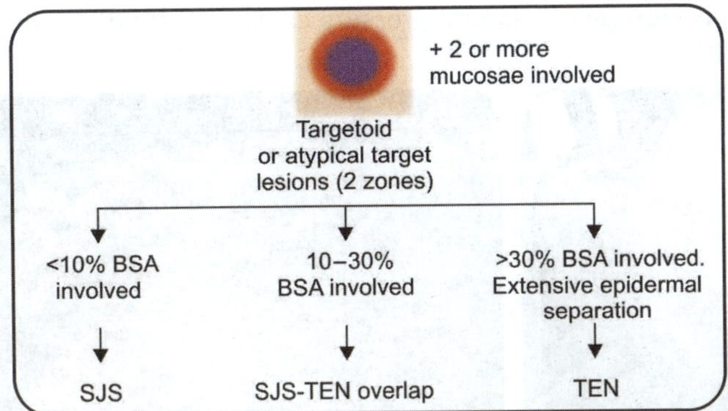

- **Skin lesions:** Dusky **macules with targetoid/atypical targets (2 zones, instead of 3 zones as in classical targets of EM), epidermal necrosis and separation from underlying dermis** (SJS causes less and TEN more separation). Skin is usually tender to touch and is dusky in color (Figs. 9A and B)
- **Prominent mucosal involvement (2 or more mucosal areas involved—oral> eye> genital)** (Figs. 10A and B).

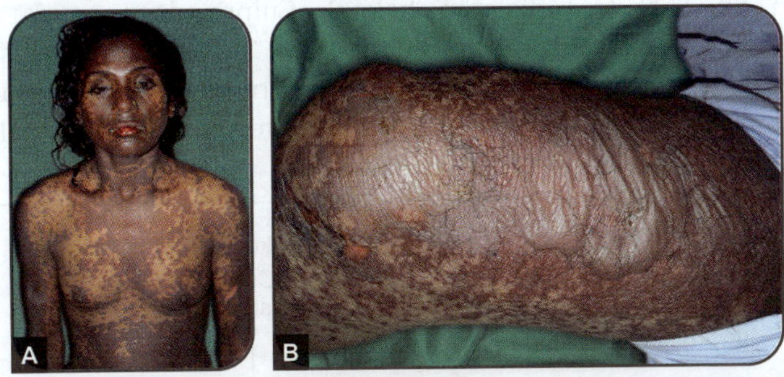

Figs. 9A and B: (A) Severe mucosal involvement (eye, oral) with dusky macules; (B) Dusky macules with flaccid blister formation

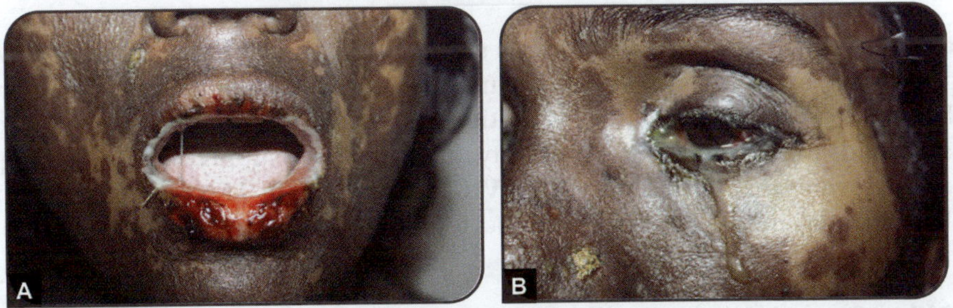

Figs. 10A and B: (A) Severe oral involvement with hemorrhagic red-black crusts on lips; (B) Severe eye involvement—can lead to vision loss

- In TEN—"Toxic" refers to toxemia which is responsible for systemic symptoms. The term "necrolysis" was obtained by combining the key clinical feature "necrosis + epidermolysis = necrolysis"

- **Positive Nikolsky sign** (gentle lateral pressure causes epidermis to slide over the dermis) (Figs. 11A and B).

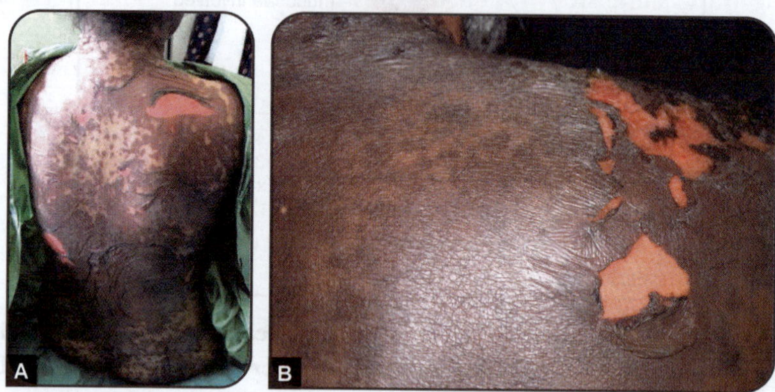

Figs. 11A and B: (A) Dusky macules in TEN. Note the wrinkling and movement of epidermis over dermis, leading to separation and erosions; (B) Positive Nikolsky sign—The raw lesion was due to lateral tangential pressure with finger separating the necrotic epidermis from the dermis

- Pathology in SJS/TEN (*see* diagram below): Culprit drug enters circulation (1). Keratinocytes express Fas receptor on their surface. This receptor binds to the drug (2) triggering keratinocyte destruction (3) which in turn leads to epidermal necrosis and separation from underlying dermis. CD8 lymphocytes in the dermis below the affected keratinocyte also contribute to the destruction (4)

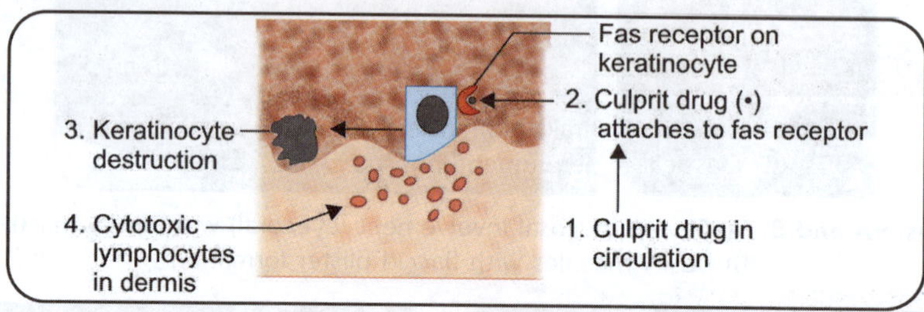

- **Treatment**—In **SJS, high dose systemic steroids** introduced early is the DOC. Another drug is **cyclosporine** (acts as a dermal lymphocyte inhibitor). If the patient progresses to TEN, there is extensive epidermal separation and raw lesions increasing the risk of infections. Steroids would cause more mortality due to immunosuppression related sepsis and hence, **intravenous immunoglobulin (IVIG) is the DOC in TEN** which acts by blocking the Fas receptor and helps stop keratinocyte destruction.

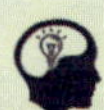

Aid to Remember

Drugs causing SJS/TEN
"Steven can soap himself"
Steven: **Stevens**-Johnson syndrome
Ca: **Ca**rbamazepine
S: **S**ulpha
O: **O**xicam NSAIDs
A: **A**llopurinol
P: **P**enicillin, **p**henytoin

Fixed Drug Eruption (FDE)

- As they **recur at the same site with each exposure to the medication**, their site on the skin is "fixed"
- Starts as red patches (Fig. 12A), may soon developing blisters (bullous FDE). **Classically, hyperpigmentation occurs after the lesion heals** (Fig. 12B)
- **On genitals, they often cause recurrent blisters and ulcers and they heal with hyperpigmentation** (Fig. 12C, Figs. 13A and B) **(Note—Similar presentation occurs in herpes genitalis but does not heal with hyperpigmentation)**
- **NSAIDs (m/c cause)**, cotrimoxazole, tetracyclines, penicillin, metronidazole, paracetamol are common causes
- Most common site—**Lips, genitals.**

High Yield Points

- If cotrimoxazole mentioned in the MCQ—mark genitals as the m/c site, if NSAIDs mentioned—mark lips as m/c site. If no drug mentioned in MCQ, mark genitals
- Pick-up word in MCQs on FDE—"recurrent blisters/ulcers on genitals healing with hyperpigmentation."

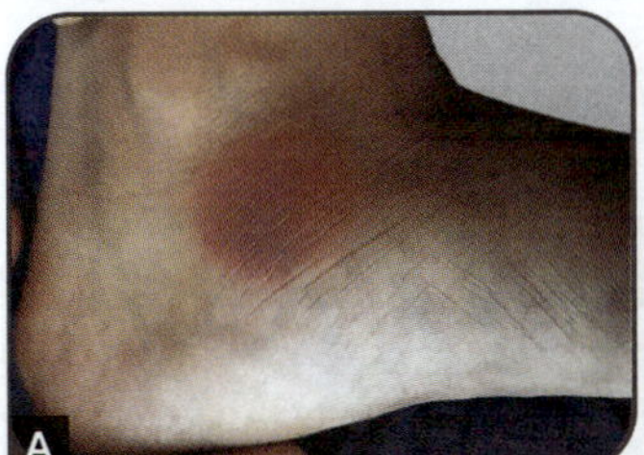

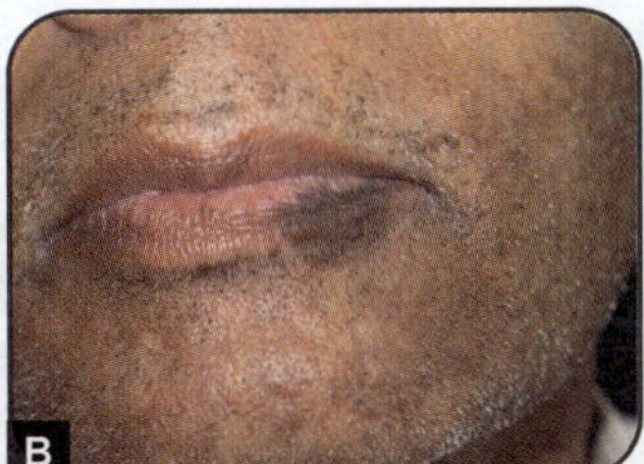

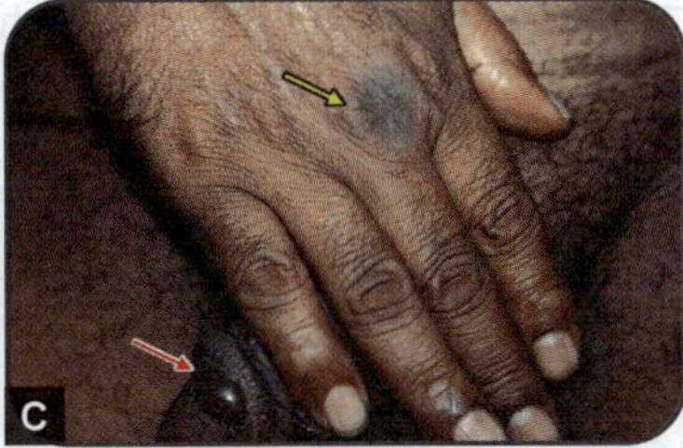

Figs. 12A to C: (A) Erythematous patch after intake of metronidazole for diarrhoea; (B) Hyperpigmentation on lips after taking NSAIDs; (C) Classical hyperpigmentation patch on skin (yellow arrow) with genital blister (red arrow)—will recur at same site with re-exposure to the drug

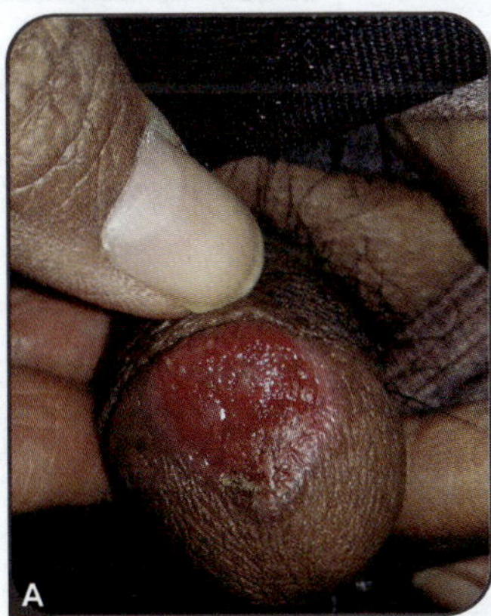

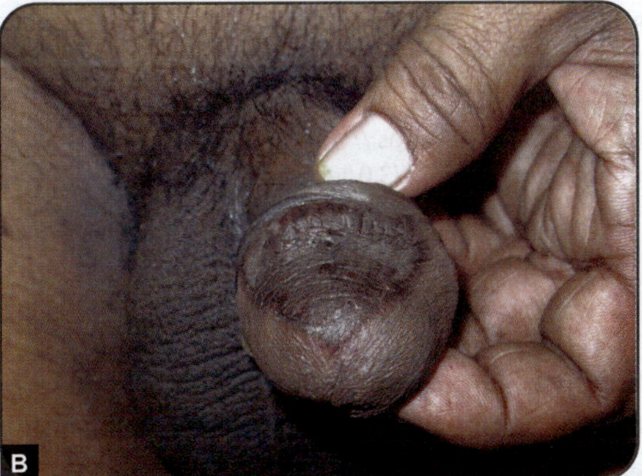

Figs. 13A and B: (A) Recurrent erosions on glans; (B) Erosions typically healing with hyperpigmentation

DRESS Syndrome (Drug Hypersensitivity Syndrome)

- **DRESS** = **D**rug **R**ash with **E**osinophilia and **S**ystemic **S**ymptoms
- It is an adverse drug reaction commonly associated with the aromatic antiepileptic drugs (AED), viz., phenytoin, carbamazepine, phenobarbital, lamotrigine, etc.
- Also was later described for other drugs like minocycline, dapsone, nevirapine, etc.
- Typical features—Rash developing > 3 weeks after start of drug ingestion, fever, multiorgan involvement (lymphadenopathy, hepatitis, myocarditis, nephritis, pneumonitis) and eosinophilia.

Drug Induced Pigmentation

See Chapter 13.

Erythema Nodosum (EN)

- Most common form of panniculitis (inflammation of panniculus, i.e. subcutaneous fat)
- Presents as **erythematous, tender, nodules and plaques, typically located on the shins. These do not ulcerate. Overlying skin is red and shiny (Figs. 14A to C)**
- Acute onset, patients often have **fever and joint pains**
- A **hypersensitivity response** to various triggers.

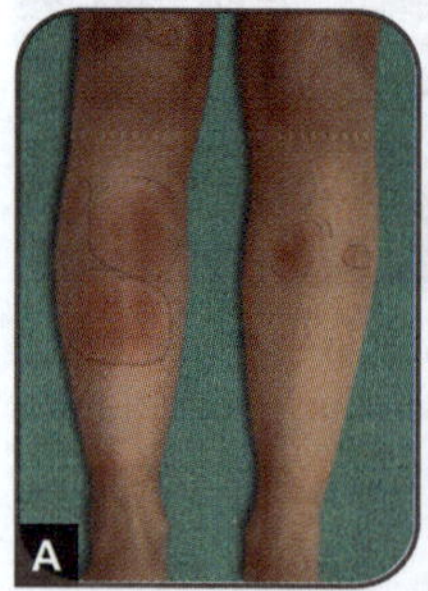

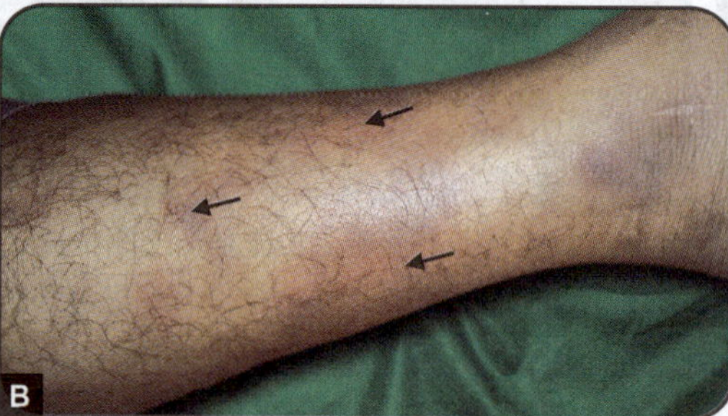

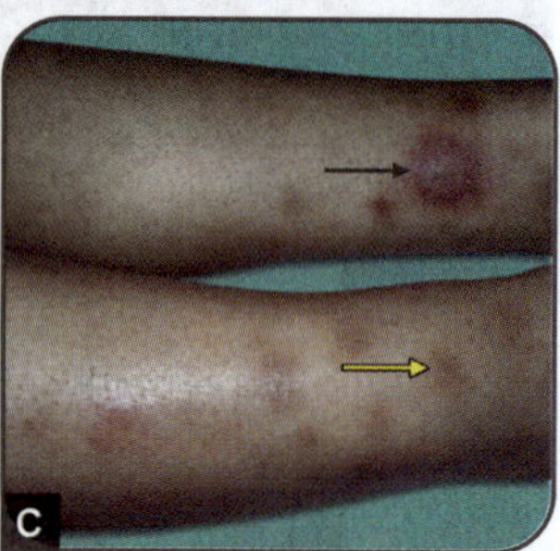

Figs. 14A to C: (A) Erythematous tender nodules on shin; (B) Close-up of dusky nodules (lesions are often more felt than seen); (C) Erythema nodosum—Red nodules (black arrow), few subsiding with bruise-like pigmentation (yellow arrow)

Source: James Heilman (https://commons.wikimedia.org/wiki/File:ENlegs.JPG), "ENlegs", https://creativecommons.org/licenses/by-sa/3.0/legalcode

- **Etiology:**
  - Idiopathic—Most common
  - Infections—**Streptococcus** (m/c infection). Others are Bacterial gastroenteritis (Yersinia, Salmonella, campylobacter) viral upper respiratory tract infections
  - Drugs (OCPs, sulfonamides, penicillin, bromides, iodides)
  - Sarcoidosis
  - Inflammatory bowel disease-IBD (Crohn's disease > ulcerative colitis)
  - Neutrophilic dermatoses (Behçet's disease, Sweet's syndrome)

- Rheumatoid arthritis
- Pregnancy
- Malignancy (acute myelogenous leukemia, Hodgkin's disease).

- **Histopathology**: Septal panniculitis with neutrophils and histiocytes, no vasculitis.
- **Treatment:**
  - Most are self-resolving in 3–4 weeks
  - Bed rest, NSAIDs, potassium iodide, corticosteroids, dapsone—for idiopathic EN
  - Colchicine for EN caused by Behcet's disease.

Aid to Remember

Causes of Erythema nodosum—"NODOSUM"

NO: **No** cause, **N**eutrophilic dermatoses (Behçet's disease, Sweet's syndrome)
D: **D**rugs (iodides, bromides, sulfonamides)
O: **O**CP
S: **S**arcoidosis
U: **U**lcerative colitis (also Crohn's)
M: **M**icrobes, **M**aternity, and **M**alignancy

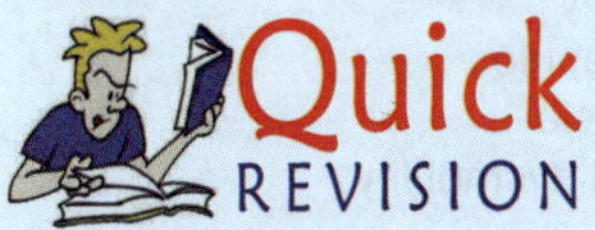

- Erythema multiforme—Target lesions (3 zones). HSV is the most common cause. Drugs-rare cause. Self-resolving, often recurrent. 2 types—EM minor, EM major
- SJS/TEN—Targetoid lesions (2 zones) + mucosal involvement + systemic features. Drug is the most common cause. HSV is not a common cause (contrast with EM). Common drugs responsible are antibiotics (sulpha group, penicillin), nevirapine, lamotrigine, NSAIDs (oxicam group), carbamazepine, phenytoin, allopurinol. SJS <10% body surface area (BSA) involved, SJS-TEN overlap cases-10–30% BSA involvement, and TEN >30% BSA involvement. Positive Nikolsky sign. Treatment (DOC): SJS-Steroids. TEN-IVIG
- Fixed drug eruption—Typically hyperpigmentation recurs at the same site on re-exposure to the drug. Common sites—lips, genitals. On genitals-recurrent blisters, erosions and ulcers healing with hyperpigmentation (contrast with herpes genitalis). NSAIDs (m/c cause), cotrimoxazole, tetracyclines are the top 3 causes of FDE
- DRESS syndrome—Drug rash with eosinophilia and systemic symptoms. Rash after 3 weeks, eosinophilia, fever, hepatitis, lymphadenopathy. Commonly with antiepileptics
- Erythema nodosum—Hypersensitivity to various triggers. Idiopathic (m/c), Streptococcus, TB, sarcoidosis, drugs (OCPs, sulfonamides, penicillin, bromides, iodides), IBD, pregnancy, Behcet's disease. Presents as red, tender nodules on shins. Histopathology: septal panniculitis without vasculitis.

QUESTIONS

1. All are manifestations of SLE *except:*
a. Discoid lesions
b. Butterfly rash
c. Photosensitivity
d. Sex ratio in nearly equal

2. Which of the following autoantibodies shows a strong association with Gottron's papule and heliotrope rash?
a. Anti-Mi-2
b. Anti Jo-1
c. Anti P155/P140
d. Anti Scl-70

3. A 40-year-old woman presented with a 8 months history of erythema and swelling of the periorbital region and papules and plaques on the dorsolateral aspect of forearms and knuckles with ragged cuticles. There was no muscle weakness. The most likely diagnosis is:
a. SLE
b. Dermatomyositis
c. Systemic sclerosis
d. Mixed connective tissue disorder

4. Shawl sign is seen in:
a. Neonatal lupus
b. Cutaneous scleroderma
c. SLE
d. Dermatomyositis

5. Gottron's papules are:
a. Erythematous papules on cheeks
b. Erythema seen over elbows and knees
c. Periorbital lesions
d. Violaceous papules over knuckles

6. "Gottron's papules" seen in dermatomyositis are:
a. Vesicular
b. Psoriatic
c. Lichenoid
d. Pustular

7. Heliotrope rash is seen in:
a. Psoriasis
b. Dermatomyositis
c. Discoid lupus erythematosus
d. Pemphigus

8. All are dermatological manifestations of dermatomyositis *except:*
a. Gottron's patches
b. Mechanic's hands
c. Periungual telangiectasia
d. Salmon rash

9. Localized scleroderma is:
a. Shagreen patch
b. Morphoea
c. Heliotrope erythema
d. Gottron's papule

10. All are cutaneous manifestations of systemic sclerosis, *except:*
a. Sclerodactyly
b. Gottron's papule
c. Telangiectasia
d. Esophageal dysmotility

11. Most specific antibody for SLE is:
a. SS-A (Ro)
b. Anti-Sm
c. Anti ds-DNA
d. Antihistone

12. Scarring alopecia not seen in:
a. SLE
b. DLE
c. Trichotillomania
d. Lichen planus

13. All are causes of erythroderma *except:*
a. Psoriasis
b. Seborrheic dermatitis
c. Cutaneous lymphoma
d. SLE

14. All are true regarding SLE *except:*
a. Anti-ds DNA correlates with disease activity
b. Anti-Sm correlates with disease activity
c. Anti-ribosomal antibody correlates with psychosis
d. None of the above

15. A 23-year-old lady develops pigmentation on cheeks with photosensitivity. Diagnosis is:

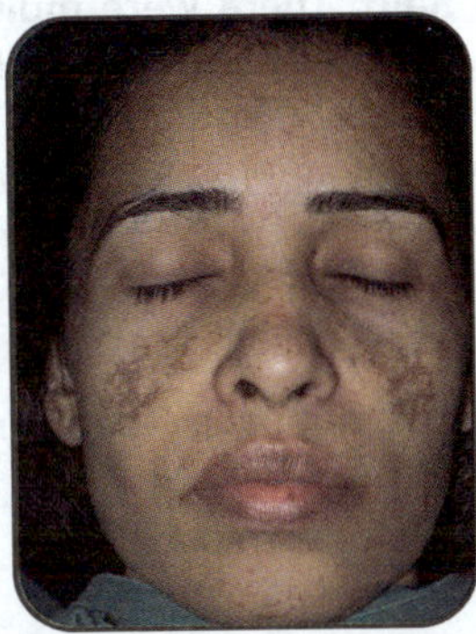

a. Melasma b. SLE
c. Photodermatitis d. Rosacea

16. Carpet tack sign is seen in:
a. Lupus vulgaris b. Lupus pernio
c. DLE d. SLE

17. All are classically seen in dermatomyositis *except:*
a. Calcinosis cutis b. Heliotrope rash
c. Shawl sign d. Gottron's rash

18. Toxic epidermal necrolysis involves body surface area:
a. <10% b. 10–20%
c. 20–30% d. >30%

19. The patient came with history of bullae involving >30% body surface area along with erosions of the lips and other mucosae for the past 7 days. What is the most probable underlying etiology? *(AIIMS May 2015)*

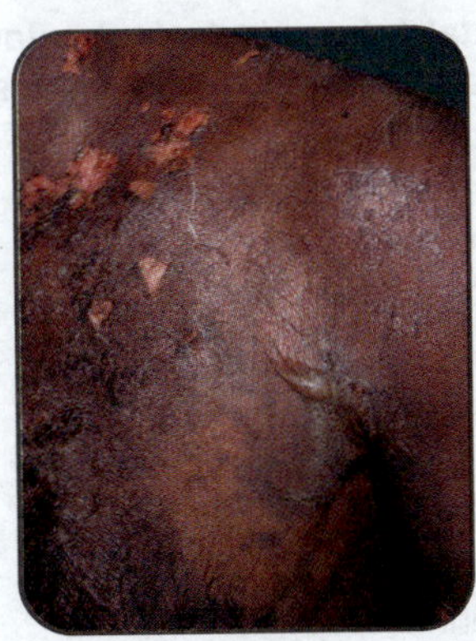

a. Drugs
b. Bacterial infection
c. Viral infection
d. Malignancy

20. A 20-year-old patient with neurocysticercosis develops generalized peeling of skin (except palms and soles) and severe oral and genital involvement starting after taking seizure medication. Diagnosis is: *(AIIMS Nov 2015)*
a. Stevens-Johnson syndrome
b. Toxic epidermal necrolysis
c. Fixed drug eruption
d. Pemphigus vulgaris

21. A patient is presenting with nonpruritic painless vesicles surrounded by an erythematous halo on face and hand. There is history of drug intake for fever 2 weeks back. The patient is suffering from:

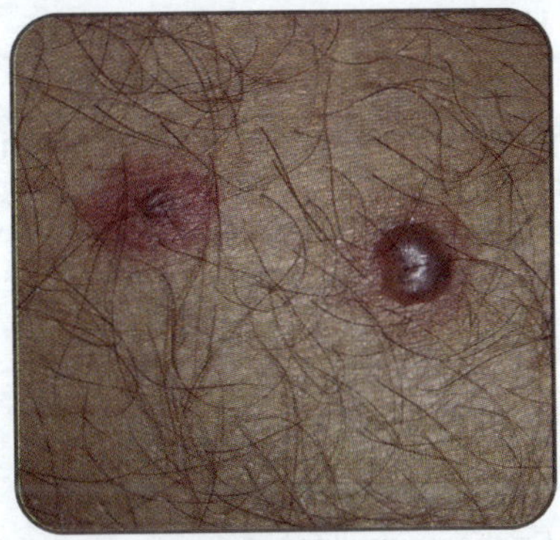

a. Bullous pemphigoid
b. Erythema multiforme
c. Herpes zoster
d. Dermatitis herpetiformis

22. Target lesion on acral areas is seen in:
a. Stevens-Johnson syndrome
b. Erythema multiforme
c. Toxic epidermal necrolysis
d. Lichen planus

23. Stevens-Johnson syndrome is caused by:
a. Herpes simplex
b. CMV
c. Chickenpox
d. Toxoplasma

24. A 27-year-old sexually active male develops a vesiculobullous lesion on the glans soon after taking tab paracetamol for fever. The lesion healed with hyperpigmentation. The most likely diagnosis is:

a. Behcet's syndrome
b. Herpes genitalis
c. Fixed drug eruption
d. Pemphigus vulgaris

25. Recurrent erythematous plaques on glans in a 19-year-old sexually active male which heals with residual hyperpigmentation is suggestive of?

a. Balanitis
b. Fixed drug eruption
c. Herpes gestationis
d. Chlamydia

26. All cause erythema multiforme *except:*

a. HSV b. Drugs
c. Idiopathic d. HPV

27. Erythema multiforme is most often related to:

a. Herpes-zoster infection
b. Herpes simplex infection
c. Molluscum contagiosum infection
d. Human papilloma virus infection

28. Target or iris lesion seen in:

a. Urticaria
b. Erythema multiforme
c. Scabies
d. Lichen planus

29. Regarding erythema multiforme all are true *except:*

a. No vesicles
b. Target lesions are seen
c. Involves face and neck regions
d. Sign of internal malignancy

30. What is not true about Erythema multiforme? *(NEET Pattern)*

a. Associated with Herpes simplex
b. Involves distal parts of extremities
c. No vesicle
d. Target lesions

31. A 60-year-old patient presented with several bullous lesions for the last 3 days; each bulla was surrounded by an erythematous halo. There were multiple target lesions. Patient also had oral erosions. The most likely diagnosis is:

a. Chickenpox
b. Herpes simplex
c. Herpes zoster
d. Erythema multiforme

32. All are true about erythema multiforme *except*:

a. Due to herpes simplex
b. Due to sulphonamide
c. Lesion are symmetrical
d. Mucous membrane is usually involved

33. Which of these statements is false for lesions of erythema nodosum?

a. They are considered as hypersensitivity reaction
b. The skin overlying the lesion is red, smooth and shiny
c. They are usually non tender
d. They can be associated with tuberculosis

34. Erythema nodosum is seen in all *except:*

a. SLE b. TB
c. Pregnancy d. Sulfonamide use

35. Erythema nodosum is seen in all of the following *except:*

a. SLE
b. TB
c. Pregnancy
d. Chronic pancreatitis

36. Neonatal fat necrosis (subcutaneous fat necrosis of newborn) resembles:

a. Erythema induratum
b. Post steroidal panniculitis
c. Lupus panniculitis
d. Lipodermatosclerosis

37. Erythema nodosum is seen in all of the following *except*:

a. Rheumatoid arthritis
b. Tuberculosis
c. Enteric fever
d. Aspirin therapy

38. The most common site of fixed drug eruption is:

a. Face
b. Extremity
c. Trunk
d. Glans penis

39. Drug causing fixed drug eruption:

a. Sulfonamide
b. Erythromycin
c. Aminoglycoside
d. None of the above

40. A 23-year-old male complains of recurrent lesions on glans penis. It always occurred at the same site and healed with hyperpigmentation. What is the most likely diagnosis?

a. Fixed drug eruption
b. Herpes
c. Candidal balanoposthitis
d. Behcet's disease

41. DRESS syndrome is associated with all *except:*

a. Drug reaction
b. Eosinophilia
c. Myocarditis
d. Encephalitis

42. Erythema nodosum is seen in:

a. Tuberculoid leprosy
b. Lepromatous leprosy
c. Rheumatic fever
d. Cutaneous TB

43. Erythema nodosum is due to all *except:*

a. Contraceptive pills
b. Barbiturates
c. Penicillin
d. Sulphonamides

44. A patient presented with rashes in >30 percentage skin with hemorrhagic crusting on lip. The cause would be:

a. Drugs *(AIIMS Nov 18)*
b. Virus
c. Malignancy
d. Bacterial infection

45. A 25-year-old male having fever and malaise since 2 weeks, arthritis of ankle joint and tender erythematous nodules over the shin. Diagnosis is:

a. Erythema nodosum
b. Hansen's disease
c. Weber-Christian disease
d. Nodular vasculitis

46. A young female presents with a history of fever and nodular lesion over the shin. Histopathology reveals foamy histiocytes with neutrophilic infiltration. There is no evidence of vasculitis. Most probable diagnosis is:

a. Sweet's syndrome
b. Erythema nodosum
c. Erythema nodosum leprosum
d. Behcet's syndrome

47. Erythema multiforme is associated with *(NEET pattern)*

a. Antimalarial drugs
b. Celiac disease
c. Idiopathic thrombocytopenic purpura
d. Leukemia

48. Pigmentation of nail is caused by all drugs *except:* *(AIIMS Nov 16)*

a. Cyclophosphamide
b. Chlorpromazine
c. Chloroquine
d. Amiodarone

49. Which is a correct combination?

a. Erythema infectiosum: TB
b. Erythema marginatum: Parvovirus
c. Erythema multiforme: Sarcoidosis
d. Erythema chronicum: Lyme's disease

50. Which of the following skin lesions is associated with nonhematological malignancy?

a. Erythema nodosum
b. Pyoderma gangrenosum
c. Acanthosis nigricans
d. Splinter hemorrhages

51. A patient comes with fever and joint pains. He was given NSAIDs. He subsequently developed a brown colored macular eruption on nose. The diagnosis is: *(AIIMS May 17, May 18)*

a. Dengue
b. Chikungunya
c. Fixed drug eruption
d. Melasma

52. **The following diseases can cause bullous lesions in skin *except*:**
a. Pemphigus
b. Impetigo
c. Toxic epidermal necrolysis
d. Pityriasis Rosea

53. **A male with erythematous patch over penis after taking an over-the-counter medicine. This would be associated with:**

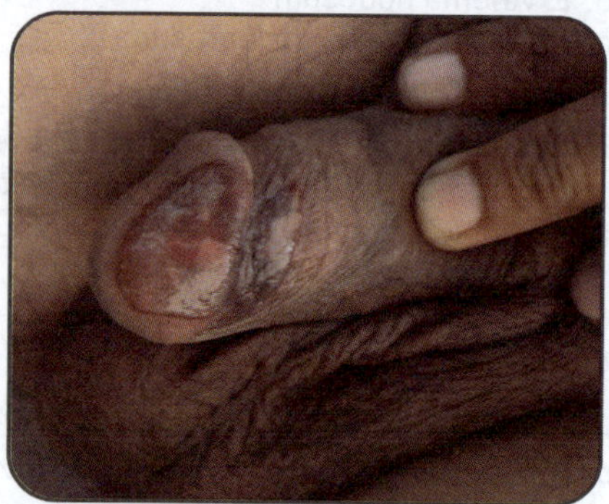

a. Azithromycin
b. Terbinafine
c. Doxycycline
d. Aceclofenac

New Questions

54. **Pick true/false statements regarding erythema multiforme:**
a. Most commonly due to herpes virus
b. Targetoid lesions are seen
c. Koebner's phenomenon is seen
d. Steroids are the drug of choice
e. Antimalarials can cause

55. **Arrange the following drugs on their risk for causing Stevens-Johnson syndrome (from most to least):**
1. Nevirapine
2. Macrolides
3. Paracetamol
4. Thiazides

a. 1, 2, 3, 4
b. 4, 1, 2, 3
c. 2, 1, 3, 4
d. 1, 2, 4, 3

56. **Assertion: Intravenous immunoglobulin is used in Toxic epidermal necrolysis Reason: CD4-T cells are involved in the pathogenesis of Toxic epidermal necrolysis**
a. Both Assertion and Reason are true and Reason is correct explanation of Assertion
b. Both Assertion and Reason are true but Reason is not correct explanation of Assertion
c. Assertion is true and Reason is false
d. Assertion is false and Reason is true
e. Both Assertion and Reason are false

57. **Photosensitivity is seen with:**
a. Lupus erythematosus
b. Scleroderma
c. Dermatomyositis
d. DRESS syndrome
1. If a, b, c are correct
2. If a and c are correct
3. If a and d are correct
4. If all four (a, b, c, & d) are correct

58. **Match the items of column A with best alternative in column B:**

Column A	Column B
1. Erythema nodosum	a. Nikolsky sign positive
2. Fixed drug eruption	b. Shin nodules
3. Stevens-Johnson syndrome	c. Dermal hyperpigmentation
4. Systemic sclerosis	d. Heliotrope rash
	e. Target lesion
	f. Salt and pepper pigmentation

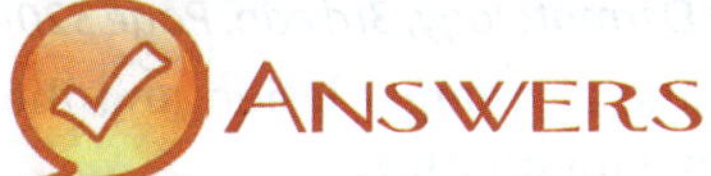

1. **Ans. (d) Sex ratio in nearly equal** (See page 332 for explanation)
2. **Ans. (a) Anti-Mi-2** *(Ref: Rook's Textbook of Dermatology, 9th edn, Page 53.11)*
3. **Ans. (b) Dermatomyositis** *(Ref: Rook's Textbook of Dermatology, 9th edn, Page 53.5)*

   Absent muscle involvement is seen in a subset of dermatomyositis with only skin involvement called as "clinically amyopathic dermatomyositis."
4. **Ans. (d) Dermatomyositis** *(Ref: Rook's Textbook of Dermatology, 9th edn, Page 53.5)*
5. **Ans. (d) Violaceous papules over knuckles** (See page 334 for explanation) *(Ref: Rook's Textbook of Dermatology, 9th edn, Page 53.6)*
6. **Ans. (c) Lichenoid** *(Ref: Rook's Textbook of Dermatology, 9th edn, Page 53.6)*
7. **Ans. (b) Dermatomyositis** *(Ref: Rook's Textbook of Dermatology, 9th edn, Page 53.5)*
8. **Ans. (d) Salmon rash** *(Ref: Rook's Textbook of Dermatology, 9th edn, Page 53.5-7)*
9. **Ans. (b) Morphoea** *(Ref: Andrew's Textbook, 11th edn, Page 169)*
10. **Ans. (b) Gottron's papule** (See page 335 for explanation)
11. **Ans. (b) Anti-Sm** *(Ref: Rook's Textbook of Dermatology, 9th edn, Page 51.34)*
12. **Ans. (c) Trichotillomania**
13. **Ans. (d) SLE** (See page 297-Chapter 12 for explanation)
14. **Ans. (b) Anti-Sm correlates with disease activity** *(Ref: Rook's Textbook of Dermatology, 9th edn, Page 51.33-34)*
15. **Ans. (a) Melasma**

    The word pigmentation indicates a disorder of melanin (e.g. melasma). SLE, rosacea, photodermatitis all have erythema not pigmentation.
16. **Ans. (c) DLE** *(Ref: Andrew's Textbook, 11th edn, Page 155)*
17. **Ans. (a) Calcinosis cutis**

    Calcinosis cutis is calcium deposits in skin and is not a classical feature of DM.
18. **Ans. (d) >30%** *(Ref: Andrew's Textbook, 11th edn, Page 114)*
19. **Ans. (a) Drugs** *(Ref: Rook's Textbook of Dermatology, 9th edn, Page 119.15-16)*

    >30% involvement with blisters along with 2 mucosal involvements suggests TEN which is most commonly drug induced.
20. **Ans. (b) Toxic epidermal necrolysis** *(Ref: Fitzpatrick's Textbook, 8th edn, Page 442)*

    Generalized skin involvement (would indicate >30%), severe oral and genital involvement points to TEN. Palm and sole involvement (acral involvement) is a feature classically of erythema multiforme and not TEN (which has more truncal involvement).

21. Ans. (b) Erythema multiforme *(Ref: Bolognia Dermatology, 3rd edn, Page 320)*

Erythematous halo would point to the outermost red zone of a target lesion and the central vesicle would point to the blister of bullous erythema multiforme.

22. Ans. (b) Erythema multiforme *(Ref: Bolognia Dermatology, 3rd edn, Page 320)*

23. Ans. (a) Herpes simplex *(Ref: Fitzpatrick's Textbook, 8th edn, Page 440)*

Drugs are the cause in 85% cases of SJS. In the rest 15% cases, infection (e.g. mycoplasma, HSV) and immunization is found.

24. Ans. (c) Fixed drug eruption *(Ref: Andrew's Textbook, 11th edn, Page 118)*

Blister on genitals healing with hyperpigmentation is typical of FDE. Similar blister not healing with hyperpigmentation would be herpes genitalis. Behcet's disease would cause aphthous ulcer and not blisters on genitals. Pemphigus vulgaris causes mucosal erosions but would not heal with hyperpigmentation.

25. Ans. (b) Fixed drug eruption *(Ref: Andrew's Textbook, 11th edn, Page 118)*

26. Ans. (d) HPV (See page 339 for explanation)

27. Ans. (b) Herpes simplex infection *(Ref: Bolognia Dermatology, 3rd edn, Page 320)*

28. Ans. (b) Erythema multiforme (See page 338 for explanation)

29. Ans. (a) No vesicles

Bullous/vesicular EM will have blisters.

30. Ans. (c) No vesicle

31. Ans. (d) Erythema multiforme

The bullous lesions with surrounding erythematous halo suggests bullous EM with bullous target lesions. One mucosa (usually oral) can be involved in EM major which would be the diagnosis here.

32. Ans. (d) Mucous membrane is usually involved

The commonest type of EM is EM minor which does not have mucosal involvement. EM Major which does have mucosal involvement is rarer.

33. Ans. (c) They are usually non tender (See page 344 for explanation)

34. Ans. (a) SLE *(Ref: Bolognia Dermatology, 3rd edn, Page 1498)*

35. Ans. (d) Chronic pancreatitis *(Ref: Rook's Textbook of Dermatology, 9th edn, Page 99.20)*

Both SLE and chronic pancreatitis would be the correct answers here. Since, EN can have a rare association with an "SLE-like syndrome due to C4 deficiency", better answer is D.

36. Ans. (b) Post steroidal panniculitis *(Ref: Bolognia Dermatology, 3rd edn, Page 1650)*

37. Ans. (d) Aspirin therapy *(Ref: Rook's Textbook of Dermatology, 9th edn, Page 99.19-20)*

38. Ans. (d) Glans penis *(Ref: Fitzpatrick's Textbook, 8th edn, Page 454)*

39. Ans. (a) Sulfonamide *(Ref: Fitzpatrick's Textbook, 8th edn, Page 455)*

40. Ans. (a) Fixed drug eruption (See page 342 for explanation)

41. Ans. (d) Encephalitis *(Ref: Rook's Textbook of Dermatology, 9th edn, Page 119.5)*

CNS is usually not involved (even when involved, it causes cerebral vasculitis and not encephalitis).

42. Ans. (d) Cutaneous TB (See page 345 for explanation)

43. Ans. (b) Barbiturates *(Ref: Rook's Textbook of Dermatology, 9th edn, Page 99.20)*

44. Ans. (a) Drugs

The diagnosis is TEN.

45. Ans. (a) Erythema nodosum (See page 344 for explanation)

46. Ans. (b) Erythema nodosum

47. Ans. (a) Antimalarial drugs

48. Ans. (d) Amiodarone *(Ref: Rook's Textbook of Dermatology, 9th edn, Page 82.25)*

49. Ans. (d) Erythema chronicum: Lyme's disease (See text for explanation)

For details about erythema chronicum migrans, refer to the chapter on "protozoal, arthropod and parasitic infections."

50. Ans. (c) Acanthosis nigricans

Erythema nodosum and splinter hemorrhages can both be associated with a hematological malignancy (though it is rare). Pyoderma gangrenosum is associated with AML. Common cause of malignancy induced acanthosis nigricans is adenocarcinoma of stomach.

51. Ans. (b) Chikungunya

Chikungunya is febrile viral illness with severe joint pain. Hyperpigmentation (nose and face) mimics melasma and develops as the fever subsides. This nose pigmentation is called the "chik sign'. Fixed drug eruption would be bluish-grey not brown.

52. Ans. (d) Pityriasis Rosea

53. Ans. (d) Aceclofenac

NSAIDs are common causes of FDE.

New Answers

54. Ans. a-True; b-False; c-True; d-False; e-True

55. Ans. (a) 1, 2, 3, 4

56. Ans. (c) Assertion is true and Reason is false

57. Ans. (2) If a and c are correct

58. Ans. 1-b; 2-c; 3-a; 4-f

CHAPTER 15

Disorders of Hair and Nail

HAIR DISORDERS

Types of Hair

Depending on diameter of hair	Depending on whether follicles have androgen receptors (AR)
Lanugo hair—fine hair present on the body of the fetus.	**AR present—Androgen dependent**
Vellus hairs/Terminal hairs—After birth, lanugo is replaced by vellus and terminal hairs. Vellus hairs are fine, barely visible and light-colored. Terminal hairs are thick and dark.	**AR absent—Androgen independent**

Anatomy of Hair Follicle

- **Upper segment**—Area between attachment of hair bulge (bulge is at the point of attachment of arrector pilorum muscle onto hair follicle) to the skin surface. Upper segment is further subdivided into **infundibulum** (area between attachment of sebaceous duct and skin surface) and **isthmus** (area between attachment of sebaceous duct and the hair bulge).
- **Lower segment**—Area between hair bulge and hair bulb.

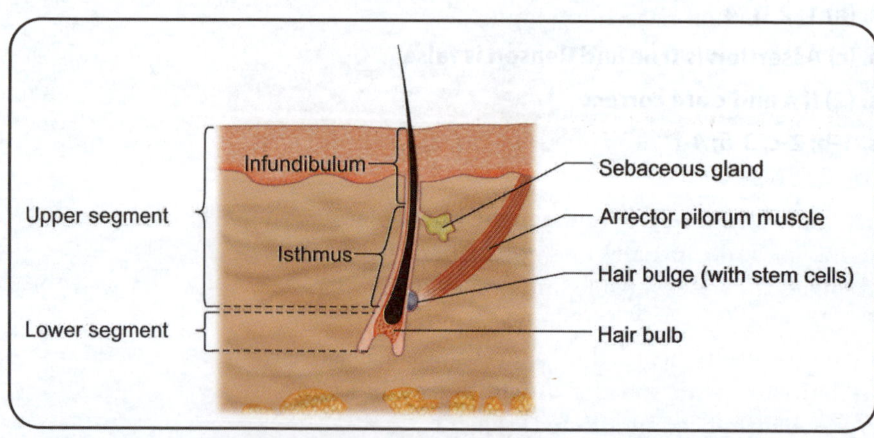

Stages of Scalp Hair Cycle

Three stages of hair on scalp (see diagram below):

1. **Anagen hairs**—growing hairs (growth phase lasts for 1,000 days, 86% of all scalp hairs are in this phase). Upper segment (US) and Lower segment (LS) are well formed. Hair bulb is black.
2. **Catagen**—Transitional hair from the growing to the resting stage (lasts for an average of 10 days, constitute 1% of all scalp hairs). In this phase, LS shortens and hair bulb rises up
3. **Telogen ("club" hairs)**(MCQ)—resting hairs (lasts for 100 days, 13% of all scalp hairs are in this phase). In this phase, LS is lost and hair bulb (which has become white) will rest at the level of hair bulge (only US remains). Telogen hairs fall down (average 100–150 hairs fall/day) and the follicle enters back into the anagen phase by reforming the LS.

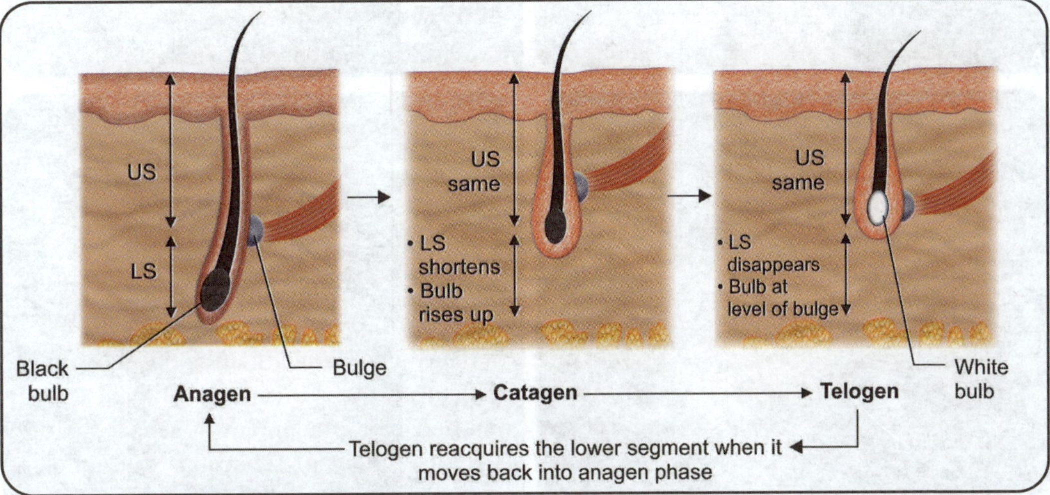

Hair Loss (Alopecia)

- **Non-cicatricial (Non-scarring) alopecia**—Noninflammatory-reversible permanent
- **Cicatricial (scarring) alopecia**—Inflammatory-usually irreversible.

NON-CICATRICIAL ALOPECIA

Alopecia Areata

- **Autoimmune lymphocytes damage** the **black pigmented anagen hair bulbs**(MCQ) **(since antigen is melanin in hair)** and consequent hair loss. Hair bulge having **stem cells is not involved** (hence reversible and non-scarring alopecia)
- Often suddenly noticed **smooth hairless patch**(MCQ) in one or more round or oval patches, usually on the scalp, bearded area, eyebrows, eyelashes (Figs. 1A and B)
- **Patchy hair loss with sparing of white/grey hairs in the patch** (no bulb melanin-in white/grey hair hence not affected) (Figs. 1C and D).

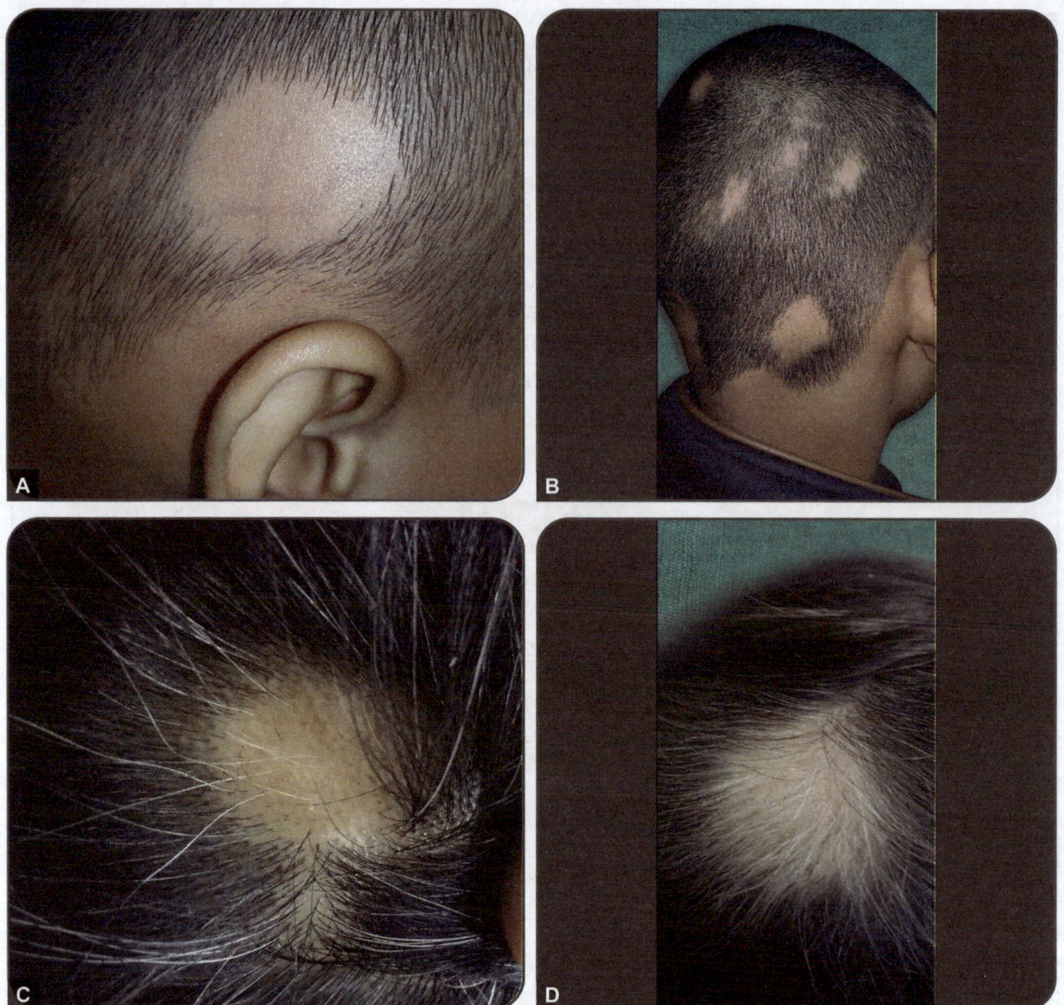

Figs. 1A to D: (A) Localised smooth surfaced oval patch of hair loss; (B) Multiple smooth surfaced alopecia patches; (C and D) Sparing of white hairs

- Nail-**Regular pitting (transverse and longitudinal pits)** (see Figure 7B in the nail disorder topic next), **Trachyonychia (20 nail dystrophy)** (see Figures 8A and B in the nail disorder topic next).
- Severe variants—**Alopecia totalis** (loss of complete scalp hairs), **Alopecia universalis** (loss of complete body hairs) (Figs. 2A and B).
- **Ophiasis**—Patches of hair loss on temporal or occipital hairline (Fig. 3A)
- **Exclamation hairs**—Instead of hairs tapering at the top in normal individuals, in alopecia areata hair increases in size as it rises up, tapers in the middle and the hair bulb is at the bottom (like an exclamation mark) (Fig. 3B). It is seen on margins of the patch and **indicates active expanding disease**.

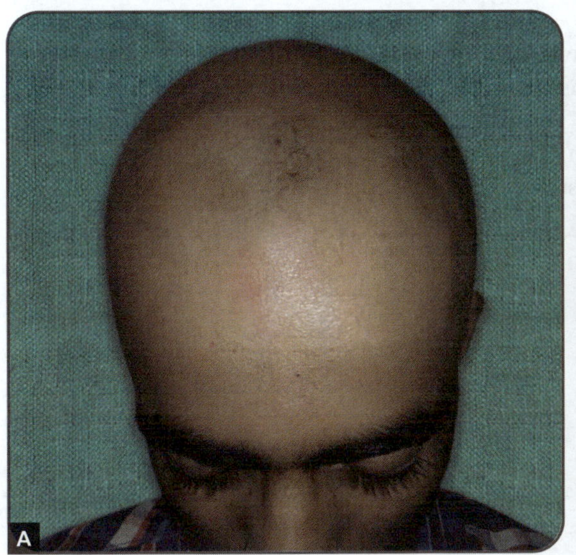

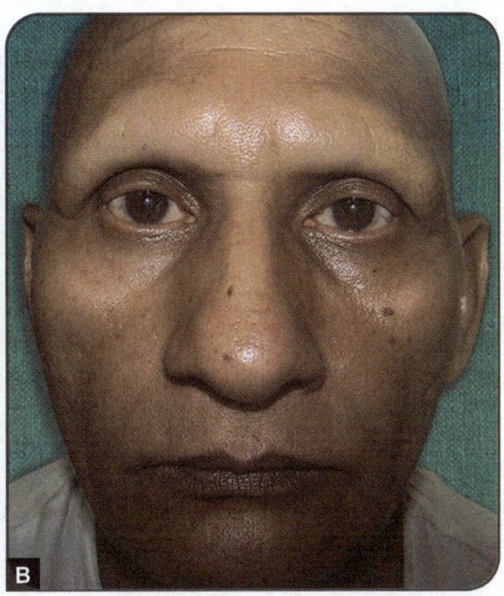

Figs. 2A and B: (A) Alopecia totalis—Loss of complete scalp hairs (note eyebrows are normal); (B) Alopecia universalis—Loss of complete body hairs. Note loss of scalp hairs, eyebrows, eyelashes, facial hairs

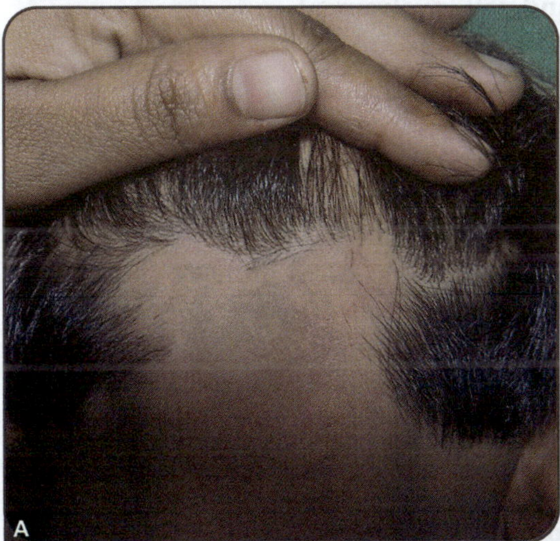

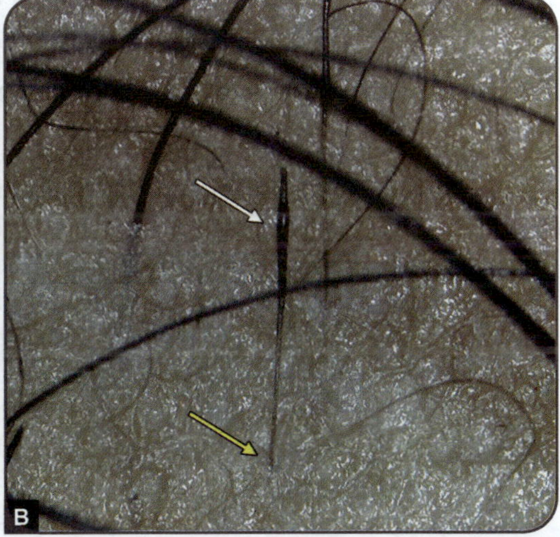

Figs. 3A and B: (A) Ophiasis-areata at occipital hairline; (B) Exclamation hair—Note narrow at skin surface (yellow arrow) and broader at top (white arrow). The hair bulb part of the exclamation mark is under the skin surface and is not seen here

- Histopathology—Lymphocytes around the bulb appear like "swarm-of-bees".
  Associations—Atopy

- **Treatment:**
  - Some patches will regrow in a few weeks **without any treatment.**
  - **Intralesional injection of corticosteroid is the treatment of choice**(MCQ) when <50% scalp affected
  - **Topical minoxidil**, topical anthralin can also be used
  - Phototherapy works as an immunosuppressive therapy.

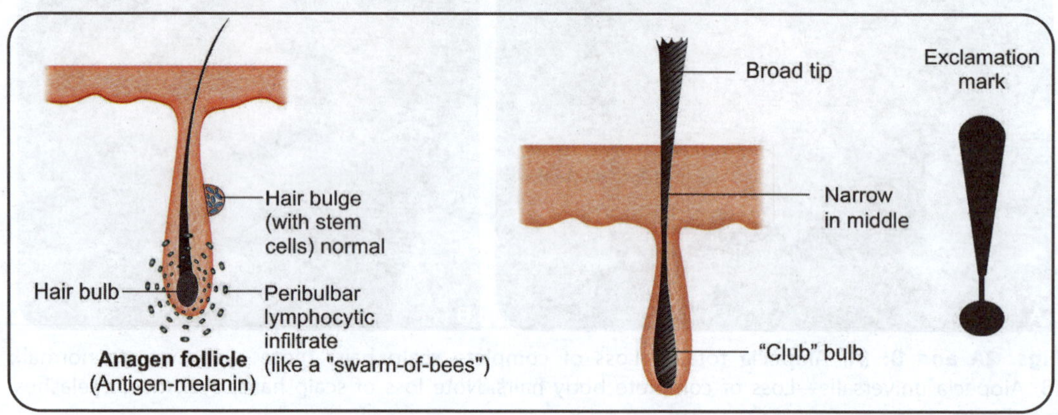

- **Poor prognostic factors for alopecia areata—Atopic dermatitis,** childhood onset, extensive disease, ophiasis, long duration **and nail involvement.**

Androgenetic Alopecia—AGA (Patterned Hair Loss)

- Androgenetic alopecia—The word is derived from **"andro" meaning androgens** are primarily responsible and **"genetic" indicating a genetic predisposition**
- The hair effects of androgens are mediated through androgen receptor (AR) which is present on androgen dependent hairs (frontal and vertex areas in males) and absent on androgen independent hairs (lateral and posterior scalp areas). Testosterone is the major circulating androgen, but its effect on hair is by its more potent metabolite dihydrotestosterone (DHT). The conversion of testosterone to DHT is catalysed by the enzyme 5α-reductase. DHT causes thinning and ultimately fall of the androgen dependent hairs. Finasteride, being a 5α-reductase inhibitor is used for treatment.
- The term **"patterned hair loss"** describe a fixed pattern of hair loss classically characterized by a **gradual decline in scalp hair diameter (called miniaturization). Vellus hairs (thin hairs) increase.**
- **Two patterns—Male pattern and female pattern**
- **Male pattern AGA (Figs. 4A and B)**
  - **First sign—Frontal hair line recession**
  - **Loss of frontal and vertex hairs** (see diagram next)
  - **Sparing of posterior and lateral scalp hairs**
  - Grading scale—**Norwood-Hamilton classification** (Stages I to VII)

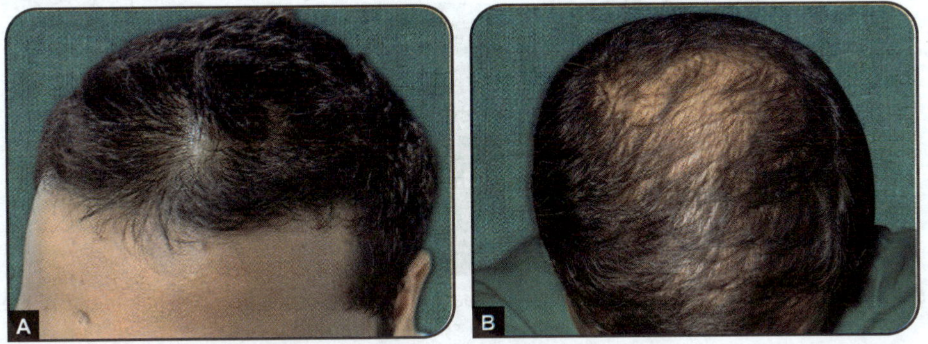

Figs. 4A and B: (A) Frontal hair line recession; (B) Vertex thinning (miniaturization), normal lateral and posterior scalp hairs

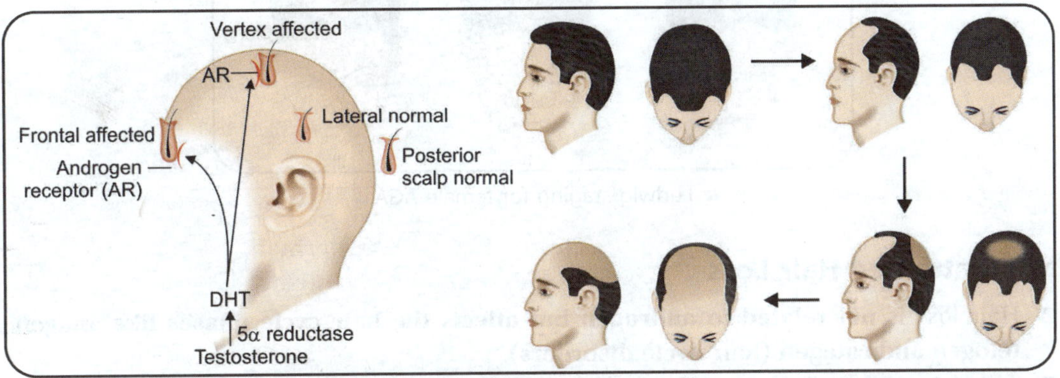

Male pattern AGA

- **Treatment**—Topical minoxidil (FDA-approved), oral finasteride (5α-reductase type 2 inhibitor), oral dutasteride (5α-reductase type 1 and 2 inhibitor), hair transplant in late stages. Treatment is lifelong.

- **Female pattern AGA (Figs. 5A and B)**
  - **No loss of frontal hairline**
  - **Loss of mid-frontal scalp hairs (gradual increase of central parting—Christmas-tree pattern)**(MCQ)
  - **Sparing of temporal and occipital hairs**
  - May be associated with underlying hyperandrogenic situations like PCOD
  - Grading scale—**Ludwig classification** (Stages I to III)
  - **Treatment**—Topical minoxidil(MCQ) (FDA-approved), Oral antiandrogen therapy(MCQ) with androgen receptor blockers (AR blockers)—cyproterone acetate, spironolactone, flutamide. If underlying hyperandrogenism (e.g. PCOD) is present- AR blockers are more effective than minoxidil and if such a factor is absent, minoxidil > AR blockers. Finasteride may be used but is not very effective and is also contraindicated in pregnancy. Treatment is life-long.

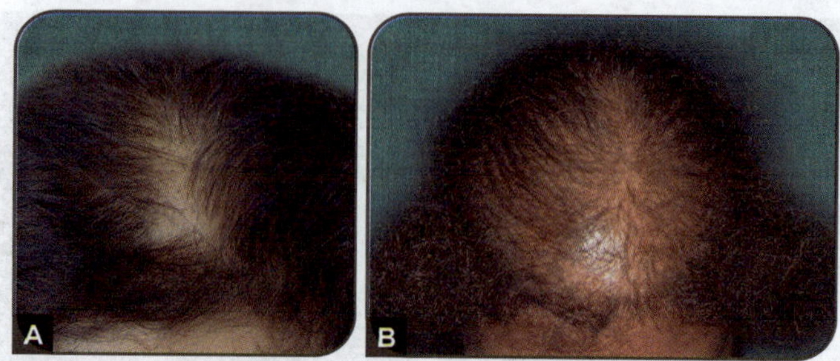

Figs. 5A and B: (A) Increase of mid-frontal scalp "parting" area. Normal anterior hairline; (B) Extensive female pattern hair loss still sparing of anterior hair line

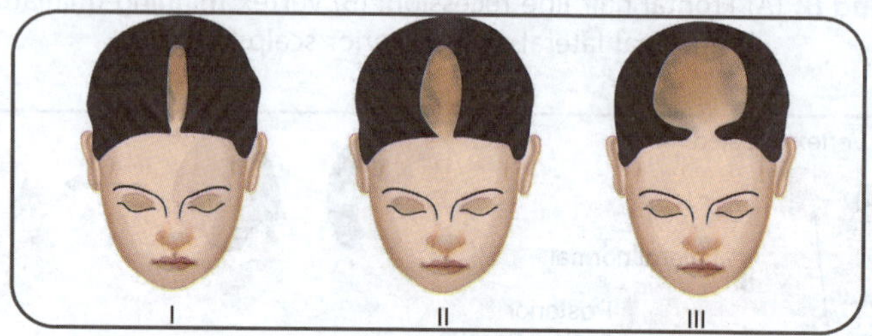

Ludwig staging for female AGA

Non-Patterned Hair Loss

- Hair loss is **not related to androgen but affects the hair cycle phases like anagen, telogen and catagen (hair cycle disorders)**.
- Two types occur: **Telogen effluvium and Anagen effluvium**

A. Telogen effluvium

- Telogen effluvium is defined as an **increase in the shedding of telogen hairs**
- **The pull test (trichogram) is positive** (large number of hairs can be dislodged on pulling)
- **Acute Telogen effluvium (ATE)**(MCQ)—Normally, hair follicles pass from anagen to telogen one by one. But sometimes, all anagen hairs pass into telogen phase at the same time **(e.g. with severe fevers, severe psychological trauma** which would divert growth factors towards this new emergency, away from anagen forcing them to go into the resting telogen phase). **Also during pregnancy**, there is a prolonged anagen and after delivery, sudden conversion to telogen occurs. In both situations, there would be large number of telogens on scalp. **As telogen lasts for 3 months and then they are shed, all these telogen hairs are shed simultaneously after 2–3 months of fever/child-birth/severe psychological trauma, creating sudden, dramatic hair losses ("effluvium" means fall)**. Normally, under 100 hairs are lost. In ATE, 100-1,000 hairs may be shed simultaneously. No treatment is required and normal hair cycle soon returns.
- **Chronic Telogen effluvium:**(MCQ) The same process can happen with numerous **chronic insults** like thyroid disorders (both hyper- and hypothyroidism), anemia, crash-dieting, zinc deficiency, malnutrition, metabolic disorders like liver and kidney diseases, SLE.

B. Anagen effluvium (AE)

- AE is a result of a disturbance of **anagen phase of hair follicle**. The hair falls out 7–14 days after the initiating event.
- It can happen with **anti-growth agents like chemotherapy** (responsible for the commonly encountered chemotherapy induced hair loss), **radiation**, toxins, severe PEM. **Anagen hairs can be identified by its black pigmented bulb.**
- Hair regrows after the offending agent is stopped.

Trichotillomania(MCQ)

- The term "trichotillomania" is derived from the Greek ***thrix***, hair; ***tillein***, pulling out; and ***mania***, madness
- An **"impulse control disorder"**
- **Patients have an urge to pluck hair**, resulting in localized or full alopecia of the scalp
- Plucking cause hair shaft fractures. **Some hairs are broken short, some long (due to the different force of pull on different days)—responsible for the typical feature of "varying lengths of hairs inside area of hair loss"** (Fig. 6B)(MCQ)
- **Hair is never completely lost in the patch** (in contrast with alopecia areata).
- **Orentreich/Friar-tuck/tonsure sign**(MCQ)—Loss of central area (easier to pull) and sparing of margins of scalp (Fig. 6A).

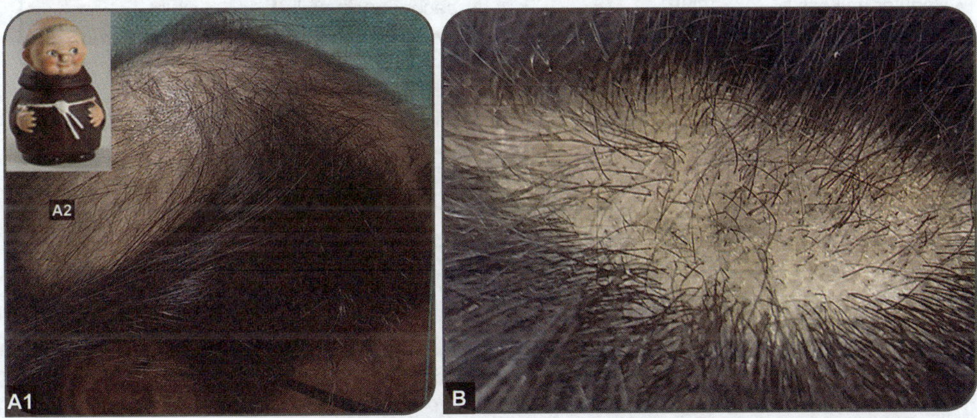

Figs. 6A and B: (A1) Loss of hair in accessible areas on scalp-vertex, sparing of margins (tonsure sign), (A2) The mythical character called friar-tuck in Robinhood stories who had similar hair (inset); (B) Close up of an localized area—Note varying lengths of hair

- Histopathology—No/little peribulbar inflammation (in contrast to alopecia areata), **Pigmented deposits in the follicle and perifollicular hemorrhage (due to plucking)**(AIIMS Nov 16) are useful markers.
- Treatment—Clomipramine, selective serotonin reuptake inhibitors (SSRIs), hypnosis, behavioral modification therapy, psychotherapy.

Aid to Remember

Mnemonic for causes of non-scarring alopecia—'TOPHATS'

T: **T**inea capitis (grey patch/black dot types)
O: **O**ut of iron, zinc, proteins
P: **P**hysical—Trichotillomania
H: **H**ormonal—**H**ypothyroidism, Androgenetic alopecia
A: **A**nagen effluvium, **A**utoimmune—Alopecia areata, SLE
T: **T**elogen effluvium
S: **S**econdary syphilis (moth-eaten alopecia)[PGI 04]

High Yield Points

How to make a diagnosis in MCQs on non-scarring alopecia

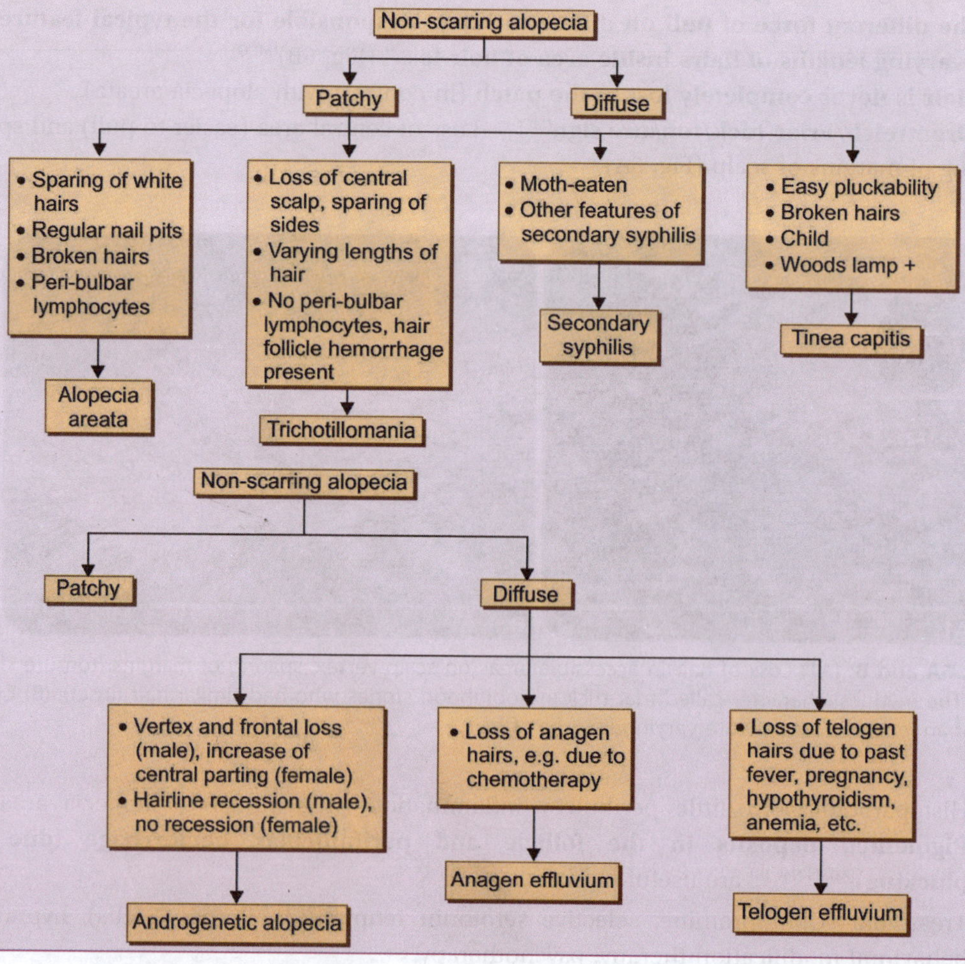

- Non-scarring alopecia
  - Patchy
    - • Sparing of white hairs • Regular nail pits • Broken hairs • Peri-bulbar lymphocytes → Alopecia areata
    - • Loss of central scalp, sparing of sides • Varying lengths of hair • No peri-bulbar lymphocytes, hair follicle hemorrhage present → Trichotillomania
    - • Moth-eaten • Other features of secondary syphilis → Secondary syphilis
    - • Easy pluckability • Broken hairs • Child • Woods lamp + → Tinea capitis
  - Diffuse

- Non-scarring alopecia
  - Patchy
  - Diffuse
    - • Vertex and frontal loss (male), increase of central parting (female) • Hairline recession (male), no recession (female) → Androgenetic alopecia
    - • Loss of anagen hairs, e.g. due to chemotherapy → Anagen effluvium
    - • Loss of telogen hairs due to past fever, pregnancy, hypothyroidism, anemia, etc. → Telogen effluvium

Scarring/Cicatricial Alopecia

- Lichen planopilaris—See Chapter 10 for details
- DLE
- SLE (can cause both scarring and non-scarring alopecia)
- Tinea capitis—can cause both scarring (Kerion and Favus types) and non-scarring—(Grey patch and black dot types) alopecia—See Chapter 5 for details
- Lupus vulgaris
- Sarcoidosis

Aid to Remember

Aid to remember causes of scarring alopecia

- 3L—Lichen planus, Lupus erythematosus (DLE), Lupus vulgaris
- 2F—Folliculitis, Favus (tinea capitis)
- 2S—Sarcoidosis, SLE

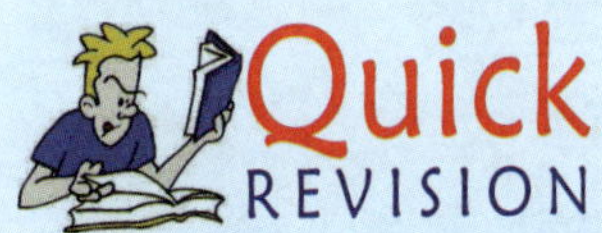

- Three stages of scalp hairs—Anagen (growing hairs—lasts for 1,000 days, 86%), catagen (transitional hair-lasts for 10 days, 1%), Telogen (resting hairs-lasts for 100 days, 13%)
- Non-scarring alopecia (non-cicatricial alopecia)
  - Alopecia areata—Autoimmune damage to pigmented hair bulbs. Bulge is normal—hence, non-scarring reversible hair loss. Presents as smooth patches of complete hair loss with sparing of white/grey hairs. Severe variants—Alopecia totalis and universalis. Poor prognosis—Nail pitting, exclamation hairs, long duration, ophiasis pattern. Intralesional steroids—DOC. Other agents—minoxidil, anthralin. For extensive disease, contact immunotherapy with DNCB, SADBE, DPC.
  - Androgenetic alopecia (patterned hair loss)—Cause is genetic and hormonal (DHT). Male pattern—Recession of anterior hairline and vertex thinning. Normal lateral and posterior scalp. Hamilton-Norwood grading. Treatment—Topical minoxidil, Oral finasteride. Female pattern—Normal hairline. Loss of mid-frontal area. Widening of central parting. Association with hyperandrogenism (e.g. PCOD). Ludwig's grading. Treatment—Topical minoxidil, oral androgen receptor blockers
  - Telogen effluvium—Acute: After 2–3 months of fever, child-birth, psychological trauma. Self-resolving. Chronic: After continuous body insults like malnutrition, thyroid disorders, anemia, starvation.
  - Anagen effluvium—Anagen hair loss with chemotherapy, radiation, toxins
  - Trichotillomania—Impulse control disorder of hair plucking. Loss of central scalp, sparing of argins (tonsure sign), hairs of varying lengths
  - Other causes—SLE, Tinea capitis (grey patch/Black dot)
- Scarring alopecia (cicatricial alopecia)

  Causes—SLE, Tinea capitis (Favus/Kerion), Lichen planopilaris. DLE, Linear morphoea, chronic folliculitis.

NAIL DISORDERS

Anatomy of Nail

- Nail matrix is the birth place of nail and is responsible for nail plate production. Proximal part of the matrix makes the upper (dorsal) nail plate while distal matrix makes the lower (ventral) nail plate

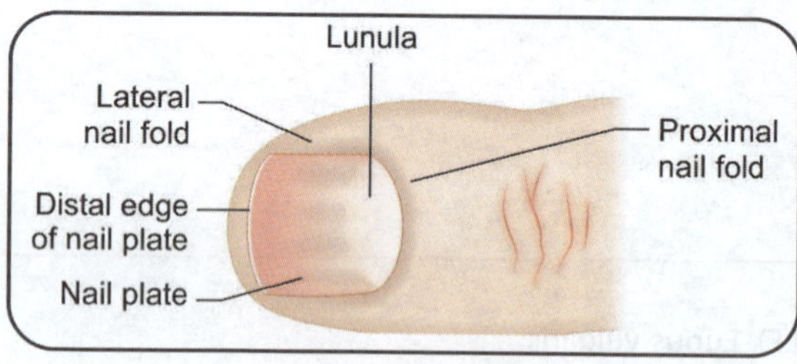

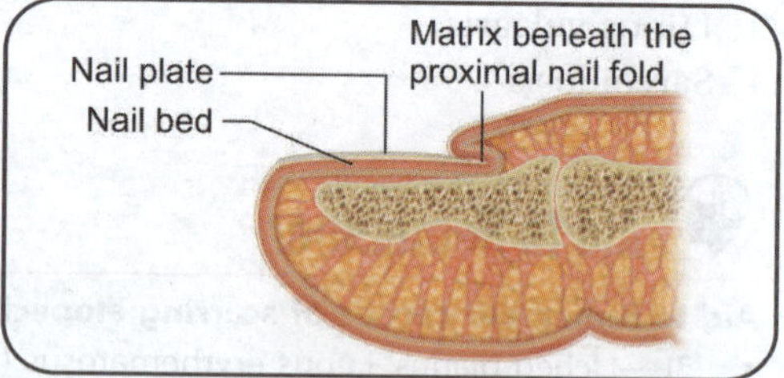

- Proximal nail fold covers the nail and protects the nail matrix underneath
- Nail plate covers the nail bed
- Nail growth rate: Fingernails: 3 mm/month, Toenails: 1 mm/month.

Diseases of Nail

1. **Pitting**
   - Depressions on nail plate **due to proximal nail matrix involvement**(MCQ)
   - Seen in **psoriasis, eczema, alopecia areata**
     - **Psoriasis**—Randomly distributed, deep, irregular, large (**RIDL- Random, irregular, deep, large**) (Fig. 7A)
     - **Alopecia areata**—Geometric pitting—**Small, superficial, regular pits in vertical and horizontal pattern (grid-like)** (Fig. 7B)
     - **Eczema**—irregular, mild and localized
   - Rare causes—SLE, dermatomyositis, sarcoidosis, pemphigus
   - Extensive pitting combined with other nail plate irregularities results in a very rough nail called **trachyonychia (20 nail dystrophy)** (Figs. 8A and B).

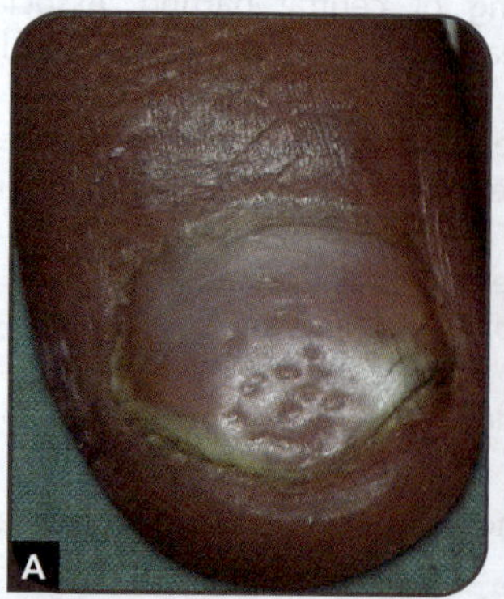

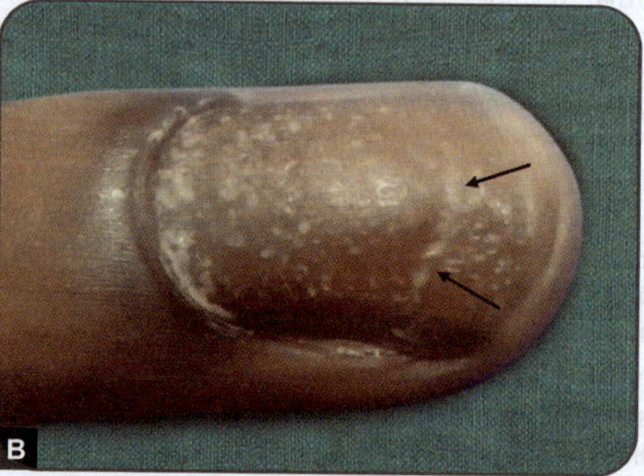

Figs. 7A and B: (A) Irregular, deep pits in psoriasis; (B) Regular horizontal pits in alopecia areata

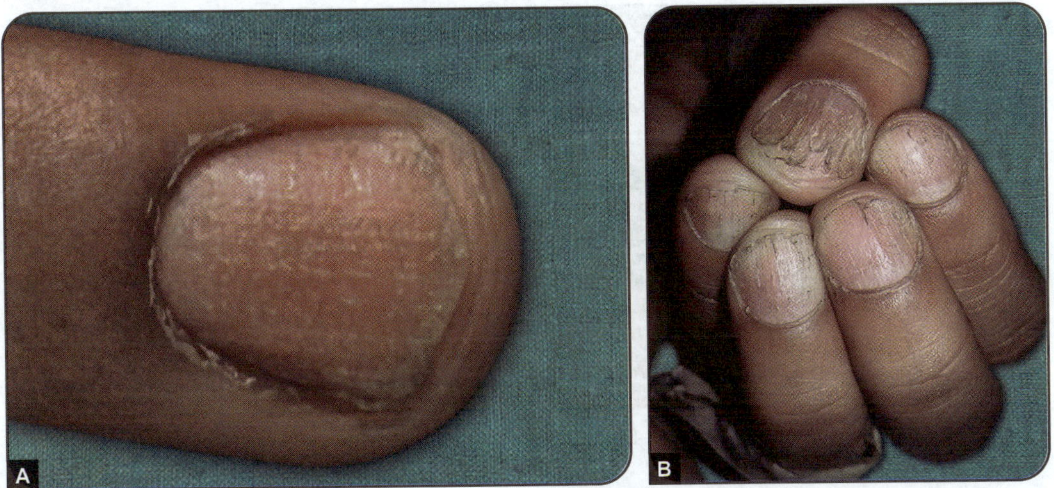

Figs. 8A and B: (A) Roughened sandpaper-like nail; (B) 20 nails affected (20 nails dystrophy)

2. **Trachyonychia (20 nail dystrophy/Sandpaper nails)** (Figs. 8A and B)
   - Typically diffusely roughened nail plates (like sandpaper)

   Causes: **Alopecia areata (commonest cause),**(MCQ) **lichen planus, psoriasis and eczema**.
3. **Beau's line**(MCQ)
   - **Horizontal grooves** on nail plate due to temporary interruption of the activity of the proximal nail matrix (Fig. 9)
   - Can occur with any major systemic disease or injury, e.g. drugs, fever.

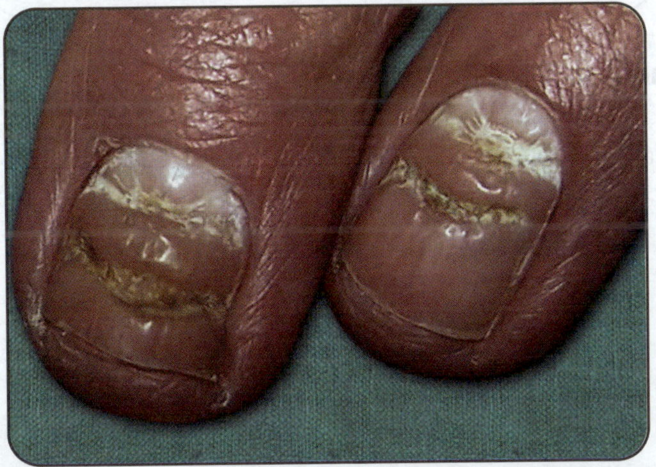

Fig. 9: Horizontal grooves on nail plate (Beau's lines)

4. **Half and half nail (Lindsay's nails)**(MCQ) (Fig. 10)
   - Proximal nail plate is white, distal 50% is brown
   - It is due to **increase in melanin** and capillary wall thickening.

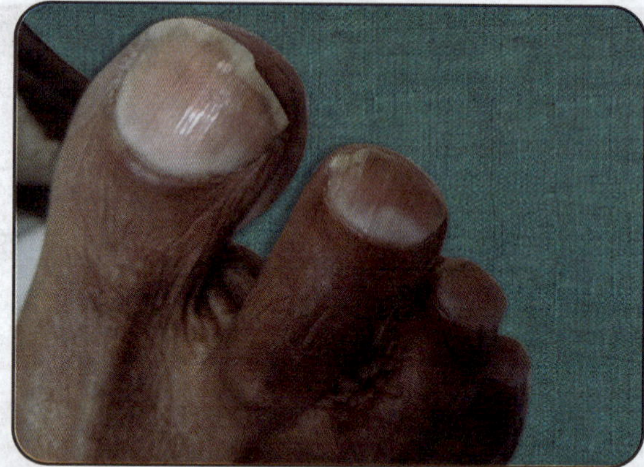

Fig. 10: Half and half nail—Distal red brown half and the proximal white half

Schematic Representation

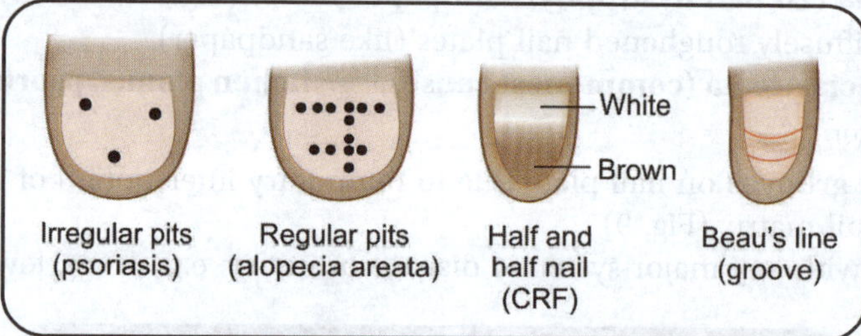

Nail Involvement in Specific Diseases

- Nail psoriasis—See Chapter 10 for details
- Nail lichen planus—See Chapter 10 for details.

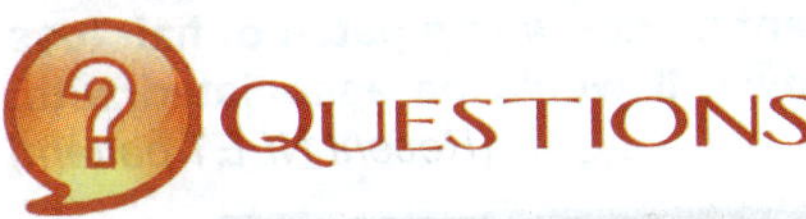

QUESTIONS

1. **A female patient presents with diffuse alopecia to you. She had suffered from typhoid fever 3 months back. Most probable diagnosis is:**
   a. Androgenetic alopecia
   b. Telogen effluvium
   c. Anagen effluvium
   d. Alopecia areata

2. **A 30-year-old female developed diffuse hair loss 3-month after delivery of her first child. The probable diagnosis is:**
   a. Androgenetic alopecia
   b. Endocrinal alopecia
   c. Telogen effluvium
   d. SLE

3. **Diagnosis of a female with hair loss involving crown and frontal scalp with maintenance of frontal hair line:**

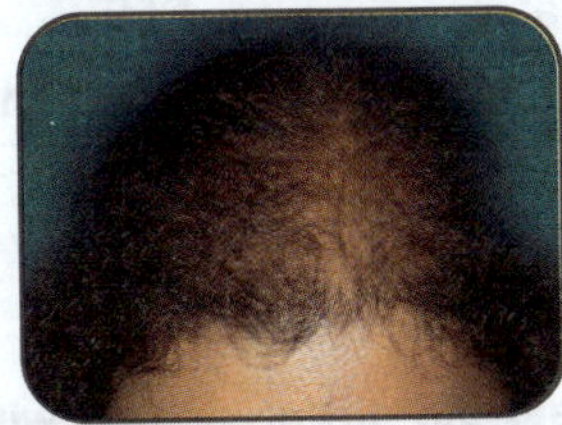

   a. Alopecia areata
   b. Anagen effluvium
   c. Male pattern baldness
   d. Female pattern baldness

4. **A male patient presents with patchy loss of hair on scalp, eyebrows and beard. He has also history of rapid graying of hair in a few areas. The likely diagnosis is:**

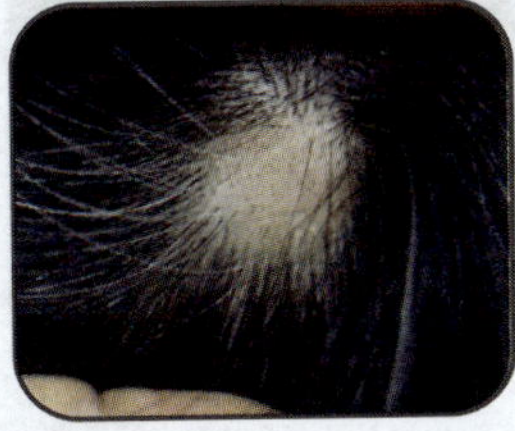

   a. Alopecia areata
   b. Anagen effluvium
   c. Telogen effluvium
   d. Androgenetic alopecia

5. **An 8-year-old child has localized non cicatricial alopecia over scalp with itching and scales. The diagnosis is:**
   a. Tinea barbae
   b. Alopecia areata
   c. Tinea capitis
   d. Lichen planus

6. **A male presents with focal alopecia and boggy swelling on scalp and easily pluckable hair. Diagnosis is:**
   a. Alopecia areata
   b. Patterned baldness
   c. Telogen effluvium
   d. Tinea capitis

7. **Anagen phase of the hair indicates:**
   a. The phase of activity and growth
   b. The phase of transition
   c. The phase of resting
   d. The phase of degeneration

8. **Growth phase of hair is:**
   a. Anagen
   b. Metagen
   c. Telogen
   d. None

9. **This phase in hair cycle determines the length to which hair in different body areas can grow:**
   a. Anagen
   b. Catagen
   c. Telogen
   d. Kenogen

10. **Eyebrows do not grow beyond certain length as they have a short:**
    a. Anagen phase b. Telogen phase
    c. Catagen phase d. Exogen phase

11. **Cicatricial alopecia is seen in:**
    a. DLE b. Psoriasis
    c. Alopecia areata d. Lichen planus
    e. SLE

12. All of the following are causes of cicatrizing alopecia *except:*

a. Lichen planus
b. Discoid lupus erythematosus
c. Alopecia areata
d. Lupus vulgaris

13. Scarring alopecia is seen in:

a. Tinea capitis
b. Androgenetic alopecia
c. Alopecia areata
d. Lichen planus

14. Which of the following conditions causes alopecia without scarring?

a. DLE
b. Herpes zoster
c. Alopecia areata
d. Lichen plano pilaris

15. Cicatricial alopecia seen in:

a. Tinea capitis b. Psoriasis
c. DLE d. Alopecia areata

16. Scarring alopecia seen in all *except*:

a. Trichotillomania
b. Lichen planus
c. Trauma
d. Discoid lupus erythematous
e. Sarcoidosis

17. Exclamation mark hair is a feature of:

a. Telogen effluvium
b. Androgenetic alopecia
c. Alopecia areata
d. Alopecia mucinosa

18. Alopecia areata is not associated with which of the following condition?

a. Exclamation sign
b. Atopy
c. Pitting nails
d. Geographical tongue

19. A child presenting with localized patch of complete hair loss with normal appearance of scalp. Diagnosis is:

a. Tinea capitis
b. Cradle cap
c. Alopecia areata
d. Telogen effluvium

20. A patient comes with a patch of hair loss as shown. It would be associated with: *(Recent NEET pattern)*

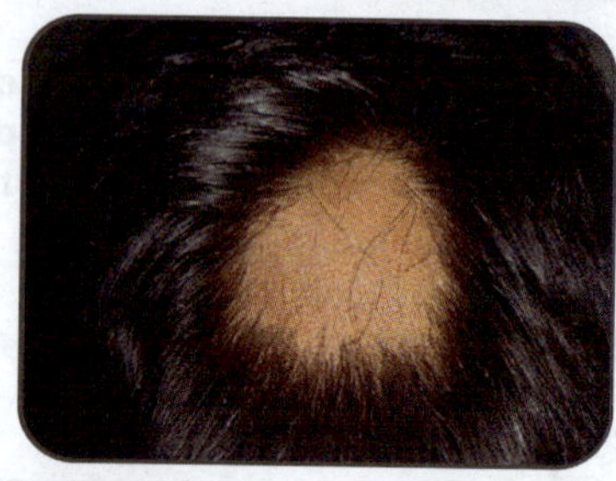

a. Paronychia
b. Pitting of nail
c. Pterygium of nail
d. Onychomycosis

21. Nail is involved in:

a. Psoriasis b. Lichen planus
c. Fungal infection d. Alopecia
e. Viral infection

22. Nails are involved in all *except:*

a. Psoriasis b. Lichen planus
c. Tinea d. DLE

23. Pitting nail dystrophy is seen in:

a. Dermatophytic infection
b. Psoriasis
c. Lichen planus
d. Seborrheic dermatitis

24. A 12-year-old girl presented with painful boggy swelling of scalp, multiple sinuses with purulent discharge, easily pluckable hairs and lymph node senlarged in occipital region. Which one of the following would be most helpful for diagnostic evaluation?

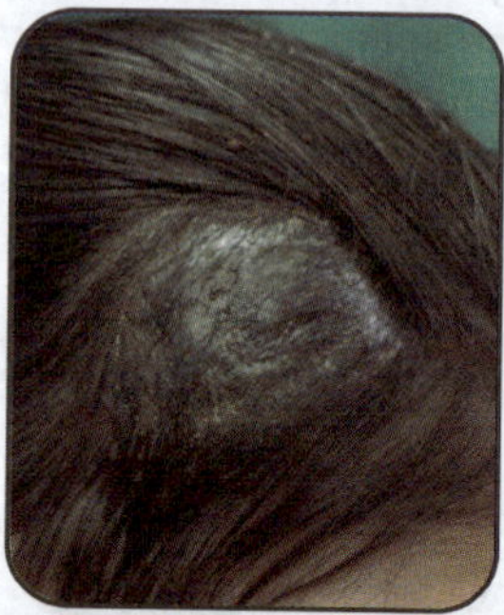

a. Bacterial culture b. Biopsy
c. KOH mount d. Patch test

25. A 35-year-old male comes with complaints of baldness. On examination well defined bald patches were seen with no scarring. Small broken hairs were seen in the area. What is the likely diagnosis? *(AIIMS May 16)*

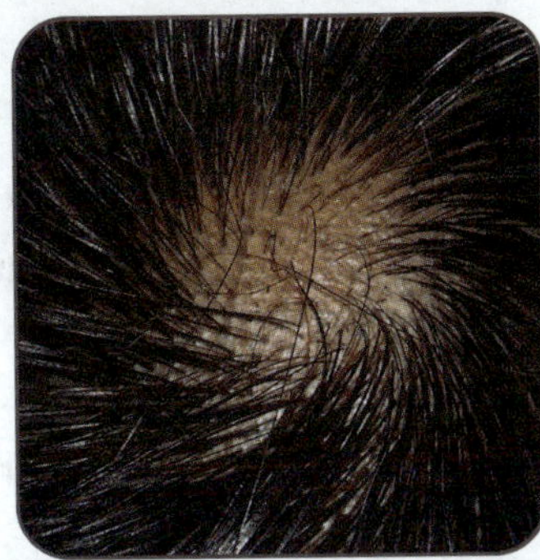

a. Androgenetic alopecia
b. Alopecia areata
c. Anagen effluvium
d. Telogen effluvium

26. Causes of cicatricial alopecia include:

a. DLE
b. Telogen effluvium
c. Lichen planus
d. Androgenetic alopecia
e. Trichotillomania

27. A patient has thinned nails and onycholysis. What else is expected?

a. Anemia
b Longitudinal ridging of nails
c. Leukoplakia
d. Oil drop sign

28. Nail pitting in psoriasis indicates involvement of:

a. Nail bed
b. Proximal nail matrix
c. Distal nail matrix
d. Hyponychium

29. Not a sign of lichen planus:

a. Pterygium
b. Trachyonychia
c. Thickening of nail
d. Tented nail

30. A 24-year-old female presents with patchy hair loss in the right temporal and occipital region. Examination reveals non-scarring alopecia with multiple small broken hairs. Scrapings from scalp show mild inflammation, peri-follicular hemorrhage and surrounding lymphocytic infiltration. What is the likely diagnosis? *(AIIMS Nov 16)*

a. Alopecia areata
b. Androgenic alopecia
c. Loose anagen hair
d. Trichotillomania

31. Pigmentation of nail is caused by all of these drugs *except*: *(AIIMS Nov 16)*

a. Chlorpromazine b. Zidovudine
c. Chloroquine d. Amiodarone

32. A 30-year-old lady comes with a 2 months history of non-scarring patchy alopecia as shown in the image. There was no erythema. The diagnosis is: *(AIIMS May 2017)*

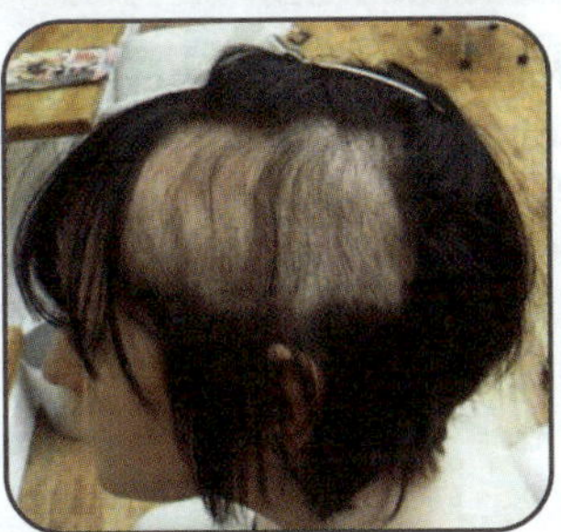

a. Alopecia areata
b. Trichotillomania
c. Telogen effluvium
d. Androgenetic alopecia

33. A child comes with a circular scaly patchy hair loss with itching in the lesions. The investigation of choice is: *(AIIMS May 2017)*

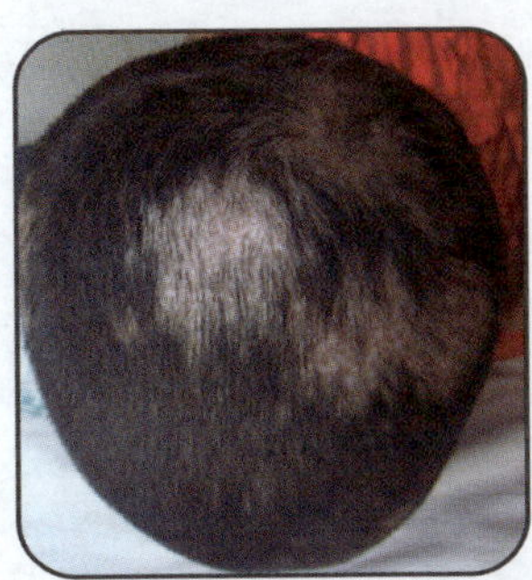

a. Slit skin smear b. KOH
c. Gram-stain d. Tzanck smear

34. A 4-month-old child presents with yellow greasy flakes in hair and crusted lesions in flexures. The diagnosis is:
(Recent- May 2017)

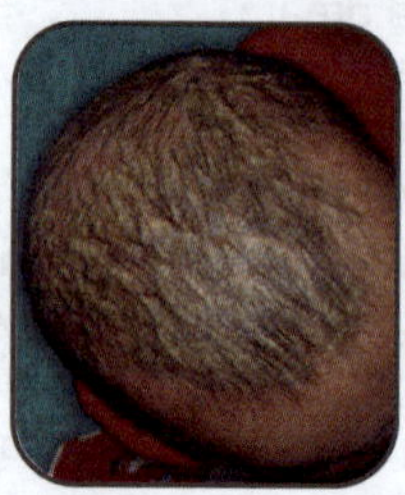

a. Atopic dermatitis
b. Seborrheic dermatitis
c. Impetigo
d. Psoriasis

New Questions

35. The following statements are true/false regarding poor prognostic factors in alopecia areata:

a. Exclamation hairs
b. Ophiasis
c. Adult onset
d. Atopic individual
e. White hairs

36. Cicatricial alopecia is seen in:

a. Lichen planus
b. SLE
c. Sarcoidosis
d. Morphea

1. If a, b, d are correct
2. If a and b are correct
3. If c and d are correct
4. If all four (a, b, c, & d) are correct

37. Match the items of column A with best alternative in column B:

Column A	Column B
1. Loss of frontal-parietal hair line 2. Chemotherapy induced hair loss 3. Hairs of varying lengths in alopecia patch 4. Peribulbar inflammation	a. Alopecia areata b. Telogen effluvium c. Trichotillomania d. Anagen effluvium e. Androgenetic alopecia f. Lichen planopilaris

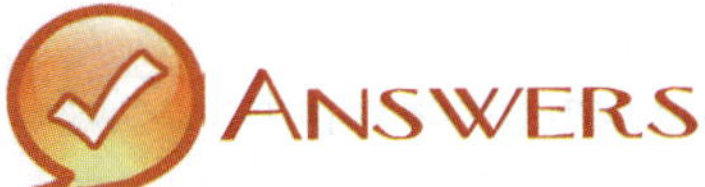

1. **Ans. (b) Telogen effluvium** *(Ref: Rook's Textbook of Dermatology, 9th edn, Page 89.25)*
2. **Ans. (c) Telogen effluvium** *(Ref: Rook's Textbook of Dermatology, 9th edn, Page 89.25)*
3. **Ans. (d) Female pattern baldness** *(Ref: Fitzpatrick's Textbook, 8th edn, Page 982)*
4. **Ans. (a) Alopecia areata** *(Ref: Rook's Textbook of Dermatology, 9th edn, Page 89.31)*

   Patchy loss suggests alopecia areata. Graying of hair indicates sparing of grey hairs in this disease.
5. **Ans. (c) Tinea capitis**

   Localized hair loss with itching and scaling indicates tinea capitis (grey patch). Alopecia areata has smooth patchy hair loss without itching and scaling. Lichen planus has scarring alopecia.
6. **Ans. (d) Tinea capitis**

   Boggy swelling and easily pluckable hairs suggests kerion (tinea capitis).
7. **Ans. (a) The phase of activity and growth** *(Ref: Bolognia Dermatology, 3rd edn, Page 1073)*
8. **Ans. (a) Anagen**
9. **Ans. (a) Anagen**
10. **Ans. (a) Anagen phase**
11. **Ans. (a, d, e) DLE; Lichen planus; SLE** (See page 366 for explanation)
12. **Ans. (c) Alopecia areata** *(Ref: Rook's Textbook of Dermatology, 9th edn, Page 89.35)*
13. **Ans. (d) Lichen planus** *(Ref: Rook's Textbook of Dermatology, 9th edn, Page 89.35)*

    Both tinea capitis and lichen planus cause scarring alopecia. Since, tinea capitis can cause non-scarring alopecia as well, lichen planus will be a better answer here.
14. **Ans. (c) Alopecia areata** *(Ref: Rook's Textbook of Dermatology, 9th edn, Page 89.35)*
15. **Ans. (c) DLE**

    Tinea capitis causes both scarring and nonscarring alopecia while DLE would cause only scarring alopecia.
16. **Ans. (a) Trichotillomania**
17. **Ans. (c) Alopecia areata** *(Ref: Fitzpatrick's Textbook, 8th edn, Page 991)*
18. **Ans. (d) Geographical tongue** (See page 357–358 for explanation)
19. **Ans. (c) Alopecia areata** (See page 356 for explanation)
20. **Ans. (b) Pitting of nail**
21. **Ans. (a, b, c, d, e) Psoriasis, Lichen planus, Fungal infection, Alopecia, Viral infection**

    Viral warts can affect nail bed, nail folds.
22. **Ans. (d) DLE**
23. **Ans. (b) Psoriasis**

24. Ans. (c) KOH mount

Easily pluckable hairs, boggy swelling, sinuses all indicate kerion (tinea capitis).

25. Ans. (b) Alopecia areata

Well defined hair loss, absence of scarring, broken hairs all suggests alopecia areata.

26. Ans. (a, c) DLE, Lichen planus (See page 366 for explanation)

27. Ans. (b) Longitudinal ridging of nails (See page 251-Chapter 10 for explanation)

(Refer to topic of lichen planus in chapter "papulosquamous disorders").

Thinned nails and onycholysis indicates lichen planus.

28. Ans. (b) Proximal nail matrix *(Ref: Fitzpatrick's Textbook, 8th edn, Page 1014)*

29. Ans. (c) Thickening of nail (See page 251-Chapter 10 for explanation)

(Refer to topic of lichen planus in chapter "papulosquamous disorders").

30. Ans. (d) Trichotillomania (See page 362 for explanation)

Non-scarring alopecia, short broken hairs and perifollicular hemorrhage suggests diagnosis of trichotillomania.

31. Ans. (d) Amiodarone (See page 344-Chapter 14 for explanation)

(For more on drugs causing nail pigmentation, refer to the drug reaction topic in Chapter 14).

32. Ans. (b) Trichotillomania

Patchy hair loss will be seen in Alopecia areata and Trichotillomania. Telogen effluvium and androgenetic alopecia will have diffuse hair loss. You can see incomplete hair loss in the patch. Alopecia areata would have a smooth surfaced patchy loss, not incomplete loss.

33. Ans. (b) KOH

Scaly, itchy, localised patchy hair loss in a child is tinea capitis. KOH smear is done from loose hairs. SSS is for leprosy and leishmaniasis. Tzanck smear is for herpes, pemphigus, etc.

34. Ans. (b) Seborrheic dermatitis

Yellow greasy scales point to a diagnosis of cradle cap (seborrheic dermatitis).

New Answers

35. Ans. a-True; b-True; c-False; d-True; e-False

36. Ans. (4) If all four (a, b, c, & d) are correct

37. Ans. 1-e; 2-d; 3-c; 4-a

CHAPTER 16

Skin Tumors, Vascular Lesions, Skin and Endocrinal Disorders

CUTANEOUS LYMPHOMA

Mycosis fungoides (MF)

- **Most common form of primary cutaneous T-cell lymphoma**
- The disease has an **indolent course with a good prognosis in early stages** but in later stages the lymph nodes and the visceral organs get involved and prognosis worsens.

Sézary syndrome (SS): Sézary syndrome is a distinctive **(leukemic) form of cutaneous T-cell lymphoma (CTCL) with poor prognosis** in which patients have significant blood involvement with a triad of Sezary cells in skin and blood, generalized lymphadenopathy and erythroderma (>90%) skin involvement.

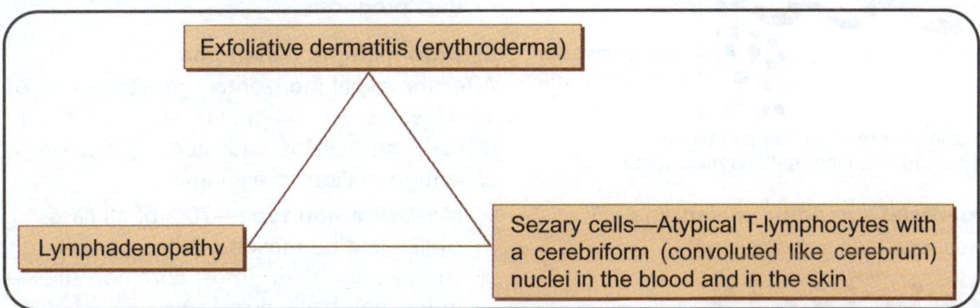

Sèzary syndrome

Investigations:

- Histopathology—Tendency of atypical T cells to enter the epidermis in large numbers (**epidermotropism**). When these atypical cells cluster into a group in the epidermis, the collection is called **Pautrier's microabscess**
- Immunohistochemistry—**CD4+**, CD7 -ve, CD26 -ve.

MALIGNANT MELANOMA

- Malignant cells originate from melanocytes at the dermoepidermal junction and either disperse horizontally in epidermis (**called radial growth stage**) or invade the dermis (**called vertical growth phase**)
- **Depth of invasion** is the single most important factor for prognosis

- **Risk factors**
  - Light-skinned people
  - UV radiation—very important factor
  - An increased risk of pre-existing nevi—Either quantitatively (large number of nevi >100) or qualitatively (atypical nevi, giant congenital nevi >20 cm)
- **ABCDE criteria** is used for clinical diagnosis

A	Asymmetry in lesions
B	Border (irregular)
C	Color (multiple)
D	Diameter >6 mm
E	Evolution of lesions

Types of Melanoma

(a) Lentigo maligna (melanoma-in-situ) and Lentigo maligna melanoma 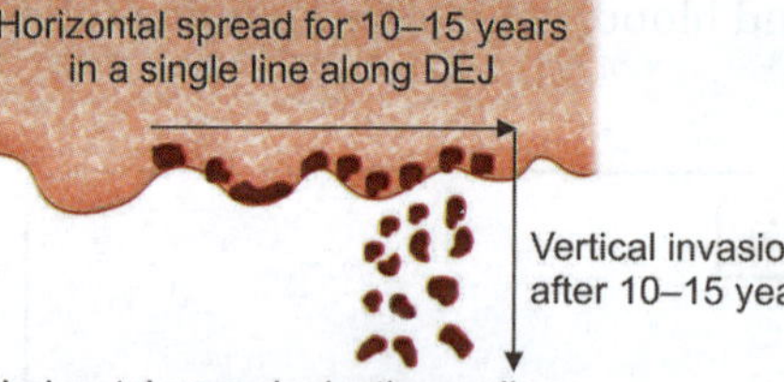 	**Lentigo Maligna (melanoma-in-situ)** • Indicates early melanoma with only the horizontal spread of melanoma cells in a single layer along the DEJ. • Presents as hyperpigmented macules that slowly extends peripherally over 10–15 years • Occurs on sun damaged skin, e.g. face • Best prognosis **Lentigo maligna melanoma** After the radial (horizontal) growth period of 10–15 years, vertical growth phase of invasive the disease can develop and then the disease is called as lentigo maligna melanoma
(b) Superficial spreading melanoma 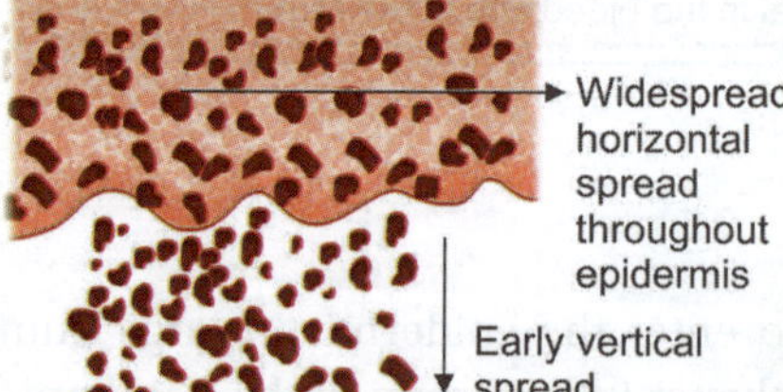 	• **Most common type**—70% of all cases • Unlike lentigo maligna, it has no preference for sun-damaged skin (most common sites—legs in females, back in males) • Horizontal spread is widespread throughout the epidermis (contrast to the single file along DEJ in lentigo maligna) • Early and more extensive vertical growth phase
(c) Nodular melanoma 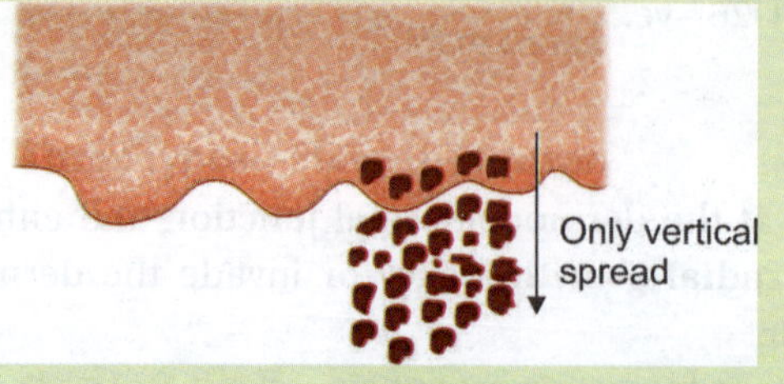 	• **No radial growth phase, only a vertical downward growth phase** • **ABCDE criteria does not apply to this melanoma** • Presents as a tumourous nodular mass • **Poorest prognosis**

Contd...

Contd...

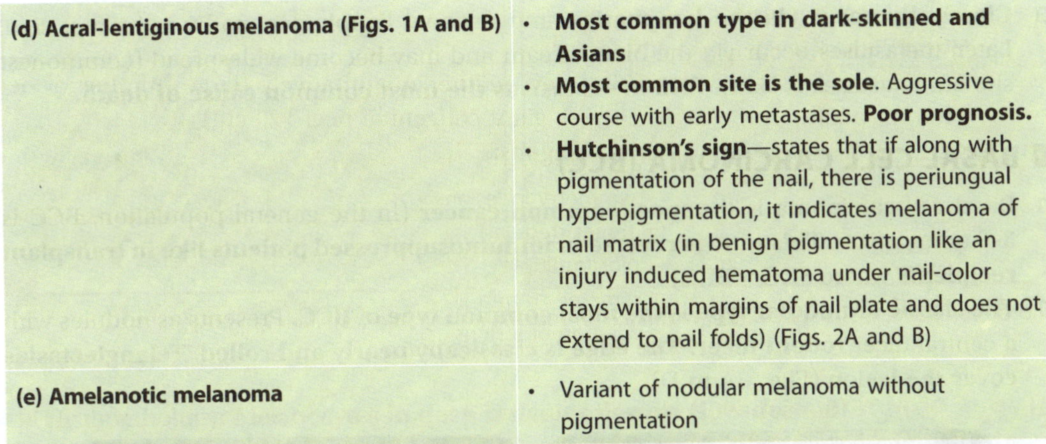

(d) Acral-lentiginous melanoma (Figs. 1A and B)	• **Most common type in dark-skinned and Asians** • **Most common site is the sole**. Aggressive course with early metastases. **Poor prognosis.** • **Hutchinson's sign**—states that if along with pigmentation of the nail, there is periungual hyperpigmentation, it indicates melanoma of nail matrix (in benign pigmentation like an injury induced hematoma under nail-color stays within margins of nail plate and does not extend to nail folds) (Figs. 2A and B)
(e) Amelanotic melanoma	• Variant of nodular melanoma without pigmentation

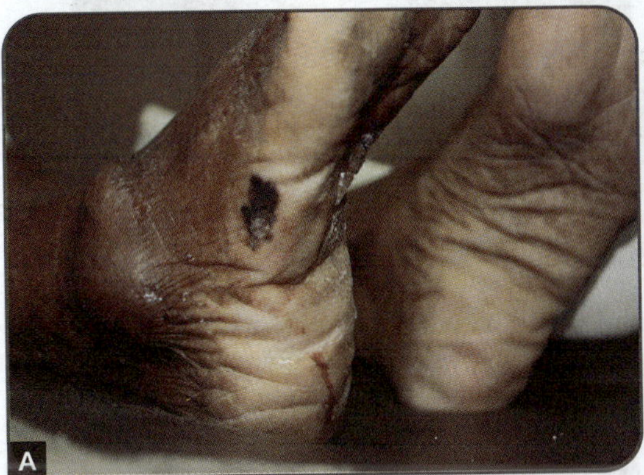

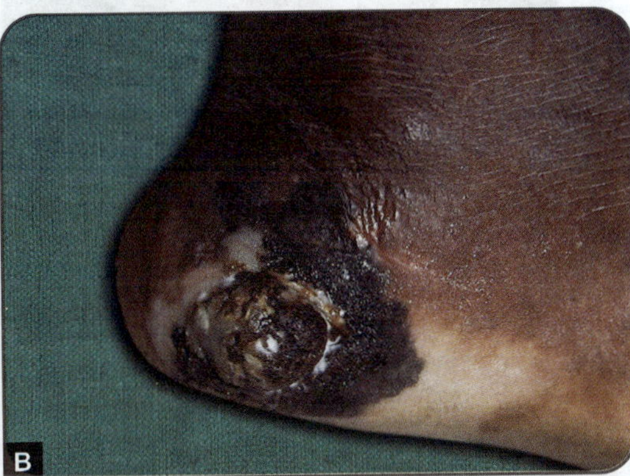

Figs. 1A and B: Acral lentiginous melanoma (A) Note the fulfillment of ABCD criteria—asymmetry, irregular borders, multiple colors, diameter >6 mm, on acral location; (B) Note the acral location, irregular pigmentation, asymmetry, nodule-indicating the vertical growth phase

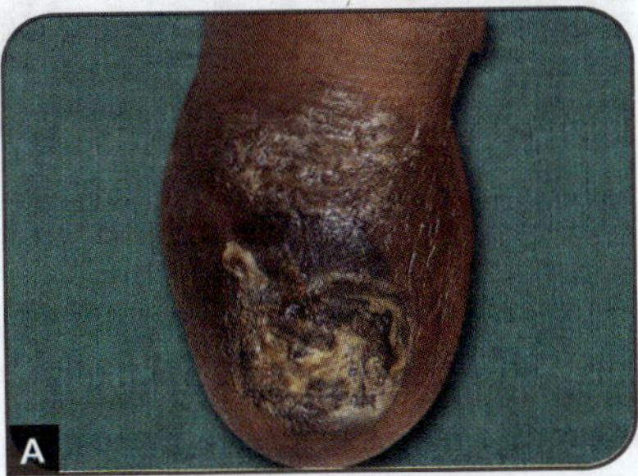

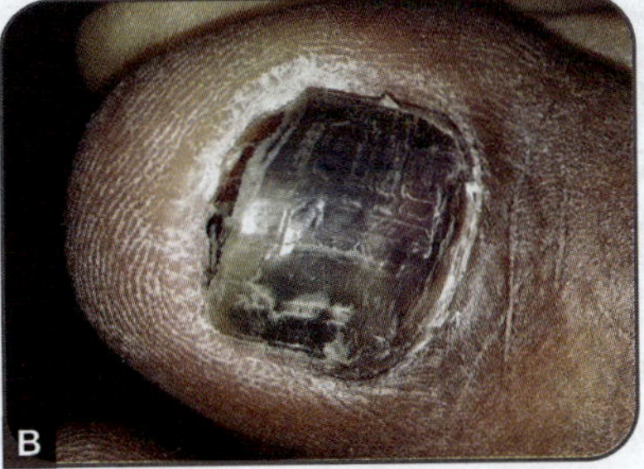

Figs. 2A and B: (A) Hutchinson's sign positive—involvement of periungual skin with dystrophy and loss of the nail plate secondary to the tumor; (B) Hutchinson's sign negative (not a melanoma)—trauma and bleed under nail—note color not extending on periungual area

Metastases

- **Classically occur via the lymphatics,** and regional lymphadenopathy is its first sign. Later, metastases occur via the bloodstream and may become widespread (commonest site of metastases is skin). **CNS metastasis is the most common cause of death.**

BASAL CELL CARCINOMA (BCC)

- Basal cell carcinoma is the **most common cancer** (in the general population, BCC is 3–6 times > SCC. **This ratio is reverse in immunosuppressed patients like in transplant recipients** where SCC > BCC)
- **The classic or nodular type is the most common type of BCC.** Presents as nodules with a central ulcer **rodent ulcer. The edge is classically pearly and rolled. Telangiectasias cover the lesion** (Figs. 3A to D)

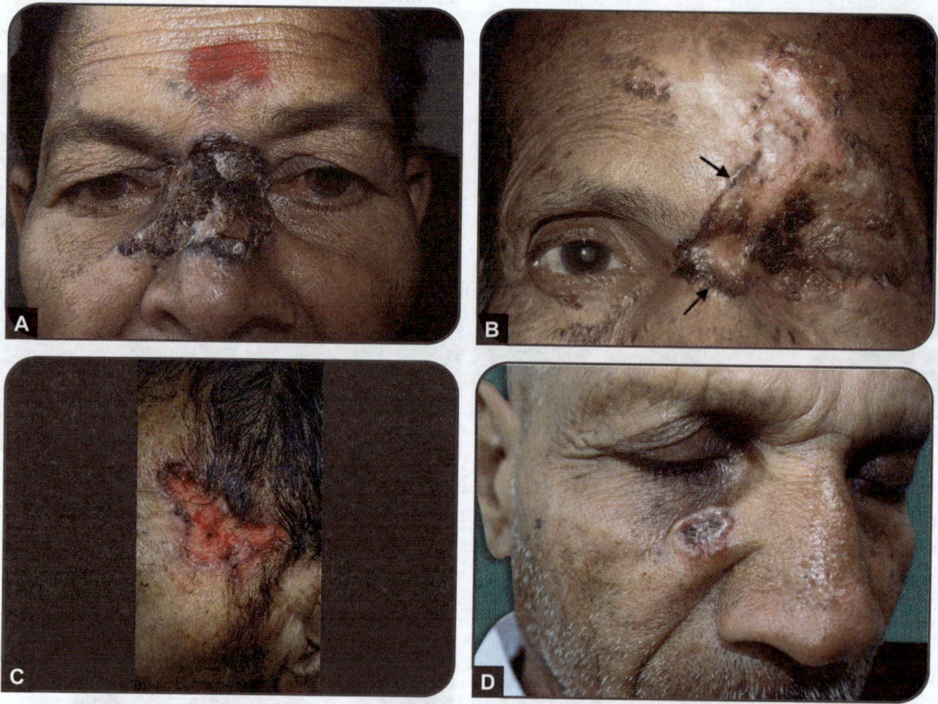

Figs. 3A to D: (A) Classical locally destructive BCC; (B) Note local tissue destruction and beaded, rolled margins (black arrows); (C) Ulcerated plaque—Note the rolled borders; (D) Nodulo-ulcerated lesion with rolled borders

- **Pathogenesis**: UVB radiation (290–320 nm)
- **Most common site is the face (most common site on face is the nose)**. The forehead, ears, periocular areas, and cheeks are also favored sites.
- **Metastasis is extremely rare** and if it occurs, regional lymph nodes are the most frequently involved followed by the lung, bone, skin and liver

SQUAMOUS CELL CARCINOMA

- **2nd most common cause of skin cancer (However, most common type in immunosuppressed transplant recipients)**
- **Etiology**—UV radiation is major predisposing factor—hence, face, scalp, neck, dorsal hands are common sites involved, though it can occur in other sites
- **Other risk factors**—High-risk genital HPV (HPV-16, 18, 31 and 35) involved in genital SCC, chronic ulcers
- Typical presentation is a solitary, hard, eroded papule/nodule/ulcer with **indurated everted edges (note BCC has a pearly rolled margin), "Majority of lower lip cancers are SCC and present as ulcers"** (Figs. 4A and B).

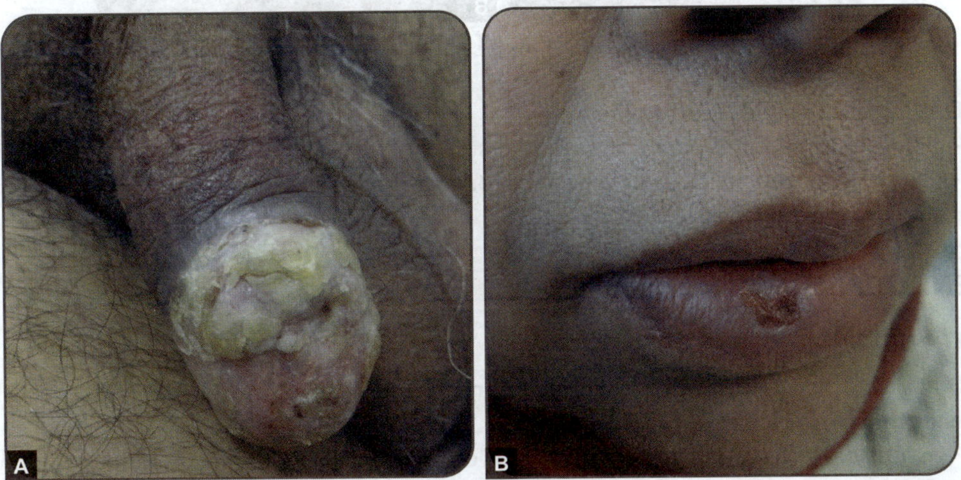

Figs. 4A and B: (A) SCC: Verrucous plaque on glans; (B) SCC: Lower lip ulcer

High Yield Points

- Most common skin cancer (overall)—BCC
- Most common in organ transplant recipients—SCC
- Most common site on lip and hands—SCC

PREMALIGNANT SKIN DISEASES

a. **Oral leucoplakia (OL)**
   - **Most common precancerous lesion of the oral mucosa**
   - Presents as a white non-removable plaque (Figs. 5A and B)
   - Potentially malignant (0–20% risk of conversion to malignancy)
   - OL is in the same clinical spectrum of disease as oral erythroplakia (OE)—OE has more chances of malignant conversion as compared to OL
   - Non-homogenous OL (speckled OL) is more risky than homogenous OL
   - Risk factors—Tobacco, alcohol use, HPV

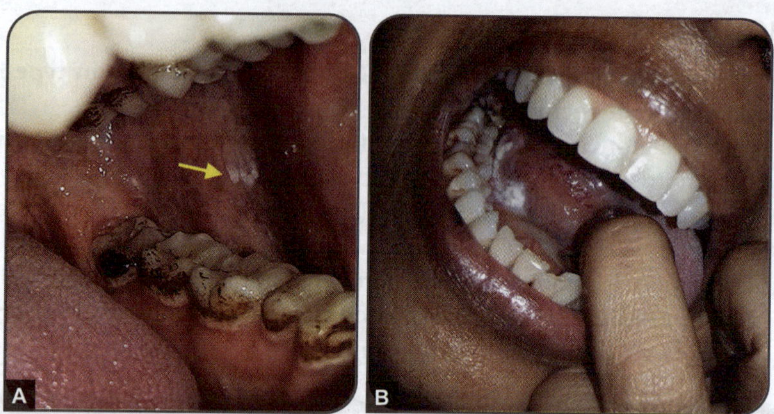

Figs. 5A and B: (A) Leukoplakia on buccal mucosa; (B) Leukoplakia on floor of mouth and tongue

b. **Oral erythroplakia/Erythoplasia**
   - Persistent red fixed patch on mucosal surface
   - **Least common of all oral precancerous lesions** but with the **maximum potential** to convert to malignancy

ENDOCRINOLOGY AND SKIN

Skin Signs of Diabetes Mellitus

a. **Dry skin (xerosis) and itching—most common manifestation**
b. **Acanthosis nigricans**:
   - **Symptoms**: Velvety hyperpigmentation of the intertriginous/flexural area (Fig. 6A).
   - **Etiology**:
     1. Commonly associated with insulin resistance—obesity (pseudo-acanthosis nigricans)
     2. Androgen excess conditions (e.g., PCOD)
     3. Drug-related (nicotinic acid, testosterone, diethylstilbestrol, oral contraceptives, glucocorticoids)
     4. Idiopathic
     5. Malignancy (gastric adenocarcinoma)
   - When the palms are involved, the rough appearance of palms is called **tripe palms** and is usually then associated with lung cancer
   - **Pathogenesis:**
     Insulin resistance → Release of insulin-like growth factor (ILGF) → excess growth factor will then stimulate epidermal keratinocytes → epidermal thickening of acanthosis nigricans
   - **Histopathology**—Even though the disease is named as "acanthosis" "nigricans"—there is **no acanthosis on histopathology**. Instead there is papillomatosis (upward finger like projections of dermal papilla) and hyperkeratosis. Also the dark skin color is not due to melanin but the visual appearance of hyperkeratosis.

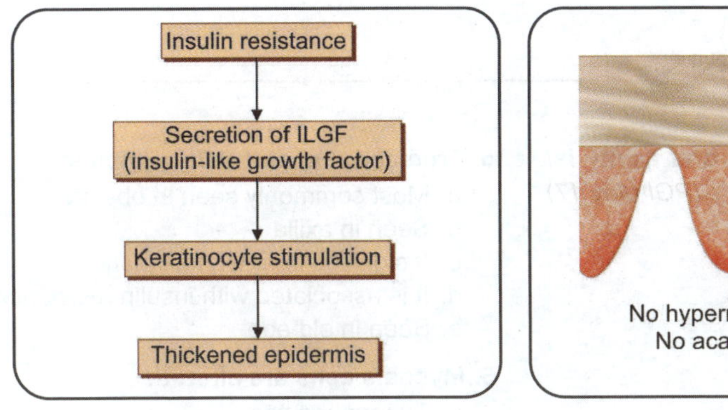

Pathogenesis

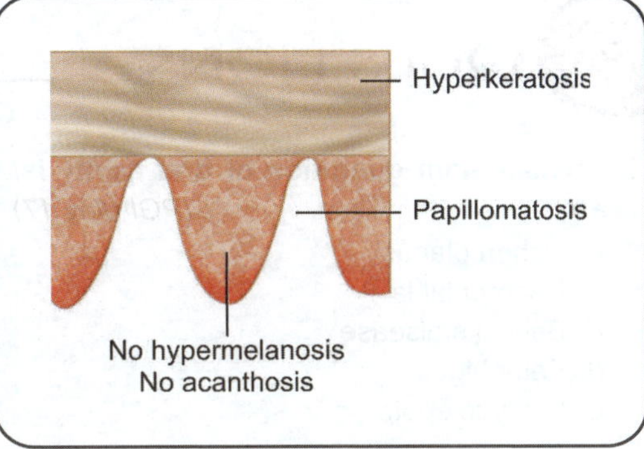

Histopathology

c. **Necrobiosis lipoidica**—Yellow wrinkled atrophic patches on the shins, may ulcerate. It is characterized by well-circumscribed, depressed, waxy, yellow-brown plaques on the anterior shin. Two-third are insulin-dependent diabetics (Fig. 6C). The reason may be due to microangiopathy secondary to diabetes. Treatment is superpotent topical steroids. Topical calcineurin inhibitors (e.g. tacrolimus), intralesional injections of triamcinolone are also effective.

d. **Generalized granuloma annulare (GA)**—GA is an annular, erythematous, non-scaly plaque (similar to tinea, but tinea is scaly) typically on dorsum of hands. Generalized GA may be a feature of diabetes (Fig. 6B).

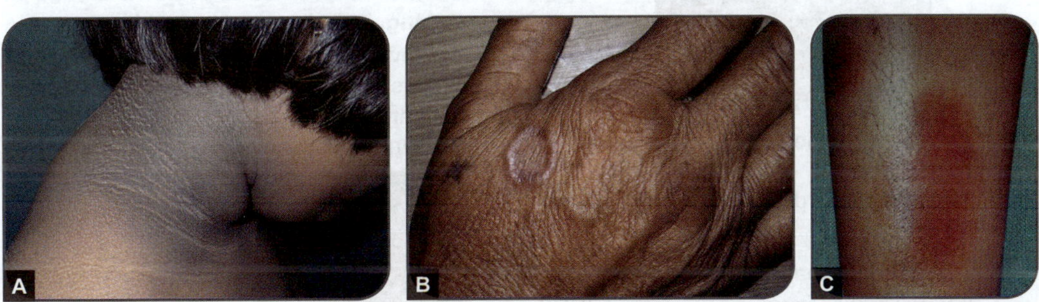

Figs. 6A to C: (A) Acanthosis nigricans—velvety plaque in neck flexure in an obese child; (B) Granuloma annulare—Annular non-scaly plaque at a typical site; (C) Necrobiosis Lipoidica—Yellowish brown atrophic shin plaque with telangiectasia

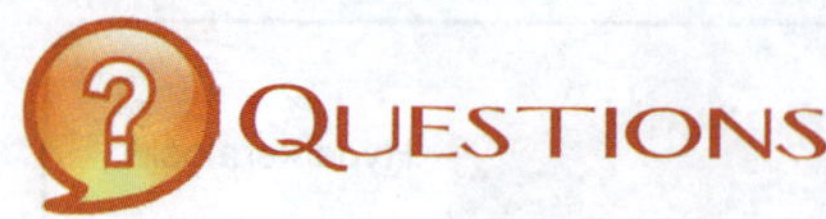

1. Premalignant condition of oral cavity is/ are: *(PGI May 17)*
a. Lichen planus
b. Erythroplakia
c. Behcet's disease
d. Pemphigus
e. Fordyce spots

2. A 40-year-old man with diabetes has the following lesions in axilla. The diagnosis is: *(Recent NEET pattern)*

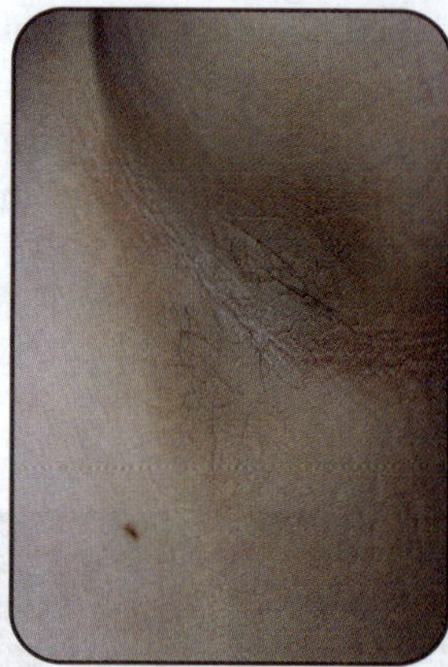

a. Acanthosis nigricans
b. Lichen planus
c. Allergic contact dermatitis
d. Melasma

3. Acanthosis nigricans is associated with:
a. Internal malignancy *(PGI)*
b. Endocrine disorder
c. Bloom's syndrome
d. Pigmentation of neck, face, etc.
e. All are correct

4. False regarding acanthosis nigricans is:
a. Prognostic indicator
b. Velvety plaques with dirty hyperpigmentation
c. Sign of malignancy
d. Gastric adenocarcinoma is commonest malignant association
e. Indicate hyperandrogenic state

5. True about acanthosis nigricans:
a. Most commonly seen in obesity
b. Seen in axilla
c. It signifies internal malignancy
d. It is associated with insulin resistance
e. Seen in old age

6. Mycosis cells are altered:
a. T-Lymphocytes
b. Monocytes
c. B-Lymphocytes
d. Eosinophils

7. Which of the following statement about mycosis fungoides is not true?
a. It is the most common skin lymphoma
b. Pautrier's microabscesses are common
c. It has a indolent course and good prognosis
d. It usually presents with diffuse erythroderma

8. A patient comes with a history of lesion on the nose since 2 years. It bleeds on itching. The diagnosis would be:
a. Nevus *(AIIMS Nov 17)*
b. Basal cell carcinoma
c. Marjolin's ulcer
d. Dermatofibroma

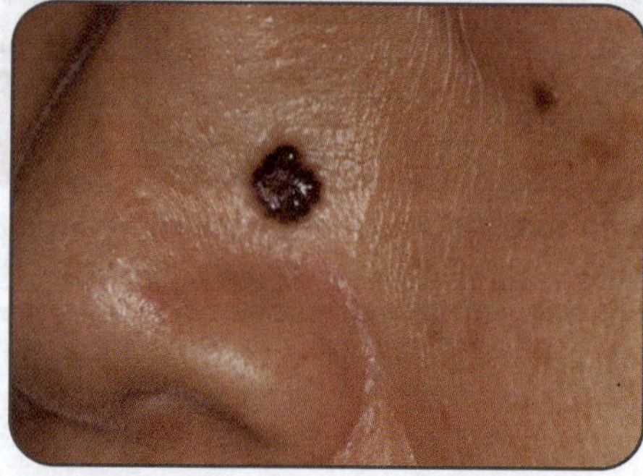

9. Which nevi commonly predispose to malignant melanoma?
a. Dermal
b. Junctional
c. Congenital
d. Lentigo

10. Predisposing factors for skin cancer are:

a. Smoking
b. UV light
c. Chronic ulcer
d. Infrared light
e. Arsenic

11. Predisposing factors for skin cancer are:

a. Lichen planus
b. Bowen's disease
c. Psoriasis
d. Behcet's disease
e. UV rays

12. Least propensity for lymphatic spread would be in: *(AIIMS May 18)*

a. Basal cell cancer
b. Squamous cell cancer
c. Malignant melanoma
d. Merkel cell carcinoma

13. A patient presents with the lesions as shown. Which condition would you rule out? *(AIIMS Nov 17)*

a. Diabetes
b. Hyperthyroidism
c. Hypothyroidism
d. Sarcoidosis

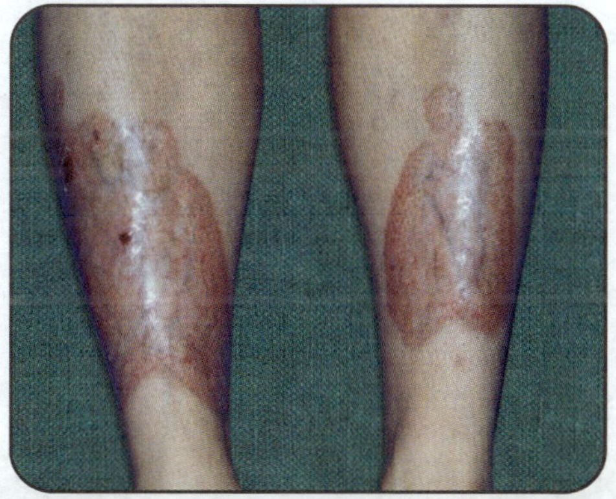

14. A 70-year-old female presents with a lesion on cheek with pearly raised border and telangiectasia on surface of lesion. Diagnosis is: *(AIIMS May 2016)*

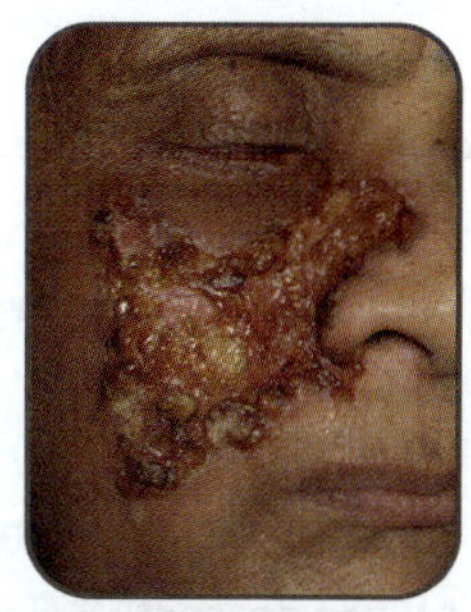

a. Basal cell carcinoma
b. Squamous cell carcinoma
c. Actinic keratosis
d. Wart

15. Which oral condition is not premalignant? *(PGI Nov 15)*

a. Lichen planus
b. Oral submucous fibrosis
c. Erythroplakia
d. Leukoplakia
e. Aphthous ulcer

New Questions

16. The following statements are true/false regarding Basal cell carcinoma:

a. Most common skin cancer in organ transplant patients
b. Everted edge
c. Most common site is nose
d. Bleeds on manipulation
e. Metastasis is common

17. Assertion: Acanthosis nigricans is seen in obesity
Reason: Insulin resistance is seen in obesity

a. Both Assertion and Reason are true and Reason is correct explanation of Assertion
b. Both Assertion and Reason are true but Reason is not correct explanation of Assertion
c. Assertion is true and Reason is false
d. Assertion is false and Reason is true
e. Both Assertion and Reason are false

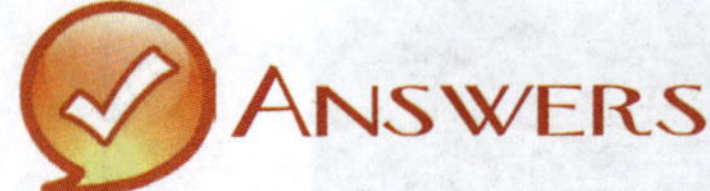

1. **Ans. (a, b) Lichen planus, Erythroplakia.** *(Ref: Andrew's Textbook, 11th edn, Page 727)*
   Lichen planus especially of the ulcerative/erosive type and erythroplakia have premalignant potential.
2. **Ans. (a) Acanthosis nigricans**
3. **Ans. (e) All are correct** *(Ref: Andrew's Textbook, 11th edn, Page 568)*
   Bloom's syndrome is a rare cause of acanthosis nigricans.
4. **Ans. (a) Prognostic indicator** (See page 383 for explanation)
5. **Ans. (a, b, c, d) Most commonly seen in obesity; Seen in axilla; It signifies internal malignancy; It is associated with insulin resistance** (See page 383 for explanation)
6. **Ans. (a) T-Lymphocytes** (See page 376 for explanation)
7. **Ans. (d) It usually presents with diffuse erythroderma**
   Mycosis fungoides usually presents as patches and plaques. Erythroderma is later in the course of the disease.
8. **Ans. (b) Basal cell carcinoma**
   Note the lesion is having pearly nodular edge, ulcer and is on the nose- all favoring BCC. It can bleed on touch
9. **Ans. (c) Congenital** *(Ref: Rook's Textbook of Dermatology, 9th edn, Page 143.2)*
10. **Ans. (a, b, c, e) Smoking; UV light; Chronic ulcer; Arsenic**
11. **Ans. (a, b, e) Lichen planus; Bowen's disease; UV rays**
12. **Ans. (a) Basal cell cancer**
13. **Ans. (a) Diabetes**
    This condition is necrobiosis lipoidica.
14. **Ans. (a) Basal cell carcinoma**
    Pearly raised border with telangiectasia suggests BCC.
15. **Ans. (e) Aphthous ulcer**
    Oral lichen planus (of the ulcerative variety) is premalignant.

New Answers

16. **Ans. a-False; b-False; c-True; d-True; e-False**
17. **Ans. (a) Both Assertion and Reason are true and Reason is correct explanation of Assertion**

CHAPTER 17

Important Short Topics

MAST CELL DISORDERS

Urticaria (Hives)

- Classical lesion is a **wheal**—a vascular reaction due to mast cell rupture leading to local **dermal edema**, red flare and itching
- Wheals are typically **transient** and **subside within 24 hours** only to occur at a new site
- **Pathogenesis:**

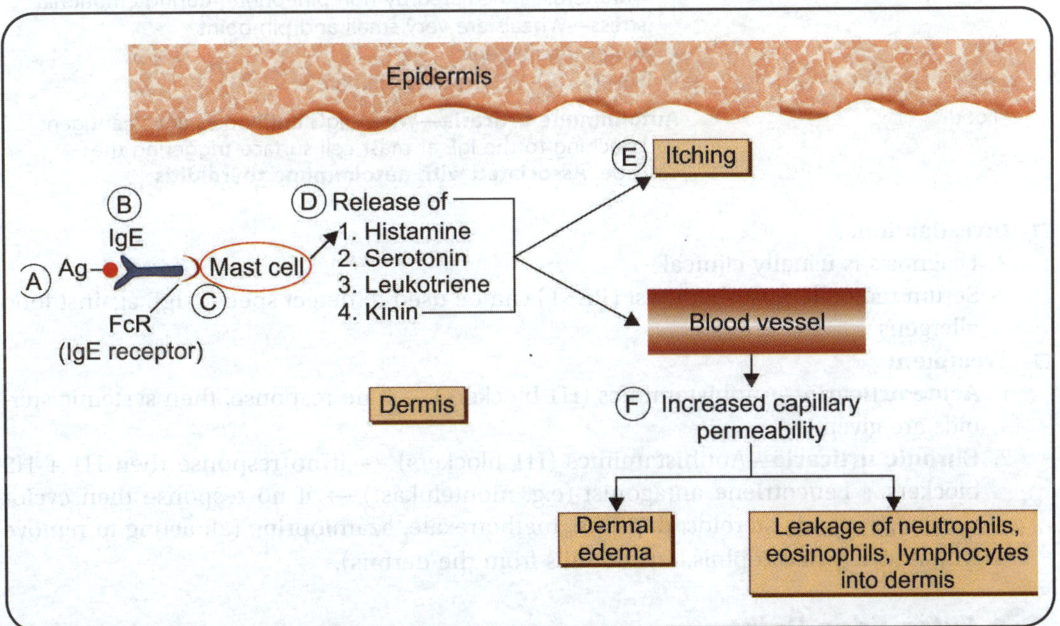

A trigger antigen Ag • (A), attaches to the IgE antibody on the surface of the mast cells (B), in superficial dermis, which in turn attaches to the Fc receptor (IgE receptor) (C), at the mast cell surface. This triggers mediator release from mast cells (D), causing itching (E), and increased capillary permeability (F)

- **Classification**

Acute urticaria (<6 weeks)	Chronic urticaria (>6 weeks)
Drugs (m/c)—Penicillin and related antibiotics (m/c), opiates, radiocontrast dye, aspirin, other NSAIDs	**Idiopathic (m/c)** (Fig. 1A)
Infections—upper respiratory Infections (streptococcal)	Physical—Due to physical factors, e.g.: • Cold urticaria—in response to cold temperature (may be associated with underlying cryoglobulinemia) • **Cholinergic:** Due to action of acetylcholine on mast cells—**due to increase in core body temperature and sweating**, such as during a warm bath, exercise, fever. Wheals are very small and pin-point • **Scratching (Dermatographism)—m/c form** of physical urticaria. Linear wheals as a result of firm stroking of the skin. **Fades within 30 minutes** (Fig. 1B) * Note: white dermatographism is not a feature of urticaria but seen in atopic dermatitis (Fig. 1D) • Adrenergic—mediated by norepinephrine during emotional stress—Wheals are very small and pin-point • Water (Acquagenic) • Sun (Solar)—in exposed skin areas
Food	**Autoimmune urticaria**—Where IgG antibodies act as antigens → attaching to the IgE at mast cell surface triggering the cascade. **Associated with autoimmune thyroiditis**

- **Investigation:**
  - Diagnosis is usually clinical
  - Serum radioallergosorbent test (RAST) can be used to detect specific IgE against food allergens
- **Treatment**
  1. **Acute urticaria**—Antihistaminics (H1 blockers) → if no response, then systemic steroids are given
  2. **Chronic urticaria**—Antihistaminics (H1 blockers) → if no response then H1 + H2 blockers + Leucotriene antagonist (e.g. montelukast) → if no response then cyclosporine, systemic steroids, dapsone, methotrexate, azathioprine (all acting to remove lymphocytes, neutrophils, eosinophils from the dermis).

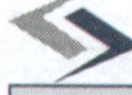

Extra-Edge Point

Omalizumab—Anti-IgE monoclonal antibody is used for refractory cases

Angioedema (Quincke Edema)

- Pathology is similar to urticaria, but **not in the superficial dermis like in urticaria but in the deeper dermis**, subcutaneous tissue and submucosal tissue.
- **Seen clinically not as itching but as swelling in the most distensible tissues, such as the eyelids and lips** (Fig. 1C).

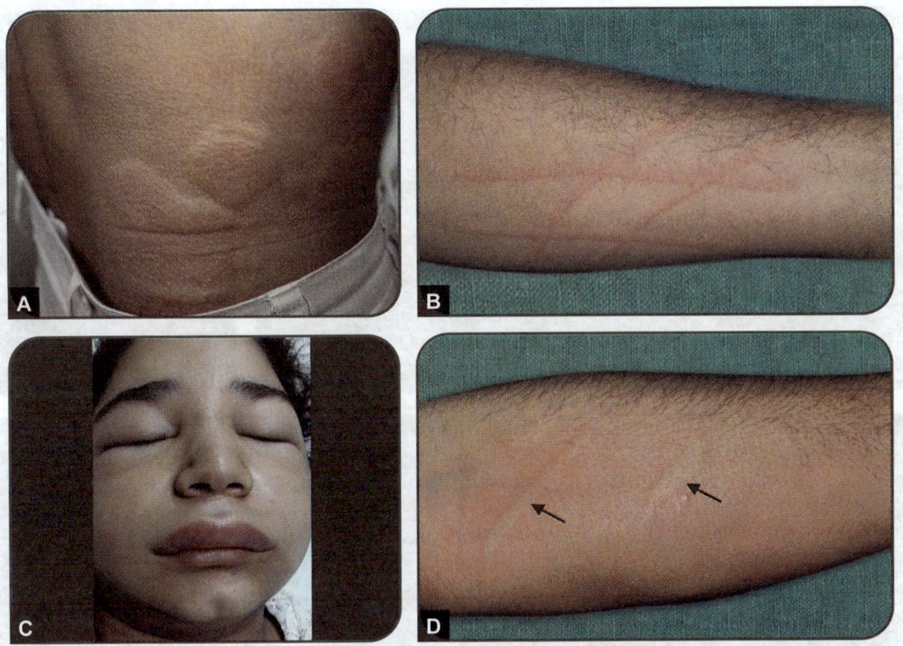

Figs. 1A to D: (A) Urticaria—edematous, itchy, evanescent plaques; (B) Dermatographism—Linear red wheals after scratching; (C) Angioedema—swollen eyelids and lip; (D) White dermatographism—on scratching there are white marks due to vasoconstriction. No relation to urticaria—seen in atopic dermatitis

- The mucous membranes of the mouth, tongue, or larynx may also be involved causing sudden respiratory distress and airway obstruction.
- **ACE inhibitor** drugs may also cause angioedema.
- Treatment—**Epinephrine (DOC)**, injectable hydrocortisone

Anaphylaxis

An acute immunological distress presenting as itching, urticaria or angioedema along with systemic features (bronchospasm, laryngeal edema, hypotension). It may be life threatening.

Mastocytosis

- **The hallmark:** Pathologic accumulation of mast cells in tissues—skin or systemic or both (Fig. 2D)
- Mutations in **c-kit gene** appear to play a central role in adult forms of mastocytosis
- The **most common form in children is urticaria pigmentosa** where cutaneous deposits of numerous mast cells occur—**clinically, the eruption usually begins as itchy pigmented macules mainly on trunk** (Figs. 2A and B).
- Diagnosis: **Darier's sign** (Figs. 2C).

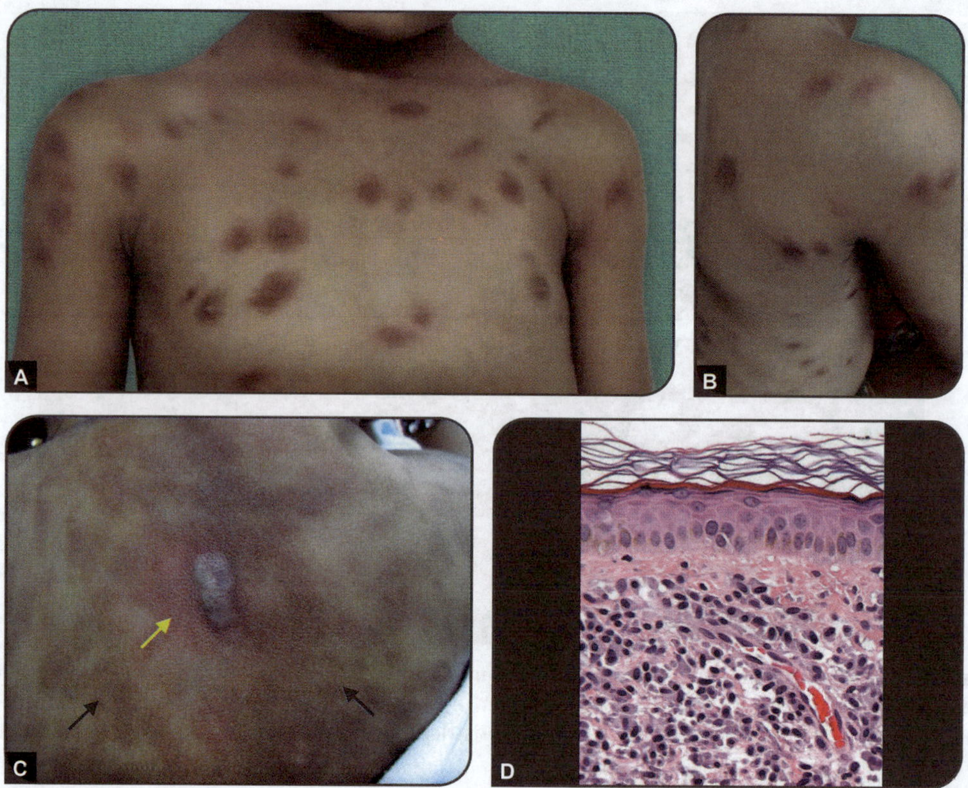

Figs. 2A to D: (A) Urticaria pigmentosa—hyperpigmented macules on anterior trunk in a child; (B) Hyperpigmented macules on posterior trunk in the same child; (C) Darier's sign positive—on rubbing the hyperpigmented lesions (black arrows), red edematous urticarial lesion develops (yellow arrow); (D) Mastocytosis histology: Note the numerous dermal mast cells

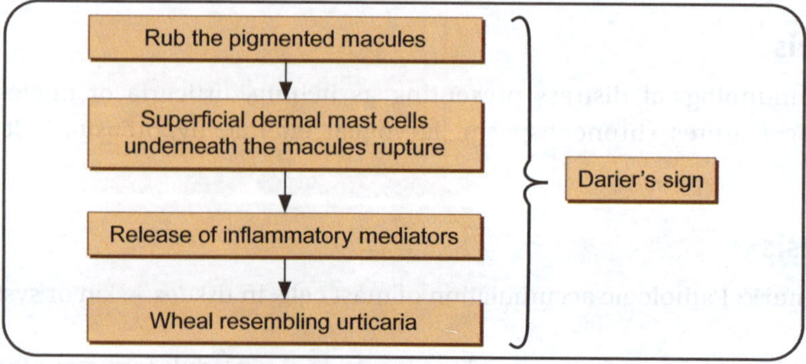

- Histopathology: Numerous mast cells are seen under the pigmented macules
- Treatment: Lesions resolves by adulthood in most patients. Till then symptomatic relief occurs with anti-histaminics, topical steroids, topical tacrolimus, phototherapy

Aid to Remember

Urticaria pigmentosa—Reverse the words. You would get **pigmentosa** → **urticaria**, i.e. it is a pigmented lesion which on rubbing becomes an urticaria-like wheal (Darier's sign)

LICHEN NITIDUS

- Chronic disease typically presents as tiny (1–2 mm), shiny, **pin-point uniform papules** in children
- Lesions are asymptomatic, especially on the **penis, forearms, and dorsal hands** (Figs. 3A and B).
- Koebner phenomenon may occur

Pick-up words in MCQs on lichen nitidus
Pin-point papules on dorsum of hands and penis

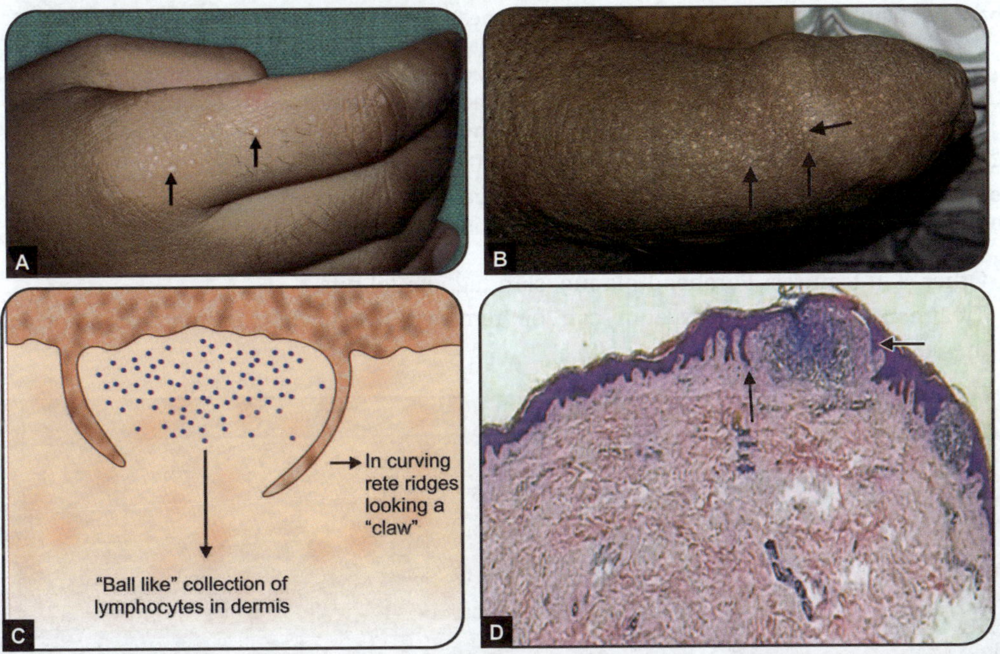

Figs. 3A to D: (A) Pin-point papules on dorsum of hands; (B) Pin-point papules on shaft of penis (black arrows); (C) Schematic diagram for histology of lichen nitidus; (D) Histology of lichen nitidus (black arrow points to the claw-like rete ridges)

- Histopathology—Classically called as "**clutching the ball**" appearance—Papillae are elongated, curved downwards and holds a collection of dermal lymphocytes and histiocytes within it (as if a clutch is holding a ball within its grasp) (Figs. 3C and D).
- No treatment is required as lesions are **self-resolving**

TUBEROUS SCLEROSIS (EPILOIA, BOURNEVILLE DISEASE)

- **Epiloia** (**epi** = epilepsy, **loi** = low intelligence, **a** = adenoma sebaceum).
- Hamartomatous growths of glial and neuronal tissue produce **potato-like nodules** in the cerebral cortex (**potato is a type of tuber, hence the name tuberous sclerosis**). When these nodules calcify they can be picked up by X-ray, CT, MRI.
- The skin features are listed below

Ash-leaf macule	• **Hypopigmented** macules (not depigmented) (Figs. 4A and B) • **First to occur** (at birth), **most common manifestation** (90% of patients) • **Wood's light makes it more prominent** • >3 is significant (<3 can even be seen in normal people)
Adenoma sebaceum	• Papules symmetrically over the cheeks, nose, and forehead. • 75–90% patients (Fig. 5B) • Onset: 2–5 years
Shagreen plaque	• Literal meaning of **shagreen = named after a type of rough leather**, resembling shark skin. Such leathery plaques are seen on the lumbosacral area (Fig. 4A). • Histopathologically, they are masses of collagen (**collagenoma**) • Onset: First decade of life
Koenen tumors (periungual angiofibromas)	• **Periungual tumors** (Fig. 5A) • Onset: Puberty

- Other skin features: Forehead plaque, skin tag, dental pits
- Treatment: Adenoma sebaceum can be removed by shaving, dermabrasion, or laser therapy.

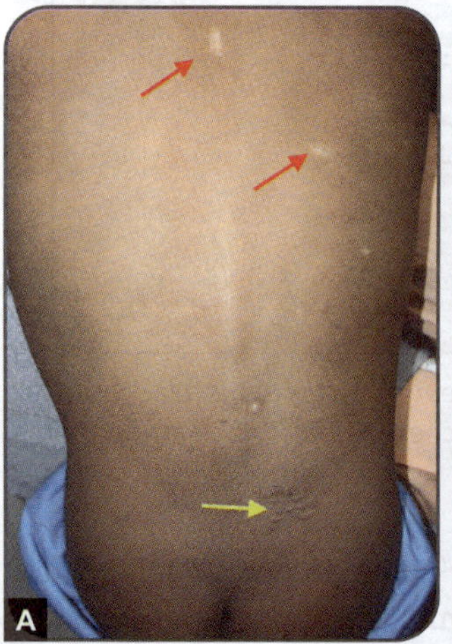

Figs. 4A and B: (A) Ash-leaf macules (Red arrows), Shagreen plaque (yellow arrow); (B) Close-up of the hypopigmented ash leaf-shaped macule

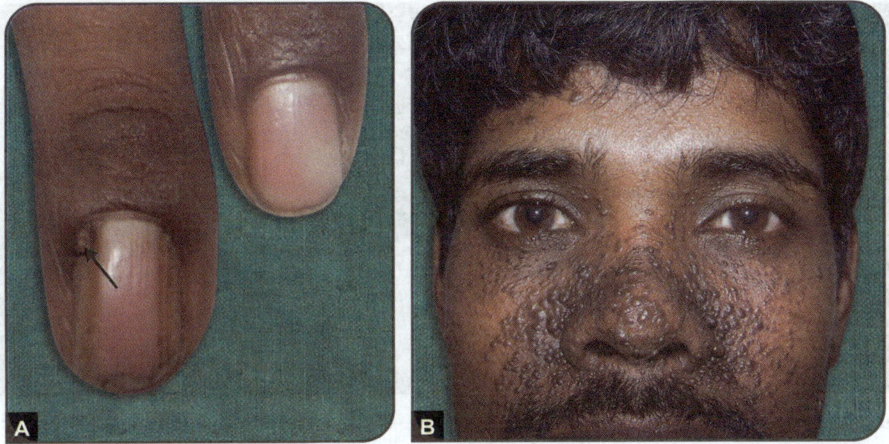

Figs. 5A and B: (A) Koenen's tumor—Periungual location; (B) Adenoma sebaceum—symmetrical papules on face

NEUROFIBROMATOSIS (NF)

- Autosomal—dominant with nervous system, bone, and skin manifestations
- **Type 1 NF (Von Recklinghausen's disease)**
  a. **Neurofibromas**—The neurofibromas are such soft tumors that they can be easily pushed down into the subcutaneous fat by pressure with the finger ("**buttonhole sign**") and springs back when released (Figs. 6A, B, and D)
  b. **Café au lait spots** (First manifestation, often at birth, uniformly pigmented, smooth edged, brown macule, ≥6 at least 1.5 cm in adults is diagnostic) (Fig. 6B)
  c. **Axillary freckles (Crowe's sign)—Pathognomic** (Fig. 6C)
  d. **Lisch nodules** (pigmented iris hamartomas)—Pathognomic
- Type 2 NF—Usually no skin features but have bilateral acoustic neuromas

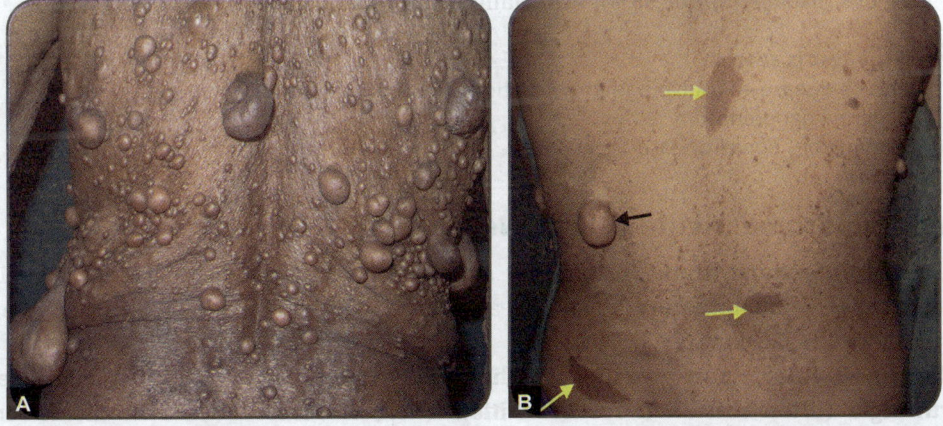

Figs. 6A and B: (A) Multiple neurofibromas; (B) Neurofibroma (black arrow) with accompanying café-au-lait spots (yellow arrows)

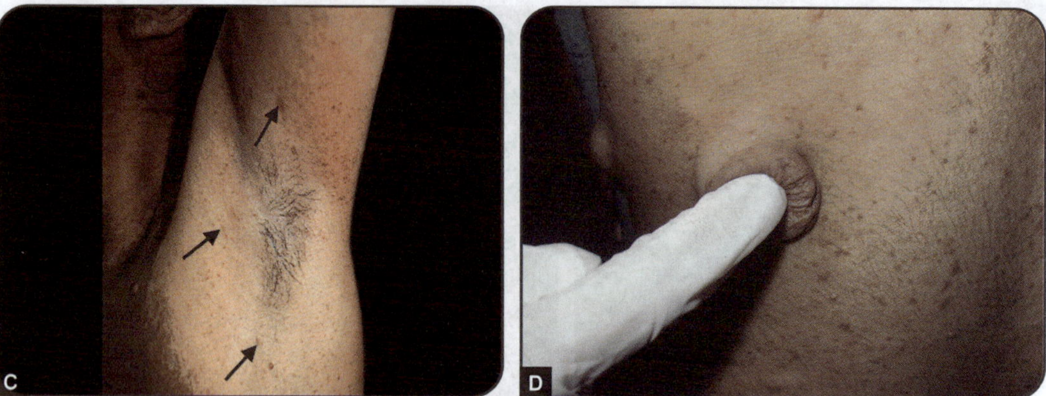

Figs. 6C and D: (C) Crowe's sign (axillary freckles)—hyperpigmented small macules in axilla (black arrows); (D) Button hole sign positive in neurofibroma

NEUTROPHILIC DERMATOSES

- A group of diseases, with common histopathological features of diffuse **neutrophilic infiltrates in skin** and **often associated with internal diseases**
- Hypersensitivity reaction to an internal or external trigger
- There are many disease under the umbrella term of neutrophilic dermatoses viz- **dermatitis herpetiformis (discussed in detail in Chapter 9), Sweet's syndrome, Pyoderma gangrenosum, Behcet's disease**
- **Pathergy test—A papule/pustule occurs in response to minor trauma like a needle prick (with a blunt needle) at 48 hours at the site of the prick.**
  Pathogenesis of pathergy phenomenon: Skin injury caused by needle prick apparently triggers a cutaneous inflammatory response and creates a new papule/pustule. This suggests an increased or aberrant release of cytokines from keratinocytes or other cells in the epidermis or dermis. The specificity of skin pathergy reaction is very high especially in Behcet's disease (about 99%), especially when it is positive at 48 hours.

Pathergy test is seen in
1. Behcet's disease—Positive pathergy reaction is very important for diagnosis
2. Pyoderma gangrenosum
3. Inflammatory bowel disease

Sweet's Syndrome (Acute Febrile Neutrophilic Dermatosis)

- **Etiology: Infections** (upper respiratory streptococcus, gastrointestinal tract infection), Other causes—inflammatory bowel disease, underlying malignancy (AML), pregnancy, drug induced, vaccination
- **Clinical: Tender, non-pruritic, erythematous plaques or papules with fever, arthralgia (often mistaken for cellulitis).** There is severe edema in the lesions—giving an appearance of blistering but on pricking with a needle—**no fluid is found (pseudo-vesicular appearance)** (Figs. 7A and B).

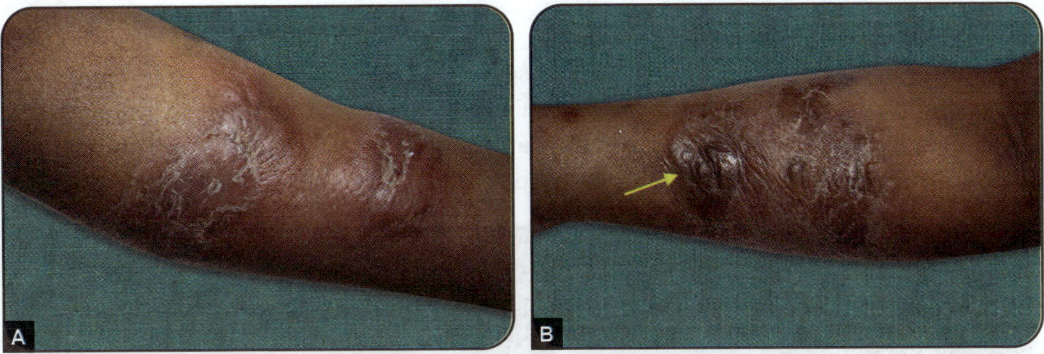

Figs. 7A and B: (A) Edematous, tender plaques on extremity; (B) Severe edema can give pseudo-vesicular appearance (yellow arrow)

Pyoderma Gangrenosum

- Chronic, recurrent, **very painful, ulcerative disease** typically on lower legs (Figs. 8A and B).
- The leg ulcers are typically **undermined, painful, with a blue or purple (violaceous) border**

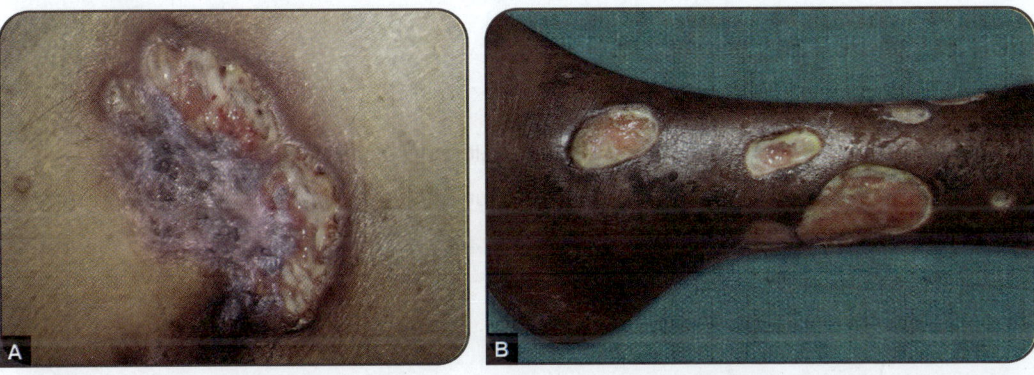

Figs. 8A and B: (A) Painful ulcer: Note the purple/violaceous margin; (B) Painful, undermined leg ulcers

- **50% of patients have an underlying systemic disease (m/c inflammatory bowel disease, hematologic disorder—IgA monoclonal gammopathy, AML, CML)**
- Treatment—Oral steroids—DOC

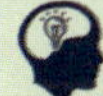

Aid to Remember

"Pyoderma gangrenosum is associated with:
Three B's—BLOOD, BOWEL, and BONES"

Behcet's Disease

- A multisystem, remitting and relapsing disease
- **Aphthous ulcer** (typically round/oval with **a red halo** around it) is a major criterion and is the first symptom (Fig. 9A). The **genital aphthous ulcers** involve primarily the scrotum and penis in men and the vulva in women (Fig. 9B).

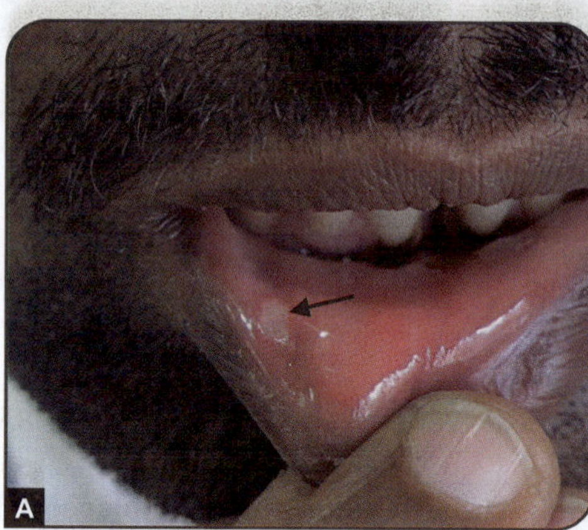

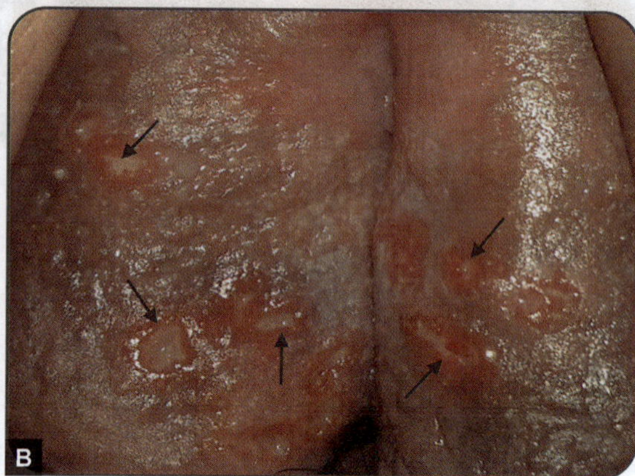

Figs. 9A and B: (A) Small, round oral aphthous ulcer with a red halo; (B) Aphthous ulcers on the labia in a female with Behcet's disease

- Association with HLA-B51

1 point	Oral aphthosis
1 point	Skin manifestations pustules illiculitis, skin aphthosis
1 point	Vascular lesions, Thrombosis, aueurysm
1 point	Positive pathergy test, aneurysm, arterial thrombosis
2 points	Genital aphthosis
2 points	Ocular lesions

Diagnosis of Behcet's disease is made with a score of 3 points

- **Treatment**—Colchicine and dapsone work best for aphthous ulcers. Oral steroids, thalidomide, azathioprine work systemically

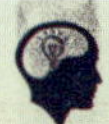

Aid to Remember

PROSE
Pathergy Test
Recurrent genital ulceration
Oral ulceration (recurrent)
Skin lesions (e.g. erythema nodosum, subcutaneous thrombophlebitis)
Eye lesions (e.g. iridocyclitis, chorioretinitis)

PHOTOTHERAPY

- Either UVA therapy or UVB therapy is given.
- **Psoralens** (e.g. 8-methoxypsoralen) are agents that enter cells and then absorb photons of UV light to produce photochemical reactions that can repair disease processes in skin.
- **Mechanism of action:**

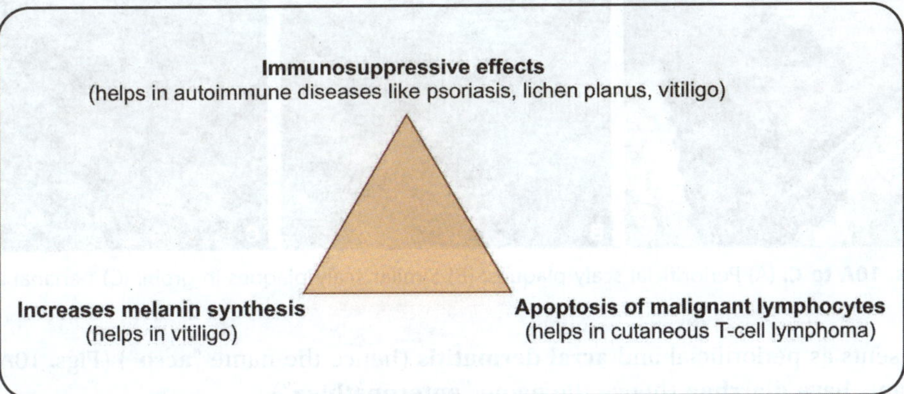

- **Indications**
  - Psoriasis
  - Vitiligo
  - Lichen planus
  - Cutaneous T-cell lymphoma
  - Atopic dermatitis
- **Types of phototherapy**

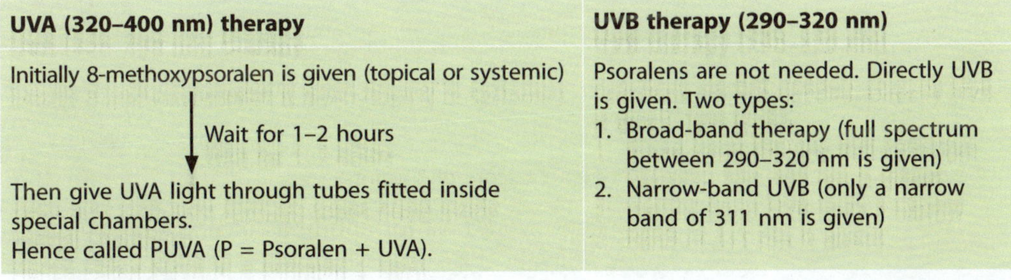

UVA (320–400 nm) therapy	UVB therapy (290–320 nm)
Initially 8-methoxypsoralen is given (topical or systemic) ↓ Wait for 1–2 hours Then give UVA light through tubes fitted inside special chambers. Hence called PUVA (P = Psoralen + UVA).	Psoralens are not needed. Directly UVB is given. Two types: 1. Broad-band therapy (full spectrum between 290–320 nm is given) 2. Narrow-band UVB (only a narrow band of 311 nm is given)

ACRODERMATITIS ENTEROPATHICA

- Autosomal-recessive, inherited disorder of mutations in the gene that encodes the protein for transport of zinc from the gut to tissues.
- Human breast milk has adequate zinc supply till weaning and then clinical zinc deficiency symptoms start

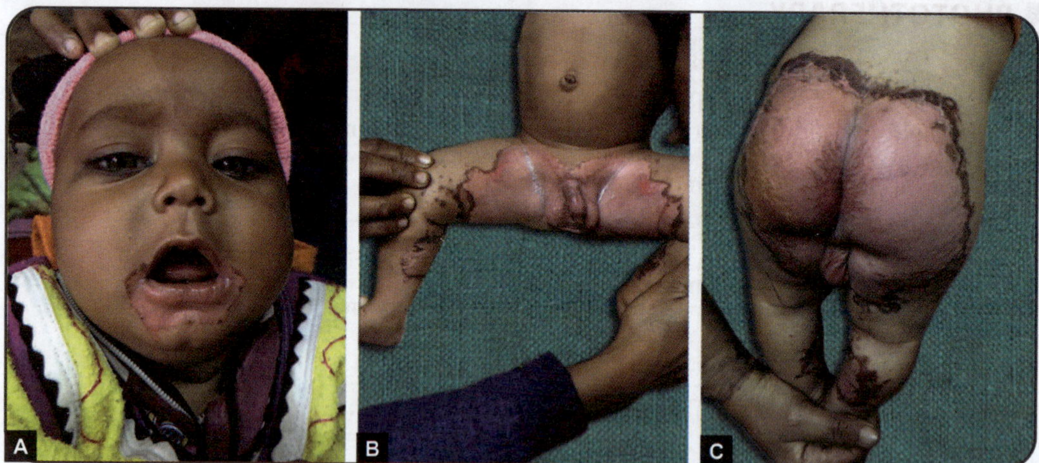

Figs. 10A to C: (A) Periorificial scaly plaques; (B) Similar scaly plaques in groin; (C) perianal area

- Presents as periorificial and **acral dermatitis** (hence the name "**acro**") (Figs. 10A to C). Infants have **diarrhea** (hence the name "**enteropathica**")
- Diagnosis—Low serum zinc levels
- Treatment—Life-long oral zinc supplementation

QUESTIONS

1. A patient gets recurrent urticaria while doing exercise and on exposure to sunlight. Which of the following is the most likely cause? *(AIIMS)*

a. Chronic idiopathic urticaria
b. Dermographism
c. Cholinergic urticaria
d. Photodermatitis

2. A 22-year-old woman developed small itchy wheals after physical exertion, walking in the sun, eating hot spicy food and when she was angry. The most likely diagnosis is:

a. Chronic idiopathic urticaria
b. Heat urticaria
c. Solar urticaria
d. Cholinergic urticaria

3. Following is a type of physical urticaria:

a. Dermographism
b. Urticaria pigmentosa
c. Urticarial vasculitis
d. Auto-immune urticaria

4. A child scratches his hand with a pen. A red wheal appears which persists for 30 minutes. What would be the diagnosis?

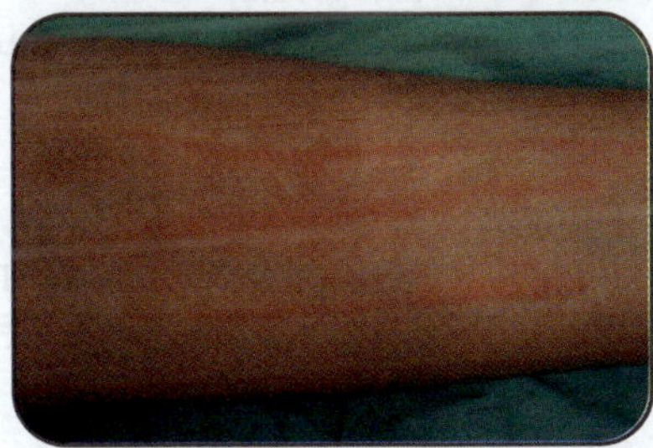

a. Atopy
b. Contact urticaria
c. Cold urticaria
d. Dermographic urticaria

5. Urticarial lesions are best described as:

a. Non-pruritic
b. Bullous
c. Evanescent
d. Macular

6. Darier's sign is seen in:

a. Darier's disease
b. Urticaria pigmentosa
c. Allergic vasculitis
d. Atopic dermatitis

7. A 5-year-old male child has multiple hyperpigmented macules over the trunk. On rubbing the lesion with the rounded end of a pen, he developed an urticarial wheal confined to the border of the lesion. The most likely diagnosis is:

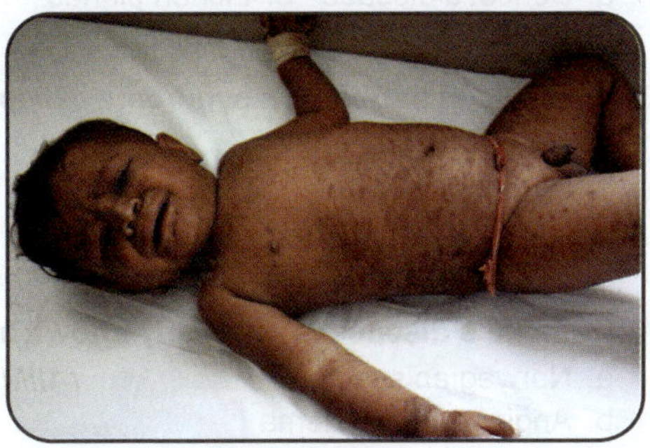

a. Fixed drug eruption
b. Lichen planus
c. Urticaria pigmentosa
d. Urticarial vasculitis

8. A 9-year-old has multiple itchy erythematous wheals all over the body for 2 days. There is no respiratory difficulty. Which is the best treatment?

a. Anthelmintics
b. Systemic corticosteroids
c. Antihistamines
d. Adrenaline

9. A man takes peanuts and develops, tongue swelling, neck swelling, stridor, hoarseness of voice. What is the probable diagnosis?

a. Angioneurotic edema
b. Foreign body in bronchus
c. Parapharyngeal abscess
d. Foreign body in larynx

10. Immediately after eating, a man develops swelling of face and lips, respiratory distress, intense pruritus, hypotension and feeling of impending doom. The most likely diagnosis:
a. Angioneurotic edema
b. Anaphylaxis
c. Myocardial infraction
d. Food stuck in throat

11. Pathergy test is used for diagnosis of:
a. Reiter's syndrome b. Behcet's syndrome
c. Lichen planus d. Atopic dermatitis

12. Oculo-oro-genital ulcers are a feature of: *(NEET Pattern)*
a. Behcet's disease b. Lichen planus
c. SLE d. Psoriasis

13. All are seen in Behcet's syndrome *except:*
a. Genital ulcers
b. Uveitis
c. Oral ulcers
d. Pyoderma gangrenosum

14. Quincke's disease is popularly known as: *(AIIMS)*
a. Norwegian scabies
b. Angioneurotic edema
c. Seborrheic dermatitis
d. Saddle nose

15. A patient gives a history of recurrent oral ulcers. The ulcers are small with a yellow floor surrounded by an erythematous halo on the lips. He also has multiple, tender nodules on the shin. He most likely has:
a. Behcet's syndrome
b. Herpes labialis
c. Fixed drug eruption
d. Pemphigus vulgaris

16. Recurrent oral ulcers with pain and erythematous halo around them. Diagnosis is:

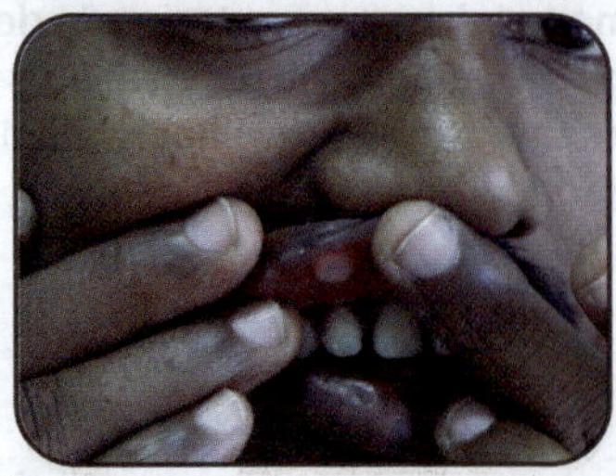

a. Aphthous ulcer b. Herpes
c. Chicken pox d. Measles

17. Acute febrile neutrophilic dermatosis is:
a. Sweet's syndrome
b. Kasabach-Merritt syndrome
c. Behcet's syndrome
d. Mucha-Habermann disease

18. A child with fever presents with multiple tender erythematous skin lesions. On microscopic examination, the skin lesions have neutrophilic infiltration in the dermis. What is the diagnosis?
a. Sweet's syndrome
b. Behcet's syndrome
c. Pyoderma gangrenosum
d. Juvenile dermatosis

19. A 24-year-old female presented with complaints of rash on exposure to sun, after exercise, when she gets angry or on eating spicy food. What is the likely diagnosis? *(AIIMS May 16)*
a. Atopic dermatitis
b. Solar keratosis
c. Cholinergic urticaria
d. Chronic idiopathic urticaria

20. Which of the following is false about acrodermatitis enteropathica?
a. Triad of diarrhoea, dementia and dermatitis
b. Low serum zinc levels
c. Symptoms improve with zinc supplementation
d. Autosomal recessive

21. A young 8-year-old boy presents with multiple discrete, shiny, pin-head papules on dorsal aspect of hand, forearms and shaft of penis. The diagnosis is:
a. Molluscum contagiosum
b. Scabies
c. Lichen planus
d. Lichen nitidus

22. Button hole sign is seen in:
a. Neurofibromatosis
b. Tuberous sclerosis
c. Lichen planus
d. Syphilis

23. Pyoderma gangrenosum true is: *(JIPMER May 15)*

a. Associated with staph aureus
b. Associated with underlying systemic condition
c. Gangrenous tissue
d. Presents with nodules

24. A female presents with recurrent wheals. Which statement/s is/are true? *(PGI May 17)*

a. IgE mediated
b. Stress is a precipitating cause
c. Long term therapy with agents suppressing IgE
d. Mast cells have no role
e. Transient lesions

25. Which one of the following statements is correct?

a. Omalizumab is an antileukotriene
b. Omalizumab is a blocking antibody that neutralises IgE
c. Omalizumab is a newer long acting anticholinergic agent
d. Omalizumab is once a day long acting beta-2 agonistic

26. Darier's sign seen in: *(Recent May 17)*

a. Urticaria pigmentosa
b. Idiopathic urticaria
c. Darier disease
d. Morphea

27. An infant presents with perioral and perianal lesions. The likely diagnosis is: *(Recent May 17)*

a. Biotin deficiency
b. Acrodermatitis enteropathica
c. Seborrheic dermatitis
d. Psoriasis

New Questions

28. Arrange the steps in the flow of pathogenesis of urticaria (from earliest to last):

1. Histamine release
2. Neutrophil
3. Fc Receptor stimulation
4. IgE attachment

a. 4, 3, 1, 2 b. 4, 2, 1, 3
c. 3, 4, 2, 1 d. 3, 4, 1, 2

29. Assertion: Omalizumab is an effective drug in psoriasis
Reason: Omalizumab is an anti-IgE monoclonal antibody

a. Both Assertion and Reason are true and Reason is correct explanation of Assertion
b. Both Assertion and Reason are true but Reason is not correct explanation of Assertion
c. Assertion is true and Reason is false
d. Assertion is false and Reason is true
e. Both Assertion and Reason are false

30. Arrange the clinical features of tuberous sclerosis as per the time on onset after birth (from earliest to last):

1. Koenen's tumor
2. Ash leaf macule
3. Adenoma sebaceum
4. Shagreen patch

a. 2, 1, 3, 4 b. 2, 4, 1, 3
c. 2, 3, 4, 1 d. 2, 4, 3, 1

31. Match the items of column A with best alternative in column B:

Column A	Column B
1. Behcet's disease 2. Pyoderma gangrenosum 3. Dermatitis herpetiformis 4. Sweets syndrome	a. Tender edematous extremity plaques b. Aphthosis c. Eczematous plaques d. Lacy oral lesions e. Painful deep undermined ulcers f. Itchy vesicles

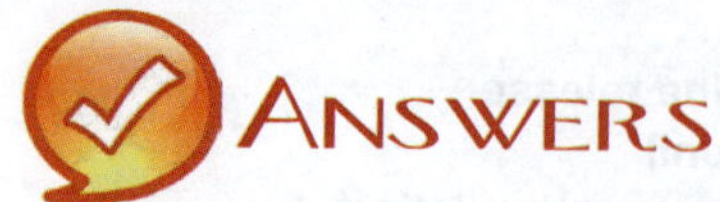

1. **Ans. (c) Cholinergic urticaria** *(Ref: Andrew's Textbook, 11th edn, Page 151)*
Exercise and exposure to sunlight increases body temperature. Sweating then occurs. Urticaria as a consequence will be cholinergic urticaria. Photodermatitis is sun induced but not an urticaria.
2. **Ans. (d) Cholinergic urticaria** *(Ref: Andrew's Textbook, 11th edn, Page 151)*
Physical exertion, walking in the sun, eating hot spicy food and anger triggers sweat and cholinergic urticaria.
3. **Ans. (a) Dermographism** *(Ref: Andrew's Textbook, 11th edn, Page 152)*
4. **Ans. (d) Dermographic urticaria** (See page 394 for explanation)
5. **Ans. (c) Evanescent** (See page 393 for explanation)
Urticarial lesions are typically transient (evanescent) and disappear in a few minutes to hours only to occur at a new location.
6. **Ans. (b) Urticaria pigmentosa** *(Ref: Andrew's Textbook, 11th edn, Page 606)*
7. **Ans. (c) Urticaria pigmentosa**
The description is of Darier's sign in urticaria pigmentosa.
8. **Ans. (c) Antihistamines**
The case describes acute urticaria. No respiratory difficulty indicates no added angioedema. Treatment is removal of offending factors (infections, drug, etc.) and antihistaminics. Antihelminthics have no role. Systemic steroids and adrenaline would be given in angioedema.
9. **Ans. (a) Angioneurotic edema**
Peanut is a food trigger for angioedema.
10. **Ans. (b) Anaphylaxis**
Angioedema does not itch. Swelling of face and lips, respiratory distress, pruritus and hypotension suggests anaphylaxis.
11. **Ans. (b) Behcet's syndrome** *(Ref: Fitzpatrick's Textbook, 8th edn, Page 2038)*
12. **Ans. (a) Behcet's disease** *(Ref: Fitzpatrick's Textbook, 8th edn, Page 2036)*
13. **Ans. (d) Pyoderma gangrenosum** *(Ref: Fitzpatrick's Textbook, 8th edn, Page 2036)*
14. **Ans. (b) Angioneurotic edema** (See page 394 for explanation)
15. **Ans. (a) Behcet's syndrome** (See page 403 for explanation)
Small oral ulcers with an erythematous halo suggest aphthous ulcers. Tender nodules on shin indicate erythema nodosum (for details on erythema nodosum, see Chapter 14). Both together indicate a diagnosis of Behcet's disease.
16. **Ans. (a) Aphthous ulcer**
17. **Ans. (a) Sweet's syndrome** *(Ref: Fitzpatrick's Textbook, 8th edn, Page 362)*

18. Ans. (a) Sweet's syndrome

Tender skin lesions with a neutrophilic infiltrate in dermis indicates a neutrophilic dermatosis. Behcet's disease presents as orogenital aphthous ulcers and not as tender skin lesions. Hence Sweet's syndrome which presents as tender, cellulitis-like lesions would be the diagnosis here.

19. Ans. (c) Cholinergic urticaria (See page 394 for explanation)

20. Ans. (a) Triad of diarrhoea, dementia and dermatitis (See page 410 for explanation)

The triad is seen in pellagra not in acrodermatitis enteropathica.

21. Ans. (d) Lichen nitidus *(Ref: Fitzpatrick's Textbook, 8th edn, Page 313)*

Pin point, shiny, papular lesions on dorsal aspect of hand, forearms and penis is typical of lichen nitidus.

22. Ans. (a) Neurofibromatosis *(Ref: Andrew's Textbook, 11th edn, Page 503)*

23. Ans. (b) Associated with underlying systemic condition (See page 402 for explanation)

24. Ans. (a, b, e) IgE mediated; Stress is a precipitating cause; Transient lesions

Recurrent wheals point to urticaria. It is an IgE mediated disorder. Stress precipitates adrenergic urticaria. Long term treatment is with anti-H1 antihistamines, leukotriene antagonists or lymphocytes/neutrophil/eosinophil inhibitors, not with IgE inhibitors.

Mast cells are central to pathology. Lesions of urticaria are always transient

25. Ans. (b) Omalizumab is a blocking antibody that neutralises IgE

26. Ans. (a) Urticaria pigmentosa

27. Ans. (b) Acrodermatitis enteropathica

New Answers

28. Ans. (a) 4, 3, 1, 2

29. Ans. (d) Assertion is false and Reason is true

30. Ans. (c)

31. Ans. 1-b; 2-e; 3-f; 4-a

Index

Page numbers followed by *f* refer to figure.

A

B

C

D

E

H

M

N

Q

R

S

T